AF834284

Shaken Baby Syndrome

Shaken Baby Syndrome

Investigating the Abusive Head Trauma Controversy

Keith Findley
University of Wisconsin–Madison Law School

Cyrille Rossant
Institute of Neurology, University College London

Kana Sasakura
Konan University Faculty of Law

Leila Schneps
National Centre for Scientific Research, Sorbonne University

Waney Squier
Formerly John Radcliffe University Hospital Oxford

Knut Wester
University of Bergen

CAMBRIDGE
UNIVERSITY PRESS

CAMBRIDGE
UNIVERSITY PRESS

Shaftesbury Road, Cambridge CB2 8EA, United Kingdom

One Liberty Plaza, 20th Floor, New York, NY 10006, USA

477 Williamstown Road, Port Melbourne, VIC 3207, Australia

314–321, 3rd Floor, Plot 3, Splendor Forum, Jasola District Centre, New Delhi – 110025, India

103 Penang Road,#05–06/07, Visioncrest Commercial, Singapore 238467

Cambridge University Press is part of Cambridge University Press & Assessment, a department of the University of Cambridge.

We share the University's mission to contribute to society through the pursuit of education, learning and research at the highest international levels of excellence.

www.cambridge.org
Information on this title: www.cambridge.org/9781009384766

DOI: 10.1017/9781009177894

© Cambridge University Press & Assessment 2023

This publication is in copyright. Subject to statutory exception and to the provisions of relevant collective licensing agreements, no reproduction of any part may take place without the written permission of Cambridge University Press & Assessment.

First published 2023 (version 2, July 2023)

Printed in the United Kingdom by TJ Books Limited, Padstow Cornwall, July 2023

A catalogue record for this publication is available from the British Library.

Library of Congress Cataloging-in-Publication Data
Names: Findley, Keith, editor, contributor. | Rossant, Cyrille, contributor. | Sasakura, Kana, 1978– contributor. | Schneps, Leila, contributor. | Squier, Waney, contributor. | Wester, Knut, contributor.
Title: Challenging shaken baby syndrome : how invalid science informs diagnoses and verdicts / [edited by] Findley Keith ; [contributors] Rossant Cyrille, Sasakura Kana, Schneps Leila, Squier Waney, Wester Knut.
Description: Cambridge, United Kingdom ; New York, NY : Cambridge University Press, 2023. | Includes bibliographical references and index.
Identifiers: LCCN 2022043098 (print) | LCCN 2022043099 (ebook) | ISBN 9781009177887 (paperback) | ISBN 9781009177894 (ebook)
Subjects: MESH: Shaken Baby Syndrome – diagnosis | Child Abuse – legislation & jurisprudence | Diagnostic Errors – legislation & jurisprudence | Intracranial Hemorrhage, Traumatic | Sudden Infant Death – diagnosis | Mandatory Reporting
Classification: LCC HV6626.5 (print) | LCC HV6626.5 (ebook) | NLM WS 430 | DDC 362.76–dc23/eng/20221209
LC record available at https://lccn.loc.gov/2022043098
LC ebook record available at https://lccn.loc.gov/2022043099

ISBN 978-1-009-38476-6 Hardback

Cambridge University Press & Assessment has no responsibility for the persistence or accuracy of URLs for external or third-party internet websites referred to in this publication and does not guarantee that any content on such websites is, or will remain, accurate or appropriate.

Every effort has been made in preparing this book to provide accurate and up-to-date information that is in accord with accepted standards and practice at the time of publication. Although case histories are drawn from actual cases, every effort has been made to disguise the identities of the individuals involved. Nevertheless, the authors, editors, and publishers can make no warranties that the information contained herein is totally free from error, not least because clinical standards are constantly changing through research and regulation. The authors, editors, and publishers therefore disclaim all liability for direct or consequential damages resulting from the use of material contained in this book. Readers are strongly advised to pay careful attention to information provided by the manufacturer of any drugs or equipment that they plan to use.
Updates and errata can be found on the book's website: https://shakenbaby.science and comments can be sent to contact@shakenbaby.science

This book might never have been written were it not for John Plunkett. John was an inspiration and a mentor to many of us, both editors and contributors. Those of us who had the pleasure of spending time with him will remember his warmth and humour, keen intelligence, scientific curiosity, and absolute unwillingness to tolerate any kind of nonsense, especially nonsense masquerading as 'science'. As a forensic pathologist he was one of the first to sound the alarm of wrongful convictions based on the shaken baby syndrome (SBS) in the 1980s. He was responsible, with colleagues, for overturning many convictions of innocent parents based on faulty scientific evidence and was personally involved in some 50 such cases. His willingness to challenge the generally accepted dogma inevitably led to personal and professional criticism, and he was charged with 'false swearing' in 2005 but soon acquitted. In 2016 he was the recipient of the Innocence Network's Lifetime Achievement Award.

He galvanised a generation of doctors and lawyers. He set up an online forum that brought together physicians, biomechanicians, and other scientists to exchange information and foster critical appraisal of the voluminous literature on SBS.

John Plunkett said, 'People need to know that families are being destroyed because doctors don't understand injury mechanisms.' We hope that this book will show how the determination of SBS does indeed destroy families and that it will provide the science to help us understand injury mechanisms. We therefore dedicate this book to the memory of our valued friend and mentor, John Plunkett.

Contents

Foreword

After a Quarter of a Century, Have Any Lessons Been Learned from the Trial of Louise Woodward?

Barry Scheck

Twenty-five years ago, the Louise Woodward trial in Boston (the 'nanny murder case') thrust shaken baby syndrome (SBS) into headlines across the globe, raising worldwide consciousness about the hypothesis that infants and toddlers could be seriously brain injured, even killed, by violent shaking. Although the case was tried in the early days of SBS prosecutions, the underlying science was fiercely disputed and litigated at trial. A quarter of a century later, although science has advanced, the issues remain just as hotly disputed and poorly understood, and yet parents and caregivers continue to be prosecuted and families torn apart based on the hypothesis.

This exquisitely conceived, comprehensively documented, interdisciplinary book advances a sensible, science-based, international effort to evaluate how deaths and serious brain injuries suffered by infants ought to be analysed and investigated. As the Prologue to this book warns, notwithstanding careful evidence-based analyses of relevant disciplines in 26 chapters, with contributions of 32 professionals from 8 countries in 16 different specialties, there is good reason to fear that this effort will be reflexively dismissed by many specialists in child abuse paediatrics and denounced as an effort to create medical and scientific controversies where none exist for the purpose of confusing judges and juries. Specifically, in 2018 the Society for Pediatric Radiology (SPR) published a 'consensus statement' in a medical journal – *Pediatric Radiology* [1]. They claimed there is now a 'consensus view' about SBS and abusive head trauma (AHT) as medical 'diagnoses' and that courts should limit or exclude expert testimony that challenges the reliability of the 'diagnoses'. They asserted the validity of the whole enterprise of inferring from a collection of intracranial and other findings (retinal haemorrhages (RH), subdural haematomas (SDH), oedema of the brain, among others) the occurrence of unwitnessed mechanisms of injury – either violent shaking alone or violent shaking and a violent impact to the head with force roughly equivalent to what occurs in a car accident or from a baby being dropped from a height of two stories.

Reflexive dismissal of this textbook would be tragic. The stakes are very high. Wrongful convictions of any kind traumatise families for generations, especially in cases involving the death of a child, and have resulted in death sentences and lengthy imprisonment of the innocent. Wrongfully separating children from their parents, siblings, or caregivers is harrowing and causes enduring harm to all concerned, including those medical professionals who initiated the process as 'mandatory reporters'. On the other hand, as paediatric physicians acknowledge, correctly identifying child abuse, protecting children, counselling families, and holding abusers accountable is an extraordinarily important, complex, and demanding task [2].

This book had to be written because the debate over SBS/AHT has reached a stage of cognitive rigidity and entrenchment [3]. In this climate, it is difficult to incorporate new information and alter perspectives [4, 5]. The reaction to negative feedback – that is, challenges to the SBS/AHT hypothesis – has been doubling down and increased overconfidence on the part of its proponents [6]. What the international medical, scientific, and legal community needs now when it comes to the SBS/AHT debate is a re-set, an intentional effort to create what Nobel Prize winner Daniel Kahneman and psychologist Gary Klein have described as a 'learning environment', a 'high validity environment' where there are stable relationships and prolonged study of objectively identifiable cues and subsequent events and outcomes [7]. This book engages that process.

Certain domains of medicine can be comparatively 'high-validity' environments. Feedback is relatively rapid and unequivocal from objectively identifiable cues in a diagnosis (symptoms and signs) and subsequent events (the tumour was benign or malignant), or between cues and the outcomes of possible actions (a therapeutic intervention either did or did not prevent the spread of cancerous cells). As Kukucka and Findley point out in Chapter 13, however, the experience-based opinions of child abuse physicians about SBS/AHT are made in an 'open-loop system' where they rarely receive feedback on their subjective judgements and therefore cannot learn from experience. There is no objective feedback system to inform child abuse physicians and their teams whether a child's injuries resulted from intentional or accidental conduct or even natural processes, whether their SBS/AHT 'diagnosis' was accurate, or what mechanism caused the intracranial findings. Accordingly, a child abuse team of physicians and other experts could consistently 'diagnose' SBS/AHT for decades and be wrong in every instance but would never know it 'because there are no ready checks on erroneous clinical judgements about SBS/AHT to reveal errors and prompt corrective action'.

That must change. One indispensable step towards creating a 'learning environment' in the SBS/AHT debate is to acknowledge error and to study, as objectively as possible, the history of how those errors came to pass. In Chapter 9 Dr Marvin Miller takes such a step. He succinctly makes 13 observations that challenge or undermine the SBS/AHT diagnosis with helpful references to other chapters of this book. He provides an overview of the new scientific evidence that has emerged over the past 25 years. All of Dr Miller's observations have merit, but I would like to focus in this foreword on 6 of them that help illuminate important lessons that can be learned from the trial of Louise Woodward a quarter of a century ago.

The Biomechanics of Shaken Baby Syndrome. Biomechanical analysis has shown that shaking alone cannot produce sufficient forces to cause the 'triad' of intracranial findings (RH, SDH, and oedema of the brain) associated with SBS/AHT (Chapter 14). Moreover, the categorical assertion of SBS proponents for decades that short falls could not produce these findings is demonstrably false (Chapter 15). Indeed, even after Dr John Plunkett, the courageous forensic pathologist to whom this book is dedicated, discovered a well-authenticated videotape of an accidental fatal short fall producing the triad, a 'lucid interval', and death, those findings and Dr Plunkett were attacked for years.

The Pathogenesis of Retinal Haemorrhages. Shaken baby syndrome proponents have asserted for decades that violent shaking causes RHs and that RHs are 'pathognomonic' of child abuse – meaning no other clinical situations can cause them. In fact, due to the work of Dr Patrick Lantz and his method for detecting RHs at the time of autopsy, as well as research cited in the ground-breaking study by the Swedish Agency for Health Technology Assessment known as SBU (Chapter 10), there is now a significant body of data showing that non-birth-related RHs in infants can be secondary to a traumatic or non-traumatic aetiology. Retinal haemorrhages are likely associated with raised intracranial pressure (ICP), and isolated shaking is unlikely to cause RHs independently of other intracranial pathology.

History Provided by Alleged Perpetrator. A basic tenet of sound medical practice is taking a comprehensive history as a starting point for laboratory and imaging testing to reach a diagnosis. However, in cases where the triad is found, the history offered by the last person with the infant is frequently dismissed because child abuse paediatricians believe that RHs and other intracranial findings are diagnostic of SBS.

The Neuropathology of Shaken Baby Syndrome. Gross and microscopic neuropathology findings at autopsy in alleged SBS cases appear counter to what violent shaking would produce (Chapter 3). The neuropathology of most alleged SBS cases is not diagnostic of trauma but consistent with multiple different causes of hypoxia which lead to a cascade of changes that cause increased ICP.

The Multidisciplinary Teams in Child Abuse Investigations. Almost all child abuse investigations are evaluated by a multidisciplinary team (MDT) typically consisting of an abuse paediatrician, paediatric radiologist, paediatric ophthalmologist, social worker, child protection worker, detective, and related hospital staff. Shaken baby syndrome proponents claim that the MDT ensures fair and impartial evaluations of cases infants who present with an unexplained triad. Dr Miller pushes back and says that, in his experience, the various members of the MDT all have 'similar thinking': unless there is some history of confirmed trauma, the finding of the triad will generally lead the MDT team to agree on a diagnosis of SBS. He calls it a classic example of 'groupthink', citing Kukucka and Findley (Chapter 13).

Problematic Use of Confessions and 'Admissions' as Proof of Shaken Baby Syndrome. Confessions have been relied upon as scientific proof of the SBS/AHT 'diagnosis' and the presumed mechanisms of inflicting injury – violent shaking alone or violent shaking and violent impact. Such proof, however, is circular and subjective (Chapter 12). It is now clear that many of these confessions are induced during plea bargaining or elicited or coerced during interrogation (Chapter 12). Frequently a caregiver will 'admit' to gently shaking an infant who was found unresponsive as an attempt to revive the infant, and then that benign statement is extrapolated into an admission of violent shaking because the 'triad' – the signs of the SBS 'diagnosis' – have been found. Or worse, a guilt-presumptive interrogation will be conducted where the parent or caregiver will be manipulated or explicitly coerced into making admissions to violent shaking or slamming because the interrogators believe that's what the medical findings show.

The Louise Woodward case Twenty-five years ago, in October 1997, Louise Woodward, an 18-year-old British au pair, was tried for the murder of 8-month-old Matthew Eappen, the son of two doctors, Sunil and Debbie Eappen. I was one of the defence attorneys in the case. The trial was televised every day in the United States and the United Kingdom. It attracted enormous publicity. It stirred deep passions about cultural issues involving gender, class, and the childcare choices of professionals. Most of all, as Clyde Haberman wrote 7 years ago in a 'Retro Report' about the case: 'Perhaps no crime staggers the mind, or turns the stomach more, than the murder of a baby, so it is not a surprise when law enforcement comes down hard on the presumed killers' [8].

Over the past 25 years, the Woodward case has gained significance within the medical, scientific and legal communities. It represented the very first time the scientific underpinnings of SBS were challenged by many of the leading scientists in the world, whose research had previously been cited by SBS proponents as foundational to the diagnosis [8]. The prosecution claimed that Ms Woodward violently slammed Matthew's head against a hard surface and shook him violently with his head snapping back and forth between 2 and 6 hours before she called 911 and Matthew was admitted to the hospital. The defence offered powerful proof from the CT scans that there was no swelling from the alleged violent slamming of the head at the site of the skull fracture and no physical evidence (bruising, neck injury) from violent shaking just hours before admission. The defence also presented neuroimaging and neuropathology proof that Matthew's skull fracture and SDH were about 3 weeks old and that the SDH re-bled, creating a slowly evolving mass effect which led to brain stem compression, massive cerebral swelling, hypoxic-ischemic injury, and ultimately death.

The Biomechanics of Shaken Baby Syndrome/Abusive Head Trauma

In the Woodward case, Dr Madsen, the neurosurgeon who operated on Matthew the day of his admission, testified that Matthew Eappen was the victim of abuse: 'Retinal haemorrhages with a subdural haematoma and subarachnoid bleeding is the paradigmatic triad for a non-accidental injury' [9].[1] Dr Madsen then proceeded to tell the grand jury that 'to get this degree of injury in an accident, it might require a high-speed automobile accident, or a fall from a very high distance', such as 'from a second or third story balcony' [10]. Madsen testified that the skull fracture and SDH occurred 'either two or three hours, or at most, six hours prior to admission to the hospital' [11]. The rest of the MDT – Dr Eli Newberger, the chief paediatrician; Dr Patrick Barnes, the chief neuroradiologist; and Dr Lois Smith, the chief ophthalmologist – all supported Madsen's analysis. Such testimony about the biomechanical forces involved in SBS shaking or impact being analogous to high-speed car accidents or falls from second or third stories was extremely common, albeit admittedly derived from anecdotal literature and 'experience'.

The defence called Dr Lawrence Thibault, at the time perhaps the pre-eminent expert in biomechanical engineering in the world. Dr Thibault held appointments at the University of Pennsylvania as chief of the Department of Bioengineering, director of the Head Injury Center, and founder of the Laboratories for Injury Research and Prevention [12]. Dr Thibault also advised the National Highway Traffic and Safety Administration as the chairman of the Head and Neck Injury Committee, advised the Joint Chiefs of Staff, and was science advisor to the Centers for Disease Control's National Center for Injury Prevention and Control [13].

Citing biophysics data, Dr Thibault eviscerated the Commonwealth's position, opining that slamming Matthew's head against a hard surface with the force of a fall from two stories would have resulted in a depressed comminuted skull fracture and splitting of skin – neither of which was present in this case [14]. It was undisputed that at admission Dr Mandl carefully examined Matthew's head and felt no swelling, and the pre-surgical CT scan 'bone window' showed no swelling at the site of the skull fracture. Dr Thibault testified that a skull fracture produced with

[1] Repeated references by prosecution witnesses to the conclusiveness of the 'triad' for 'diagnosing' SBS lays bare another myth that has arisen in the years since the Woodward trial. As scientific advances have made clear that the 'triad' is not pathognomonic for abuse – because a long and growing list of non-abusive accidental and natural factors can produce it – child abuse physicians have taken to claiming that no one ever 'diagnosed' SBS on the basis of the 'triad' and that it is a defence construct, a straw man created by defence lawyers and experts so it can be destroyed in court. Published articles from the era, and countless transcripts of expert testimony in SBS cases, including the Woodward case, prove the contrary – the 'triad' was indeed created by and relied upon by prosecution experts for years, as it still is today.

force equivalent to a drop from 31 inches, much less the 15-foot drop claimed by the prosecution, would produce soft tissue swelling visible on a CT scan 4–6 hours later [15]. This biomechanical testimony provided strong support for the defence position that the skull fracture and SDH were old injuries, approximately 3 weeks old, and certainly did not arise from a violent slamming and shaking 2–6 hours prior to admission as alleged by the prosecution.

Dr Thibault was also the co-author of a foundational 1987 paper, 'Shaken Baby Syndrome', with his former student Dr Duhaime [16]. He repeatedly testified that the paper had concluded that shaking alone without impact could not generate the forces necessary to cause the triad without injury to the neck or spine (there was no injury to Matthew's neck or spine). He was also unequivocal in asserting that the impact generated by short falls of less than 3 feet could result in the triad. Dr Thibault's mentor, the much-honoured neurosurgeon Dr Ayub Ommaya, whose models and theoretical work were fundamental to understanding the biomechanics of traumatic brain injury, testified for the defence and agreed with Dr Thibault's biomechanical analysis. Defence witnesses Dr Alisa Gean, the chief neuroradiologist at San Francisco General Hospital, neuropathologist Dr Jan Leestma, neurosurgeon Dr Ron Uscinski, and medical examiner Dr Michael Baden all concurred, offering additional observations from the perspective of their disciplines. No biomechanical expert was called by the prosecution on its direct case or rebuttal and I doubt today any reasonably objective expert in biomechanics would disagree with the assessments of Drs Thibault and Ommaya of the evidence in the Woodward case.

The Pathogenesis of Retinal Haemorrhages

Dr Thibault offered extensive and extraordinary testimony about the biomechanical mechanisms by which RHs and peri-macular folds occurred due to sudden increases in ICP, not severe shaking [17]. His testimony presages the research of Dr Lantz and the conclusions of the SBU cited in Chapter 10.

Dr Lois Smith testified for the prosecution that post-surgical ophthalmoscopic examination revealed peri-macular folds and deep RHs. She admitted, however, that she assumed that drawings of *pre-surgical* ophthalmoscopic examination by a colleague that did not show the peri-macular folds and deep RHs were 'wrong' because those injuries 'had to be there' [18]. She further said the peri-macular folds were produced when Matthew's eyeballs slammed against the bony orbits of the eye, although she conceded that mechanism is not described in the literature [19]. Dr Smith asserted that the RHs and peri-macular folds couldn't be caused by a dramatic increase in ICP and were pathognomonic of violent shaking [20]. Dr Thibault rejected this mechanism, nowhere identified in the literature, saying that the connective and muscle tissue that 'virtually pack that cone-shaped orbit the eyeball sits in front of' would prevent the eyeball from slamming into the bony socket [21]. Dr Smith agreed, by the way, that, as far as she knew, no one had greater expertise about the biomechanics of SBS/AHT than Dr Thibault [22]. Interestingly, she also agreed she would have expected to see swelling in the bone window of the CT scan, a skin split, or an abrasion if there had been a high-velocity impact like a fall from 15 feet onto a hard surface [23].

History Provided by Alleged Perpetrator

With respect to taking a history, Dr Madsen was asked:

Q: So, would you agree that one reason it would be important to know that the hours and morning before admission of an infant such as in this case, whether that infant had been lethargic, had been unusually sleepy and sleeping for unusually long periods of time, had been difficult to arouse, had experienced in waking states unusual irritation, crankiness and crying, and a loss of appetite, and the reason that those things taken together might be important is that they could be clinical signs of a gradually evolving bleeding in the subdural space, putting pressure on the brain stem; that's something you'd want to know.

A: If there has been a history suggesting that that was the case, you might want to know that, yes [24].

Dr Mandl, the emergency room physician, also agreed that such a history would be consistent with a slowly evolving mass effect from a re-bleed of an old SDH [25].

What neither of them knew was that Louise Woodward had given that exact history to Debbie Eappen on the evening Matthew came to the hospital, as reflected in Dr Eappen's own handwritten notes [26]. In short, just as Dr Miller observed, in cases where the triad is found, the history offered by the last person with the infant is frequently ignored or dismissed because child abuse paediatricians believe the elements of the triad are diagnostic of SBS. If the MDT at Children's Hospital had followed traditional tenets of sound medical practice and used the comprehensive history given by Louise as a starting point for testing to reach a diagnosis, they might have noticed the lack of swelling in the CT scans, and they might have been more conscientious about preserving and examining the neuropathology evidence.

The Neuropathology of SBS

The defence called Dr Jan Leestma, a giant in his field and the sole author of a neuropathology textbook that was, at the time of the trial, the only textbook in the field [27]. Dr Leestma's examination of slides from the dura in the subdural area and the skull fracture identified critical evidence of healing (calcium deposits, fibroblasts, osteoid, and osteoblasts), all findings that the SDH and skull fracture were weeks old [28]. These neuropathology findings strongly supported the defence position that the brain swelling was from a hypoxic-ischemic injury associated with a re-bleed of an old SDH, not shearing of the white matter of the brain from violent shaking.

Yet so certain were members of the MDT about their presumption of abuse that they failed to follow standard protocols that could have revealed additional evidence that Matthew's injuries were old. Dr Madsen agreed that the rules of Children's Hospital required that '[a]ll specimens removed during surgical procedures are sent to the Pathology Lab for evaluation. The surgical staff and pathologists will decide on the rare exceptions to this rule'. Nonetheless, Madsen admitted he did not preserve the blood clot that 'squalled' out of Matthew Eappen's skull at the time of the craniectomy. Madsen conceded that, if the clot had been cut into sections, an analysis could have been made as to its age [29].

Dr Leestma testified that it was 'standard' that the clot should have been preserved and sent to the pathology lab for analysis. He said it was 'very common' to get a specimen from a neurosurgeon that contains a subdural clot that, based on naked eye examination, the pathologist labelled an 'acute subdural haematoma'. However, Dr Leestma testified that, when he examines the clot under the microscope, he finds 'that it is often older than that. I find membrane and organizational characteristics within the clot that the surgeon did not appreciate' [30]. He explained:

A: The process of subdural formation and healing is a dynamic one. The process begins to form a membrane and capillaries. Those capillaries can bleed. The bleeding can be minimal, or it can be extensive, in which case you have superimposition of a more acute process on an older process. If that bleeding, or re-bleeding, as you want to use the word, is massive, it can overshadow the underlying process.

Q: And in your experience, has that been a factor in failure to identify membranes at surgery?

A: In my opinion, yes [31].

This is a critical lesson to be learned from the Woodward case. Very careful attention must be paid to collection and analysis of neuropathology specimens to ensure that timing of injuries can be analysed and that re-bleeds from older injuries are not misdiagnosed as acute or hyper-acute injuries that resulted from trauma. As suggested in Chapter 3, and as happened in the Woodward case, the reflexive assumption that violent shaking and/or impact were the mechanisms that created a SDH, RHs, and oedema of the brain has diverted the attention of child abuse teams away from evidence of older pathology, re-bleeds, and hypoxic-ischemic injuries. This is particularly troublesome because the clinical assessment of symptoms, lab testing, and neuroimaging has its limits. As Dr Ommaya observed, 'Pathology is always the final truth' [32].

Just as parts of the dura were thrown away, notwithstanding a directive from the medical examiner to preserve all specimens, the skull was not saved and the medical team did not perform 'histology', a microscopic examination of the tissue. Dr Cleveland, an expert in fractures called by the prosecution, said such an examination 'would get maybe your best data on exactly when the healing process might have started' [33].

Even more troubling was the sudden disclosure of exculpatory autopsy photographs of the skull fracture turned over the last day of trial. On direct examination, at the beginning of the trial, Dr Feigin, the medical examiner, used a photo of the skull fracture in his testimony that he said showed 'no rounding or smoothing whatsoever', which would be evidence the fracture was old and healing [34]. At the end of trial, however, the medical examiner turned over photos that Dr Baden, the defence expert, said clearly showed 'lipping and rounding' of the fracture, indicating healing and that the injury was old [35].

The Multidisciplinary Teams in Child Abuse Investigations

The use of MDTs plainly has advantages in child abuse investigations; proper assessment of such cases requires the participation of practitioners from several complex specialities. But the danger of 'groupthink' identified by Dr Miller, and exposure to sources of cognitive bias as described by Kukucka and Findley (Chapter 13) (organisational allegiance, base rate or prevalence effects, stress, exposure to irrelevant contextual information such as extraneous facts or theories, including peer opinion), can produce serious errors in perceptions and judgement, even amongst leading medical experts. Indeed, cognitive bias is an innate and subconscious phenomenon, and errors that arise from it do not necessarily reflect incompetence, malfeasance, or deliberate prejudice. It affects all people, especially when information is ambiguous and subjective judgements are made. The great challenge facing the medico-legal community and forensic scientists is developing best practices to mitigate and identify the effects of cognitive bias.

The Blind Reading

Remarkably and fortuitously, the Woodward case provides a great example of such a best practice – a blind reading of the radiology by Dr Alisa Gean. As we were feverishly preparing for trial under a very tight schedule, the defence team consulted with Dr Charles Fitz, a highly respected paediatric radiologist at the University of Pittsburgh. Unbeknownst to us, Dr Fitz sent the CT scans to Dr Gean, whom he later told us was the most brilliant neuroradiologist he knew. Dr Gean testified that she did a 'blind reading' of the CT scans – that is, she read the scans without any knowledge about the clinical history, including the age of the patient or any diagnostic hypothesis. All she knew was that this was a 'trauma case'. She did not know if it was for a patient or a legal case. Based solely on the images in the scan, she stated: 'My reading was that this was evidence of a re-bleed into a pre-existing subdural haematoma' [36].

Dr Gean went on to say that such blind readings and consultations were not unusual in her field because patients who present with trauma often can't give a history. 'And sometimes it actually improves diagnosis, because without that historical input, one has a broader differential diagnosis, and one might exclude other entities if one narrows it to just some specific points. So it actually improves the distillation, if you will, of the ultimate diagnosis, starting out with something that's objective, just what you have from the pictures' [36]. Dr Gean's 'blind reading' permitted her to conduct an analysis of the medical evidence free of the contextually biasing information attendant to a child-death case that included the triad.

Dr Gean was not an expert who testified in legal cases, and she rarely testified in SBS/AHT cases afterwards. Her contributions to the Woodward defence, however, were extraordinary. She pointed out the critical CT scan evidence showing no swelling at the site of the skull fracture, a finding that refuted the prosecution's core contention that Louise had slammed the baby's head on a fixed surface with a force of 20 miles per hour (mph) 2–6 hours prior to calling 911. Why did the neuroradiologists, paediatricians, and medical examiner overlook the evidence in the CT scan? One possible explanation is found in the Fawver et al. study cited in Chapter 13, where radiologists read case notes that were either accurate or misleading. Diagnostic accuracy decreased 40% among those who read the misleading case notes: 'It appears that the radiologists who read the misleading case notes did notice the relevant diagnostic information but failed to interpret it correctly.'

Similarly, Dr Gean's testimony suggests the MDT was susceptible to a cognitive bias known as the base-rate or prevalence effect. She noticed on the CT scans 'a very classic teaching example' of 'anoxia', meaning total oxygen deprivation [37]. It's quite possible the MDT missed this evidence of hypoxic-ischaemic injury because they were so used to diagnosing SBS/AHT cases, assuming severe impact and shaking.

Dr Gean's 'blind reading' is a good example of a technique known as linear sequential unmasking – expanded (LSU-E) (Chapter 13). Linear sequential unmasking has been recommended and used for years as a best practice in fingerprint analysis and DNA testing. It minimises the risks of error from cognitive biases by revealing case information to analysts sequentially so each step of the analytical process can be conducted under conditions that enable a 'blind' read to the greatest extent possible.

Linear sequential unmasking – expanded adapts the method to the medical context. First, the experts should form (and document) their initial opinion based solely on the raw data/evidence. Then experts may consider other relevant information and, in so doing, they should prioritise information that is more relevant, more objective, and/or lower in biasing power. This is precisely what Dr Gean did, starting with her 'blind reading' of the CT scans in the Woodward case.

Doubling Down, Overprecision, and Excessive Certainty

Cognitive scientists warn that in response to disconfirming feedback that 'poses a salient threat to expert identities', experts often respond by 'doubling down and exhibiting overprecision, or excessive certainty regarding the accuracy of one's beliefs' [6]. This 'doubling down' and denial of critical objective facts by Dr Newberger, the leader of the MDT of Harvard's Children's Hospital, was on disturbing display in the Woodward case.

After relying on the 1987 Duhaime–Thibault paper, and after acknowledging that he was not an expert in biomechanics and had not made a specific study of tolerance criteria for injury to the neck or spine, Dr Newberger insisted that Matthew Eappen was 'violently shaken back and forth for at least a minute with the head uncontrollably snapping back and forth'. But, he claimed, such violent shaking was 'not likely to break a neck'; 'would not cause any damage to the ligaments of the spinal cord'; 'would not cause any displacement of vertebrae'; and 'would not cause any injuries to the muscles of the neck'. He lectured a grand juror who thought the severe shaking Newberger described would have likely broken Matthew's neck that 'in virtually all cases of shaken baby syndrome you don't see bone injury. I *suspect* that it has something to do with the way the neck is constructed, that nature has given us the ability to move our neck without fracturing bones' [38].

After saying the force of the impact that caused the skull fracture was equivalent to the baby being dropped on his head from a two-story building onto concrete, a speed at impact he agreed was about 20 mph [39], and being confronted with the fact that Dr Mandl (the ER physician) found no swelling on the head, Dr Newberger testified that Dr Mandl 'may have missed' the swelling [40]. After being shown that there was no swelling at the site of fracture on the CT scan, Dr Newberger then suggested that, when 'the heart may not be pumping right', it 'takes time for swelling to develop, there might not be the usual inflammatory process that causes soft tissue swelling' [41]. He made that statement, however, without recalling that Matthew's heart rate and blood pressure from the time he was taken from his home to the time he arrived at the hospital were 'within normal limits' [41].

Twenty-five years later, it is hard to pick the most distressing aspect of Dr Newberger's 'doubling down' testimony and actions.

- Is it his science-free speculation in response to a grand juror that 'in virtually all cases of shaken baby syndrome you don't see bone injury to the neck because nature has given us the ability to move our neck without fracturing bones'?
- Is it the glib suggestions that Dr Mandl, who testified to carefully examining Matthew's head for swelling because he knew it was important, simply 'missed it'?
- Is it his sudden pivot to the 'no swelling happened' position when confronted by the lack of swelling in the CT scan?
- Is it his insistence that the lack of swelling was caused by the 'heart not pumping right' when the medical records he supposedly reviewed showed that the heart rate and blood pressure were within normal limits? (Note that, if Matthew's head had, in fact, been slammed against a fixed hard surface at a speed equivalent to 20 mph, and, if he had died when his heart stopped beating right after impact, that might have accounted for less-than-expected swelling at the site of the skull fracture, but not for the absence of split skin or a fracture that was depressed or comminuted.)
- Is it his continued failure to acknowledge the history Louise gave Debbie Eappen about Matthew's behaviour the day he collapsed, a history Drs Mandl and Madsen agreed on

cross-examination could be consistent with the defence theory of a re-bleed of an old SDH?
- Is it Newberger's arrogant, demeaning speculation that Dr Thibault was the 'junior author' of the article he wrote with his former student Dr Duhaime, and that, because Dr Thibault was not a clinician, he did not 'formulate the questions and very provocative and interesting conclusions of that article' [43]?

All of that testimony was deeply troubling, but in terms of the impact it had on the trial, I believe the most significant instance of denial and rejection of disconfirming information was his inexplicable insistence the fluid Dr Madsen described as 'serum' that spurted out of Matthew Eappen's head during the craniectomy could not have been serum.

The Serum That Wasn't Serum

Dr Madsen, the neurosurgeon who actually operated on Matthew, described in his contemporaneous notes a 'yellowish-clearish fluid' that spurted out when he opened the dura. He said unequivocally this was serum, which had a yellowish hue caused by the breakdown of old blood. This was not cerebrospinal fluid (CSF) because 'CSF is even a clearer fluid than serum would be' [43]. All the defence experts, particularly Drs Thibault, Gean, and Leestma, provided detailed explanations as to why the initial spurting out of serum followed by blood meant that the SDH represented a re-bleed of an older injury.

The presence of serum posed a serious problem for Dr Newberger. He agreed that if serum spurted out, it meant that the SDH was an old injury. Clinging to his opinion that this was not an old injury, he insisted that it wasn't serum:

Q: And if this were, in fact, serum, would that not indicate the existence, the possibility of an older injury?

A: Yes.

Q: There would be a possibility of an older injury if that were, in fact, serum. And serious consideration would have to be given if that were, in fact, serum, to the question as to whether this was an older injury, fair enough?

Q: Yes, but it wasn't [44].

Dr Patrick Barnes had the same total denial reaction to the disconfirming serum evidence – despite Dr Madsen's description it was serum, he insisted it couldn't have been serum.

The Problematic Use of Confessions or Admissions As Proof of Shaken Baby Syndrome

There was no confession in the Woodward case. In fact, there was general agreement between the prosecution and the defence as to what Louise said about events on the day before she called 911. Debbie Eappen produced written notes of what Louise said when Matthew was admitted. The problem was that Drs Madsen, Newberger, Barnes, and Mandl all said they were not aware of that history. Dr Mandl agreed on cross-examination that this history would be consistent with the effects of the re-bleed of an old SDH – the defence theory of the case [25]. In short, the history Louise gave to Debbie Eappen soon after Matthew collapsed was powerful exculpatory evidence because it is extremely unlikely she could have anticipated or known about symptoms consistent with the re-bleed of an old

SDH. Her statements constitute proof of what lawyers call 'consciousness of innocence' rather than tell-tale admissions demonstrating 'consciousness of guilt'.

Nonetheless, the prosecution used Dr Newberger's belief that the 'triad' was 'virtually pathognomonic of shaken baby syndrome' and his certainty about the mechanisms that must have caused Matthew's injuries to make the history Louise gave sound like admissions, purposeful understatements and evasions showing consciousness of guilt:[2]

> Q: Doctor, do you have an opinion to a reasonable degree of medical certainty whether a gentle shaking at approximately 2:45 PM on February 4th to arouse or revive Matthew because he appeared sick and unresponsive, would have caused Matthew's eye, brain, and skull injuries that were observed to be present in Matthew?
>
> A: Yes.
>
> Q: What is your opinion, Doctor?
>
> A: My opinion is that a 'gentle shaking', as you described, could not have brought forward, produced the injuries which I saw in my examination [45].

Dr Newberger then swore to a 'reasonable degree of medical certainty' that tossing Matthew onto a bed just prior to admission to the hospital could not 'have caused his eye, brain, and skull injuries' and that Matthew 'being dropped onto towels covering a tile bathroom floor' could not 'have caused the injuries to his eyes, brain, and skull' [45]. While no one, and certainly not Louise, was claiming those actions on the day Matthew collapsed were the cause of his collapse, the prosecution cynically presented Louise's statements about what happened that day as if the defence were claiming that explained Matthew's death.

This approach of using an unshakably certain inference about the unwitnessed mechanisms of severe shaking and impact based solely on the 'triad', and then contrasting these unequivocal assertions by a respected doctor to whatever inadequate explanation the last caregiver provides, is a classic, formulaic, and a very effective way to try a shaken baby case.

The Most Important Lessons

The most important lesson to be learned from the trial of Louise Woodward is that the defence proved its case. This was an old SDH, about 3 weeks old, that re-bled, causing a mass effect and a herniation of the brain. The history taken down by the mother, Debbie Eappen, from Louise, accurately described the symptoms of the evolving re-bleed. That was not known by the key members of the MDT whose testimony quickly led to Louise's indictment for murder based on the presumed mechanisms SBS/AHT 'diagnosis' – a violent slamming and severe shaking a few hours before admission to the hospital. That was the charge. I thought the medical and scientific evidence was overwhelming at the time of trial that the violent slamming and shaking never happened. As this book demonstrates, new understandings of the science in this area only make that conclusion stronger for those who are willing to examine the case. I believe, and the defence argued at trial, that the old skull fracture and SDH were probably the result of an accidental fall weeks earlier. The prosecution's expert witnesses insisted short accidental falls could not cause such 'triad' injuries. We now know that is completely wrong.

Twenty-five years ago, the presumption of abuse on the basis of unvalidated science and the rush to infer or interpret away any medical findings and evidence inconsistent with

---

[2] See footnote 1. This is another example of prosecution witnesses embracing the 'triad' as pathognomonic of SBS.

abuse were deeply troubling to me. It was also deeply troubling to Judge Hiller B. Zobel, who presided at the Woodward trial. Shortly after the jury rendered its murder verdict – which would have sent Louise to prison for life – Judge Zobel, declaring the outcome of the case a 'miscarriage of justice', courageously used his discretionary powers to reduce her conviction to involuntary manslaughter and her sentence to time served so she could be discharged from custody immediately, after spending 279 days in an American jail. I think Judge Zobel thought Louise was innocent, that it was an old injury that re-bled and there was no violent slamming and shaking. The prosecutors have stated publicly they agree that Judge Zobel thought she was innocent.

In retrospect, the rush to judgement was also troubling to at least one of the prosecution's most adamant experts at the trial – Dr Patrick Barnes, the prosecution's paediatric neuroradiologist. Dr Barnes was troubled by an accusatory remark I made during cross-examination when he refused to 'assume' facts for purposes of a hypothetical question ('Were you there, Dr Barnes?'). He subsequently set about re-examining the scientific evidence base for the positions he had so firmly embraced at trial [8]. In the end, he concluded that he had been wrong and that the SBS hypothesis simply was not supported by high-quality research. Almost 10 years later, in 2007, Dr Barnes testified in post-conviction proceedings on behalf of Audrey Edmunds, a Wisconsin woman convicted of killing an infant in her care based on the old triad-based medical hypothesis. Dr Barnes testified that the evidence base for SBS was woefully inadequate under accepted evidence-based medicine standards. The courts ultimately vacated Edmunds's conviction and the prosecution dismissed the charges, making her the first person to be exonerated on the basis of shifting understandings of the medical science underlying the SBS/AHT hypothesis. Dr Barnes went on to become a vocal critic of SBS/AHT.

As this book demonstrates, while scientists have learned a great deal in the years since the Woodward case, and while, accordingly, child abuse physicians have backed off from some of their more extreme and dogmatic positions, the same patterns that were on display in the Woodward trial are repeated today in SBS/AHT prosecutions across vast portions of the world. The science remains unresolved and justice remains elusive. This book launches a new chapter in the advancement of both science and law by opening a rigorous inquiry into SBS/AHT and the prosecution of child abuse. We can only hope that this book arrives at a moment when the medical and legal communities are ready to move past the cognitive rigidity and entrenchment that has so marked this field for the past decades into a 'high-validity environment' that enables real learning and, in the end, better justice.

References

1. Choudhary AK, Servaes S, Slovis TL et al. Consensus statement on abusive head trauma in infants and young children. *Pediatric Radiology*. 2018 Aug;48 (8):1048–65.
2. Leventhal JM, Asnes AG, Pavlovic L, Moles RL. Diagnosing abusive head trauma: The challenges faced by clinicians. *Pediatric Radiology*. 2014;44(4):537–42.
3. Dane E. Reconsidering the trade-off between expertise and flexibility: A cognitive entrenchment. *Academy of Management Review*. 2020;35(4):579–603.
4. Furr N, Cavarreta F, Garg S. Who changes the course? The role of domain knowledge and novel framing in making technology changes. *Strategic Entrepreneurship Journal*. 2012;6:236–56.
5. Staats BR, Diwas KC, Gingo F. Maintaining beliefs in the face of negative news: The moderating role of

experience. *Management Science*. 2018;64 (2):804–24.

6. Kang S, Kim JW. The fragility of experts: A moderated-mediation model of expertise, expert identity threat, and overprecision. *Academy of Management Review*. 2022;65(2):577–605.
7. Kahneman D, Klein J. Conditions for intuitive expertise: A failure to disagree. *American Psychologist*. 2009;64 (6):515–26.
8. Haberman C. Shaken baby syndrome: A diagnosis that divides the medical world. 2015, 13 September. www.nytimes.com/2015/09/14/us/shaken-baby-syndrome-a-diagnosis-that-divides-the-medical-world.html.
9. Transcript of Trial Vol. 3:50, *Commonwealth* v. *Woodward*, No. 97-433 (Sup. Ct. Middlesex Cnty., Mass. 8 Oct. 1997).
10. Transcript of Trial Vol. 3:48–9, *Commonwealth* v. *Woodward*, No. 97-433 (Sup. Ct. Middlesex Cnty., Mass. 8 Oct. 1997).
11. Transcript of Trial Vol. 3:55–6, *Commonwealth* v. *Woodward*, No. 97-433 (Sup. Ct. Middlesex Cnty., Mass. 8 Oct. 1997).
12. Transcript of Trial Vol. 11:161, *Commonwealth* v. *Woodward*, No. 97-433 (Sup. Ct. Middlesex Cnty., Mass. 21 Oct. 1997).
13. Transcript of Trial Vol. 11:164, *Commonwealth* v. *Woodward*, No. 97-433 (Sup. Ct. Middlesex Cnty., Mass. 21 Oct. 1997).
14. Transcript of Trial Vol. 11:192–6, *Commonwealth* v. *Woodward*, No. 97-433 (Sup. Ct. Middlesex Cnty., Mass. 21 Oct. 1997).
15. Transcript of Trial Vol. 11:198, *Commonwealth* v. *Woodward*, No. 97-433 (Sup. Ct. Middlesex Cnty., Mass. 21 Oct. 1997).
16. Duhaime AC, Gennarelli TA, Thibault LE et al. The shaken baby syndrome. A clinical, pathological, and biomechanical study. *Journal of Neurosurgery*. 1987;66 (3):409–15.
17. Transcript of Trial Vol. 11:213–23, *Commonwealth* v. *Woodward*, No. 97-433 (Sup. Ct. Middlesex Cnty., Mass. 21 Oct. 1997).
18. Transcript of Trial Vol. 6:62, *Commonwealth* v. *Woodward*, No. 97-433 (Sup. Ct. Middlesex Cnty., Mass. 14 Oct. 1997).
19. Transcript of Trial Vol. 6:52, *Commonwealth* v. *Woodward*, No. 97-433 (Sup. Ct. Middlesex Cnty., Mass. 14 Oct. 1997).
20. Transcript of Trial Vol. 6:54, *Commonwealth* v. *Woodward*, No. 97-433 (Sup. Ct. Middlesex Cnty., Mass. 14 Oct. 1997).
21. Transcript of Trial Vol. 11:219, *Commonwealth* v. *Woodward*, No. 97-433 (Sup. Ct. Middlesex Cnty., Mass. 21 Oct. 1997).
22. Transcript of Trial Vol. 6:2, *Commonwealth* v. *Woodward*, No. 97-433 (Sup. Ct. Middlesex Cnty., Mass. 14 Oct. 1997).
23. Transcript of Trial Vol. 6:96–9, *Commonwealth* v. *Woodward*, No. 97-433 (Sup. Ct. Middlesex Cnty., Mass. 14 Oct. 1997).
24. Transcript of Trial Vol. 3:45, *Commonwealth* v. *Woodward*, No. 97-433 (Sup. Ct. Middlesex Cnty., Mass. 8 Oct. 1997).
25. Transcript of Trial Vol. 2:180–3, *Commonwealth* v. *Woodward*, No. 97-433 (Sup. Ct. Middlesex Cnty., Mass. 7 Oct. 1997).
26. Transcript of Trial Vol. 2:204–5, *Commonwealth* v. *Woodward*, No. 97-433 (Sup. Ct. Middlesex Cnty., Mass. 7 Oct. 1997).
27. Transcript of Trial Vol. 9:45–6, *Commonwealth* v. *Woodward*, No. 97-433 (Sup. Ct. Middlesex Cnty., Mass. 17 Oct. 1997).
28. Transcript of Trial Vol. 9:144–6, *Commonwealth* v. *Woodward*, No. 97-433

(Sup. Ct. Middlesex Cnty., Mass. 17 Oct. 1997).

29. Transcript of Trial Vol. 3:85–8, *Commonwealth* v. *Woodward*, No. 97-433 (Sup. Ct. Middlesex Cnty., Mass. 8 Oct. 1997).

30. Transcript of Trial Vol. 9:178–80, *Commonwealth* v. *Woodward*, No. 97-433 (Sup. Ct. Middlesex Cnty., Mass. 17 Oct. 1997).

31. Transcript of Trial Vol. 9:182–3, *Commonwealth* v. *Woodward*, No. 97-433 (Sup. Ct. Middlesex Cnty., Mass. 17 Oct. 1997).

32. Transcript of Trial Vol. 12:57, *Commonwealth* v. *Woodward*, No. 97-433 (Sup. Ct. Middlesex Cnty., Mass. 22 Oct. 1997).

33. Transcript of Trial Vol. 3:199, *Commonwealth* v. *Woodward*, No. 97-433 (Sup. Ct. Middlesex Cnty., Mass. 8 Oct. 1997).

34. Transcript of Trial Vol. 4:138, *Commonwealth* v. *Woodward*, No. 97-433 (Sup. Ct. Middlesex Cnty., Mass. 9 Oct. 1997).

35. Transcript of Trial Vol. 14:140–2, *Commonwealth* v. *Woodward*, No. 97-433 (Sup. Ct. Middlesex Cnty., Mass. 27 Oct. 1997).

36. Transcript of Trial Vol. 10:169–70, *Commonwealth* v. *Woodward*, No. 97-433 (Sup. Ct. Middlesex Cnty., Mass. 20 Oct. 1997).

37. Transcript of Trial Vol. 10:198–9, *Commonwealth* v. *Woodward*, No. 97-433 (Sup. Ct. Middlesex Cnty., Mass. 20 Oct. 1997).

38. Transcript of Trial Vol. 7:106–8, *Commonwealth* v. *Woodward*, No. 97-433 (Sup. Ct. Middlesex Cnty., Mass. 15 Oct. 1997).

39. Transcript of Trial Vol. 7:91, *Commonwealth* v. *Woodward*, No. 97-433 (Sup. Ct. Middlesex Cnty., Mass. 15 Oct. 1997).

40. Transcript of Trial Vol. 11:53–4, *Commonwealth* v. *Woodward*, No. 97-433 (Sup. Ct. Middlesex Cnty., Mass. 21 Oct. 1997).

41. Transcript of Trial Vol. 7:95–6, *Commonwealth* v. *Woodward*, No. 97-433 (Sup. Ct. Middlesex Cnty., Mass. 15 Oct. 1997).

42. Transcript of Trial Vol. 7:76–7, *Commonwealth* v. *Woodward*, No. 97-433 (Sup. Ct. Middlesex Cnty., Mass. 15 Oct. 1997).

43. Transcript of Trial Vol. 3:76–8, *Commonwealth* v. *Woodward*, No. 97-433 (Sup. Ct. Middlesex Cnty., Mass. 8 Oct. 1997).

44. Transcript of Trial Vol. 7:124, *Commonwealth* v. *Woodward*, No. 97-433 (Sup. Ct. Middlesex Cnty., Mass. 15 Oct. 1997).

45. Transcript of Trial Vol. 7:27–38, *Commonwealth* v. *Woodward*, No. 97-433 (Sup. Ct. Middlesex Cnty., Mass. 15 Oct. 1997).

About This Book

This book tackles a highly controversial subject at the intersection of medicine, science, and law. We therefore want to make clear from the outset what this book is about and what it does and does not put into question.

Child abuse is a pervasive societal issue that has only recently received the consideration it deserves. Effective child protection systems are essential to detect and protect abused children.

Shaking is a form of physical child abuse that predominantly affects children under two years of age. Half a century ago, the British paediatric neurosurgeon Dr Norman Guthkelch noticed that many parents and caregivers were shaking their infants as a means of discipline [5]. Abusive shaking is assumed to be widespread around the world [8]. Sometimes parents and caregivers inflict intentional head trauma on infants and cause severe injuries.

The Importance of Clear Definitions

This book is not about child abuse in general; it is about the scientific reliability of a causal link between abusive shaking and a constellation of intracranial findings in infants. We wish to be precise with our definitions in order to facilitate rational discussion. In this book we employ the following definition: 'Shaken baby syndrome' (SBS) is the medical hypothesis according to which, with a few rare exceptions, all infants presenting with retinal and subdural haemorrhage possibly associated with bridging vein thrombosis with no history or evidence of major trauma are presumed to have been violently shaken moments before showing neurological compromise [1].

The medical establishment distanced itself from the term 'shaken baby syndrome' in the early 2010s and has instead been promoting an alternative terminology and definition: 'Abusive Head Trauma (AHT) is the current most appropriate and inclusive diagnostic term for infants and young children who suffer from inflicted intracranial and associated spinal injury' [2].

The Danger of Ambiguous Terms

Because they conflate a criminal act with a constellation of medical findings, both terms are highly ambiguous and lead to confusion. As Guthkelch himself declared 40 years after propounding his shaking hypothesis, the use of a more neutral term, such as 'retino-dural haemorrhage of infancy' (RDHI), is recommended. This term describes medical findings without presuming a unique aetiology [6]. The newer term 'abusive head trauma' (AHT) continues to purport to 'diagnose' abuse yet widens the range of associated medical findings and their potential causes (not only shaking but also impact) to such a degree as to be unhelpful.

This book uses the term SBS because it is specific and it encapsulates the very kernel of the issue: the claim that certain intracranial findings can alone (with no or minimal evidence of external trauma) be used as proof that shaking has occurred and that it was an intentional (or knowing or reckless or negligent) and hence abusive act. Our definition of SBS makes clear why it is at the intersection of medicine (retino-dural haemorrhage is a medical finding), science (a causality hypothesis that would require robust evidence), and law (the observation of specific medical findings indicates with near certainty that a crime has occurred).

The Core Issue: 'Triad'-Based Medical Determinations of Abuse

Many physicians believe they can reliably determine that abuse has occurred based solely on the presence of RDHI. The term 'triad' is sometimes used to refer to the association of the two medical findings of RDHI with encephalopathy.

This belief relies on the false assumption that subdural and retinal haemorrhage are almost always traumatic in infants. Yet, as this book will show, the evidence base of a causal link between abusive shaking and RDHI is weak.

Furthermore, many other explanations for these medical findings (differential diagnoses) have been demonstrated over the years. The oft-repeated claim that these 'rare' causes are always meticulously excluded before concluding abuse as a default determination is misleading [3]. Few of these medical conditions are commonly accepted or examined but, most importantly, a determination by exclusion is dangerous as it ignores all potential explanations yet unidentified by medical science. It is this idea of a systematic default determination of abuse based on specific intracranial findings, now denied by some of the very same authors who supported it in the past, that we challenge in this book [7].

We also challenge the more general claim that medicine can reliably 'diagnose' child abuse. This usurps the role of the courts; abuse is a legal determination, not a medical diagnosis [4]. This book does not dispute that physical abuse is a likely determination in children with multiple unexplained traumatic injuries. That uncontroversial claim is not our focus.

A Legitimate Controversy

We recognise that many would prefer not to see the publication of this book, claiming that challenges to SBS by 'denialists' are dangerous and create the risk of encouraging abusive caregiver behaviour.

We do not deny that child abuse occurs.

We do not want anyone to read this book as presenting any claim that violently shaking or abusing a child is safe. Abusive behaviours are dangerous and must be prevented. Perpetrators must be criminally prosecuted.

We do not want anyone to believe this book could help actual perpetrators be exculpated. Rather, this book should help courts make the most informed decisions in each case by comprehending the real state of current scientific knowledge regarding RDHI, SBS, and AHT.

We do maintain that failure to engage in legitimate scientific inquiry and debate, and to rely prematurely on an inadequately supported hypothesis to remove children from their parents or send caregivers to prison, is itself abusive, unscientific and dangerous.

There are those who claim that challengers of SBS are attempting to create a medical controversy where there is none, in order to confuse judges and juries [2]. According to them, there is a near-universal consensus on the validity of SBS/AHT, a 'diagnosis' that is purportedly supported by dozens of professional societies around the world.

We do assert there is a legitimate controversy about SBS [4, 7]. As this book will show, many professionals do not agree with the 'consensus'. More importantly, even a true medical consensus would not compensate for the dearth of valid, high-quality science to support SBS. Unfortunately, the lack of reliable scientific evidence is only apparent via a comprehensive, if not systematic, review of the thousands of relevant publications in the medical literature, especially outside of the narrow field of child abuse paediatrics.

The few who have had the time and energy to thoroughly review the literature have come to challenge the very hypothesis they initially believed in. Many of them have participated in writing this book in the hope of helping their colleagues comprehend the controversy with an open and critical mind.

Structure of the Book

This book provides careful, evidence-based analyses of the relevant disciplines in 26 chapters with the contributions of 32 professionals from 8 countries in 16 different specialties and 18 additional professionals from 12 other countries in the international chapter.

Section 1 Prologue

After Chapter 1, which exposes the difficulties in challenging long-held beliefs related to the science of SBS/AHT, and Chapter 2, which provides an historical overview of the controversy, the four main sections of the book are as follows.

Section 2 Medicine

In Chapter 3, we provide a thorough review of the neuropathology of the medical findings associated with SBS/AHT. Chapter 4 explains why radiology and pathology must be correlated in order to increase the accuracy of imaging diagnosis of infant head trauma, and how some imaging findings thought to indicate specific pathology have never been verified or even been shown to be incorrect. Chapter 5 tackles benign external hydrocephalus (BEH), a medical condition that is associated with RDHI and that may be frequently misdiagnosed with SBS/AHT, as shown in Chapter 6.

Other conditions associated with these findings include sudden infant death syndrome, which has strong epidemiological links to SBS/AHT as explored in Chapter 7, and many other rare conditions and intrinsic risk factors, as briefly reviewed in Chapter 8. Because the list of potential causes of RDHI is ever growing and essentially unknowable, such a list is not included in this book. In Chapter 9 a paediatrician reveals how he changed his mind on the validity of SBS/AHT.

Section 3 Science

Chapter 10 presents a systematic review performed by the Swedish Agency for Health Technology Assessment (SBU) and the critical response that followed. This study showed that the evidence base of SBS/AHT is weak due to serious methodological shortcomings (such as circular reasoning) and that it relies particularly on confessions. Chapter 11 explains how police interrogation may lead to false confessions, which, as shown in Chapter 12, is a major reason confessions have such a low scientific value. Physicians typically claim they rely on their clinical experience and judgement to confidently diagnose abuse, but Chapter 13 shows how any medical expert may make serious mistakes due to cognitive biases.

At the same time, Chapter 14 shows that biomechanical data have failed to support the idea that shaking could cause RDHI. On the contrary, short falls can, and Chapter 15 explains why statistical arguments made to refute this idea are false. Chapter 16 explores the epidemiology of SBS/AHT in Sweden. Finally, in Chapter 17, methodological shortcomings in the clinical literature are demonstrated by a mathematical model.

Section 4 Law

Chapter 18 tackles issues with mandatory reporting and child protection policies, particularly in the United States and in New Zealand. Chapter 19 discusses the admissibility of SBS/AHT evidence in American courts, while Chapter 20 exposes challenges in exonerating wrongly convicted parents and caregivers in the US criminal justice system.

Section 5 International

Shaken baby syndrome/abusive head trauma is an issue in many countries. The last section of this book provides a detailed report on the situation in the United Kingdom (Chapter 21), France (Chapter 22), Sweden (Chapter 23), Japan (Chapter 24), and Australia (Chapter 25). Finally Chapter 26 presents a short compilation of the situation in many more countries: Argentina, Brazil, Canada, Chile, China, Colombia, Costa Rica, Denmark, Ecuador, Estonia, Germany, India, Israel, Luxembourg, Mexico, New Zealand, Norway, Peru, Portugal, Romania, Saudi Arabia, South Africa, South Korea, Spain, Switzerland, Taiwan, Turkey, and Vietnam.

Section 6 Postface

The book ends with challenges to frequenty-repeated claims about SBS/AHT along with references to the relevant chapters.

Updates and errata can be found on the book's website: https://shakenbaby.science and comments can be sent to contact@shakenbaby.science

References

1. Chadwick DL, Kirschner RH, Reece RM et al. Shaken baby syndrome: A forensic pediatric response. *Pediatrics*. 1998 Feb 1;101(2):321–3.
2. Choudhary AK, Servaes S, Slovis TL et al. Consensus statement on abusive head trauma in infants and young children. *Pediatric Radiology*. 2018 Aug;48 (8):1048–65.
3. David TJ. Non-accidental head injury: The evidence. *Pediatric Radiology*. 2008 38: S370–7.
4. Findley KA, Risinger DM, Barnes PD et al. Feigned consensus: Usurping the law in shaken baby syndrome/abusive head trauma prosecutions. *Wisconsin Law Review*. 2019:1211–67.
5. Guthkelch AN. Infantile subdural haematoma and its relationship to whiplash injuries. *British Medical Journal*. 1971 May 22;2(5759):430–1.
6. Guthkelch AN. Problems of infant retino-dural hemorrhage with minimal external injury. *Houston Journal of Health Law and Policy*. 2012 12:201–8.
7. Papetti R, Kaneb P, Herf L. Outside the echo chamber: A response to the Consensus Statement on Abusive Head Trauma in Infants and Young Children. *Santa Clara Law Review*. 2019 59:299–366.
8. Runyan DK. The challenges of assessing the incidence of inflicted traumatic brain injury: A world perspective. *American Journal of Preventive Medicine*. 2008 Apr 1;34(4):S112–S115.

Abbreviations

AAP	American Academy of Pediatrics
ADC	Apparent Diffusion Coefficient
AE	Anoxic Encephalopathy
AHT	Abusive Head Trauma
ALTE	Acute/Apparent Life-Threatening Event
βAPP	beta-Amyloid Precursor Protein
ASDH	Acute Subdural Haematoma
AT	Accidental Trauma
ATD	Anthropomorphic Test Device
AVM	Arteriovenous Malformation
BCS	Battered Child Syndrome
BEH	Benign External Hydrocephalus
BESS	Benign Enlargement of Subarachnoid Space
BFA	Biomechanical Forensic Analysis
BN	Bayesian Network
BRUE	Brief Resolved Unexplained Event
BV	Bridging Veins
CAP	Child Abuse Paediatrician
CAT	Child Abuse Team
CML	Classic Metaphyseal Lesions
CNS	Central Nervous System
COCAN	Council on Child Abuse and Neglect
CPR	Cardio-pulmonary Resuscitation
CPT	Child Protection Team
CSC	Cervical Spinal Cord
CSDH	Chronic Subdural Haematoma
CSF	Cerebrospinal Fluid
CSVT	Cerebral Sinovenous Thrombosis
CT	Computed Tomography
CVST	Cerebral Venous Sinus Thrombosis
CVT	Cortical Vein Thrombosis
DAI	Diffuse Axonal Injury
DWI	Diffusion-Weighted Imaging
EBM	Evidence-Based Medicine
EDH	Epidural Haemorrhage
EDS	Ehlers–Danlos Syndrome
FEM	Finite-Element Modelling
GA1	Glutaric Aciduria Type 1
GMC	General Medical Council (UK)
GOR	Gastro-oesophageal Reflux
HAS	Haute Autorité de Santé (France)
HC	Head Circumference
HIE	Hypoxic-Ischaemic Encephalopathy
HII	Hypoxic-Ischaemic Injury
HU	Hounsfield Unit
IASDH	Infantile Acute Subdural Haematoma
ICH	Intracranial Haemorrhage
ICI	Intracranial Injury
ICP	Intracranial Pressure
IDH	Intradural Haemorrhage
IEAFS	Increased Extra-axial Fluid Spaces

IHI	Inflicted Head Injury
ISPCAN	International Society for the Prevention of Child Abuse and Neglect
IUD	Intrauterine Death
IVH	Intraventricular Haemorrhage
IVT	Intracranial Venous Thrombosis
MDT	Multidisciplinary Team
MRI	Magnetic Resonance Imaging
NAHI	Non-accidental Head Injury
NAI	Non-accidental Injury
NAT	Non-accidental Trauma
OI	Osteogenesis Imperfecta
ONSH	Optic Nerve Sheath Haemorrhage
RBC	Red Blood Cell
RDHI	Retino-dural Haemorrhage of Infancy
RH	Retinal Haemorrhage
RICP	Raised Intracranial Pressure
SAH	Subarachnoid Haemorrhage
SBS	Shaken Baby Syndrome
SBU	Swedish Agency for Health Technology Assessment and Assessment of Social Services (Sweden)
SCI	Spinal Cord Injury
SDH	Subdural Haematoma
SIDS	Sudden Infant Death Syndrome
SES	Socioeconomic Status
SGA	Small for Gestational Age
SSS	Superior Sagittal Sinus
SUDI	Sudden Unexpected Death in Infancy
TAI	Traumatic Axonal Injury
US	Ultrasound
VAI	Vascular Axonal Injury
VT	Vitreo-retinal Traction
VWD	von Willebrand Disease
WBC	White Blood Cell
WM	White Matter

Chapter 1

Maintaining the Orthodoxy and Silencing Dissent

Chris Brook

Retreating to ivory towers [1]. Armchair experts [2]. Pseudo-scientists [3]. Naysayers [4]. Nonbelievers [5]. Biased [6]. Denialists [7]. Deceitful, dishonest, unethical [8]. Evil [9]. These terms have all been used to describe those who challenge the science behind shaken baby syndrome (SBS), those who challenge the way abuse of infants is 'diagnosed'.

Name-calling is used to delegitimise those with opposing views and to defend the legitimacy of the orthodoxy [10].[1] In psychology, legitimacy is a 'property of an authority, institution, or social arrangement that leads those connected to it to believe that it is appropriate, proper, and just. Because of legitimacy, people feel that they ought to defer to decisions and rules, following them voluntarily out of obligation rather than out of fear of punishment or anticipation of reward' [11].

The defence of the orthodox approach to SBS and the efforts to delegitimise and silence those with opposing views have gone beyond name-calling. Legal threats have been made to pressure editors to retract a properly peer-reviewed journal article that questioned an SBS diagnosis [12]. An entire edition of an academic journal, which was to publish a debate by proponents and challengers of SBS, foundered after pressure was placed on the publisher [13]. Experts have been charged with perjury or subjected to complaints to medical boards after testifying for the defence [14]. They have faced censorship by medical associations. Workplace harassment and threats to employment have been endorsed and encouraged through calls for wholesale sackings and de-registration of doctors who question SBS orthodoxy [8].

No other contemporary medicolegal issue has seen the level of controversy of SBS. Indeed, no other field of forensic science (or forensic medicine) has seen such controversy nor departed so severely from the norms of scientific discourse. Forty years after writing his 1971 article [15] that hypothesised shaking as a cause of subdural haemorrhage in infants, Dr Norman Guthkelch lamented that, 'while controversy is a normal and necessary part of scientific discourse, there has arisen a level of emotion and divisiveness on shaken baby syndrome/abusive head trauma that has interfered with our commitment to pursue the truth' [16]. The dispute over SBS has been described as 'tribal warfare' [13].

1.1 Delegitimising and Silencing Dissent

Perhaps the most famous battle over SBS took place in 1997 in Boston, where Louise Woodward, a 19-year-old au pair from England, was tried for the murder of an 8-month-old boy in her care. Prosecution witnesses, including Dr Eli Newberger, Dr Gerald Feigin,

1 Worthlessness is being portrayed by 'pseudo-science' and 'armchair expert', while depravity is portrayed in terms such as 'dishonest', 'unethical', and 'naysayers'.

Dr Joseph Madsen, and Dr Patrick Barnes, testified that the infant had been violently shaken. Defence witnesses Dr Jan Leestma, Dr Michael Baden, and Dr Ronald Uscinski testified that the infant had an old, chronic subdural haemorrhage that had re-bled. The trial made daily headlines on both sides of the Atlantic. Woodward was found guilty but the judge who presided over her trial quickly exercised his discretionary authority to serve the interests of justice and reduced her conviction from second-degree murder to manslaughter and imposed a sentence of time served, leading to her immediate release from custody.

After the case the battle spilled into the literature, where supporters of the SBS hypothesis attacked the defence witnesses, calling the possibility of re-bleed a 'courtroom diagnosis' rather than a medical diagnosis, and declared that the 'triad' of brain swelling, subdural haemorrhage, and retinal haemorrhage were 'virtually unique' diagnostic features of SBS [17].

Subsequent to the trial, prosecution witness Dr Patrick Barnes changed his mind about SBS, having moved beyond the child abuse literature to look instead at the science of traumatic head injury written by specialists in those fields. This led to Barnes being included in an 'axis of evil' doctors who questioned the SBS orthodoxy, alongside defence witnesses from the Woodward case Leestma and Uscinski as well as others such as Dr Janice Ophoven and Dr John Plunkett [9].

In 2001, Plunkett published a seminal article showing that short falls could cause the findings associated with SBS [18]. Later the same year, Plunkett gave testimony at the murder trial of Lisa Stickney, a day care worker accused of shaking to death a 14-month-old boy in her care. Stickney claimed that the boy had fallen from a chair. Plunkett testified that such a fall could explain the boy's death, contradicting the opinions of doctors who had testified for the prosecution. After Stickney was acquitted, the district attorney charged Plunkett with 'false swearing'. The other defence expert in the case, pathologist Dr John Antonius, was the subject of a complaint to the state board of medical examiners.

Both Plunkett and Antonius were eventually cleared, but at considerable personal cost in terms of time, money, and stress. The prosecutor contacted other prosecutors in SBS cases in other jurisdictions to inform them that Plunkett was being investigated for perjury. Lawyers for Dr Plunkett asserted that the charges were a 'blatant attempt to discredit Dr Plunkett to prevent him from testifying for the defence'. The message sent to those who challenged the SBS orthodoxy in court was also clear. '"It's scary," said Chicago neuropathologist Dr Jan Leestma, who had testified for the defence in several SBS cases, "and there comes a point where you start to ask yourself, 'Do I want to keep on doing this?'"'[14].

It was also 2001 when Dr Jennian Geddes and her collaborators published two ground-breaking articles that transformed our understanding of the findings associated with SBS [19, 20]. Geddes made detailed microscopic studies of the brains of infants who had been diagnosed with non-accidental injury and found that the majority do not have torn nerve fibres, which had been the assumed mechanism of encephalopathy in SBS cases. Instead, Geddes found that they predominantly had hypoxia, a failure of oxygen supply. This was truly a paradigm shift and showed that both the brain swelling and subdural haemorrhages that had been associated with shaking or trauma could in fact have a range of causes, including non-traumatic ones (see Chapters 3 and 4).

In a 2003 article, Geddes proposed a 'unified hypothesis', describing a scenario in which a lack of oxygen caused a cascade of events resulting in not only brain swelling and subdural haemorrhages but also retinal haemorrhages, thus explaining all three elements of the so-called triad of SBS findings [21]. As a lack of oxygen can have many causes, from cardiac issues to choking, this hypothesis had enormous implications for SBS cases.

Rather than being lauded for her breakthrough scientific achievements, Geddes's questioning of orthodox views provoked antagonism from doctors from the UK and the United States and she became the subject of forceful attacks in expert reports, lectures, and public presentations [22]. In 2005, an appeal was held against three shaken-baby convictions. During the trial, the prosecutors made a calculated attack on Geddes's integrity. It was 'horrendous', she recalled. 'I was there for two days being cross-examined. It was an attempt to shut my theory down, to prove my research was rubbish and that I was dishonest' [23]. During her testimony, Geddes admitted that, at that stage, the unified hypothesis was just that, a hypothesis, and pointed out that the orthodoxy about the mechanism of SBS was also just a hypothesis.

Proponents of SBS claimed that Geddes recanted the unified hypothesis during the 2005 trial, a claim that Geddes has emphatically denied, publishing her denial in the literature in 2009 [24]. Yet claims that Geddes recanted her hypothesis persist to this day. Proponents also cite the 2005 appeals court judgment as showing that Geddes's hypothesis should be discounted, as though a legal judgment should be used to inform the opinion of experts. Geddes took early retirement from neuropathology largely because of the toll taken by these attacks.

Efforts to silence Dr Waney Squier, who also questioned the science behind SBS, are further expository. Squier has been described as 'one of the world's foremost experts in babies' brains' [25] and 'probably the person [who] has done the best science in pathology [over] the last two decades' [26]. After giving testimony for the defence in which she disagreed with conventional assumptions and questioned the scientific foundation of the SBS theory, police instigated a complaint to the General Medical Council (GMC). The GMC brought Squier before the Medical Practitioners Tribunal, where a panel consisting of a retired military commander, a former policeman, and a retired geriatric psychiatrist heard testimony from a band of doctors who support the SBS orthodoxy. The GMC argued that Squier had 'failed in her overriding duty to the court to remain objective and to assist the court'. The tribunal sided with the establishment, finding that Squier had provided 'deliberately misleading' and 'dishonest' evidence in court. The GMC struck her from the medical register.

Considering that the Tribunal's panel lacked the appropriate educational background to differentiate the claims regarding science, it was clear that the decision rested on the number, authority, and credentials of the witnesses, illustrating a key problem at the interface between law and science: a court's reliance on authority.

Squier, who had formed her opinions by critically assessing what could and could not be learned from the published studies [27], appealed to the High Court. In reinstating Squier's registration, High Court Justice Mitting found that she had not misstated facts from research papers and had not acted dishonestly. Nevertheless, Justice Mitting found that Squier had 'cherry-picked' from articles to support her arguments, stating that she 'did not misstate the facts which she sought to extract from the four research papers; but her citation was so selective as to misrepresent each of [the articles]' [28].

As an example, Squier had challenged the prosecution's assertion that retinal haemorrhages were diagnostic of abuse. To support her position, she referred to limitations of that assertion identified in a 2005 study by Matthieu Vinchon. Justice Mitting found that, although Squier had correctly cited from the study, she had omitted 'the authors' clear conclusion about the coincidence of abusive injury and retinal haemorrhage in small babies'. The omission referred to was Vinchon's conclusion that 'the specificity of . . . severe retinal haemorrhage for the diagnosis of child abuse was 100%' [29].

Squier was not wrong to challenge the premises underlying these conclusions. No properly trained scientist would accept a result that claims 100% specificity, a big red flag for methodological flaws and circular reasoning. Vinchon himself has admitted that 'we were a bit disturbed to find a 100% positive predictive value . . . because this figure does not look like a scientific result; however, from a legal perspective, we think that this is precisely what a judge hopes for' [30]. Indeed, Vinchon had excluded findings related to retinal haemorrhages from his diagnosis model 'because of the circularity bias'.

Justice Mitting's reliance on a 'conclusion' of the Vinchon study, without comprehending its methodology or the significance of the limitations, illustrates a second key problem at the interface between science and law: judges are not scientists, are not trained to critically appraise scientific literature or clinical publications, and do not understand the fields over which they are adjudicating.

The High Court banned Squier from providing evidence in court for 3 years. The police, prosecutors, and medical establishment had successfully removed a major roadblock to gaining convictions.[2] The ramifications were broader still. Courts in the UK have acknowledged that, subsequent to the Squier case, it became very difficult to find doctors willing to testify for the defence [31].

1.2 The Interface of Science, Law, and Medicine

It is not hard to understand how the court's problem of lacking scientific expertise leads to the problem of reliance on credentials and authority. Nor is it hard to understand the potential for reliance on authority to become entrenched within fields of forensic sciences. It is therefore not entirely surprising that the science–law interface has long been so problematic.

However, this is not the only clash of cultures at play. Shaken baby syndrome sits not only at the interface between science and law but also at the interface between science and medicine. Squier was opining that, while the GMC and many doctors may consider SBS medicine, it is not science.

But surely medicine is scientific? A history of evidence-based medicine is instructive. In medicine, 'clinical practice was historically viewed as the "art of medicine". Expert opinion, experience, and authoritarian judgment were the foundation for decision making. The use of scientific methodology, as in biomedical research, and statistical analysis, as in epidemiology, were rare in the world of medicine' [32]. The birth of evidence-based medicine has been attributed to 'an increasing awareness of the weaknesses of [these] standard clinical practices' [32]. Dr Gordon Guyatt first called this new movement scientific medicine, which was not well received due to the implication that mainstream medicine was anything short of scientific. Guyatt subsequently referred to the movement as evidence-based medicine.

Haven't we now moved on from authoritative medicine? Is there still such a divide between medicine and science? While there has been a dramatic increase in scientific

---

[2] This was a co-ordinated effort to block Squier from testifying, as outlined by Detective Inspector Colin Welsh from New Scotland Yard at a National Centre for Shaken Baby Syndrome conference. Heather Kirkwood's notes of the presentation are available at https://bit.ly/3WxvfnB. Also see BBC FILE ON 4 'SHAKEN BABIES'. 15 February 2011 (bbc.in/3t2aTW3).

methods being applied to medicine, the nature of much (not all) medicine remains different from science. Scientific research is highly specialised, while most medical doctors need to know and synthesise a broad range of topics in order to make diagnoses and provide treatments. By necessity, the training in and learning of these types of knowledge is different.

In order to synthesise and disseminate such volumes of knowledge, a system of medical guidelines exists that aims to guide decisions and provide criteria regarding diagnosis, management, and treatment in specific areas of healthcare. Modern guidelines are authored by a group of experts in each particular field. Although these guidelines should be and often are based on evidence and science, they represent a divide between the science and the doctors who rely upon the guidelines.

> It is ironic that we now find ourselves in the situation where the dramatic increase in science that should enable us to move from authority-based medicine to evidence-based medicine has reached a point where physicians are increasingly reliant on others to synthesize the science, but most 'statements that include recommendations intended to optimize patient care' are developed by consensus-based guideline panels that actually move us back toward authority-based medicine. [33]

1.3 Scientific Reference Standards

So why does Squier believe that, even though SBS is widely accepted by many medical practitioners and authorities, 'there is no scientific evidence to support it and there never has been' [34]? It boils down to this: studies that claim to support the SBS hypothesis do not have robust reference standards.

In studies of diagnostic accuracy, reference standards are used to categorise participants as having or not having the relevant medical condition. This categorisation must be independent of the diagnostic index test and it must be accurate in making the classifications [35]. For example, a biopsy can provide accurate evidence for skin cancer and thus can be used as a reference standard. If one were to use a set of findings such as the evolving appearance, asymmetry, and blurred edges of a mole as a method to diagnose skin cancer, one can determine the accuracy of that diagnostic method by comparing it to the results of the reference standard – that is, the biopsy.

To assess the accuracy of using the findings of encephalopathy and subdural and retinal haemorrhages as an index test for diagnosing abuse, an accurate reference standard is required.[3] Even when a differential diagnosis is included in the diagnostic process, attempting to exclude all other possible causes, that process needs to be assessed for accuracy, and this requires a reference standard. Controlled experiments cannot be done by shaking infants to categorise infants as abused, a common ethical problem in medicine: one cannot give someone a disease to see how it progresses. Other reliable reference standards are therefore required.

Independently witnessed shaking events represent a possible reference standard, but in the 50 years since the SBS hypothesis was proposed, there are virtually no documented, independently witnessed shaking events that have resulted in the findings associated with

[3] Or any other constellation of injuries used as indicative of abuse, including extensive, multi-layered retinal haemorrhages.

SBS. Witnessed shaking events do occur; they just do not result in SBS-associated findings [36].

The vast majority of research on SBS instead uses reference standards that invoke the very findings that are used in the diagnostic index test, either directly by using criteria such as 'no history accounting for patient's serious head injury' or indirectly by using conclusions of medical or multidisciplinary teams or results of legal judgments, which have themselves used elements of the diagnostic index test in their determination [37].[4] Using diagnostic test results as a reference standard for testing the accuracy of a diagnostic test leads to unreliable results based on circular reasoning [38] (see Chapter 10).

Attempts to circumvent these problems have used confessed cases as the reference standard [39]. These attempts have been hopelessly inadequate as they ignore the wealth of research into false confessions and interrogation and interview methods. These issues are examined in detail in Chapters 11 and 12.

Again, differences between science and medicine can explain, in part, the different perspectives taken on this methodology. In a medical setting, when there is no sound reference standard, a panel of experts may be invited to assign a reference diagnosis for use in research [40]. The accuracy of such diagnostic methods can then be assessed by following their implications for the treatment and recovery of the patients [41]. If the diagnosis was correct, the patient will respond to the treatment, so there is a feedback loop providing information about the accuracy of the diagnosis. In SBS, however, no such feedback loop exists, so there is no way of determining the accuracy of the classification of abused versus non-abused, as made by a multidisciplinary or medical panel. Without such a feedback loop providing a measure of accuracy, the risk of bias and circularity is high.

This problem of inadequate reference standards has been known for decades [19], yet researchers of SBS continue to use the same flawed methods [42].[5] A key to science is the insight that 'human knowledge is constantly threatened by error. Error may arise as the result of mistakes, false assumptions, entrenched traditions, belief in authorities, superstition, wishful thinking, prejudice, bias, and even fraud' [43]. Science has a strong focus on detecting and eliminating these sources of error [43]. The SBS community, by contrast, has allowed inadequate research standards and the resulting bias to remain the cornerstone of their methodology for decades.

1.4 A Clash of Reviews

In 2016, the Swedish Agency for Health Technology Assessment and Assessment of Social Services (SBU), an independent national body that evaluates methods used by medical and social services, reported that there was only 'very low quality' evidence that the 'triad' of

[4] See also Feldman KW, Bethel R, Shugerman RP et al. The cause of infant and toddler subdural hemorrhage: A prospective study. *Pediatrics*. 2001;108:636–46, 'Multiple injuries, incompatible with normal, unintentional childhood injury', criteria also used in Bhardwaj G, Jacobs MB, Martin FJ et al. Photographic assessment of retinal hemorrhages in infant head injury: The Childhood Hemorrhagic Retinopathy Study. *Journal of the American Association for Pediatric Ophthalmology and Strabismus*. 2017.

[5] See also Thamburaj K, Soni A, Frasier LD et al. Susceptibility-weighted imaging of retinal hemorrhages in abusive head trauma. *Pediatric Radiology*. 2019;49:210–16; Gencturk M, Tore HG, Nascene DR et al. Various cranial and orbital imaging findings in pediatric abusive and non-abusive head trauma, and relation to outcomes. *Clinical Neuroradiology*. 2019 Jun;29(2):253–61.

findings associated with SBS is diagnostic of shaking [44]. The systematic review had excluded research that did not have scientifically rigorous reference standards. A 2003 systematic review by an Australian physician reached similar conclusions after giving similarly low weight to research with poor reference standards [45]. Considering that guidelines for systematic reviews mandate risk of bias assessment for study inclusion, it is not *scientifically* controversial to assess studies with poor reference standards as having a high risk of bias [46]. Yet both the 2003 and 2016 reviews became very controversial in the *medical* community, which railed against both reports and called for retraction [3]. This is explored in detail in Chapter 10.

Seemingly in response to the findings of the SBU systematic review, and with an eye on the *Daubert* standard for admission of forensic evidence in US courts, a consensus statement was released in 2018 in support of the SBS orthodoxy [47]. In contrast to the Swedish report, however, the authors of the consensus statement made no attempt to follow methodological guidelines [48]. No system was outlined or followed for the creation of the panel of authors. There was no author with expertise in methodology, nor even a methodology section. No quality assessment was made or criteria outlined for the inclusion of studies [49]. These methodological omissions and flaws mean that the consensus statement is not a document of *scientific* significance. However, the statement was endorsed by multiple medical societies, which provided it with an air of authority. Indeed, the consensus statement has proven to be a document with *medical* and *judicial* significance.

1.5 The Biggest Controversy Surrounding Shaken Baby Syndrome

In courtrooms, believers in the SBS orthodoxy continue to portray a degree of certainty in their 'diagnosis' of abuse that is regularly interpreted by judges and juries as being 'beyond reasonable doubt'. And therein lies the real controversy that surrounds SBS: not the name-calling, nor the retraction of articles, not the intimidation, complaints, and legal proceedings brought against those who question the SBS orthodoxy. The real controversy is that thousands of parents and caregivers throughout the world have been accused of abusing children, been convicted and given long jail sentences or even been sentenced to death, while thousands more have had their children removed from their care based on the testimony of highly credentialed medical expert witnesses who believe in the SBS orthodoxy, but who lack a scientific foundation for those beliefs.

Dissenting opinions are crucial to science. According to Nobel Prize–winning physicist Richard Feynman,

> [I]t is imperative in science to doubt; it is absolutely necessary, for progress in science, to have uncertainty as a fundamental part of your inner nature. To make progress in understanding, we must remain modest and allow that we do not know. If we investigate further, we find that the statements of science are not of what is true and what is not true, but statements of what is known to different degrees of certainty. [50]

Those challenging the orthodoxy argue that there remains far too much uncertainty in the accuracy of diagnostic methods in shaken baby cases to conclude that abuse has occurred.

This book is a testament to the difficulty of silencing dissenting voices in science. In the book, those who question the SBS orthodoxy provide detailed, compelling reasons to severely doubt the orthodoxy and provide directions for future research to make progress in our understanding of the causes of the syndrome that should be known as retino-dural haemorrhage of infancy.

References

1. Bilo RAC. The Swedish Agency for Health Technology report about traumatic shaking: Much ado about nothing? *Forensic Science, Medicine, and Pathology.* 2018;14:541–4.
2. Vedelago C, Mannix L. Legal threats and police searches. *The Age.* 19 May 2021. bit.ly/3sZZjur.
3. Debelle GD, Maguire S, Watts P et al. Abusive head trauma and the triad: A critique on behalf of rCPCH of traumatic shaking. The role of the triad in medical investigations of suspected traumatic shaking. *Archives of Disease in Childhood.* 2018;103(6):606–10.
4. Binenbaum G, Forbes BJ, Topjian AA, Twelves C, Christian CW. Patterns of retinal hemorrhage associated with cardiac arrest and cardiopulmonary resuscitation. *Journal of the American Association for Pediatric Ophthalmology and Strabismus.* 2021;25(6):324.e1–324.e4. https://doi.org/10.1016/j.jaapos.2021.06.005.
5. Tully J. Abusive head trauma: Mechanisms, myths and mysteries. Seminar at the Victorian Forensic Paediatric Medicine Service, 19 March 2017. Royal Children's Hospital, Melbourne.
6. Dyer C. Child death expert provided 'misleading and biased' evidence, panel hears. *BMJ.* 2015;351:h5400. www.bmj.com/content/351/bmj.h5400.
7. Hymel KP. Denying the abusive head trauma denialists their day in court, one step at a time. *Pediatric Radiology.* 2019;49:1710–11.
8. Strouse PJ. Child abuse: We have problems. *Pediatric Radiology.* 2016;46:587–90.
9. Fitzsimmons J. Abusive head trauma evidence: Admissibility at Trial 2 presentation for the National District Attorneys Association's National Center for Prosecution of Child Abuse. 2010.
10. Benet-Martínez V, Waller NG. From adorable to worthless: Implicit and self-report structure of highly evaluative personality descriptors. *European Journal of Personality.* 2002;16:1–41.
11. Tyler TR. Psychological perspectives on legitimacy and legitimation. *Annual Review of Psychology.* 2006;57(1):375–400.
12. Brook C, Lynøe N, Eriksson A, Balding D. Retraction of a peer reviewed article suggests ongoing problems with Australian forensic science, Forensic Science International. *Synergy.* 2021;3. https://doi.org/10.1016/j.fsisyn.2021.100208.
13. McDonald S. The shaken baby debate. *Prometheus: Critical Studies in Innovation.* 35(5):1–191.
14. Hanson M. Battle of the expert. *ABA Journal.* 2005;91:52.
15. Guthkelch AN. Infantile subdural haematoma and its relationship to whiplash injuries. *BMJ.* 1971;430(2):430–1.
16. Guthkelch AN. Problems of infant retino-dural hemorrhage with minimal external injury. *Houston Journal of Health Law and Policy.* 2012;201(12):201–8.
17. Chadwick DL, Kirschner RH, Reece RM et al. Shaken baby syndrome: A forensic pediatric response. *Pediatrics.* 1998;101:321–3.
18. Plunkett J. Fatal pediatric head injuries caused by short-distance falls. *American Journal of Forensic Medicine and Pathology.* 2001;22(1):1–12.
19. Geddes JF, Hackshaw AK Vowles GH, Nickols CD, Whitwell HL. Neuropathology of inflicted head injury in children. I. Patterns of brain damage. *Brain.* 2001;124:1290–4.
20. Geddes JF, Vowles GH, Hackshaw AK et al. Neuropathology of inflicted head injury in children. II. Microscopic brain injury in infants. *Brain.* 2001;124:1299–1306.
21. Geddes JF, Tasker RC, Hackshaw AK et al. Dural haemorrhage in non-traumatic infant

deaths: Does it explain the bleeding in 'shaken baby syndrome'? *Neuropathology Applied Neurobiology*. 2003;29:14–22.

22. Jennian Geddes in statement given in *Squier v GMC*, 2016, EWHC 2739.
23. Storr W. 'We believe you harmed your child': The war over shaken baby convictions. *The Guardian*. 8 December 2017.
24. Geddes JF. Nonaccidental trauma: Clinical aspects and epidemiology of child abuse. *Pediatric Radiology*. 2009;39 (759):457–60.
25. Rumbelow H. Why I denied shaken baby syndrome. *The Times*. 16 November 2016.
26. Aspelin P. Keynote address: Can a sign or occult finding predict a causal relationship? How to reason about possible child abuse. *University of Michigan Journal of Law Reform*. 2017;50:749–62.
27. Greenhalgh T. How to read a paper: Getting your bearings (deciding what the paper is about). *BMJ*. 1997;315:243–6.
28. *Squier v GMC* [2016] EWHC 2739 @53.
29. Vinchon M, Defoort-Dhellemmes S, Desurmont M, Dhellemmes P. Accidental and nonaccidental head injuries in infants: A prospective study. *Journal of Neurosurgery*. 2005;102(4 Suppl):380–4.
30. Vinchon M. Response to Lynøe: Questions about isolated trauma shaking and confessions. *Child's Nervous System*. 2017;33(9):1423–4.
31. Baker J (2013) *Judgment*, Re L and M (Children) EWHC 1569 (Fam).
32. Sur RL, Dahm P. History of evidence-based medicine. *Indian Journal of Urology*. 2011;27(4):487–9.
33. LeFevre M. From authority- to evidence-based medicine: Are clinical practice guidelines moving us forward or backward? *Annals of Family Medicine*. 2017;15(5):410–12. https://doi.org/10.1370/afm.2141.
34. Sweeney, J. Should Waney Squier have been struck off over shaken baby syndrome? BBC Newsnight. 17 October 2016.
35. For example, Cohen JF, Korevaar DA, Altman DG et al. STARD 2015 guidelines for reporting diagnostic accuracy studies: Explanation and elaboration. *BMJ Open*. 2016;6(11):e012799.2016.
36. For example, Thiblin I, Andersson J, Wester K et al. Medical findings and symptoms in infants exposed to witnessed or admitted abusive shaking: A nationwide registry study. *PLoS One*. 2020;15(10): e0240182.
37. Recce RM, Sege R. Childhood head injuries. *Archives of Pediatric and Adolescent Medicine*. 2000;154:11–15.
38. For example, Eva Lai Wah F, Tz Sung RY, Nelson EAS et al. Unexplained subdural hematoma in young children: Is it always child abuse? *Pediatrics International*. 2002;44(1):37–42.
39. For example, Adamsbaum C, Grabar S, Mejean N, Rey-Salmon C. Abusive head trauma: Judicial admissions highlight violent and repetitive shaking. *Pediatrics*. 2010;126(3):546–55.
40. For example, Reitsma JB, Rutjes AWS, Khan KS, Coomarasamy A, Bossuyt PM. A review of solutions for diagnostic accuracy studies with an imperfect or missing reference standard. *Journal of Clinical Epidemiology*. 2009;62:797–806.
41. For example, Handels, RLH, Wolfs, CAG, Aalten P et al. Optimizing the use of expert panel reference diagnoses in diagnostic studies of multidimensional syndromes. *BMC Neurology*. 2014;14(190). https://doi.org/10.1186/s12883-014-0190-3.
42. For example, Sidpra J, Jeelani NUO, Ong J et al. Skull fractures in abusive head trauma: A single centre experience and review of the literature. *Child's Nervous System*. 2021;37:919–29.
43. Hoyningen-Huene P. Systematicity: The nature of science. *Philosophia*. 2008;36:167–80.
44. Elinder G, Eriksson A, Hallberg B et al. Traumatic shaking: The role of the triad in medical investigations of suspected traumatic shaking. *Acta Paediatrica*. 2018;107:3–23.

45. Donohoe M. Evidence-based medicine and shaken baby syndrome. Part 1: Literature review, 1996–1998. *American Journal of Forensic Medicine and Pathology*. 2003;24 (3):239–42.

46. For example, Guyatt GH, Oxman AD, Vist GE et al. GRADE: An emerging consensus on rating quality of evidence and strength of recommendations. *BMJ*.2008;336:924–6.

47. Choudhary AK, Servaes S, Slovis TL et al. Consensus statement on abusive head trauma in infants and young children. *Pediatric Radiology*. 2018;48 (8):1048–65.

48. Belton I, MacDonald A, Wright G, Hamlin I. Improving the practical application of the Delphi method in group-based judgment: A six-step prescription for a well-founded and defensible process. *Technological Forecasting and Social Change*. 2019;147:72–82.

49. Liberati A, Altman DG, Tetzlaff J et al. The PRISMA statement for reporting systematic reviews and meta-analyses of studies that evaluate health care interventions: Explanation and elaboration. *PLoS Medicine*. 2009;6(7): e1000100. https://doi.org/10.1371/journal.pmed.1000100.

50. Feynman R. The relation of science and religion. *Engineering and Science*. 1956;19(5):21.

Chapter 2

The History of Shaken Baby Syndrome

Randy Papetti

'If history and science have taught us anything, it is that passion and desire are not the same as truth'.

Edward O. Wilson, Consilience *[1]*

This chapter summarises the history of a forensic medical concept known as shaken baby syndrome (SBS). This is no small task: the medical and forensic beliefs that came to be known as SBS date back to 1971 – more than 50 years ago [2].

Though the history of SBS is now in its sixth decade, the controversy surrounding it emerged more recently. Few viewed SBS in its initial form as controversial, and so SBS became firmly embedded in paediatric and forensic medicine by the mid-1980s without much debate. It wasn't until the early 2000s that investigators from various disciplines – medical, scientific, and legal – started raising questions about the reliability of the SBS tenets. Once those investigations began, serious controversy emerged. That controversy has now raged for two decades.

Given the consequences of an SBS determination, it is fair to ask why no consensus has been reached in the medical and scientific communities as to whether the 'diagnosis' and its various foundational premises are reliable – and even whether it is truly a 'diagnosis' at all. If the debate involved merely an objective determination of whether SBS has been scientifically validated, that determination would have occurred long ago – the issues are complex, but they are not *that* complex. Shaken baby syndrome, however, is not just a medical or scientific concept. The determination and its functions involve a complicated mix of medicine, science, law, and social policy. For this reason, understanding the history and politics surrounding this purported medical and scientific concept is critical to understanding the controversy.

2.1 The Role of Physicians in Protecting Children from Abuse

Physicians today play an active role in identifying and reporting suspected abuse. But that was not always true (see Chapter 18). Until the early 1960s, physicians rarely reported suspected abuse and generally did so only when the abuse was extreme. As one commentator later put it: 'Child abuse was not a medical problem, it was a social problem that was often ignored' [3]. There were several reasons for this: past practice, a mistaken view that only deeply disturbed individuals would abuse children, inadequate training in how to recognise abuse, concerns over being sued, and a reluctance to become involved in what society still largely perceived as a family issue. In addition, in many jurisdictions, child protective agencies did not exist or had limited authority and resources, so it was often unclear to whom a report should be made or what, if anything, would be done about it. This appears to have been the case in nearly every country.

In 1962, an American professor and paediatrician named C. Henry Kempe and his colleagues published an extraordinarily influential article. In 'The Battered-Child Syndrome', Kempe argued that child abuse was a significant cause of childhood disability and death yet was 'frequently not recognized or, if diagnosed, is inadequately handled by the physician because of hesitation to bring the case to the attention of the proper authorities' [4]. Kempe urged physicians to accept that, when they see abuse, they have a duty and responsibility to protect the child from further harm.

Kempe's message was powerful. But the article suggested a diagnostic approach that perhaps sowed the seed of the problems later to come with SBS. The article appeared to counsel physicians to *presume* abuse from particular medical findings, even though the findings might have multiple explanations or were incompletely understood. This approach would help physicians, in the words of the article's abstract, 'guarantee that no expected repetition of trauma will be permitted to occur'.

'The Battered-Child Syndrome' was immediately impactful. It seemed to release a wave of pent-up sentiment within the paediatric community around the world that more needed to be done to protect children from abuse. By way of example, in 1962, there were no laws in the United States requiring physicians to report child abuse. By 1967, all 50 states had enacted mandatory reporting laws. To further encourage reporting, the laws gave reporting physicians immunity from civil liability. The campaign to persuade legislatures to enact reporting laws and to expand services to protect children was led by paediatricians such as Kempe. This all inspired a massive increase in the study of the medical and social aspects of child abuse.

With the mandatory reporting laws in place, and society and the medical profession more alert to the child abuse problem, reported cases of suspected abuse grew exponentially. This, in turn, required governments to dedicate enormous resources to investigate the reports, remove children from abusive homes, and prosecute perpetrators. Soon, physicians began to specialise in child abuse and to work integrally with similarly focused police officers, social workers, and prosecutors in detecting, investigating, studying, preventing, and prosecuting child abuse. This was the birth of a passionate and powerful child protection community – with physicians at its centre.

2.2 Shaking Infants Is Identified As Dangerous

As part of the surge in child abuse literature, A. Norman Guthkelch, a prominent British paediatric neurosurgeon, published a paper in 1971 titled 'Infantile Subdural Haematoma and Its Relationship to Whiplash Injuries' [2]. Guthkelch sought to explain cases where infants had a subdural hematoma, a pooling of blood outside the brain, which he assumed was caused by head trauma, yet the child's head showed no sign of having been impacted. Guthkelch suggested that shaking an infant could result in subdural haemorrhage and thus explain how infants might have sustained such internal head injuries despite no external evidence of head trauma. Guthkelch expressly labelled his shaking concern a 'hypothesis'.

Guthkelch's shaking hypothesis soon caught the attention of John Caffey, an influential figure in the American child protection movement. Caffey was a paediatric radiologist, textbook author, and child protection crusader who had been writing about suspicious injuries in children since the 1940s. Caffey echoed Guthkelch's contention that shaking would explain how infants presented without obvious evidence of head trauma, yet had subdural hematoma and, in many cases, brain injury and/or rib fractures [5]. Caffey also argued that shaking would explain the retinal haemorrhages found in many abused children, which he speculated were caused by 'traction stresses' within the eye as the vitreous and the retina move at different speeds during shaking [5]. Caffey's theory that shaking can cause subdural and retinal haemorrhage and brain injury was initially referred to as whiplash–shaken infant syndrome and, by the early 1980s, as shaken baby syndrome [6]. Although Caffey admitted having 'manifestly incomplete' evidence to support his theory [6], and though little was done in the decade after Caffey's writings to validate it [7], the belief that shaking is a frequent cause of such internal findings soon became widely accepted in paediatric medicine.

2.2.1 Shaken Baby Syndrome Becomes Diagnostic

By the 1990s, SBS had come to rest on two foundational tenets. The first – which was part of the original hypothesis – was that the mechanism of shaking is very effective in inflicting brain injury and subdural and retinal haemorrhage. This biomechanical premise was often explained in the literature or in courtrooms through analogies such as that shaking inflicts forces on a child comparable to the forces present in multi-story falls or head-on automobile collisions [6]. Although this tenet had in no way been validated, there was no obvious reason for physicians or researchers to question Guthkelch's and Caffey's guidance that babies are vulnerable and that shaking can seriously hurt them. But, over time, a second foundational tenet emerged: that shaking *can* cause (1) subdural haemorrhage, (2) retinal haemorrhage, and (3) brain injury began morphing into a rather categorical medical belief that such findings *almost always mean* the baby had been shaken. In short, the internal SBS findings had become diagnostic – or at least nearly diagnostic – of child abuse.

This progression occurred as the child abuse literature increasingly advised that each of the three primary SBS findings is nearly always the result of significant trauma, typically associated with shaking or other severe rotational or shearing forces. By 1993, the child abuse literature advised that a finding of subdural haemorrhage in a young child should trigger a *presumption* of child abuse. This presumption of abuse became the official policy of the American Academy of Pediatrics (AAP). In 1993 and 2001, the AAP's Committee on Child Abuse and Neglect issued highly influential statements on SBS. These statements advised that the presence of any 'intracranial injury' in a child under one year of age, the most common form of which they identified as subdural haemorrhage, should trigger a 'presumption of child abuse' [8, 9]. The 2001 AAP statement explained: 'Although physical abuse in the past has been a diagnosis of exclusion, data regarding the nature and frequency of head trauma consistently support the need for a presumption of child abuse when a child younger than one year of age has intracranial injury.' Thus, for multiple decades, the policy of the leading paediatric medical organisation in the world was that physicians should presume child abuse merely upon a finding of subdural haemorrhage in infancy. The AAP's guidance, unsurprisingly, became dogma in paediatric and forensic medicine [10, 11].

The second internal finding said to be characteristic of SBS and abuse was retinal haemorrhage. The child abuse literature often described retinal haemorrhages as even more probative of abuse than subdural haemorrhage. A 1979 article asserted that 'retinal hemorrhage in children under 3 with or without other evidence of injury is pathognomonic of the battered child syndrome' [12]. A 1994 paper similarly urged, 'It must be embedded in the minds of the pediatric emergency room residents that retinal hemorrhage is associated with child abuse until proven otherwise' [13]. A 1998 treatise on child maltreatment taught that 'Retinal hemorrhages in an infant without a history of severe accidental trauma constitute child abuse until proven otherwise' [14].

Although the literature varied between describing retinal haemorrhages specifically as proof of shaking or more generally as proof of abuse, the prevailing explanation was that retinal haemorrhages are so probative of abuse because they reflect shaking or other severe rotational or whiplash forces [15]. For example, a 2001 treatise on SBS advised that the 'presence of retinal hemorrhages is virtually diagnostic of the violently shaken infant in the absence of severe accidental trauma' [16]. A 2002 US Department of Justice guide on investigating child abuse, still available online, advises, 'According to all credible studies in the past several years, retinal hemorrhage in infants is, for all practical purposes, conclusive evidence of shaken baby syndrome in the absence of a good explanation', with the only 'good' explanations listed in the guide as severe auto accidents and falls from several stories onto a hard surface [17].

The third finding deemed indicative of SBS was present in more serious cases, when patients presented with brain damage or dysfunction. This might take the form of cerebral oedema, neurologic collapse, or more mild or transient neurologic dysfunction such as seizures. Proponents of the SBS diagnosis attributed the brain swelling and dysfunction to diffuse axonal and tissue tears within or on the surface of the brain, which, they reasoned, reflected damage from shearing forces the brain sustained during violent shaking or other severe acceleration-deceleration trauma [18].

It is not uncommon for all three of these findings to occur together, which is why the SBS findings were referred to as a medical syndrome. Given that each finding individually was thought to be so probative of severe trauma and SBS, when a child presented with all three (or even just subdural and retinal haemorrhage), the differential diagnosis for most physicians basically was SBS or other major accidental trauma akin to an unrestrained automobile accident [19]. Frequent explanations offered by caretakers included that the baby sustained a fall or similar household accident, had recently not been well, or was found unresponsive or suffering a seizure without having had any significant recent trauma. The medical literature emphatically rejected these explanations as being capable of producing the SBS findings [9] and, in fact, frequently implored physicians to view such explanations as evidence the caretaker was lying [20].

By the 1990s, the child abuse literature referred to SBS as a clearly defined medical diagnosis, defined by a constellation of findings, including (1) subdural and/or subarachnoid intracranial haemorrhage, (2) retinal haemorrhages sometimes accompanied by other ocular lesions, and (3) brain injury or dysfunction [9]. A 1998 letter published by 72 leading child abuse specialists in paediatrics summarised the three diagnostic criteria:

> The shaken baby syndrome (with or without evidence of impact) is now a well-characterized clinical and pathological entity with diagnostic features in severe cases virtually unique to this type of injury – [1] swelling of the brain (cerebral edema) secondary to severe brain injury, [2] bleeding within the head (subdural hemorrhage), and [3] bleeding in the interior linings of the eyes (retinal hemorrhages). Let those who would challenge these diagnostic features first do so in the peer-reviewed literature, before speculating on other causes in court [21].

The three findings were often referred to as the SBS triad [22]. As the 1997 edition of the leading treatise on child maltreatment explained, 'SBS usually produces a diagnostic triad of injuries that includes diffuse brain swelling, subdural hemorrhage, and retinal hemorrhages. This triad must be considered virtually pathognomonic of SBS in the absence of documented extraordinary blunt force such as an automobile accident' [23].

2.2.2 Shaken Baby Syndrome Determinations Become the Basis for Legal Actions

By the 1980s, based on the guidance in the child abuse literature and from leading medical organisations about the forensic specificity of the triad findings, prosecutors and child protection agencies around the world began bringing SBS-based cases to court, though with special vigour in the United States. It is unknown how many such cases have been brought since, but the total is in the many thousands. That is, tens of thousands of individuals have been prosecuted for child abuse or homicide crimes or had their children taken away from them based on medical SBS determinations.

In early cases, the power physicians and prosecutors attributed to the triad findings was immense. For example, a chapter written by a leading child abuse prosecutor in a 2001 SBS text confidently stated: 'The expert who acknowledges the classic findings of SBS include subdural hematoma, retinal hemorrhage and edema, but chooses to ignore this constellation in favor of an alternative hypothesis will appear foolish' [24].

2.3 Shaken Baby Syndrome Becomes Controversial

The notion of SBS being a controversial theory first entered the public domain in 1997. Louise Woodward was an 18-year-old British citizen who came to America to work as an au pair. She moved in with a family in Massachusetts, where her duties included caring for an 8-month-old little boy named Matthew. One day she could not wake Matthew from a nap. She told police she lightly shook Matthew to try to arouse him before calling 911. At the hospital, doctors confirmed that Matthew had a healing skull fracture, retinal haemorrhages, and intracranial bleeding. When Matthew died 5 days later, prosecutors charged Woodward with murder. Shaken baby syndrome was a key part of the prosecution's case.

The prosecution's case was supported principally through the testimony of several well-credentialed experts, most of whom vouched for the forensic power of the SBS findings. Woodward, however, had well-credentialed experts of her own, who questioned the scientific basis for SBS and whether it was a reliable 'diagnosis'. The trial was televised daily in America and followed closely in the United Kingdom. The jury found Woodward guilty of murder and, as Massachusetts law required, she was promptly sentenced to life imprisonment.

The real controversy about the case, however, occurred later, when the trial judge ruled that it would be unjust to uphold the murder conviction because, in his view, Woodward's actions were 'characterized by confusion, inexperience, frustration, immaturity and some anger, but not malice (in the legal sense) supporting a murder conviction. Frustrated by her inability to quiet the crying child, she was "a little rough with him"', which may have been 'sufficient to start (or re-start) a bleeding that escalated fatally' [25]. The judge reduced her conviction to involuntary manslaughter and later resentenced her to time served – 279 days.

The defence challenges to SBS in *Woodward*, and the judge's decision rejecting the prosecution's premise that Woodward must have treated Matthew violently, incensed the child protection community. The day after the decision, a letter cosigned by 50 physicians who stated that they 'specialize in the diagnosis and treatment of victims of child abuse' was published on the Internet and sent to major newspapers. It was later reprinted in *Pediatrics*. The letter (later republished with 72 signatures) castigated the defence arguments. The physicians defended SBS as a 'well-characterized . . . entity' with 'virtually unique' 'diagnostic features'. The letter, however, drew criticism from a handful of SBS sceptics. In particular, a forensic pathologist named John Plunkett published 'Shaken Baby Syndrome and the Death of Matthew Eappen: A Forensic Pathologist's Response' [26]. Plunkett's piece – which foreshadowed several subsequent challenges to SBS – began with this quotation: 'The problem isn't with what we don't know. The problem is with what we do know that isn't so.' Plunkett urged physicians to 'differentiate between what we know to be true and what we think or hope to be true'.

But by this time, SBS was both well entrenched and well defended. Notwithstanding the public airing during and in the aftermath of the Woodward trial, SBS only became more accepted and vigorously defended in the next few years. In 2001, both the American Academy of Pediatrics and the National Association of Medical Examiners issued position papers endorsing SBS as a medically and scientifically reliable diagnosis. As for the questions that had been raised, the paediatric and broader child protection community dismissed them as stemming from a handful of defence experts willing to offer unreliable opinions to facilitate their expert witness work, as the product of irresponsible conspiracy theory by fringe commentators, or both [22, 27].

Somewhat ironically, as SBS reached peak acceptance around 2001, challenges to SBS became more frequent, more specific, and increasingly difficult to ignore. It took years for these challenges to make meaningful inroads in mainstream understanding. But, over time, they rendered SBS deeply controversial and exposed serious shortcomings in its reliability. Today, as put in a leading forensic neuropathology text, 'Virtually all the hallowed tenets of SBS have been challenged on the basis of scientific principles and been found wanting or wrong' [28]. What follows is an overview of the challenges and other developments that led to the SBS controversy.

2.3.1 Shaking Generates Low Acceleration-Deceleration Forces

As noted, one of SBS's foundational tenets was that shaking produces massive acceleration-deceleration and rotational forces akin to those in automobile accidents and multi-story falls. Indeed, SBS's central premise is biomechanical – that is, shaking generates forces sufficient to rip veins emerging from the brain (causing subdural haemorrhage), damage retinae (through shearing forces within the eye), and shear neural axons and tissue within and on the brain [29]. Paediatric doctors, however, are not biomechanical experts. They have little or no experience in measuring the forces a human can endure during a particular trauma (e.g., shaking or falling onto one's head) or predicting what injuries can or will result. They had no scientific basis for making the claims they did about the forces involved in even very violent shaking (see Chapter 14).

The literature confirms that SBS and its corollary biomechanical beliefs became accepted without any biomechanical validation. Indeed, the first biomechanical study of SBS, conducted in 1987, found that even very violent shaking produces forces well below those involved in impact injuries to the head and nothing like the forces child abuse experts assumed shaking produces [30]. Several subsequent scientific studies have been conducted since and nearly all report that shaking generates biomechanical conditions well below those thought necessary to cause the purported SBS injuries [30–32].

Even many of those who defend the SBS hypothesis now concede that it is unclear whether shaking alone is capable of causing the SBS findings [33]. Indeed, biomechanical literature advises that shaking alone may not even be capable of directly causing the constellation of findings once thought nearly diagnostic of violent shaking. At a minimum, these studies have revealed that the motor vehicle and multi-story-fall analogies that filled child abuse literature and courtrooms for decades – and that are still believed and repeated by many paediatric physicians and prosecutors – are without basis.

2.3.2 Short Falls Can Cause the Triad Findings and Death

Until the late 1980s, medical literature frequently recognised the potential of infants and young children to suffer subdural and retinal haemorrhage, brain injury, and, occasionally, death after relatively short falls and other similar accidents [34, 35]. Even Caffey observed that 'children have developed severe hematomas, often, after falls of only [two or three] feet' [36]. But as SBS rose in acceptance, its proponents attacked these studies as unreliable. In 1991, a paper by David L. Chadwick, a leading child abuse specialist, advised that these past reports should be viewed sceptically and that reports of fatal short falls likely were missed cases of abuse (see Chapter 15) [37].

Following Chadwick's paper, leading figures in child abuse paediatrics began categorically advising that an infant or young child's subdural or retinal haemorrhages, brain injury, or death could not be explained by a short fall. The 2001 AAP statement on SBS flatly advised that 'the constellation of these injuries does not occur with short falls.' The US Department of Justice similarly guided that 'studies show that children do not die from simple household heights; they do not even suffer severe head injuries from such falls' [17]. Experts frequently testified for the prosecution that a household fall or similar accident could not explain subdural or retinal haemorrhage, let alone brain injury or death [38].

In 2001, a paper by Plunkett reported on several children's deaths from corroborated accidents on play equipment [39]. Although the children were not infants, one of the cases involved the videotaped fall of a 23-month-old toddler in the carpet-covered garage of her home. While being filmed by her grandmother, the toddler fell off a platform on a plastic play structure, which was about 42 inches above the ground. Despite trying to break her fall with her outstretched arms, the baby hit her head on the floor. After the fall, she cried, drank, and talked, but soon vomited, became dazed, and eventually died. The hospital findings included the SBS triad – all from a short fall.

There was initially considerable backlash against Plunkett's paper, including questioning whether the child actually had retinal haemorrhages or speculating that perhaps she had previously been abused. But, since Plunkett's paper, 'several additional studies have been published that provide further support for the view that subdural hematomas, retinal hemorrhages, and other forms of significant head injury can result from accidental short falls' [40]. A 2018 paper reported on eight cases of witnessed accidental falls onto the back of a child's head (average age 12.5 months), which all produced subdural and retinal haemorrhage. One resulted in death [41]. The case law and the medical literature now recognise the potential for short falls and other household injuries to produce the SBS findings.

2.3.3 Shaken Baby Syndrome's Flawed Pathophysiological Premises

As of 2001, SBS was based on superficially coherent pathophysiological assumptions as to why shaking predictably causes the triad findings and, consequently, why in most cases one can reliably infer from the triad that shaking occurred. But none of those premises had been validated in this context. They turned out to be wrong or at least subject to significant uncertainty.

2.3.3.1 Subdural Haemorrhage

Recall that in its 1993 and 2001 statements on SBS, the AAP advised that a 'presumption of child abuse' is warranted whenever an infant has an intracranial injury such as subdural haemorrhage. Subdural haemorrhage was deemed reliable proof of shaking or of severe head trauma because physicians believed the haemorrhage results from displacement of the brain. More specifically, bridging veins extend at certain points from the brain through the arachnoid membrane and into the dura, another membrane encasing the brain.

Where the veins are extended, such as when the brain moves or is otherwise displaced, the veins can rupture or tear and blood that escapes from them may pool in an area of the dura adjacent to its attachment to the arachnoid membrane. Since in healthy children considerable force is usually necessary to displace a brain enough to rupture or tear bridging veins, physicians assumed that children with unexplained subdural haemorrhage had sustained significant trauma. And because the AAP and other paediatric experts promoted that violent shaking is a common and effective means of causing such brain displacement and bridging vein rupture, physicians presumed SBS when a child presented with subdural haemorrhage and no given history of major trauma. This reasoning, however, was grossly oversimplified (see Chapter 3). In a 2001 study, neuropathologist Jennian Geddes and her colleagues observed that the subdural haemorrhage they saw in very young children diagnosed as SBS victims often was very different from that seen in adults who suffer traumatic head injury [42]. The haemorrhage in the children was often trivial in amount and in the nature of 'thin film', in contrast with the more voluminous, space-occupying subdural haematomas found in older children and adults attributable to bridging vein rupture. Geddes et al. asked whether, 'given the differences between "adult"-type subdural and those seen in infants in [non-accidental injury], are the conditions or forces that produce the two necessarily the same?'

Several papers subsequently confirmed Geddes et al.'s observation that the subdural haemorrhage in many SBS cases is in the nature of thin film rather than mass hematoma. Whether one can infer bridging vein rupture from scant or thin film haemorrhage is questionable. In 2009, radiologist Julie Mack and paediatric neuropathologist Waney Squier coauthored papers demonstrating that thin film subdural haemorrhage in infancy can result from vascular leakage within the dura itself, as opposed to torn bridging veins [43, 44]. Such 'intradural' haemorrhage can occur from trauma that would be insufficient to tear bridging veins and sometimes without any trauma at all, as it can occur in natural conditions. The full list of potential traumatic and non-traumatic causes of small-quantity subdural haemorrhage in infancy is still being investigated (see Chapters 3–9).

Even in purported SBS cases involving larger subdural blood and fluid collections, several developments have undermined past beliefs about what can be gleaned from such collections. It is common in SBS cases for subdural collections to contain a mix of blood and fluid of different ages. These collections are sometimes referred to as a chronic subdural hematoma or, less frequently, as a hematoma-hygroma. The origin of these collections is often unknown and may have been perinatal, during birth, from various natural conditions, past head trauma, or some combination thereof.

Well into the 1990s, even most child abuse specialists cautioned that these chronic collections were not necessarily associated with abuse and should be interpreted with caution [45]. But, over time, given the extreme forensic significance that came to be attributed to subdural blood, child abuse specialists began advising that mixed-age subdurals usually should be interpreted as representing multiple episodes of abuse, with acute haemorrhage within the collection reflecting recent abuse [46]. However, these understandings too came into question.

It is unanimously accepted that, in adults, membranes rich with blood vessels may form around collections of subdural blood (of whatever origin) as part of a healing process and these membranes can themselves bleed or 're-bleed', a process that can become chronic and occasionally trigger seizures or even worse outcomes. A premise for the initial belief that chronic subdural hematomas indicate abuse was that this re-bleeding process does not occur in infancy. But that guidance was later shown to be mistaken. The weight of authority developed such that it is now generally accepted that the course of bleeding and re-bleeding of chronic subdural collections in infants and young children is similar to that in adults [47]. And since chronic subdurals are known to present serious risks to adults, there is no basis to rule out such outcomes in infancy. However, the child protection community now believes that distinctions often can reliably be made regarding mixed-age subdurals, and so controversy rages about how to interpret chronic subdural collections [48, 49].

2.3.3.2 Retinal Haemorrhages

Starting in the late 1970s, papers within the child abuse literature and statements from major medical organisations advised that retinal haemorrhages in a child effectively mean abuse until proven otherwise, with very few alternative explanations accepted. In 2000, a leading SBS proponent reported: 'Most authors find a zero incidence of retinal haemorrhage in accidentally head injured children less than three years of age even in the presence of severe brain injury, subdural and/or epidural haemorrhage' [50].

The belief that retinal haemorrhages are strong evidence of child abuse is based on the shaking hypothesis – that is, the haemorrhages reflect traumatic damage the eyes suffer when the vitreous and the retina shear and tug against one another during violent shaking (or other repetitive or severe trauma) [15]. This hypothesis is known as the vitreo-retinal traction theory [51]. The forensic corollary of this hypothesis is that, when retinal haemorrhages are found, one may presume (subject to certain limited exceptions) that the child was violently shaken or endured other repetitive or very serious trauma.

The alternative to the vitreo-retinal traction theory is that retinal haemorrhage in these cases does not reflect traumatic damage to the eye but is instead a secondary consequence of other pathology or pathologies, such as suddenly raised intracranial pressure, intracranial haemorrhage, fluctuations in venous pressure, bleeding or clotting dysfunction, lack of oxygen (hyp-hypoxia), metabolic collapse, and/or time on life support [29]. The forensic difference between the two approaches cannot be underestimated: if retinal haemorrhages are a secondary consequence, then they presumably can be found in a range of circumstances not involving shaking, abuse, or even any trauma. By contrast, if the haemorrhages reflect mechanical damage to the eye caused by severe acceleration-deceleration forces, then the contention that one may infer abuse from them (in the absence of major accidental trauma) is more plausible.

As the years progressed, evidence accumulated casting doubt on the vitreo-retinal traction theory and supporting the alternative hypothesis that, at least in most instances, retinal haemorrhages are a secondary consequence. As with most SBS beliefs, the vitreo-retinal traction theory and related beliefs regarding retinal haemorrhages were embraced in paediatric medicine and by prosecutors without first being validated. And they have not been confirmed in the more than 40 years since. Several rounds of animal testing have failed to validate the vitreo-retinal traction theory. For example, a 2017 study shook 50 piglets at levels similar to abusive shaking, yet reported 'no ocular injury' in any piglet [52].

Outside the child abuse context, medical understanding for the past 100 years has been that retinal haemorrhages can result from spikes in intracranial pressure, especially in the presence of intracranial haemorrhage [28, 53]. This has been experimentally shown via inducing retinal haemorrhages in a rhesus monkey by raising its intracranial pressure [54]. Moreover, if retinal haemorrhages in young children are a distinct traumatic injury, as opposed to a cascade consequence secondary to other pathology, then one would expect to see with some regularity cases where an abused child has retinal haemorrhages but no intracranial, venous, or systemic pathology. But studies have repeatedly revealed that such a picture is almost never seen [55, 56]. A recent study and review on the topic concluded that 'non-birth-related retinal haemorrhage in infants are secondary to intracranial pathology associated with raised intracranial pressure . . . and not the result of traction forces between the retina and the vitreous body acting directly on the retinal vessels' [57].

The literature now contains case reports and studies reporting retinal haemorrhages of all shapes, sizes, and locations in a wide variety of traumatic and non-traumatic circumstances, ranging from severe infection, several natural diseases, head injury sufficient to cause intracranial bleeding, crush injury, coagulopathies and bleeding disorders, aneurysms, and vascular malformations, and commonly after normal childbirth [29, 58–61].

Unfortunately, faced with two decades of developments that undermined the original hypothesis, child abuse specialists have not abandoned the child abuse construct. Instead, they have tried to rescue it with an endless series of qualifications and refinements. Typically without warning that past statements about retinal haemorrhages were overbroad or altogether wrong, SBS proponents now insist that certain appearances of retinal haemorrhages – often described as complex, multilayered, extending out to the periphery of the retina, or too numerous to count – remain specific for SBS [62].

This purported refinement – that severe retinal haemorrhages or retinal haemorrhages with particular characteristics are specific for abuse – is a refinement of a false construct. The range of experimental studies have failed to produce even a single instance of a violently shaken or accelerated animal having severe or complex retinal haemorrhages. Retinal haemorrhages of all shapes, sizes, locations, and severity have been found in children who suffered accidental trauma as well as in non-traumatic contexts, which is consistent with the retinal pathology usually reflecting the severity of underlying pathologies and, in some instances, the time they persist rather than anything specific to shaking, abuse, or even trauma.

Indeed, studies of newborns reveal retinal haemorrhages as or more severe than in many cases in which SBS is diagnosed and often are multilayered, in all four quadrants, and extend to the periphery [58, 59]. A 2017 study concluded: 'Clinicians should also know there is no pathognomonic size, distribution, or location of [retinal haemorrhages] seen only in AHT' [60]. Although certain natural pathologies produce distinct ocular findings, there is no scientific basis to claim that shaking or abuse does, or that ophthalmologists can distinguish retinal haemorrhages caused by shaking or abuse from other potential pathologies. Studies have also shown that optic nerve and optic nerve sheath haemorrhages, previously deemed additional evidence of abuse, are a non-specific finding, also a secondary consequence of other pathologies rather than a direct injury [58, 63].

2.3.3.3 Brain Injury in the Form of Cerebral Oedema or Encephalopathy

The third triad finding, not present in all cases, is brain injury in various forms, often in the form of cerebral oedema or differing degrees of encephalopathy. The assertion was that these findings in purported SBS are the consequence of traumatic brain injury. A 2001 position paper, 'Fatal Abusive Head Injuries in Infants and Young Children', published by the ad hoc Committee on Shaken Baby Syndrome of the National Association of Medical Examiners, explained that the brain swelling and encephalopathy seen in many SBS/AHT cases reflects 'shearing injury or traumatic diffuse axonal injury [DAI]' [18]. Traumatic DAI, the position paper advised, requires extreme rotational force, such as that present in motor vehicle accidents, and so the common finding of brain swelling and dysfunction in suspected SBS cases further supported the contention that SBS victims had endured extreme shearing trauma.

The assumption that the brain swelling in these children reflected traumatic DAI, however, was based on almost no evidence and held out as forensically significant without being validated [64, 65]. In 2001, Geddes et al. conducted an extensive neuropathological evaluation of the brains of suspected SBS and other abuse victims and confirmed that the axonal brain injury generally seen in the cases was not traumatic DAI [64]. Instead, the brain insult previously thought to reflect traumatic DAI is actually the result of hypoxia (lack of oxygen), which can, if prolonged, lead to diffuse brain swelling, dysfunction, DAI, and death. Hypoxia, of course, can occur for many reasons having nothing to do with abuse, especially in infancy (see Chapter 3).

The misunderstanding that the brain injury in these cases reflected traumatic DAI contributed to the false beliefs and courtroom talking points that these children had endured forces akin to those in auto accidents and multi-story falls, as well as that the brain injury in these cases is incompatible with the child having a lucid interval between the time of injury and collapse. Those beliefs, however, were false.

2.3.4 The Flawed Shaken Baby Syndrome Evidence Base

When Guthkelch offered the SBS hypothesis, there was, as he later recounted, 'not a vestige of proof . . . that shaking, and nothing else, caused the triad' [67]. A 1986 paper reviewed the status of SBS and acknowledged how little evidence had been provided to support the theory [7]. After the paediatric community prematurely accepted the general shaking hypothesis, a similar and pronounced acceptance-before-validation pattern emerged with respect to that community embracing specific hypotheses that increased the power of SBS. These beliefs included such tenets as the assertion that brain swelling in SBS cases reflects traumatic DAI, which, in turn, reflects shearing forces; short falls do not cause subdural haemorrhage or death; retinal haemorrhages do not result from accidental trauma except in accidents akin to a motor vehicle accident or multi-story fall; retinoschisis and macular folds are effectively pathognomonic of shaking; the subdural haemorrhage in SBS cases is the result of torn bridging veins; and infants with intracranial injury from shaking will not have a lucid interval [29].

When researchers belatedly began to dig into the evidence for these specific beliefs, they discovered that, like the overall shaking hypothesis, the beliefs had not been adequately validated. For example, the 2001 Geddes studies found that the scientific evidence for the established belief that shaking causes traumatic DAI was 'scanty' [64]. In 2004, Lantz examined the basis for the belief that macular folds in infancy are caused by vitreo-retinal traction during shaking and concluded that it was not supported by objective scientific evidence [66]. In 2009, Mack and Squier examined the evidence for the long-standing statement that the thin film subdural haemorrhage in alleged SBS victims reflects torn bridging veins and found it was based on assumption, not evidence [43, 44].

Most significantly, after being unable to validate SBS biomechanically or pathologically, those defending SBS/AHT frequently invoked the literature that had developed over the years reporting that the triad findings are far more associated with abuse than with accidental trauma or other causes. It is true that many papers report a strong association between subdural and retinal haemorrhaging and SBS/AHT. When the evidence base for these papers was examined, however, it became clear that they are rife with circularity and bias. The circularity is rampant since cases were classified as abuse based in whole or in part on the presence of subdural and/or retinal haemorrhage and then, unsurprisingly, indicated a strong statistical association between subdural and retinal haemorrhage and abuse [29, 67–71]. Because the studies used SBS dogma to determine whether an infant was abused, it was a self-fulfilling prophecy that they would find a high association between abuse and subdural retinal haemorrhages and a low association between accidental trauma and such haemorrhages. The circularity problem is nearly universal in the early SBS literature and remains widespread today. From a scientific perspective, the studies are methodologically unreliable [42, 67].

In 2016, the Swedish Agency for Health Technology Assessment and Assessment of Social Services assessed the SBS evidence and issued a damning report (see Chapter 10) [72]: 'There is insufficient scientific evidence on which to assess the diagnostic accuracy of the triad in identifying traumatic shaking (very low evidence).' The report advised that, given the lack of reliable evidence to support the SBS diagnosis, it would be 'incompatible with both doctors' professional duties and the regulations concerning legal certification' for a physician to give a definite opinion based on the triad findings that a child was shaken.

2.3.5 Alternative Diagnoses

In 2001, a baby presenting with the triad and no history of major trauma was almost automatically diagnosed with SBS. Essentially, the triad meant SBS until proven otherwise. Besides being medically questionable, this presumption unrealistically shifted the burden to distressed parents and caretakers to provide a sufficient alternative explanation, and SBS dogma accepted very few alternative explanations as sufficient. But as controversy grew over the shaking hypothesis, experts devoted more attention to other potential causes of the triad.

The first major breakthrough was the rediscovery that falls and other similar accidents may cause subdural haemorrhage, the triad, and even death. Then, over time, the list of confirmed and theorised non-traumatic explanations for the triad began to grow. In 2011, Barnes published a lengthy review identifying numerous alternative causes for the triad findings and questioning whether shaking should even be on the list [73].

In recent years, the literature and courtrooms have become filled with papers about conditions that can produce subdural and retinal haemorrhage and be confused with SBS/AHT. These controversies involve benign enlargement of the subarachnoid spaces (also known as benign subdural effusions, benign extra-cerebral collections, and external hydrocephalus; see Chapters 5 and 6), cerebral venous thrombosis, hypoxic injury, perinatal or birth-related injury, and several other conditions. The papers are often then met with literature, other commentary, or even whole campaigns from child abuse specialists rejecting or seeking to minimise these alternative diagnoses for SBS/AHT. Shaken baby syndrome/abusive head trauma has and continues to be diagnosed in cases where the given history and the child's physical findings are consistent with other aetiologies having nothing to do with abuse.

2.3.6 Judicial Recognition of the Controversy

For many years, the legal system seemed not to notice the advances in medical and scientific literature that undermined SBS, particularly for legal purposes. Shaken baby syndrome cases continued unabated and efforts to reopen past convictions almost always failed. In 2005, the Supreme Court of Judicature Court of Appeals in London was confronted with certain challenges to the reliability of SBS, particularly as offered by Geddes, but largely upheld the SBS construct, viewing the Geddes theory itself as a hypothesis [74].

It was not until 2008 that a published American judicial opinion recognised the evolution in the science and granted post-conviction relief [75]. Also in 2008, the government of Ontario, Canada issued a major report based on 'The Inquiry into Pediatric Forensic Pathology in Canada', which came to be known as the Goudge Report after its commissioner. The Goudge Report observed that 'one of the deepest controversies surrounding pediatric forensic pathology concerns shaken baby syndrome', and that 'systemic examination has identified this particular area of forensic pathology as one where change has raised the possibility of past error' [76].

In 2009, Professor Deborah Tuerkheimer evaluated the collapse of the SBS premises against the hundreds if not thousands of SBS-based criminal convictions. She concluded that, '[w]hen placed against the backdrop of recent scientific developments, these numbers reflect a crisis in the criminal justice system'. In 2012, Guthkelch, feted for decades as the founder of the SBS diagnosis, published an article expressing his concern that SBS was being over-diagnosed and remained unproven [77]. In 2014, a federal district court in Illinois heard from leading experts on both sides of the controversy and, near the end of its long order, expressed concern that SBS may be 'more an article of faith than a proposition of science' [78]. The Swedish report in 2016, which was prompted by the Supreme Court of Sweden expressing uncertainty on how to proceed in SBS cases, confirmed the low quality of the SBS evidence base [79].

2.4 The American Academy of Pediatrics and Other Organisations Rebrand Shaken Baby Syndrome

As these collective developments raised questions about the reliability of SBS and exposed the AAP's 2001 SBS statement as misguided, the AAP, in 2009, issued a new statement, 'Abusive Head Trauma in Infants and Children' [80]. The new statement conceded no past error, but it did conspicuously delete much of the guidance found in the AAP's 1993 and 2001 statements, including the recommendation to presume abuse from intracranial injury.

Overall, the 2009 statement provided very little guidance about how to diagnose SBS. The statement's most noteworthy element was to recommend that physicians not use the term *shaken baby syndrome* in 'their medical diagnosis and communications' and instead use the less-specific term *abusive head trauma.* According to the 2009 statement, 'Legal challenges to the term "shaken baby syndrome" can distract from the more important questions of accountability of the perpetrator and/or safety of the victim.'

The name change, which other medical organisations soon adopted, did not fix the shortcomings of SBS; it merely changed the name of the diagnosis, principally for legal purposes. The coauthor of the 2009 AAP statement, a paediatrician, explained the name change would 'provide more clarity in the courtroom' [81]. But if physicians cannot reliably diagnose shaking from the triad findings, and there is no external evidence of head impact, then it is fallacious to insist they can diagnose abuse from those findings. There is no different, more reliable AHT evidence base than the evidence base developed with SBS dogma. If that dogma was based on false or otherwise uncertain premises, then changing the name of the syndrome was mere rebranding. But, as things have turned out, the name change did serve, as intended, to reset the debate.

2.5 Shaken Baby Syndrome Today

Insofar as observers claimed that, as of 2009, SBS was on the edge of collapse, they were wrong. The scientific, medical, and legal challenges to the reliability of SBS – which have continued and only grown in force since 2009 – have somehow had little effect on paediatric physicians or child abuse specialists. A 2016 survey reported that more than 93% of child abuse paediatricians working at children's hospitals continue to view SBS as a valid diagnosis; the figure rises to 98% for paediatric ophthalmologists [82].

Physicians at American children's hospitals still overwhelmingly view shaking as posing risks akin to those in a high-velocity motor vehicle crash. The notion that a short fall could explain severe retinal haemorrhage, coma, or death was considered a fringe opinion. By contrast, the survey reported that less than 41% of responding forensic pathologists view SBS as a valid diagnosis. The survey and other evidence confirm that faith in SBS remains strong among paediatric physicians who evaluate children for potential abuse. The Swedish report met a massive campaign to discredit it [62, 83], including a purported 'Consensus Statement' intended to vouch for the diagnosis and discredit the challenges [33]. All this despite growing literature proving that abuse in the United States and some other countries has been over-diagnosed, partially based on the controversial SBS beliefs [84, 85].

Given the actual scientific understandings and uncertainties, this continuing confidence in the SBS/AHT beliefs is disconcerting [86, 87]. When juxtaposed with the evolved viewpoints of forensic pathologists and the doubts of biomechanical experts, the views of paediatric physicians and child abuse specialists appear to reflect insularity, not superior insight. However, this failure to absorb the actual scientific challenges to SBS – including challenges that have been validated – is perhaps less surprising once one considers the institutional responses to the challenges since they began.

2.5.1 The Claim There Is No Legitimate Controversy

Since the more serious challenges to SBS began in the late 1990s and early 2000s, SBS proponents have consistently retorted that there is no legitimacy to the challenges. Indeed, even today, SBS proponents claim that there is a consensus that SBS/AHT is a 'scientifically non-controversial medical diagnosis' that is made 'like any other medical diagnosis' [33] (see Chapter 1). Those who challenge SBS are routinely labelled denialists or worse, and they face an organised onslaught from child abuse specialists and prosecutors to discredit them [29, 89].

2.5.2 The Abandonment of Definition

To the extent that SBS proponents confront the substantive challenges, the most common reply is that the 'diagnosis' is allegedly based on much more sophisticated and nuanced considerations than the mere triad [33, 83, 90]. The triad, the contention goes, is a straw man argument invented by defence lawyers and experts, and so arguments that the triad is unreliable for diagnosing SBS/AHT are beside the point. The child protection community has dismissed the watershed Swedish report on this basis [33] (see Chapter 10).

Medical diagnoses, especially those that purport to be grounded in science, have objective diagnostic criteria. It is a matter of easily confirmed historic fact that, for at least three decades, the triad findings served as the principal diagnostic criteria for SBS. The triad findings were thought to be so forensically reliable that the AAP advised that SBS need not be made as a 'diagnosis of exclusion', but rather could be presumed merely from the internal findings. Shaken baby syndrome proponents argued, taught, and testified that the notion that almost anything else could explain the triad findings in a young child was foolish. The patient's given history, of course, is always considered, but, unlike with other diagnoses, here the given history is not accepted unless it includes an admission of non-accidental trauma. In 2016, Högberg et al. reported that in nearly 70% of reviewed cases, one of the criteria used to make the SBS/AHT diagnoses was that the physicians did not believe the given history [84].

The diagnostic process used in SBS/AHT cases continues to reflect faith in the triad and the subjective judgement of child abuse teams, not reliance on the given history. The literature indicates that, once a history is taken, it is deemed suspicious if SDH is discovered and very suspicious if the caretaker denies any significant trauma. An ophthalmological exam virtually confirms SBS/AHT if retinal haemorrhages are present, especially if they are extensive. Review of laboratory and imaging findings confirms the absence of one of the conditions that child abuse specialists will accept to explain the triad. Ultimately, SBS/AHT is confirmed by rejection of the caregiver's history as inconsistent with the physical findings. [79, 87]. This process incorporates a now-unspoken but nevertheless continuing presumption of abuse from the findings of subdural haemorrhage, unwarranted reliance on retinal haemorrhages, and the improper elevation of SBS/AHT to a default diagnosis.

2.5.3 The Campaign to Preserve the Diagnosis

The developments surrounding SBS/AHT justify an international effort to reassess the determination, especially as it has been and continues to be used in the courts. As challenges to SBS/AHT accumulate, they have raised the question whether courts should continue permitting SBS-based cases and testimony. But one important indicium courts consider is whether the beliefs are generally accepted in the relevant field. Those defending SBS/AHT rely heavily on this criterion and, to build a case for it, generate papers specifically to convey to courts that SBS/AHT remains generally accepted in paediatric medicine notwithstanding the challenges and the ongoing controversy [33, 91]. These papers are then cited in legal cases as proof of continuing general acceptance. As evidence of scientific reliability, such strategically generated evidence of acceptance adds little or nothing. But, as a strategy to preserve the use of the diagnosis for legal purposes, it has proven effective to this day.

2.5.4 The Need for Increased Oversight

In 2014, Tuerkheimer expressed that 'SBS has survived the demise of its foundational tenets ... due in part to the dynamics of child abuse specialization' [92]. Child abuse specialists dominate this area of medicine. They also join with prosecutors to set the agenda for pro-SBS advocacy organisations, have their own journals and treatises, and hold their own conferences. They lead the child abuse teams at children's hospitals and collaborate regularly with prosecutors and child protection agencies in investigating and prosecuting cases.

They created and fill the child abuse committees of major medical organisations and, from that perch, issue influential policy and position statements bearing those organisations' names. And, as noted, they lobbied for and created a board certification (child abuse paediatrics) that designates them as the experts in diagnosing abuse [93]. They publish an immense amount of literature specifically for legal purposes. By contrast, there is no similar institutional framework, dedicated resources, or physicians with a natural professional inclination or incentive to publish or advocate on the other side of these issues. These institutional realities best explain how SBS has persisted.

2.6 Conclusion

Since the challenges to SBS emerged, the debate has been characterised by excessive advocacy and inadequate oversight. A review of the literature defending the purported diagnosis against the challenges reveals a sometimes startling lack of objectivity, yet there is great deference, both within the medical profession and within the courts, to those constituencies associated with defending the diagnosis, such as child abuse specialists and prosecutors. For many reasons, this is understandable – both because they are largely defending the status quo and because their mission is the protection of vulnerable children. But a suspect diagnosis used as the basis for murder charges and taking children from their parents must be founded on reliable science rather than shaped and promoted for legal and social objectives.

The historic SBS presumption of child abuse in this context is rarely uttered today. But it remains alive and well in many jurisdictions. The presumption reflects child protection advocacy that is inconsistent with evidence-based medicine and reflects a mindset and diagnostic process at odds with the burdens of proof that are supposed to apply in criminal and most family court cases. The battles within the medical and scientific communities and within the courts appear destined to continue indefinitely.

References

1. Wilson EO. *Consilience: The unity of knowledge*. Vintage, 1998.
2. Guthkelch AN. Infantile subdural haematoma and its relationship to whiplash injuries. *BMJ*. 1971;2:430.
3. Jenny C. Medicine discovers child abuse. *JAMA* [Internet]. 2008;300(23):2796–7. https://doi.org/10.1001/jama.2008.842
4. Kempe CH, Silverman FN, Steel BF, Droegemueller W, Silver HK. The battered-child syndrome. *JAMA*. 1962;181 (1):17–24. https://doi.org/10.1001/jama.1962.03050270019004.
5. Caffey J. On the theory and practice of shaking infants: Its potential residual effects of permanent brain damage and mental retardation. *American Journal of Diseases of Children*. 1972;124(2):161–9. https://doi.org/10.1001/archpedi.1972.02110140011001.
6. Caffey J. The whiplash shaken infant syndrome: Manual shaking by the extremities with whiplash-induced intracranial and intraocular bleedings, linked with residual permanent brain damage and mental retardation. *Pediatrics*. 1971;54(4):396–403.
7. Dykes LJ. The whiplash shaken infant syndrome: What has been learned? *Child Abuse and Negligence*. 1986;10(2):211–21. https://doi.org/10.1016/0145-2134(86)90082-7.

8. American Academy of Pediatrics Committee on Child Abuse and Neglect. Shaken baby syndrome: Inflicted cerebral trauma. *Pediatrics*. 1993;92(6):872–5.

9. American Academy of Pediatrics: Committee on Child Abuse and Neglect. Shaken baby syndrome: Rotational cranial injuries technical report. *Pediatrics*. 2001;108(1):206–10. https://doi.org/10.1542/peds.108.1.206. ('The constellation of these injuries does not occur with short falls.')

10. Blumenthal I. Shaken baby syndrome. *Postgraduate Medical Journal*. 2002;78(926):732–5. https://doi.org/10.1136/pmj.78.926.732. ('Families of children with subdural haemorrhages should be thoroughly investigated by social welfare agencies.')

11. Sirotnak AP, Krugman RD. Physical abuse of children: An update. *Pediatrics Review*. 1994;15(10):394–9. https://doi.org/10.1542/pir.15-10-394. ('Most subdural hematomas in infancy are assumed to be caused by abuse until proven otherwise.')

12. Eisenbrey AB. Retinal hemorrhage in the battered child. *Child's Brain*. [Internet]. 1979;5(1):40–4. https://doi.org/10.1159/000119800.

13. Rosenberg NM, Singer J, Bolte R, Christian C, Selbst SM. Retinal hemorrhage. *Pediatric Emergency Care*. 1994;10(5):303–5. https://doi.org/10.1097/00006565-19941000-00017.

14. Monteleone JA, Giardino AP, Brodeur AE. Identifying, interpreting, and reporting. In *Child maltreatment: A clinical guide and reference*. 2nd ed. JA Monteleone, AE Brodeur, eds. GW Medical Publishing, 1998. p.15.

15. Dashti SR, Decker DD, Razzaq A, Cohen AR. Current patterns of inflicted head injury in children. *Pediatric Neurosurgery*. 1999;31(6):302–6. https://doi.org/10.1159/000028880.

16. Reichert KW, Schmidt M. Neurologic sequelae of shaken baby syndrome. In *The shaken baby syndrome: A multidisciplinary approach*. S Lazoritz, VJ Palusci, eds. Routledge, 2001, pp. 79–83.

17. Parrish R. *Battered child syndrome: Investigating physical abuse and homicide*. 4th ed. US Department of Justice, 2002.

18. Case ME, Graham MA, Handy TC, Jentzen JM, Monteleone JA. National Association of Medical Examiners ad hoc Committee on Shaken Baby Syndrome: Position paper on fatal abusive head injuries in infants and young children. *American Journal of Forensic Medicine and Pathology*. 2001;22(2):112–22. https://doi.org/10.1097/00000433-200106000-00002.

19. Jentzen JM. Pathological findings in fatal shaken impact syndrome. In *The shaken baby syndrome: A multidisciplinary approach*. S Lazoritz, VJ Palusci, eds. Routledge, 2001, p. 201 (stating that the 'classical findings of retinal hemorrhages, subdural hematoma, and brain swelling cannot be fully explained by any other medical entity').

20. Duhaime AC, Alario AJ, Lewander WJ et al. Head injury in very young children: Mechanisms, injury types, and ophthalmologic findings in 100 hospitalized patients younger than 2 years of age. *Pediatrics*. 1992;90(2 Pt 1):179–85 ('Most determinations of nonaccidental injury are based on the notion of "history insufficient to explain injuries"').

21. Chadwick DL, Kirschner RH, Reece RM et al. Shaken baby syndrome: A forensic pediatric response. *Pediatrics*. 1998;101(2):321–3. https://doi.org/10.1542/peds.101.2.321.

22. National Center on Shaken Baby Syndrome [Internet]. Executive summary of the third national conference on shaken baby syndrome; 2000 p. 1. www.dontshake.org/media/k2/attachments/2000-SaltLakeCityProgram.pdf ('Often referred to as the "triad", the consensus appears to be that a collection of (1) damage to the brain, evidenced by severe brain swelling and/or diffuse traumatic axonal injury; (2) bleeding under the membranes which cover the brain, usually subdural and/or subarachnoid bleeding; and, (3) bleeding in the layers of the retina, often accompanied by other ocular damage, when seen in young children or infants, is virtually diagnostic of

severe whiplash shaking of the head') (on file with the author).

23. Kirschner RH. Pathology of child abuse. In *The battered child*. 5th ed. ME Helfer, RS Kempe, RD Krugman, eds. University of Chicago Press, 1997, pp. 248–95.

24. Holmgren BK. Prosecuting the shaken infant case. In *The shaken baby syndrome: A multidisciplinary approach*. S Lazoritz, VJ Palusci, eds. Routledge, 2001.

25. *Commonwealth v Woodward*, No. Crim. 97-0433 (1997) 7 Mass. L. Rep 449; 1997 WL 694119.

26. Plunkett J. Shaken baby syndrome and the death of Matthew Eappen: A forensic pathologist's response. *American Journal of Forensic Medicine and Pathology*. 1999;20(1):17–21. https://doi.org/10.1097/00000433-199903000-00005.

27. Reece RM. The evidence base for shaken baby syndrome: Response to editorial from 106 doctors. *BMJ*. 2004;328(7451):1316–17; author reply 1317. https://doi.org/10.1136/bmj.328.7451.1316 (asserting that Geddes and Plunkett 'display a worrisome and persistent bias against the diagnosis of child abuse in general').

28. Leestma JE. *Forensic neuropathology*. 3rd ed. CRC Press, 2014.

29. Papetti R. The forensic unreliability of the shaken baby syndrome. *United States: Academic Forensic Pathology International*. 2018;55–9, 120–42, 150–6, 157–71, 201–20, 242–3.

30. Duhaime AC, Gennarelli TA, Thibault LE et al. The shaken baby syndrome: A clinical, pathological, and biomechanical study. *Journal of Neurosurgery*. 1987;66(3):409–15. https://doi.org/10.3171/jns.1987.66.3.0409.

31. Jones MD, Martin PS, Williams JM, Kemp AM, Theobald P. Development of a computational biomechanical infant model for the investigation of infant head injury by shaking. *Medicine, Science, and the Law*. 2015;55(4):291–9. https://doi.org/10.1177/0025802414564495.

32. Wolfson DR, McNally DS, Clifford MJ, Vloeberghs M. Rigid-body modelling of shaken baby syndrome. *Proceedings of the Institution of Mechanical Engineers, Part H*.2005;219(1):63–70. https://doi.org/10.1243/095441105X9237.

33. Choudhary AK, Servaes S, Slovis TL et al. Consensus statement on abusive head trauma in infants and young children. *Pediatric Radiology*. 2018;48(8):1048–65. https://doi.org/10.1007/s00247-018-4149-1.

34. Hall JR, Reyes HM, Horvat M, Meller JL, Stein R. The mortality of childhood falls. *Journal of Trauma*. 1989;29(9):1273–5. https://doi.org/10.1097/00005373-198909000-00015.

35. Aoki N, Masuzawa H. Infantile acute subdural hematoma: Clinical analysis of 26 cases. *Journal of Neurosurgery*. 1984;61(2):273–80. https://doi.org/10.3171/jns.1984.61.2.0273.

36. Caffey J. Significance of the history in the diagnosis of traumatic injury to children: Howland Award address. *Journal of Pediatrics*. 1965;67(5):Suppl:1008–14. https://doi.org/10.1016/s0022-3476(65)82098-4.

37. Chadwick DL, Chin S, Salerno C, Landsverk J, Kitchen L. Deaths from falls in children: How far is fatal? *Journal of Trauma*. 1991;31(10):1353–5. https://doi.org/10.1097/00005373-199110000-00006.

38. *People v Basuta* (2001) 114 Cal. Rptr. 2d 285 ('Dr. Alexander stated studies indicated that short falls do not cause serious brain injuries. In a small percentage of short fall cases, a minor skull fracture can occur and cause no internal injury. Short falls do not cause subdural bleeding').

39. Plunkett J. Fatal pediatric head injuries caused by short-distance falls. *American Journal of Forensic Medicine and Pathology*. 2001;22(1):1–12. https://doi.org/10.1097/00000433-200103000-00001.

40. *Commonwealth v Epps* (2016) 53 N.E.3d 1247.

41. Atkinson N, Van Rijn RR, Starling SP. Childhood falls with occipital injuries. *Pediatric Emergency Care*. 2018;34(12):837–41. https://doi.org/10.1097/PEC.0000000000001186.

42. Geddes JF, Hackshaw AK, Vowles GH, Nickols CD, Whitwell HL. Neuropathology of inflicted head injury in children. I: Patterns of brain damage. *Brain*. 2001;124 (Pt 7):1290–8. https://doi.org/10.1093/brain/124.7.1290.

43. Mack J, Squier W, Eastman JT. Anatomy and development of the meninges: Implications for subdural collections and CSF circulation. *Pediatric Radiology*. 2009;39(3):200–10. https://doi.org/10.1007/s00247-008-1084-6.

44. Squier W, Mack J. The neuropathology of infant subdural haemorrhage. *Forensic Science International*. 2009;187(1–3):6–13. https://doi.org/10.1016/j.forsciint.2009.02.005.

45. Giardino AP, Lyn MA, Giardino ER. *A practical guide to the evaluation of child physical abuse and neglect*. Springer, 1997.

46. Block RW. Child abuse: Controversies and imposters. *Current Problems in Pediatrics*. 1999;29(9):249–72. https://doi.org/10.1016/s0045-9380(99)80058-9.

47. Geddes JF. Pediatric head injury. In *Developmental neuropathology*. JA Golden, B Harding, eds. Wiley, 2006, p. 186.

48. Wittschieber D, Karger B, Pfeiffer H, Hahnemann ML. Understanding subdural collections in pediatric abusive head trauma. *American Journal of Neuroradiology*. 2019;40(3):388–95. https://doi.org/10.3174/ajnr.A5855.

49. Vaslow DF. Chronic subdural hemorrhage predisposes to development of cerebral venous thrombosis and associated retinal hemorrhages and subdural rebleeds in infants. *Neuroradiology Journal*. 2022;35 (1):53–66. https://doi.org/10.1177/19714009211026904.

50. Levin AV. Retinal haemorrhages and child abuse. In *Recent advances in paediatrics*. TJ David, ed. Churchill Livingstone, 2000, p. 151.

51. Levin AV, Alexander R, Binenbaum G, Forbes B, Jenny C. Information statement: Abusive head trauma/shaken baby syndrome [Internet]. American Academy of Ophthalmology. 2015. www.aao.org/clinical-statement/abusive-head-traumashaken-baby-syndrome.

52. Coats B, Binenbaum G, Smith C et al. Cyclic head rotations produce modest brain injury in infant piglets. *Journal of Neurotrauma*. 2017;34(1):234–47. https://doi.org/10.1089/neu.2015.4352.

53. Moshfeghi DM. Terson syndrome in a healthy term infant: Delivery-associated retinopathy and intracranial hemorrhage. *Ophthalmic Surgery, Lasers and Imaging Retina*. 2018;49(10):e154–e156. https://doi.org/10.3928/23258160-20181002-20.

54. Smith DC, Kearns TP, Sayre GP. Preretinal and optic nerve-sheath hemorrhage: Pathologic and experimental aspects in subarachnoid hemorrhage. *Transactions of the American Academy of Ophthalmology and Otolaryngology*. 1957;61(2):201–11.

55. Greiner MV, Berger RP, Thackeray JD, Lindberg DM. Dedicated retinal examination in children evaluated for physical abuse without radiographically identified traumatic brain injury. *Journal of Pediatrics*. 2013;163(2):527–31. https://doi.org/10.1016/j.jpeds.2013.01.063.

56. Thackeray JD, Scribano PV, Lindberg DM. Yield of retinal examination in suspected physical abuse with normal neuroimaging. *Pediatrics*. 2010;125(5):e1066–e1071. https://doi.org/10.1542/peds.2009-2184.

57. Thiblin I, Andersson J, Wester K, Högberg G, Högberg U. Retinal haemorrhage in infants investigated for suspected maltreatment is strongly correlated with intracranial pathology. *Acta Paediatrica*. 2022;111(4):800–8. https://doi.org/10.1111/apa.16139.

58. Callaway NF, Ludwig CA, Blumenkranz MS et al. Retinal and optic nerve hemorrhages in the newborn infant: One-year results of the Newborn Eye Screen Test Study. *Ophthalmology*. 2016;123(5):1043–52. https://doi.org/10.1016/j.ophtha.2016.01.004.

59. Eris E, Eris D, Seymen Z et al. Retinal haemorrhage rates and resolution time of retinal haemorrhage in newborns after hypothermic treatment for hypoxic-ischemic encephalopathy.

Archives of Pediatrics. 2020;27(1):29–32. https://doi.org/10.1016/j.arcped.2019.11.001.

60. Mattheij M, Venstermans C, de Veuster I et al. Retinal haemorrhages in a university hospital: not always abusive head injury. *Acta Neurologica Belgica*. 2017;117(2):515–22. https://doi.org/10.1007/s13760-017-0748-0.

61. Shuman MJ, Hutchins KD. Severe retinal hemorrhages with retinoschisis in infants are not pathognomonic for abusive head trauma. *Journal of Forensic Science*. 2017;62(3):807–11. https://doi.org/10.1111/1556-4029.13336.

62. Levin AV. The SBU report: A different view. *Acta Paediatrica*. 2017;106(7):1037–9. https://doi.org/10.1111/apa.13834.

63. De Leeuw MD, Beuls E, Jorens PG, Parizel P, Jacobs W. The optic nerve sheath hemorrhage is a non-specific finding in cases of suspected child abuse. *Journal of Forensic and Legal Medicine*. 2015;36:43–8. https://doi.org/10.1016/j.jflm.2015.08.009.

64. Geddes JF, Vowles GH, Hackshaw AK et al. Neuropathology of inflicted head injury in children. II: Microscopic brain injury in infants. *Brain*. 2001;124(Pt 7):1299–1306. https://doi.org/10.1093/brain/124.7.1299.

65. Shannon P, Becker L. Mechanisms of brain injury in infantile child abuse. *Lancet*. 2001;358(9283):686–7. https://doi.org/10.1016/S0140-6736(01)05849-4.

66. Lantz PE, Sinal SH, Stanton CA, Weaver RG Jr. Perimacular retinal folds from childhood head trauma. *BMJ*. 2004;328(7442):754–6. https://doi.org/10.1136/bmj.328.7442.754.

67. Findley KA, Barnes PD, Moran DA, Squier W. Shaken baby syndrome, abusive head trauma, and actual innocence: Getting it right. *Houston Journal of Health Law and Policy*. 2012;12(2):274–5.

68. Fung EL, Sung RY, Nelson EA, Poon WS. Unexplained subdural hematoma in young children: Is it always child abuse? *Pediatric International*. 2002;44(1):37–42. https://doi.org/10.1046/j.1442-200x.2002.01500.x.

69. Högberg G, Colville-Ebeling B, Högberg U, Aspelin P. Circularity bias in abusive head trauma studies could be diminished with a new ranking scale. *Egypt Journal of Forensic Science*. 2016;1(6):6–10. https://doi.org/10.1016/j.ejfs.2015.12.001.

70. Lynøe N, Elinder G, Hallberg B et al. Authors' overarching reply to all the responses received to the systematic literature review on shaken baby syndrome. *Acta Paediatrica*. 2017;106(7):1031. https://doi.org/10.1111/apa.13887.

71. Vinchon M, Defoort-Dhellemmes S, Desurmont M, Dhellemmes P. Accidental and nonaccidental head injuries in infants: A prospective study. *Journal of Neurosurgery*. 2005;102(4 Suppl):380–4. https://doi.org/10.3171/ped.2005.102.4.0380.

72. Swedish Council on Health Technology Assessment. Traumatic shaking. The role of the triad in medical investigations of suspected traumatic shaking: A systematic review [Internet]. Stockholm: Swedish Council on Health Technology Assessment (SBU); 2016 Oct 26. SBU Assessment No. 255. https://bit.ly/3zON5bX.

73. Barnes PD. Imaging of nonaccidental injury and the mimics: Issues and controversies in the era of evidence-based medicine. *Radiologic Clinics of North America*. 2011;49(1):205–29. https://doi.org/10.1016/j.rcl.2010.08.001.

74. Dyer C. Diagnosis of 'shaken baby syndrome' still valid, appeal court rules. *BMJ*. 2005;331(7511):253. https://doi.org/10.1136/bmj.331.7511.253.

75. *State v Edmunds* (2008) 746 N.W.2d 590.

76. Goudge S. Inquiry into pediatric forensic pathology in Ontario: Report. Ontario Ministry of the Attorney General. 2008. https://bit.ly/3NBli4q.

77. Guthkelch AN. Problems of infant retino-dural hemorrhage with minimal external injury. *Houston Journal of Health Law and Policy*. 2012;12(201):1–8.

78. *Del Prete v Thompson* (2014) 10 F. Supp. 3d 907.

79. Lynøe N, Elinder G, Hallberg B et al. Insufficient evidence for 'shaken baby syndrome': A systematic review. *Acta Paediatrica*. 2017;106(7):1021–7. https://doi.org/10.1111/apa.13760.

80. Christian CW, Block R, Committee on Child Abuse and Neglect, American Academy of Pediatrics. Abusive head trauma in infants and children. *Pediatrics*. 2009;123(5):1409–11. https://doi.org/10.1542/peds.2009-0408.

81. Pediatricians to Say 'Abusive Head Trauma', Not 'Shaken Baby Syndrome'. USA Today [Internet]. 2009, 27 April. https://bit.ly/3WBRNDR.

82. Narang SK, Estrada C, Greenberg S, Lindberg D. Acceptance of shaken baby syndrome and abusive head trauma as medical diagnoses. *Journal of Pediatrics*. 2016;177:273–8. https://doi.org/10.1016/j.jpeds.2016.06.036.

83. Saunders D, Raissaki M, Servaes S et al. Written on behalf of the European Society of Paediatric Radiology Child Abuse Task Force and the Society for Pediatric Radiology Child Abuse Committee. Throwing the baby out with the bath water: Response to the Swedish Agency for Health Technology Assessment and Assessment of Social Services (SBU) report on traumatic shaking. *Pediatric Radiology*. 2017;47(11):1386–9. https://doi.org/10.1007/s00247-017-3932-8.

84. Högberg U, Lampa E, Högberg G et al. Infant abuse diagnosis associated with abusive head trauma criteria: Incidence increase due to overdiagnosis? *European Journal of Public Health*. 2018;28(4):641–6. https://doi.org/10.1093/eurpub/cky062.

85. Riggs JE, Hobbs GR. Infant homicide and accidental death in the United States, 1940–2005: Ethics and epidemiological classification. *Journal of Medical Ethics*. 2011;37(7):445–8. https://doi.org/10.1136/jme.2010.041053.

86. Findley KA, Risinger MD, Barnes PD et al. Feigned consensus: Usurping the law in shaken baby syndrome/abusive head trauma prosecutions. *Wisconsin Law Review*. 2019;2019(5):1211–1267.

87. Papetti R, Kaneb P, Herf L. Outside the echo chamber: A response to the 'Consensus Statement on Abusive Head Trauma in Infants and Young Children'. *Santa Clara Law Review*. 2019;59(2):299–366.

88. Greeley CS. 'Shaken baby syndrome' and forensic pathology. *Forensic Science and Medical Pathology*. 2014;10(2):253–5. https://doi.org/10.1007/s12024-014-9540-0.

89. Moreno JA, Holmgren B. The Supreme Court screws up the science: There is no abusive head trauma/shaken baby syndrome 'scientific' controversy. *Utah Law Review*. 2013;2013(5):1357.

90. Lucas S, Bärtås A, Bonamy AE et al. The way forward in addressing abusive head trauma in infants: Current perspectives from Sweden. *Acta Paediatrica*. 2017;106(7):1033–5. https://doi.org/10.1111/apa.13840.

91. Narang S. A *Daubert* analysis of abusive head trauma/shaken baby syndrome. *Houston Journal of Health Law and Policy*. 2011;11(505):505–633.

92. Tuerkheimer D. *Flawed convictions: 'Shaken baby syndrome' and the inertia of injustice*. Oxford University Press, 2014.

93. Giardino AP, Hanson N, Hill KS, Leventhal JM. Child abuse pediatrics: New specialty, renewed mission. *Pediatrics*. 2011;128(1):156–9. https://doi.org/10.1542/peds.2011-0363.

Chapter 3

The Neuropathology of Shaken Baby Syndrome or Retino-Dural Haemorrhage of Infancy

Waney Squier and Tommie Olofsson

3.1 Introduction

When an infant presents with one or more findings of the 'triad' (subdural haematoma, retinal haemorrhage, and 'encephalopathy'), abuse is immediately suspected.[1] There is no question that abuse occurs or that trauma can cause these findings. The main question is whether pathology supports the hypothesis that these findings are *specific* for abuse by shaking.

> 'Shaken baby syndrome is a serious and clearly definable form of child abuse. It results from extreme rotational cranial acceleration induced by violent shaking or shaking/impact, which would be easily recognizable by others as dangerous.' [40]

The components of the triad are closely interdependent anatomically and physiologically. Encephalopathy is a loose clinical term describing some sort of brain malfunction, ranging from lethargy, poor feeding, or seizures to imminently fatal brain swelling. Brain swelling from any cause increases pressure within the skull. As the eye is essentially an extension of the brain, with the same covering membranes, changes in intracranial pressure are directly transmitted to the eye, resulting in retinal congestion and bleeding. Similarly, fluctuations in blood flow, venous drainage, and intracranial pressure cause congestion and bleeding into the dura.[2]

3.2 Subdural Haemorrhage

All subdural haemorrhage (SDH) is anatomically within the dura (Figure 3.1). Bleeding seeps into and cleaves the loosely adherent cells of the deep dural border layer where it can spread extensively as a thin film. When it is of sufficient volume it can be identified on scans or by the naked eye at autopsy and appears to be a 'subdural' collection, which is the term used here. All infant SDH is associated with bleeding into the dura (intradural haemorrhage (IDH)). By microscopy it is common to see IDH in continuity with SDH (Figure 3.2).

---

1 Throughout this chapter, selected statements made to support the shaken baby hypothesis have been highlighted in boxes adjacent to the section where their pathological basis is discussed. The term 'shaken baby syndrome' will be used although a more objective terminology is recommended that avoids the implications of either mechanism or intent – 'retino-dural haemorrhage of infancy' [1].

2 For readers who are not medical professionals, the anatomical appendix at the end of this chapter contains a description of the infant brain with all the terminology used throughout.

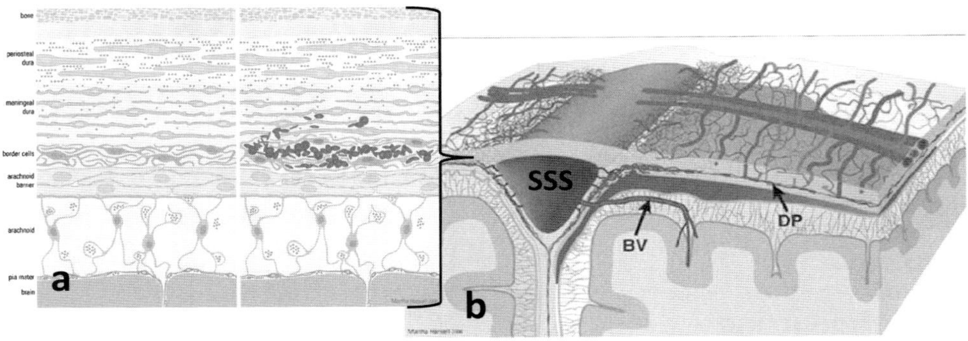

Figure 3.1 Diagrams of the meningeal membranes surrounding the brain and dural bleeding
a Diagram of detail of dural structure with blood in deep dural cell layers
b Anatomical diagram of the meninges and origin of subdural bleeding. A bridging vein (BV) drains blood from the brain, crossing the subarachnoid space and dura to enter the superior sagittal sinus (SSS). A thin film of blood leaking from the dural plexus (DP) between the dural leaflets spreads to split the dura from the arachnoid membrane. (Reproduced with kind permission [86]) (For the colour version, please refer to the plate section.)

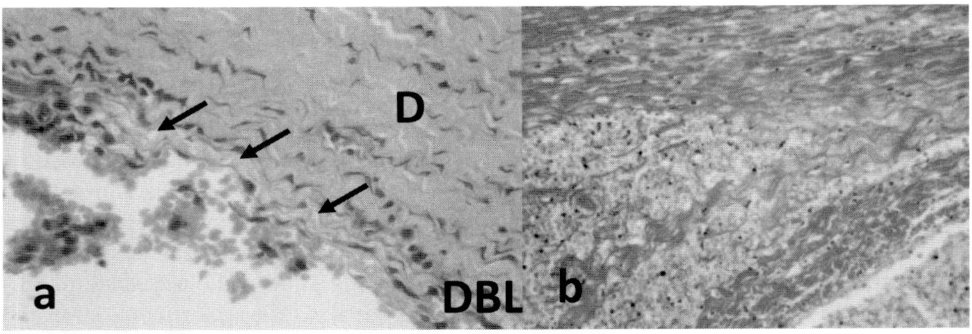

Figure 3.2 Microscopic images of infant dura
a Spinal dura (D). Note spaces between the loosely adherent cells of the deep dural border layer (DBL) (arrows). Red cells are seen between these dural cells and in the subdural compartment.
b Dura stained with Van Gieson stain; fibres of the dura are pink and red cells buff. Blood is extending between and spreading the fibres of the dura. (For the colour version, please refer to the plate section.)

Subdural haemorrhage identified on brain scans is often the first sign to raise the question of abuse. A baby may be diagnosed with a natural disease until a brain scan shows subdural bleeding. Then even the smallest films of blood, no more than 2–3 ml, are regarded as sufficient to indicate abusive head trauma (AHT).

Pathologists can identify IDH and small-volume SDH which can be missed on scans. During autopsy, it is unavoidable for blood vessels to be cut when the head is opened and leakage from these vessels may be mistaken for SDH. Care is needed to avoid damaging the bridging veins (BVs) which are one of the potential sources of SDH. Retrospective pathological reviews of the incidence and sources of SDH are unreliable because small bleeds and genuine traumatic damage to vessels can only be verified if they are specifically sought and recorded at the time of autopsy.

3.2.1 Causes of Subdural Haemorrhage

The commonest cause of infantile SDH is normal birth. Almost half of healthy newborn babies have SDH in a similar distribution to that described in SBS [2]. Trauma is another cause, and there are many natural causes – for example, coagulation disorders, meningitis, sinus or cortical vein thrombosis, vascular malformations, tumours, and metabolic diseases. Perinatal factors (multiple birth, preterm, small-for-gestational age) and male sex are associated with SDH [3, 4].

Despite wide acceptance of the suggestion by Guthkelch [5] that shaking might rupture BVs and cause subdural bleeding, this hypothesis has never been proven. On the contrary, of 30 babies observed or spontaneously confessed to have been shaken, none had SDH and one had acute subarachnoid haemorrhage [6]. A major review identified five 'independently witnessed' shaking events followed by the signs, symptoms, and radiological findings traditionally attributed to SBS/AHT [7]. Four of these cases were identified in a survey of 625 members of an international child abuse advocacy group over a 14-year period and one from 2,890 children referred for child abuse evaluations over a 15-month period. One of these cases involved a mother who tested positive for amphetamines at birth with the baby exhibiting symptoms of drug withdrawal; the shaking incident was reported by a neighbour who had just administered intravenous methamphetamines to the mother. In the four other cases, the shaking was witnessed by one parent, the alleged perpetrator being the other parent or a boyfriend of the parent; one of these cases may also have involved methamphetamines. A sixth case with neurological symptoms but no radiological findings was based on an 'anonymous report'. None of these cases meet the usual child abuse standards as 'independently witnessed'. Studies seeking to determine whether accidental low falls can produce the triad stipulate that falls must be witnessed by more than one person [8] or by 'two or more people or by a nonrelated person uninvolved in the care of the patient' [9]. Further, there is no description of the circumstances under which the witness accounts were provided. This report emphasises that witnessed accounts of shaking followed by the findings traditionally associated with shaking or abuse are rare indeed, and that 'independently witnessed' events are vanishingly rare.

3.2.2 Distribution of Subdural Haemorrhage

In the context of SBS, it is often stated that the distribution of SDH is related to its cause [10]. Both accidental and birth-related SDH may be multi-compartmental and most common in the posterior inter-hemispheric fissure [2, 4, 11, 12]. Serial imaging of infants following trauma showed that the bleeding originally was maximal near the convexity and then became evident adjacent to the sagittal sinus, falx, and tentorium, all sites adjacent to large dural sinuses. Congestion and bleeding within the falx, around the falcine plexus, is a common autopsy and imaging finding in young babies (Figure 3.3). It is considered to be due to asphyxia rather than trauma [13]. Because neither MRI nor CT scans can distinguish between intradural and thin film subdural bleeding it is easily misinterpreted on scans as inter-hemispheric SDH (Figure 3.3; see Figure 4.4).

> 'Inter-hemispheric haemorrhages and SDHs in multiple sites or of different densities were almost exclusively seen in non-accidental head injury (NAHI).' [10]

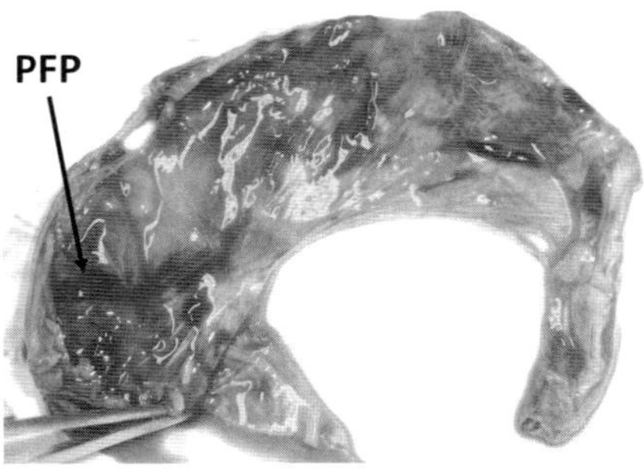

Figure 3.3 Falx at autopsy showing intense congestion. A = anterior. PFP = Posterior falcine plexus (For the colour version, please refer to the plate section.)

Blood spreads readily through the infant dura, which is loosely woven and less fibrous than in the adult. Once intradural blood has tracked into the subdural compartment it can extend widely over the brain surface, into the spinal canal and around spinal nerve roots, as discussed later in this chapter.

3.2.3 Natural History of Subdural Haemorrhage, Formation of Subdural Membranes

The dura mounts a local healing response to blood which has escaped from blood vessels (Figure 3.4). One of the earliest responses is growth of new, thin-walled blood vessels, often so wide as to be described as sinusoids, into the blood clot. Proliferation of fibrous tissue and an influx of inflammatory cells together form a thin layer or membrane over the bleeding dural surface. Over days and weeks, the layers of fibrous cells increase and the membrane becomes thicker. As delicate new blood vessels leak readily histology of healing SDH usually shows multiple foci of bleeding of different ages (Figure 3.5).

Membranes do not need to be thick to re-bleed; they may be just a few layers of cells, much thinner than the dura and difficult to see with the naked eye (Figure 3.6). They are not identifiable on brain scans unless contrast (dye) is used to highlight the new blood vessels. Fibrous tissue gradually replaces the vessels, reducing the membrane to a fibrous scar, difficult to distinguish from normal dura. The rate at which this occurs depends on a balance between fresh bleeds, which restart reactive changes, and fibrosis. The resulting fibrous scar is brown or orange due to deposition of iron from the breakdown of red blood cells. This is the most common residuum of birth injury found incidentally at infant autopsy (Figure 3.7).

Not uncommonly small vessels within a healing membrane are thrombosed (Figure 3.8), possibly as the result of the local inflammatory environment. Subdural haemorrhage has been observed radiologically to precede the development of cerebral venous sinus thrombosis (CVST) in babies [14, 15].

It is often of forensic importance to know when a subdural bleed occurred. Radiological timing is discussed in Chapter 4. Certain pathological features may indicate the age of a healing membrane [16, 17]. However, when a baby is very sick, normal reactive inflammation and healing are disturbed, so timing will be less accurate. Further, a baby maintained on life support with a severely swollen brain has impaired blood flow to the brain,

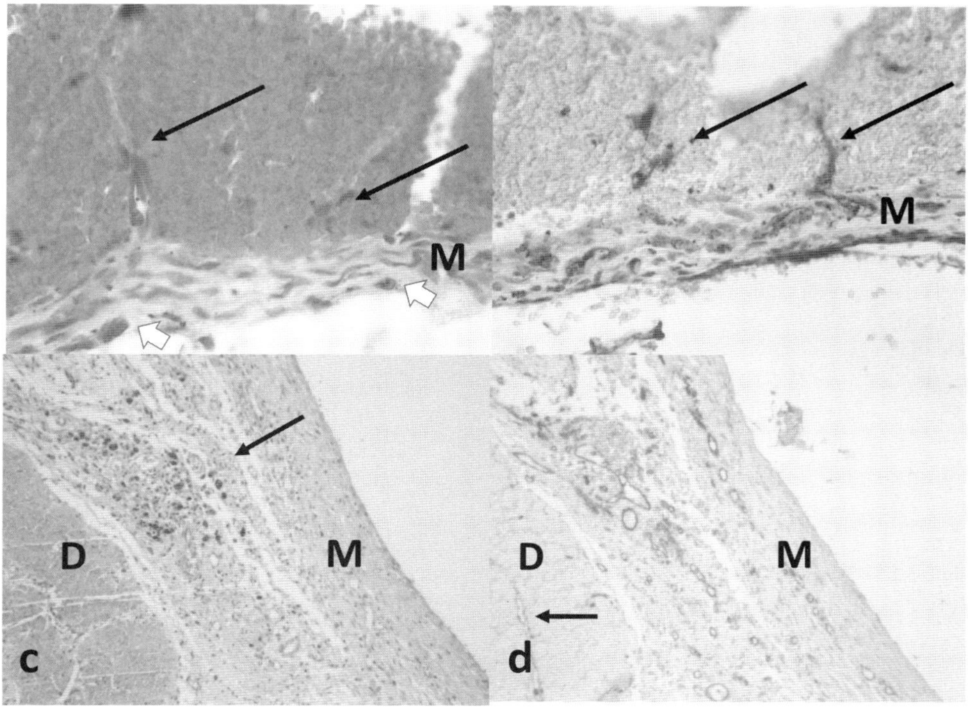

Figure 3.4 a A thin subdural membrane (M) about 6 cells deep and with a few macrophages containing brown haemosiderin (white open arrows). Blood vessels (black arrows) are growing into a mass of fresh blood above. H&E
b Same case, adjacent section stained with CD34, which stains blood vessels brown (a and b: Infant 3 months old, 3 days after trauma)
c Dura (D) bottom left with old, thick healing subdural membrane (M). The membrane is mainly fibrous, but there is a patch of cells containing haemosiderin (brown) indicating more recent bleeding (arrow) H&E
d CD 31 stains blood vessels brown. Note the many rounded profiles of large, thin-walled blood vessels (sinusoids) in the membrane and the thin vascular plexus in the normal dura (black arrow) (c and d: Male 5 months) (For the colour version, please refer to the plate section.)

inflammatory cells cannot reach the brain, and healing responses are impaired. In this circumstance, some flow may still reach the dura from extracranial vessels, so dural reactive processes may continue and allow some estimate of timing.

3.2.4 Acute and Chronic Subdural Haemorrhage, Subdural Effusions, and Hygromas

Subdural blood may be rapidly resorbed or may persist as a fluid collection.[3] The initial blood clot becomes liquid and may increase in volume; fluid leaks into it from small blood vessels damaged by inflammation (effusion). Breakdown of the haemoglobin in red cells causes the subdural fluid to become yellow or brown in colour (xanthochromia).

[3] The terms *chronic SDH*, *subdural effusion*, and *hygroma* may be used interchangeably. They are discussed in more detail in Chapter 5.

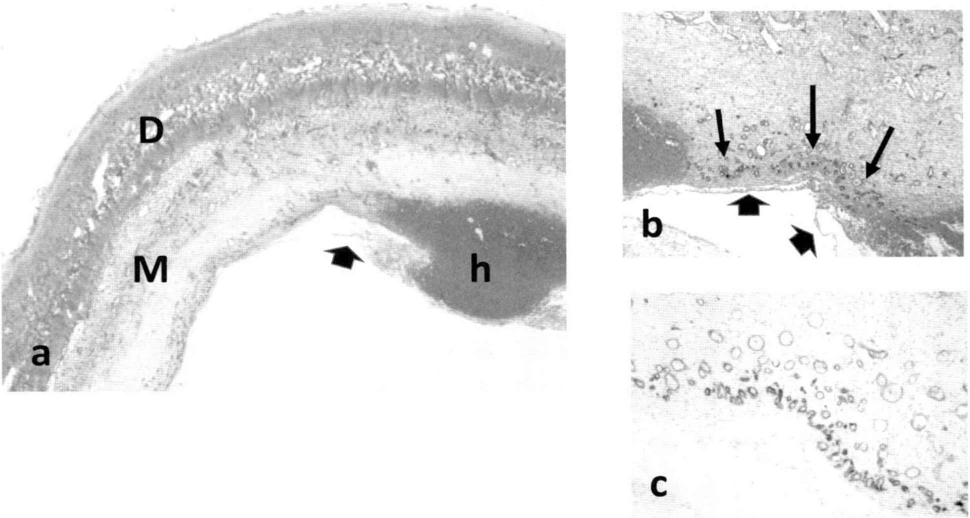

Figure 3.5 Female who had traumatic head injury at 3/12 and died in care at 7/12
a Section of dura (D) shows a thick chronic subdural membrane (M) which is pale pink and thicker than the dura itself, consistent with the 4 months since the original trauma. There is a small fresh haemorrhage (h) from the deep border of the membrane.
b Higher-power image of the edge of the membrane shows a thick layer of wide new blood vessels (arrows) which are the source of the bleeding. Fragments of deep dural border layer cells are seen adjacent to the blood clot (arrowheads).
c CD31 stain highlights the layer of new vessels close to the deep edge of the membrane.
A is stained with H&E, b with H&E and CD31, c with CD31. (For the colour version, please refer to the plate section.)

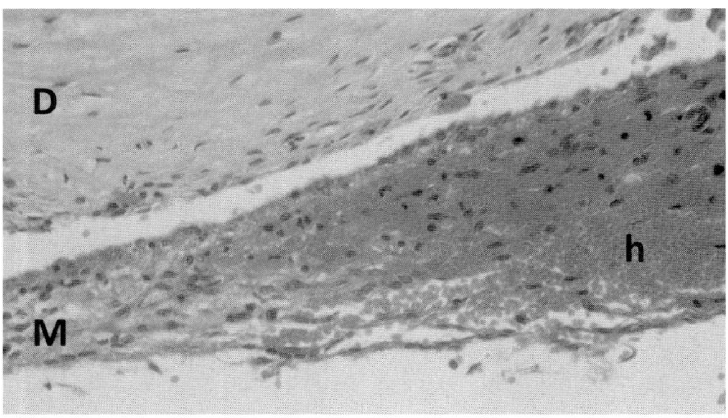

Figure 3.6 Subdural membrane (M) beneath the dura (D). The membrane has separated from the dura during tissue processing. The membrane is about 11 cells thick. There is a fresh haemorrhage (h) into the membrane. (For the colour version, please refer to the plate section.)

Recognising chronic SDH is important. Among babies suspected of having been abused, the great majority, 81%, had chronic SDH. Sixty-eight per cent of these were male, 34% were premature, and a large number had clinical and radiological findings compatible with external hydrocephalus. These appear to be a quite distinct group from babies with acute SDH [18]. This underlines the importance of consulting head circumference charts and

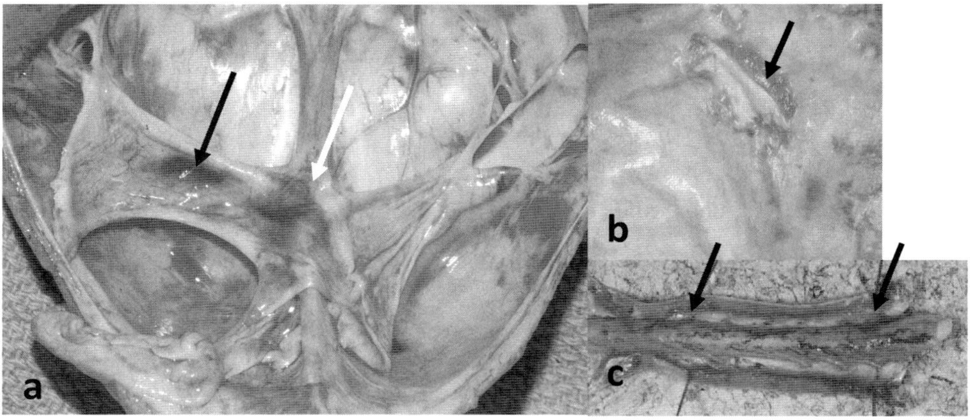

Figure 3.7 Old subdural haemorrhage
a Inner surface of the base of the skull at autopsy. The tentorium has fresh intradural bleeding (black arrow) and a patch of old, ochre-coloured subdural blood (white arrow).
b Fixed dura showing extensive pale brown subdural membrane which could easily be missed. There is a small tear (arrow) where the normal grey dura can be seen.
c Fixed infant spinal cord. The dura has been opened in the dorsal midline showing patchy yellow-brown discolouration at the thoracolumbar and sacral levels of the deep surface of the dorsal dura (arrows). (For the colour version, please refer to the plate section.)

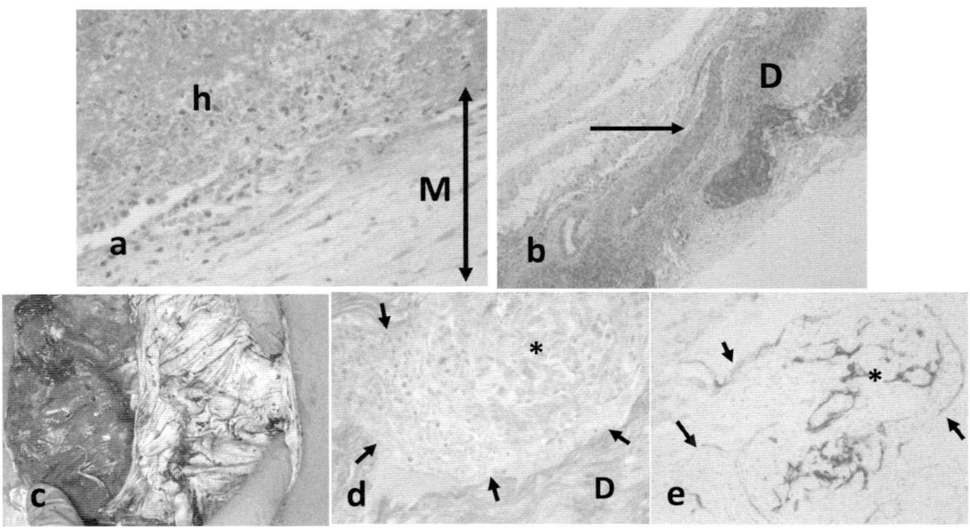

Figure 3.8 a and b: 2-month infant with venous thrombosis who collapsed 4 days following a fall and survived for 1 week
a Subdural membrane (M) and organising subdural haemorrhage (h)
b Thrombus within dural vessel (arrow). Note extensive fresh bright pink intradural bleeding.
c, d, e Male 10 years with chronic subdural haemorrhage in association with arachnoid cyst
c Fixed dura with a fluid chronic subdural haemorrhage within a membrane on the left side
d Thrombosed vein within the dura (trichrome stain) D = dura. Small arrows indicate vessel wall. *= recanalising thrombus
e CD 34 stain delineates the blood vessel wall and new vessels in the recanalising thrombus (For the colour version, please refer to the plate section.)

looking for pre-existing intracranial fluid collections which are of benign origin, but may themselves have potentially harmful effects, in order not to confuse these babies with those with traumatic SDH.

3.2.4.1 The Arachnoid Tear Hypothesis

Pathologists know that the arachnoid membrane is tough and is not readily torn but needs to be cut to access the brain surface. There is no patho-anatomical verification of the arachnoid tear hypothesis. (See also Chapter 4.)

> 'The inflicted injury (acceleration/deceleration +/− impact) can lead to tearing of convexity bridging veins at the junction of the bridging vein and superior sagittal sinus. Additionally, rupture of the arachnoid membrane allows cerebrospinal fluid to enter the subdural space, mixing with subdural blood (hematohygroma).' [29]

3.2.5 Sources of Subdural Haemorrhage

Any of the vessels within the dura, including BVs, the intrinsic blood vessels of the dura, and the new vessels of healing subdural membranes, are potential sources of dural bleeding.

3.2.5.1 Bridging Veins

Bridging veins (BVs) are terminal parts of the veins draining blood from the brain. Leaving the brain surface, they pursue a long course in the subarachnoid space before penetrating the arachnoid membrane and the deep dural layers to drain into the venous sinuses (Figure 3.1). Autopsy and imaging studies indicate that BV are few (Figure 3.9); only about 10 BVs drain into the superior sagittal sinus (SSS) on each side, although each drains a considerable volume of blood – some 5 cc of blood per minute in the adult [19]. An autopsy study in infants found 22 BVs draining the whole of each cerebral hemisphere [20] but did not specify the proportion of parasagittal BVs, those thought most likely to be damaged by shaking.

> 'Subdural bleeding is a marker for a traumatic mechanism (i.e., acceleration/deceleration, rotational and shearing forces due to violent shaking) causing rupture of the bridging veins ... Bilateral bridging vein rupture confirms violent shaking. Unilateral bridging vein rupture is suggestive of unilateral trauma.' [83]

Traditionally, SDH has been believed to occur when BVs are ruptured by shaking. However, SDH is particularly common after birth when BV rupture is rarely described. Torn BVs can sometimes be seen during craniotomy for massive, clotted SDH, but there is little evidence for this mechanism in infants where SDH is typically a thin film [12]. There is no satisfactory autopsy method to demonstrate ruptured BVs as the process of opening the dura may itself damage them. Pathology indicates that ruptured BVs cause subarachnoid bleeding [21]. The hypothesis that shaking causes rupture of BV and subdural, rather than subarachnoid, bleeding implies that shaking ruptures these vessels in their very short course across the dura, rather than in their much longer subarachnoid course. A study of four

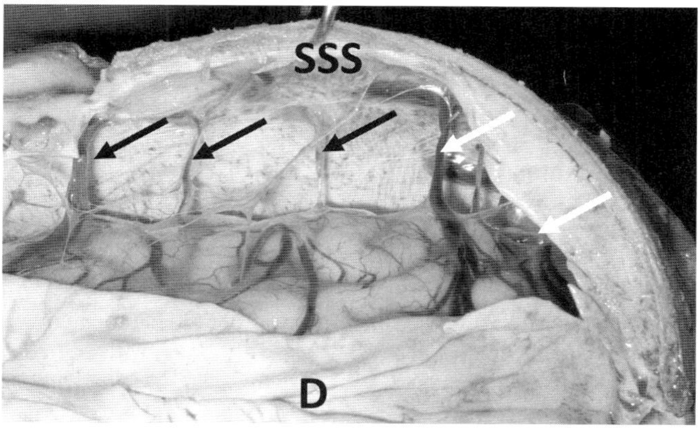

Figure 3.9 Bridging veins in infant with benign external hydrocephalus. The skull has been opened and the upper flap is lifted; the superior sagittal sinus is just below the bone (SSS). Below the dura has been folded back (D). Five bridging veins (arrows) pass from the brain surface, across a wide subarachnoid space to the SSS. The two white arrows indicate BV which are congested and possibly thrombosed. Note the acute angle as the BVs enter the SSS. (For the colour version, please refer to the plate section.)

elderly patients is often cited to suggest that the intradural section of the vein wall is weak, but the small number and age of these patients undermine the value and relevance of this study for infants [22].

3.2.5.2 The Dura

The dura is an obvious source for thin film SDH because (1) it is very vascular. It contains the large venous sinuses and an extensive plexus of small vessels between its two layers. (2) Infant thin film SDH is most commonly described adjacent to the most vascular areas of the dura: the falx, tentorium, parasagittal, and occipital dura. (3) Intradural haemorrhage is extremely common in infants and a constant finding in infants with SDH [23]. Microscopic examination often demonstrates continuity between intradural and subdural bleeding [24] (Figure 3.2).

3.2.5.3 Healing Membranes

Fresh subdural bleeding stimulates the development of a vascular membrane on the dural surface wherever blood is present. This can be a very extensive, thin membrane, hardly even visible to the naked eye and certainly beyond the resolution of brain scans, yet still capable of fresh bleeding or 're-bleeding' (Figure 3.7).

3.2.6 Effects of Subdural Haemorrhage

Infant SDH may be clinically silent or associated with signs of cerebral irritation, including seizures, vomiting, impaired consciousness or irritability which may precede evidence of increased intracranial pressure [25]. These signs are often dismissed. Seizures are difficult to detect in young babies, and vomiting and feeding difficulties are often ascribed to 'reflux'. Head circumference charts may indicate abnormal fluid collections and together with signs indicating SDH or fluid collections predating collapse will help distinguish babies with natural conditions from those with traumatic SDH.

How dural blood causes cerebral irritation is not understood. Impaired perfusion and oedema, mediated by spreading depolarisation, have been identified in the cortex adjacent to SDH [26]. Subdural blood is separated from the brain by the arachnoid membrane and subarachnoid fluid, implying a neural mechanism, possibly mediated by the trigeminal nerve [27]. Inflammation associated with dural bleeding may incite neurogenic inflammatory responses capable of potentiating the response to trauma and mediating brain swelling, subdural effusions, and poorly understood phenomena such as the 'big black brain', and syndromes involving massive brain swelling beneath a thin film SDH and both predominantly affecting the young [27].

3.3 Retinal Haemorrhage

The eye develops from the brain in early embryonic development, taking with it the same covering membranes; the white of the eye or 'sclera' is modified dura, the retina a thin layer of brain tissue whose nerve fibres form the optic nerve. The blood supply to the eye and its venous drainage are via vessels in the optic nerve surrounded by the same three layers of meninges as the brain. Changes in intracranial pressure are thus directly transmitted to the eye. If intracranial pressure increases, due, for example, to brain swelling or massive haemorrhage, the veins draining the eye are compressed and their smaller tributaries in the retina become congested and may bleed, patterns of bleeding following the anatomy of the blood vessels. Bleeding may also occur in the optic nerve sheath [28].

Retinal haemorrhages (RHs) are considered a cardinal sign of AHT and are said to occur in 85% of cases [29, 30]. However, like SDH, RH is common after birth and seen in about a third of newborn babies. Other causes include blood clotting disorders, venous thrombosis (see Figure 3.14c), anaemia, metabolic diseases, and hypoxia.

> 'Retinal haemorrhages in young children have almost become diagnostic of child abuse.' [30]

3.3.1 Mechanism

In SBS, RH is said to be due to traumatic vitreo-retinal traction, when shaking causes the vitreous body in the eye to pull on its retinal attachments, tearing retinal blood vessels. Pathological and epidemiological studies do not support this. A study of 36 infants who had been shaken showed they did not have RH or any other findings (SDH or fracture) regarded as highly specific for AHT [6]. In another study of 29 infants with RH, only one was subjected to witnessed or confessed shaking while shaking was confessed in 18% of babies without RH [31]. This study included 5 babies who had RH with chronic SDH and no fresh blood. As RHs seen in life are essentially fresh (they resolve within days or weeks), the RHs and SDHs must have occurred at different times and cannot have been caused by the same, recent violent event. This study challenges two fundamental elements of the shaking hypothesis: that the act of shaking causes vitreo-retinal traction and RH, and at the same time tears BVs, causing SDH.

An alternative mechanism is that RHs are secondary to raised intracranial pressure. This has been shown in children and is independent of age and aetiology [32]. These observations are consistent with pathological observations that RHs result from leaking through small retinal blood vessels due to increased retinal venous pressure [33]. This mechanism is the most likely explanation for birth-related RH, supported by the observation that the risk of developing RH increases with increasing duration of the second stage of labour [34]. Thiblin found all babies with bilateral RH to have intracranial pathology, mostly chronic subdural collections [28], which are usually associated with raised intracranial pressure. This confirms the association of RH with SDH in babies, which has been recognised for decades. Guthkelch [5] and Caffey [35] regarded RH as a valuable sign of clinically silent chronic SDH, and Till suggested that RHs are 'pathognomonic' of SDH, whatever its cause [25].

3.3.2 Distribution and Patterns of Retinal Haemorrhage

The distributions and patterns of RH have been used to determine their cause [36]. As with SDH, patterns of RH described in AHT, birth-related bleeding, and other conditions such as seizures, accidents, and acute life-threatening events [37] are similar and may be equally severe. In a randomised blind study, ophthalmologists were asked to determine the cause of RH from a series of photographs. Their success was only slightly better than random choice [38]. In 2020, Binenbaum, an ophthalmologist and protagonist of the shaken baby hypothesis, effectively refuted previous claims for the specificity of RH for shaking. He said that patterns that might distinguish traumatic from medical causes of RH are not perfectly correlated with abuse; 'there is generally more overlap than appreciated between abusive and accidental retinal hemorrhages' [39].

> 'The specific pattern and extent of RH help delineate the cause of the eye findings'. [36]

3.4 Spinal Cord Pathology in Shaken Baby Syndrome

Several pathologies of the spine have been associated with SBS, including spinal subdural bleeding, spinal ligamentous oedema, spinal cord parenchymal damage, and nerve root bleeding and axonal injury.

> 'On MRI 78% of these infants [victims of AHT] have spinal findings, mostly ligamentous, and up to 75% have spinal subdural hematoma that tracks from the posterior fossa.' [29]

3.4.1 The Upper Cervical Spine

The fundamental tenet of SBS is that an infant with certain symptoms was necessarily subjected to violent shaking [40]. Observations of infants injured in road traffic accidents who suffer severe whiplash demonstrate fractures or dislocations and nerve root injuries in the high cervical spine [41, 42]. However, subdural and retinal bleeding and cerebral swelling are not described in these babies. Their relatively large infant heads, poorly developed musculature, shape of the vertebral bones, orientation of their joints, and elasticity of their associated ligaments predispose these babies to maximum damage in the upper cervical levels [43]. Consequently, shaking that is sufficiently violent to cause intracranial haemorrhage would be expected also to cause damage here. There is a wide range (2–71%) in the reported incidence of neck injury in babies thought to have been shaken; spinal fractures and dislocations are rare [44, 45].

3.4.2 Spinal Subdural Blood

Subdural haemorrhage is common after birth. Cranial SDH may track and redistribute from the cranial to the spinal compartment [46] and will settle by gravity, as it does in the head, in the dorsal thoracolumbar area, the most dependant area in the supine infant. At autopsy it is common to find a patch of subdural blood lining the dorsal dura here in the absence of trauma (Figure 3.7c). It is unlikely that SDH arises locally in the spinal cord because (1) there are no bridging veins in the spinal subdural compartment and (2) the veins draining the spinal cord accompany the nerve roots and damage to the nerve roots would be clinically evident. Spinal SDH per se cannot be regarded as independent evidence of trauma.

'There is a high incidence of previously unsuspected spinal SDHs associated with intracranial collections in children with NAI.' [46]

3.4.3 Paraspinal Ligamentous Injury

Imaging studies claim that paraspinal soft tissue changes (particularly oedema) are associated with SBS [47–49]. There is limited autopsy evidence to support them: Brennan found soft tissue injuries in only 20% of babies with spinal cord pathology thought to have been victims of homicide [44]. Several studies have demonstrated a correlation between occipito-cervical ligamentous changes and cerebral hypoxic-ischaemic injury (HII) [47, 50, 51]. One potential explanation is that cerebral HII results from damage to the lower brainstem[52], which would be expected to be associated with clinical features such as cardiac and respiratory arrest and paraparesis, as well as evidence of local tissue injury. In the absence of these findings other explanations must be sought.

'Non-bony spinal abnormalities have, however, been identified in up to 2/3 of victims of AHT.' [47]

Interpretation of the pathology of the paraspinal tissues requires knowledge of the vertebral venous anatomy and physiology and its relationship to developmental stage, which has been largely ignored in standard teaching. This is that venous blood leaves the brain through the dural sinuses and then into the jugular veins in the neck to return to the heart. This is only a part of the story. It does not consider the effects of posture on venous return pathways. In normal adults in the upright position venous blood returns to the heart via the paravertebral plexus and outflow through the internal jugular veins is absent or negligible [53, 54]. This has significant implications in the first year of life when the infant goes from a predominantly supine to a predominantly upright position. The associated postural haemodynamic changes lead to morphological modifications of the posterior fossa dural sinuses, emissary veins, and jugular bulb.

When intracranial pressure is increased, flow is increased through emissary veins which connect the intracranial dural sinuses with the extracranial venous system. They are the primary venous outflow route in the upright position and are more commonly found in children. They are valveless and flow may be bidirectional; they serve the important function of equalising intracranial pressure and can act as 'safety valves' during cerebral congestion [53]. When intracranial pressure is increased, flow is increased through emissary veins and the suboccipital plexus, which can then be transmitted to the vertebral venous plexuses and the radicular vessels [55]. This is exemplified in the case illustrated in Figure 3.10.

The occipito-cervical tissues, said to show signal changes on MRI in AHT [47], are the site of the 'suboccipital cavernous sinus', an expansion of the paravertebral venous outflow pathway of the brain and subject to congestion and oedema when intracranial pressure increases. It is particularly interesting that occipito-cervical changes described by Choudhary are strongly correlated with age [47]. Seventy-eight per cent of babies with these changes, diagnosed as AHT, had a median age of 4 months, compared with 46% deemed traumatic with a median age of 15 months and only 1% aged 14 months, deemed non-traumatic. The peak incidence of paravertebral oedema as shown in this study occurs at the time when a baby begins to sit upright and venous outflow via the paravertebral system assumes a significant role.

3.4.4 Sub-scalp Bleeding and Emissary Veins

Emissary veins may provide accessory venous drainage during raised intracranial pressure as noted earlier in this chapter. In this situation blood flow may seep out through them into loose connective tissue of the deep scalp (Figure 3.10d), forming multiple rounded patches of blood. These should not be confused with contusion, particularly in the absence of superficial scalp injury.

3.4.5 Spinal Cord Parenchymal Injury

There are two major caveats when assessing pathology of the cervical spinal cord. Firstly, this is a 'watershed zone' between arterial supply from above and from ascending arteries below. In infants maintained on artificial ventilation, prolonged and severe brain swelling compromises blood flow from above, which may lead to infarction in the cervical spinal cord [56]. Preserved flow from below allows bleeding from damaged capillary vessels into the damaged tissue (reperfusion injury) and brings inflammatory cells which generate a reactive process not seen elsewhere in the terminally swollen brain. Infarction and reactive changes in the cervical cord need to be recognised as part of the 'respirator brain' and not confused with local traumatic injury.

The second caveat is to be aware of tonsillar herniation. When the brain is very swollen the cerebellar tonsils are forced out of the skull at the foramen magnum and into the upper cervical spine. Necrotic masses of displaced cerebellar tissue compress and distort the cervical cord and stretch the nerve roots and may cause local bleeding. Fragments of necrotic cerebellar cortex are often displaced around the spinal cord at all levels.

Hadley described six infants with 'whiplash-shake syndrome' [57] who had cerebral SDH and brain swelling with herniation. Five had epidural or subdural haematomas at the cervico-medullary junction and four had high cervical 'contusions'. None of the pathology as described is specific for local trauma. Epidural haemorrhage may be an artefact in infants [58] or be secondary to congestion of the paravertebral plexus; SDH may track from the cranial compartment and cervical cord 'contusions' may be a manifestation of 'respirator brain'.

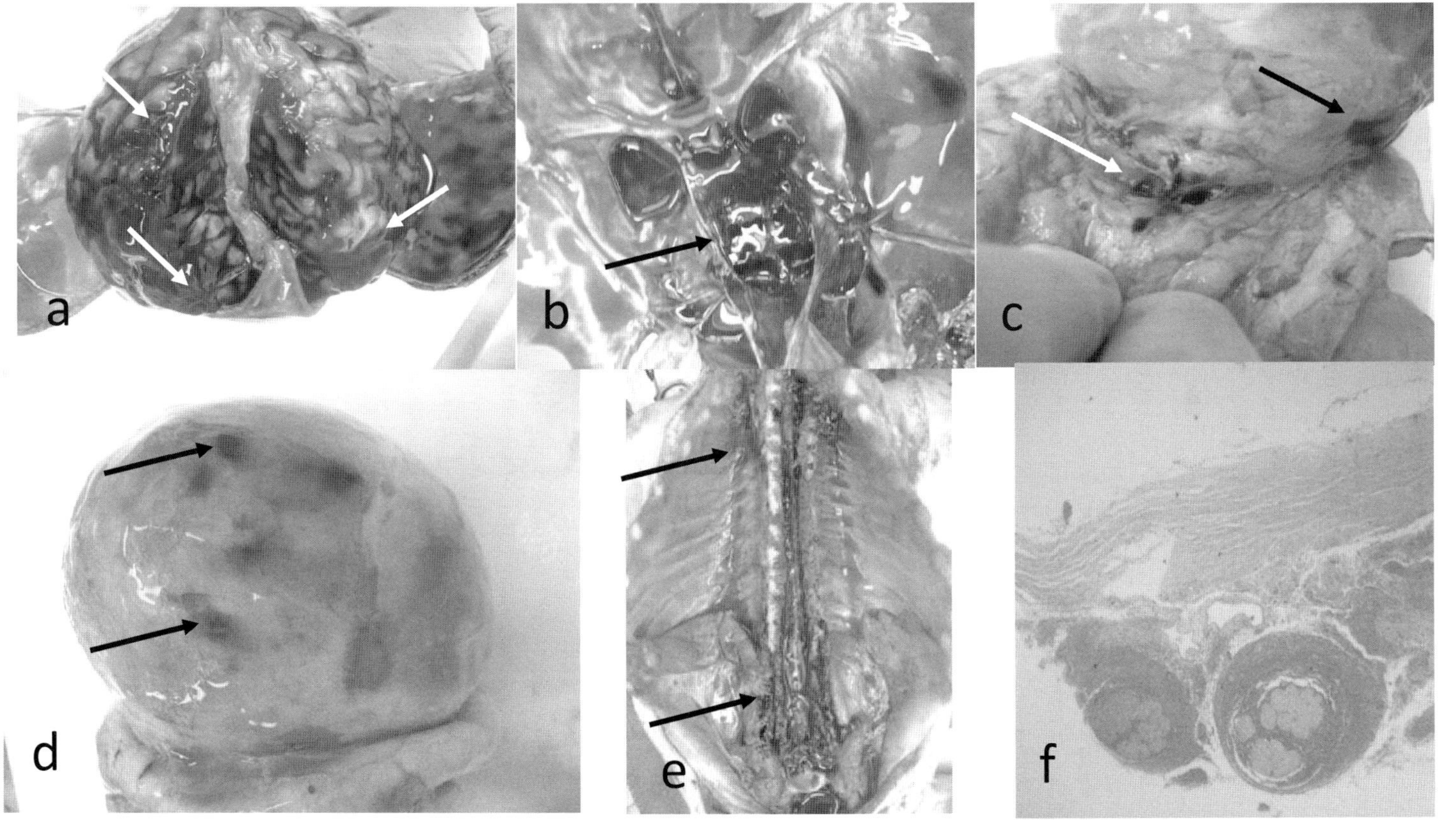

Figure 3.10 Newborn infant with displacement of the occipital bone and large cerebellar bleed following traumatic delivery
a Congested and dilated (varicose) surface and bridging veins (white arrows) over the cerebral hemispheres
b Blood clot (white arrow) occupying the posterior fossa
c The suboccipital sinus and internal vertebral venous plexus are dilated (white arrow). There is blood oozing from the right mastoid emissary vein (black arrow).
d Multiple subscalp blood patches over the vertex of the skull. Several are in sites of emissary veins (arrows).
e Extensive bleeding into nerve roots of cervical and sacral plexuses (arrows). There was no traumatic damage to adjacent soft tissues.
f Nerve roots are congested and haemorrhagic. There was no histological evidence of traumatic damage and no traumatic axonal injury. (For the colour version, please refer to the plate section.)

Kemp [59] described an association between cervical spinal injury and inflicted head trauma. Only four babies in this study with 'confirmed' shaking had cervical injuries, but we do not know whether they involved the spinal cord, nor whether the shaking was associated with impact. Brennan [44] described spinal cord damage at autopsy in 71% of babies under 2 years of age whose deaths had been determined as homicide, including AHT. The definitions of injury were very broad and included meningeal and nerve root bleeding, while parenchymal injuries were not described in sufficient detail to assess. None had fractures or dislocations of the neck bones and only one fifth had ligamentous or muscle damage. Molina [45] found neck injuries in only 2.5% of homicide deaths in children under 5 years of age. Feldman [60] found no spinal cord injuries after MRI and PM studies of 12 children with AHT.

3.4.6 Spinal Nerve Root Injury

The spinal dura extends along the spinal nerve roots, beyond the dorsal root ganglia where it blends with the sheath of the nerve roots, so blood can track along the dura into the nerve roots. This would explain the observation [61] that all babies with nerve root haemorrhage also had spinal SDH; only one baby without SDH had nerve root bleeding. Intraneural bleeding is also seen when there has been venous congestion due to raised intrathoracic pressures during resuscitation and ventilation [24] (Figure 3.10e, f).

Axonal injury in spinal nerve roots has been said to be the result of shaking and hyperflexion of the neck with stretching of nerve roots. This is sometimes claimed to be independent evidence of trauma. The characteristic finding is swellings along the nerve fibres (axons) best identified by staining for a specific protein, beta-APP (Figure 3.11). No studies have distinguished characteristics of spinal nerve root swellings which allow their cause to be determined; they appear the same whether death is due to natural causes or when there is trauma [62]. Axonal swellings take minutes or hours to develop and may persist for months or years, so must be interpreted with caution in infants, who may have suffered axonal trauma during delivery.

3.5 Encephalopathy

Encephalopathy is a broad, non-specific term which simply implies brain malfunction. It may be applied to an infant who is sleepy, irritable, or not feeding well or to one with life-threatening brain swelling. In SBS these clinical features have been ascribed to mechanical disruption of nerve fibres (axons) in the brain by shaking. This would be expected to cause an immediate loss of function with no symptom-free period or 'lucid interval' [63]. Neuropathological observations have shown this assumption to be incorrect as explained below.

> 'There is no evidence of a prolonged interval of lucidity between the injury and the onset of symptoms in children with acute subdural hematoma and brain swelling'. [63]

3.5.1 Nerve Fibre (Axonal) Injury

Axonal injury may be focal or diffuse (diffuse axonal injury (DAI)). It is recognised microscopically by swellings along axons, best identified by staining for a specific protein, beta-APP, which is normally transported along nerve fibres (Figure 3.11). Anything that

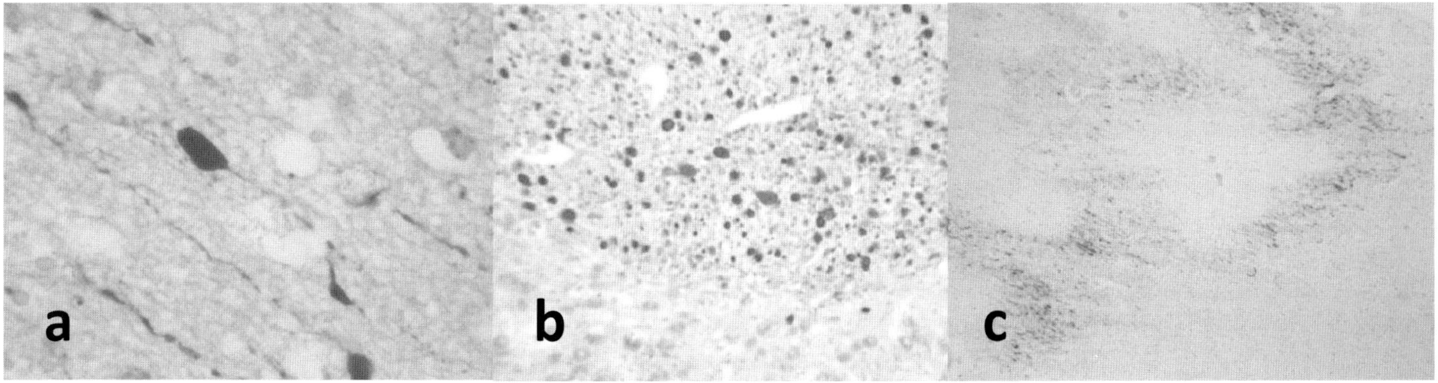

Figure 3.11 Axonal injury βAPP stain
a Single axonal swellings
b Traumatic axonal injury. A well-defined nerve fibre bundle contains many rounded, swollen axons. Note the lack of bleeding.
c Diffuse axonal injury. Irregular 'geographic' pattern of swollen axons (For the colour version, please refer to the plate section.)

disrupts normal axonal flow causes the protein to back up at the site of damage, producing beading and swelling. Many insults disrupt axonal transport – for example, hypoxia, metabolic disease, or trauma. It is not possible to accurately distinguish the cause, even with careful microscopy and special staining techniques. In adults certain patterns and distribution of axonal injury suggest the cause, but this does not appear to be the case for infants.

Traumatic axonal injury (TAI), first described in adults, refers to a specific pattern of axonal injury in the deep brain and brainstem [64] and typically associated with haemorrhages. However, it is different in infants, who rarely have haemorrhages in association with axonal injury [65]; indeed, even in infants believed to have been shaken, axonal injury is uncommon. Geddes [52, 66] showed that in 'shaken only' babies the predominant pathology was lack of oxygen and blood supply with rarely focal axonal injury in the lower brainstem and cervical nerve roots. Oehmichen [67] confirmed the absence of DAI and found similar focal axonal injury. These findings are entirely non-specific, and although they may follow blunt head trauma, they are also seen in babies after a variety of natural conditions such as heart and respiratory failure or seizures.

3.5.2 Brain Swelling (Oedema) and Hypoxic-ischaemic Injury

Deprivation of oxygen (hypoxia) may occur if the airway is obstructed – for example, if a baby chokes on food or vomit. Acute systemic hypoxia in itself initially has surprisingly little effect on the brain, but it soon affects the heart, leading to failure of blood supply (ischaemia) which does cause serious damage to the brain and other organs. Hypoxia leads to ischaemia hence the term *hypoxic ischaemic injury* (HII) is often used. When blood supply to the brain fails the toxic by-products of metabolism accumulate and cause additional cell damage. Prolonged hypoxia damages the lining cells of blood vessels and may cause them to leak.

The infant brain has a high water content and is particularly prone to swelling, which is a major cause of morbidity and mortality. Brain swelling may take time, hours or days, so a baby who has brain swelling following trauma or hypoxia may not show clinical signs immediately, in other words, the infant may demonstrate a 'lucid interval' during which the baby appears to function more or less normally between the insult and the clinical signs.

Brain swelling involves several processes; within minutes fluid in the brain redistributes, entering cells which individually swell (cytotoxic oedema), but there is no overall increase in brain fluid or brain swelling. Sometime later fluid enters the brain tissue across the damaged blood vessel walls, causing increase in weight and swelling of the brain (extracellular or vasogenic oedema). This has traditionally been considered the primary cause of swelling. A novel concept to explain early brain swelling says that accumulation of cerebrospinal fluid (CSF), which normally communicates with the perivascular glymphatic system and spaces between the cells of the brain, is the source of early and severe swelling. Within minutes of hypoxia, CSF flows rapidly into the perivascular spaces, coinciding with the onset of swelling and increased brain water content [68].

The longer the period of HII the greater will be the damage to small blood vessels, leading to leakage of fluid and brain swelling. While fluid leaks from small blood vessels, red cells rarely do. Bleeding is unusual in infant HII unless there is a further factor such as compression due to herniation or obstruction of the venous drainage. If a baby is resuscitated after severe HII, the restored blood flows through damaged blood vessels which bleed (reperfusion injury).

Both swelling and HII are very common in any baby who has suffered advanced resuscitation and been nursed on a ventilator for a period of time. This aspect of the clinical history is often overlooked in babies presenting with the triad, who not uncommonly suffer a prolonged period of hypoxia, often well over 30 minutes, between being found collapsed and receiving advanced resuscitation. Prolonged HII and resuscitation are significantly associated with RHs and brain swelling [69] and may explain the encephalopathy in babies with the triad. Caffey noted [35] that artificial respiration may induce excessively high intracranial and intraocular venous pressures, which lead to haemorrhagic brain and eye damage. In this way babies with the triad differ from cot death (sudden infant death syndrome (SIDS)) babies who are, by definition, found dead and have no pathology or intracranial bleeding. When a baby is nursed on a ventilator the heart continues to pump and breathing is maintained. The brain damaged by HII swells, increasing pressure within the skull. Blood vessels are compressed, blood flow stagnates, and toxic waste products of metabolism accumulate, causing further brain damage. The cells needed to initiate the normal reactive processes to tissue injury cannot enter the brain and healing cannot take place. For this reason, pathological interpretation of the timing and even the nature of damage can be difficult. It may be possible to find some clues of timing in the meninges, whose blood supply is from extracranial vessels and may be maintained, allowing healing responses to take place.

3.5.3 The Relationship between Hypoxic-ischaemic Injury, Brain Swelling, and the Triad

This has been the subject of considerable misunderstanding. Geddes proposed that 'These three factors, cerebral venous hypertension and congestion, arterial hypertension and brain swelling, coupled with immaturity and hypoxia related vascular fragility, provide an alternative physiological scenario for the characteristic subdural bleed of the "shaken baby syndrome"' [70]. Both Cushing, in 1905 [71], and Caffey [35] had already made this suggestion. It became the focus of a series of legal appeals in England, when this hypothesis was pitted against the shaken baby hypothesis. Geddes explained her position during the appeals: 'Paragraph 57: It is important to note that the new hypothesis did not seek to show that the triad was inconsistent with NAHI. It did, however, seek to show that it was not diagnostic' [72]. There has been a tendency to oversimplify this hypothesis to 'hypoxia causes SDH' in the literature and in the courts. This is misleading and does not consider the complexity of the physiological consequences of hypoxia, ischaemia, and reperfusion.

3.5.4 Contusions

The term *contusion* means a bruise and is pathologically defined by an area of bleeding into tissue due to leakage of red cells from blood vessels. The radiological appearances of contusions are discussed in Chapter 4. The term *contusion* carries an implication of trauma and therefore should be used cautiously. Two kinds of brain contusion are described – surface and 'subcortical contusions'. Surface contusions, characteristic of adult brain trauma, are extremely rare in the infant brain. 'Subcortical contusion' (also

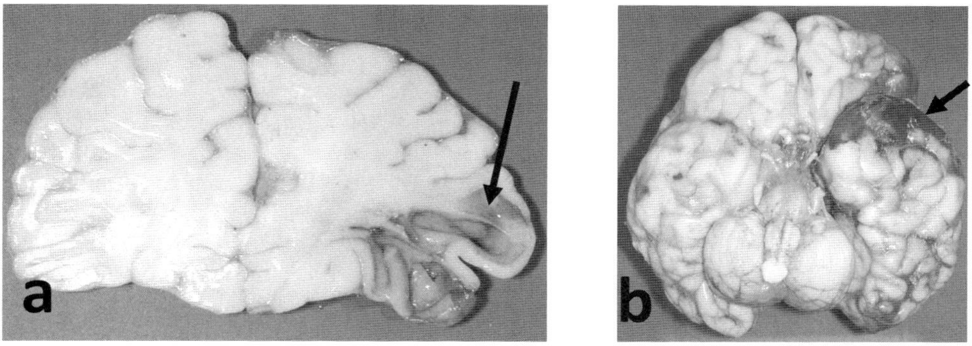

Figure 3.12 Infant brain: Subcortical cysts
a Coronal slice of fixed brain with smooth walled but blood-stained cyst (arrow) beneath an intact cortex
b Sub-pial bleed overlying the haemorrhagic cyst (For the colour version, please refer to the plate section.)

variously called gliding contusions, tears, splits, clefts, or cysts) is an incorrect and misleading term. Lesions in the immediate subcortical white matter are not infrequent in young infants with severe brain swelling; this is the watershed between the superficial and deep venous systems, the sub-plate zone which contains a hydrophilic extracellular matrix, which is prone to retain water. Pathology shows focal swelling which may be haemorrhagic or cystic and without features of trauma [73]. The overlying cortex is intact (Figure 3.12). Subcortical cysts in the parasagittal or temporal lobe location are recognised in sinus thrombosis [74, 75].

3.6 Venous Thrombosis

Cortical vein thrombosis (CVT) with or without cortical venous sinus thrombosis (CVST) is increasingly recognised as a cause of stroke and mortality in young babies. In the normal bloodstream there is a constant cycle of intravascular clot formation and lysis. When the balance of these processes is disturbed clots may form. Three factors are classically held responsible for thrombosis: stasis of flow in a blood vessel, damage to the endothelial lining of the blood vessels, or increased coagulability of the blood.

Venous drainage of the brain is via two systems, superficial and deep. The watershed territory between them is in the subcortical white matter, an area which is vulnerable to swelling and ischaemia when either drainage system is compromised. Thrombosis is more common in the superficial system. The SSS is most commonly involved with thrombosis, usually starting in the vicinity of the parietal lobe. The bridging veins here are tortuous, turning to pass through a long dural tunnel as they enter the SSS at an acute angle, against the flow in the sinus (see Figure 3.9).

3.6.1 Pathology of Cortical Vein Thrombosis

Cortical vein thrombosis and CVST (Figure 3.13) are easily missed if the dural venous sinuses, including the extensive sinuses at the base of the skull (Figure 3.14), are not carefully examined at autopsy and if the diagnosis is not borne in mind while reading the

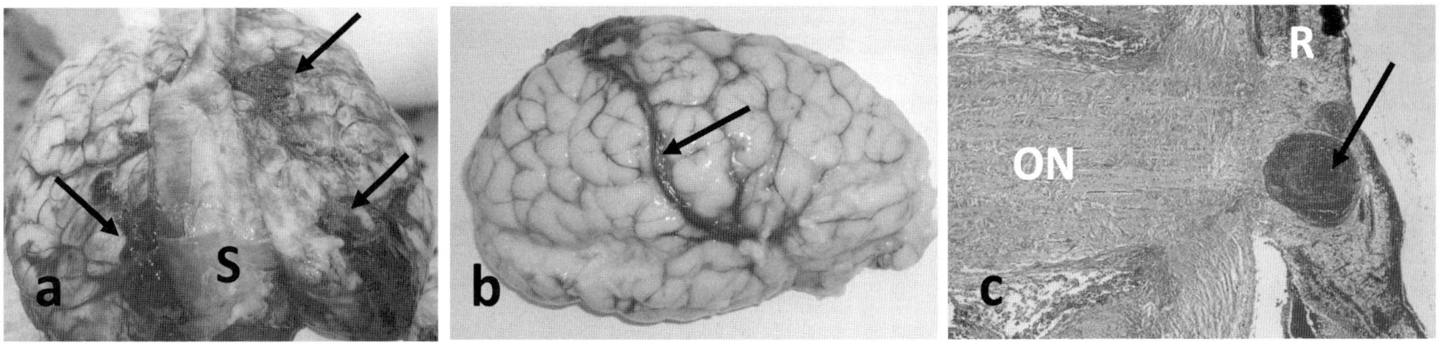

Figure 3.13 Cortical vein thrombosis in a 4-week-old baby who collapsed with seizures while in a public park
a Fresh brain with several congested, dilated, varicose veins (arrows). A midline strip of dura overlying the superior sagittal sinus (S) remains in situ
b The brain after fixation demonstrating a thrombosed superficial vein
c Central retinal vein showing a large thrombus at the optic nerve (ON) head (arrow). (R = retina) (For the colour version, please refer to the plate section.)

Dural sinuses

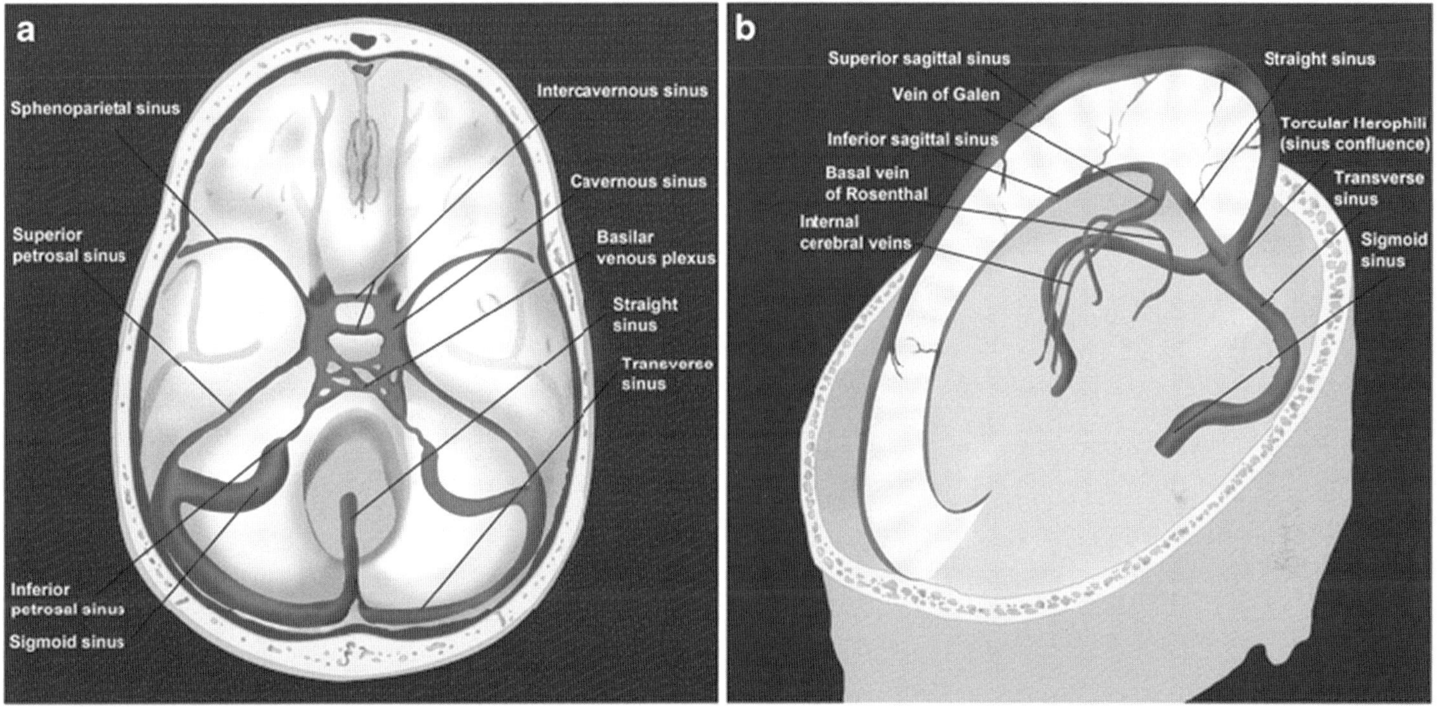

Figure 3.14 Diagram of the dural venous sinuses
(Reproduced with kind permission from [87])

histology. Evidence of head and neck infections, meningitis, and mastoiditis must be sought as these are risk factors in almost half of paediatric cases [76]. Any sick baby who has been ventilated for a period of time is likely to develop clot in the cerebral veins due to increased intracranial pressure and stasis of venous blood flow. Many also develop coagulopathy, which promotes clotting. Thrombus which has formed after death is usually soft and unattached. Microscopic examination, particularly at the sites of clot attachment, will assist in determining the age of the clot [77] and whether the clots formed before or as the result of ventilation.

Examination of the sinuses and veins may reveal nothing. A clot may cause symptoms due to metabolic disturbance without visible damage to the parenchyma, or a clot may cause parenchymal pathology and have lysed prior to imaging studies or autopsy. In longer-standing thrombosis the clot will provoke a sequence of healing and inflammatory responses; capillaries grow into the clot and form new channels to restore blood flow through the obstruction (recanalisation) (Figure 3.15). The clot gradually becomes fibrosed and shrinks down to a thin pad of fibrous tissue on the vessel lining.

Obstruction of venous outflow has a number of pathological consequences which are discussed in Chapter 4.

3.6.1.1 Varicose Veins

When thrombus forms in a vein the back pressure of the venous blood causes the vein to become congested, tortuous, stretched, and dilated (varicose) and may form a knotty mass of vessels on the brain surface exactly as varicose veins elsewhere in the body (Figures 3.13, 3.15).

3.6.1.2 Diapedesis

Venous obstruction is associated with leakage of red blood cells through the vein wall (diapedesis), which on the surface leads to focal sub-pial or subarachnoid bleeding. In the dura this leads to intra- or subdural bleeding (Figure 3.16).

3.6.1.3 Congestion and Oedema of the Parenchyma Drained by the Thrombosed Vessels

White matter oedema or haemorrhage is the commonest pathology in infants with CVST. This can be transient and reversible or lead to focal venous infarction with or without haemorrhage. Because the venous anatomy is variable and there may be extensive collaterals, there may be poor topographical correlation between the pathology and the site of thrombosis. There is sometimes generalised brain swelling. This pathology is sometimes erroneously labelled ‘non-haemorrhagic contusion’.

3.6.1.4 Sub-pial Haemorrhage

This is an under-recognised feature of venous outflow obstruction. The perivascular compartment of the cortical veins is in direct continuity with the sub-pial compartment and blood leaking from congested cortical veins can track back to the sub-pial compartment. This forms sometimes extensive bleeding beneath the arachnoid membrane but can be distinguished from subarachnoid haemorrhage by its sharply delimited margins. Microscopically, the pia is lifted by the bleeding above an apparently intact superficial cortical layer and scanty collections of red cells (diapedesis) are seen around small cortical vessels beneath it (Figures 3.17 and 3.18).

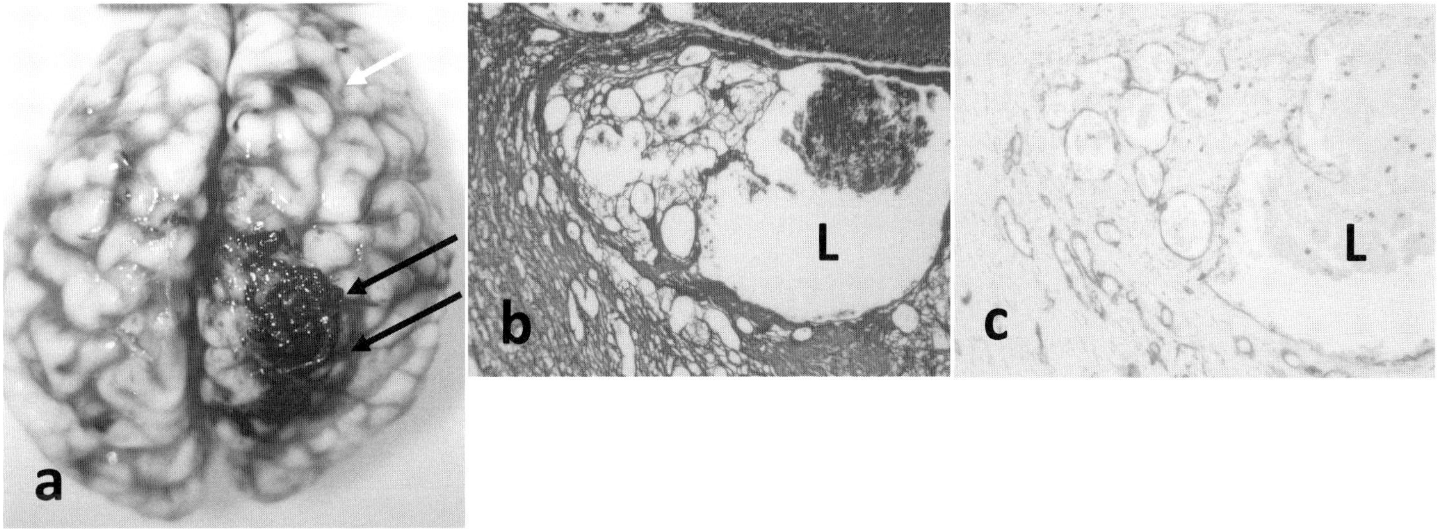

Figure 3.15 a Thrombosed surface veins. A single thrombosed vein (white arrow) and a mass of tortuous, congested, varicose veins (black arrows) are indicated.
b Thrombosed vein with organisation and recanalisation. The lumen of the vessel remains partly patent (L). The left half of the lumen is occupied by profiles of newly formed vessels which replace the original thrombus (reticulin stain).
c CD31 stains the walls of the new blood vessels brown. (For the colour version, please refer to the plate section.)

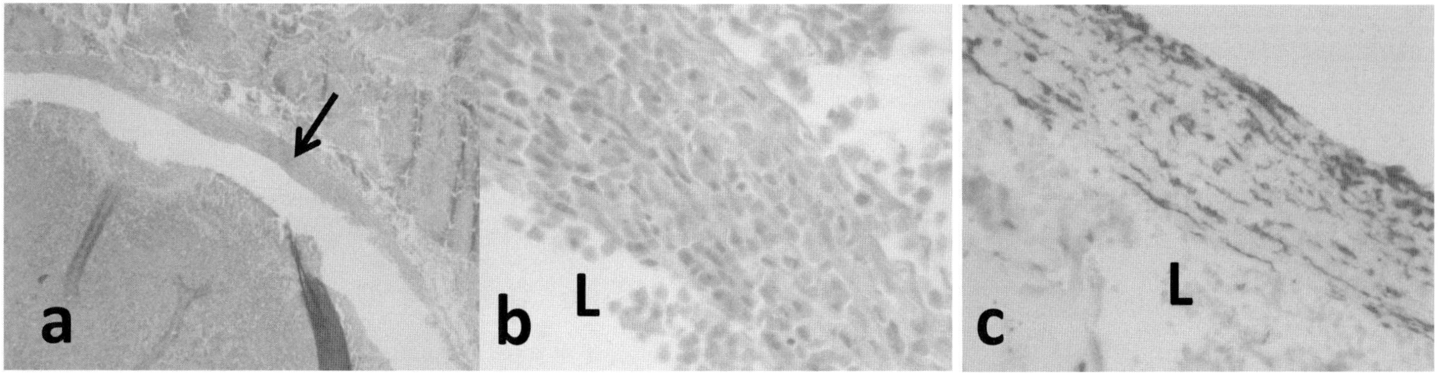

Figure 3.16 Cortical vein thrombosis – diapedesis

a Trichrome stain. Thrombus in a vein is stained pink. The clot has shrunk from the vein wall and cracked during tissue processing. The arrow indicates a point where red cells (buff colour) are passing between the cells of the vein wall (blue) to leak into the dura (intradural haemorrhage).

b Higher power shows the red cells (stained buff) between the cells of the vein wall (blue).

c Cells of the vein wall stained with smooth muscle actin (SMA) showing their separation by red cells (pale grey) lumen (L) (For the colour version, please refer to the plate section.)

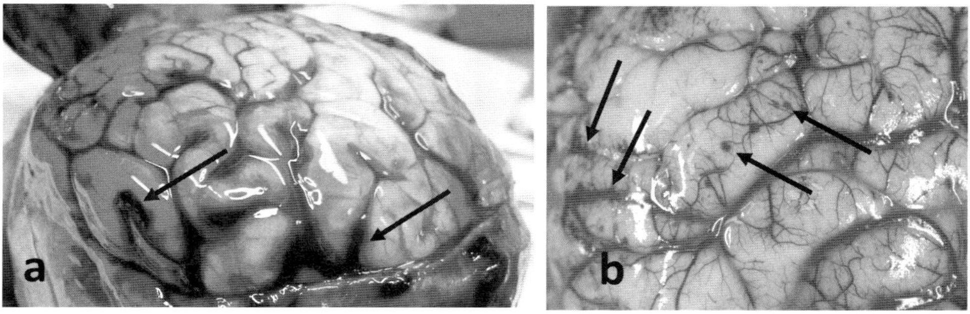

Figure 3.17 Cortical vein thrombosis – sub-pial bleeding
a Surface of fresh brain showing thin diffuse film of subarachnoid blood and well defined perivenous sub-pial blood
b Surface of fixed brain showing discrete rounded spots of sub-pial blood and localised perivenous blood (arrows)
(For the colour version, please refer to the plate section.)

3.6.1.5 Intraventricular Haemorrhage

Intraventricular haemorrhage (IVH) is typically seen in very premature babies due to bleeding from the immature germinal matrix. In babies after this premature stage the most common cause of IVH is thrombosis of the deep cerebral veins. It is seen in a third of neonates with CVST [78]. This diagnosis should be considered in any baby with IVH.

3.6.2 Bridging Vein Thrombosis

The frontal, parietal, and occipital bridging veins take a tortuous course with a long intradural tunnel to enter the SSS. This may explain their predisposition to thrombosis. It has been suggested that thrombosis of BVs is a marker of BV rupture, and thus abuse [79]. Pathological observations do not support this hypothesis [80]. The clotting process takes time, up to a few hours [81]. During this time bleeding would continue, so rupture would be accompanied by significant bleeding. An autopsy study of SDH due to ruptured BV found between 30 and 250g of clot, the average being 125g [82]. Yet there are those [81, 83] who propose that shaking causes BV thrombosis, relying on autopsy observations in babies after prolonged periods of ventilation. Without histological verification the thrombosis cannot be assumed to have preceded collapse.

'The diagnosis of non-accidental head injury caused by shaking is certain in case of: multifocal SDH with blood clots at the convexity (vertex) evidencing ruptures of the bridging veins'. [79]

Conclusion

A major textbook – *DiMaio's Forensic Pathology* [84] – notes, 'Thus the authors have grave reservations as to the existence of SBS as was expressed in the first edition of this book. Since then, there has not been a cause to change this opinion but rather to solidify it. There is just no conclusive evidence that this entity exists.'

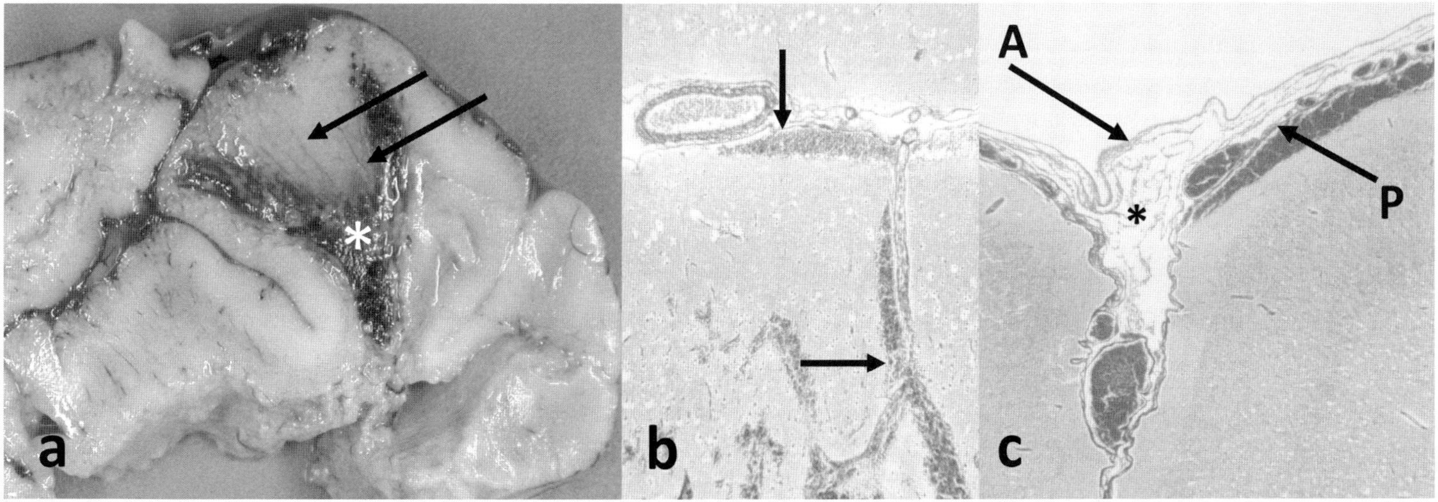

Figure 3.18 Cortical vein thrombosis – sub-pial bleeding
a Part of a slice of a fixed brain of a 3-month-old with venous thrombosis following a fall and skull fracture. There is a very thin surface sub-pial bleed. The cortex is mostly intact. Thin streaks representing veins (arrows) extend at right angles to the brain surface from a large subcortical haemorrhage (*).
b Brain surface showing blood around a vein in the subcortical white matter (arrows) tracking towards the surface. At the top a small collection of sub-pial blood (dark brown) lifts the fine pial membrane (arrow) (reticulin stain).
c Higher power of the sub-pial blood (dark brown). P = pia, A = arachnoid barrier membrane, * = subarachnoid space (For the colour version, please refer to the plate section.)

A review of the neuropathology of infants said to have been shaken, as presented in this chapter similarly fails to provide evidence to support the shaken baby concept. This hypothesis appears to have been developed with the laudable clinical desire to identify and prevent child abuse and to explain intracranial pathology, traditionally associated with trauma, in infants where no evidence of trauma is found. The explanations of the shaking hypothesis currently offered mainly misunderstand or misinterpret infant neuropathology. Others rely on confessions and consensus which rank low in the hierarchy of scientific evidence. We hope that a better understanding of pathology and science will lead to more accurate diagnosis and fairer assessment of cases in the courts.

Appendix: Anatomy and Pathophysiology in the First Year of Life

Recognising disease processes (pathology) depends on knowledge of normal anatomy. In assessing infant neuropathology acknowledging the immaturity of the anatomy and physiology is critical; we cannot simply extrapolate from adults to babies. The human brain is immature at birth and undergoes a phenomenal growth spurt in the first year of life, tripling in weight. Most of this weight gain is due to myelination. The immature brain and its coverings are equipped to cope with these challenges; the skull bones are soft, the junctions between them are unfused to allow skull compression during birth and subsequent re-expansion and rapid growth. Brain growth makes great metabolic demands and requires a correspondingly large blood supply. To accommodate this the channels in the dura draining the blood are larger and more numerous than in later life.

A further challenge is the change in predominant posture from lying to sitting and standing which is accompanied by alterations in the pattern of venous drainage from the brain in the neck and modifications in the related vascular anatomy in the head and neck.

Another change in the first year of life is the reduction of the water content of the brain, which is very high at birth. The infant brain is prone to severe water retention with a predilection for fluid to accumulate in the layer of white matter just beneath the cortex.

The brain consists of the nerve cells (grey matter) and their supporting cells, the glia. The cerebral cortex is a layer of nerve cells forming the surface layer of the brain, further masses of nerve cells form the basal ganglia in the deep parts of the brain (Figure 3.19). Nerve cells communicate with one another and with other tissues of the body via long processes, axons, and dendrites, which largely constitute the white matter. Nerve cells communicate by the release of chemical signals (neurotransmitters) which pass from the nerve terminal to the recipient cell. Neurotransmitters are synthesised in the nerve cell body and are among the proteins (including beta-APP) which are constantly transferred along their lengths. This process is initiated and controlled by electrical impulses which pass along the membrane of the fibre to its terminal. To increase the speed and efficiency of impulse transmission the axons are wrapped in layers of an insulating membrane, myelin, which gives the white matter its colour. This process begins in mid gestation but is most active in the first year of life.

Glial cells mainly make and maintain myelin and support and protect neurons by contributing to cell barriers surrounding the brain, lining the ventricles, on the brain surface beneath the meninges and around every blood vessel within the brain.

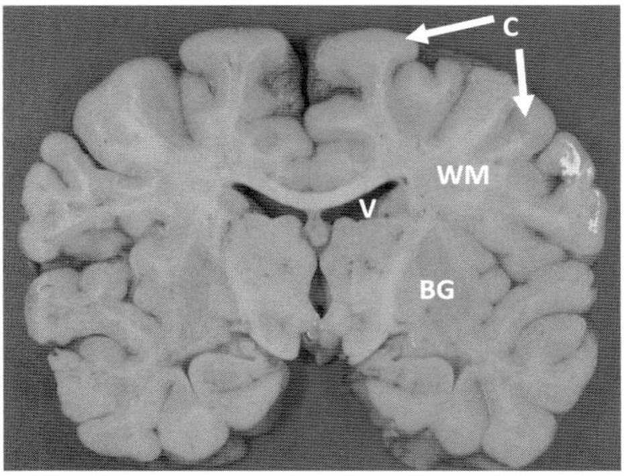

Figure 3.19 Anatomy of the infant brain after fixation. The orientation is coronal – that is, as if the cut were from one ear to the other.
C = Cortex, WM = white matter, BG = basal ganglia, V = ventricle

Four arteries supply the blood to the brain, anteriorly the carotid arteries and posteriorly the vertebral arteries. The arteries ultimately lead to the capillaries, the smallest vessels nurturing the brain tissue. Brain capillaries are highly specialised, their endothelial walls have tight junctions, and they are everywhere surrounded by fluid and a glial barrier. This constitutes the blood-brain barrier, which maintains the highly protected environment of the brain and prevents access of toxins or infections in the bloodstream. The blood and CSF are similarly separated by a barrier and the arachnoid barrier membrane maintains the integrity of the CSF in the subarachnoid space.

The CSF is formed in the ventricles of the brain and permeates between the cells of the brain, providing essential materials for them and removing metabolic waste products. The CSF is part of the glymphatic system and flows along perivascular pathways, communicating with the subarachnoid space where it covers and cushions the brain. The CSF is absorbed via dural lymphatic vessels and along spinal nerve roots.

Meninges

Three layers of membrane surround the brain (Figure 3.1). The outer membrane is the dura. It has two fibrous layers; the outer one lines the skull and is tightly bound to it. Between the outer and inner layers is a plexus of blood vessels which include the wide channels (sinuses) which collect all the blood draining from the brain and convey it to the blood vessels in the neck and then the heart. The inner layer is adherent to the second membrane surrounding the brain, the arachnoid barrier membrane, a thin but strong membrane forming a sac surrounding the brain (the subarachnoid space) which contains the CSF. Fine spidery processes extend from the arachnoid barrier membrane across the subarachnoid space and attach to the finest and innermost layer of membranes, the pia. This delicate membrane closely covers the brain surface, following its folds. The large blood vessels bringing blood into and out of the brain run in the subarachnoid compartment.

The major dural sinuses (Figure 3.14) are the superior and smaller inferior sagittal sinuses, which run along the midline of the head from front to back in the upper part of the falx, a fold of dura that extends between the hemispheres. It converges with other large sinuses, the straight and transverse sinuses in the tentorium, a fold of dura which extends as a shelf between the cerebrum and the cerebellum. Within the posterior part of the falx is a large plexus of veins (Figure 3.3).

Spinal Cord

The spinal dural tube is formed by a continuation of the inner, meningeal leaflet of the cranial dura. There is no venous plexus within the spinal dura, and it contains few blood vessels. Intradural bleeding is therefore uncommon. There are no BVs; the spinal cord is drained by radicular veins which run in the nerve roots. The dural tube is surrounded by a wide epidural compartment containing fat and the internal paravertebral venous plexus.

The vertebral venous system is composed of two venous plexuses, the internal within the vertebral canal and the external surrounding the vertebral column. The two are connected via intervertebral veins and the radicular veins. The external venous plexus connects with veins draining the chest and abdomen and is subject to changes in intrathoracic or intra-abdominal pressure which may cause epidural congestion and bleeding.

The upper part of the vertebral venous plexus expands into the suboccipital plexus (also called the suboccipital cavernous sinus) and surrounds the vertebral arteries as they enter the cranial compartment just as the cavernous sinus surrounds the internal carotid arteries. These specialised venous plexuses draining blood from the brain have an intimate relationship with the incoming arterial blood with physiological roles involving regulation of intracranial pressure and accessory venous drainage [85].

References

1. Guthkelch AN. Problems of infant retino-dural hemorrhage with minimal external injury. *Houston Journal of Health Law and Policy*. 2012;12:201–8.
2. Rooks VJ, Eaton JP, Ruess L et al. Prevalence and evolution of intracranial hemorrhage in asymptomatic term infants. *American Journal of Neuroradiology*. 2008;29(6):1082–9.
3. Högberg U, Andersson J, Squier W et al. Epidemiology of subdural haemorrhage during infancy: A population-based register study. Palazón-Bru A, editor. *PLoS One*. 2018;13(10):e0206340.
4. Vinchon M, Noizet O, Defoort-Dhellemmes S, Soto-Ares G, Dhellemmes P. Infantile subdural hematomas due to traffic accidents. *Pediatric Neurosurgery*. 2002;37(5):245–53.
5. Guthkelch AN. infantile subdural haematoma and its relationship to whiplash Injuries. *BMJ*. 1971;2(5759):430–1.
6. Thiblin I, Andersson J, Wester K et al. Medical findings and symptoms in infants exposed to witnessed or admitted abusive shaking: A nationwide registry study. *PLoS One*. 2020;15(10):e0240182.
7. Feldman KW, Melville JD, Johnson KL et al. Abusive head trauma follows witnessed infant shaking. *Child Abuse Review* [Internet]. 2022. https://onlinelibrary.wiley.com/doi/10.1002/car.2739.
8. Keenan HT, Runyan DK, Marshall SW, Nocera MA, Merten DF. A population-based comparison of clinical and outcome characteristics of young children with serious inflicted and noninflicted traumatic brain injury. *Pediatrics*. 2004;114(3):633–9.
9. Williams RA. Injuries in infants and small children resulting from witnessed and corroborated free falls. *Journal of Trauma: Injury, Infection, and Critical Care*. 1991;31(10):1350–2.
10. Datta S. Neuroradiological aspects of subdural haemorrhages. *Archives of Disease in Childhood*. 2005;90(9):947–51.
11. Nikam RM, Kandula VV, Yue X et al. Birth-related subdural hemorrhage: Prevalence and imaging morphology. *Pediatric Radiology*. 2021;51(6):939–46.

12. Vinchon M, Desurmont M, Soto-Ares G, De Foort-Dhellemmes S. Natural history of traumatic meningeal bleeding in infants: Semiquantitative analysis of serial CT scans in corroborated cases. *Child's Nervous System*. 2010;26(6):755–62.

13. Friede RL. Hemorrhages in asphyxiated premature infants. In *Developmental neuropathology* [Internet]. Heidelberg, 1989, pp. 44–58. https://bit.ly/3NBlSPE.

14. Anderst J, Carpenter S, Frazier T et al. Subdural hemorrhage in a cohort with cerebral sinovenous thrombosis: Application to abusive head trauma. *Child Abuse and Neglect*. 2021;117:105119.

15. Vaslow DF. Chronic subdural hemorrhage predisposes to development of cerebral venous thrombosis and associated retinal hemorrhages and subdural rebleeds in infants. *Neuroradiology Journal*. 2021;197140092110269.

16. Menkes JH, Sarnat HB, Maria BL, editors. *Child neurology*. 7th ed. Lippincott Williams & Wilkins, 2006.

17. Van den Bos D, Zomer S, Kubat B. Dare to date: Age estimation of subdural hematomas, literature, and case analysis. *International Journal of Legal Medicine*. 2014;128(4):631–40.

18. Andersson J, Wikström J, Högberg U, Wester K, Thiblin I. External hydrocephalus as a cause of infant subdural haematoma: Epidemiological and radiological investigations of infants suspected of being abused. *Pediatric Neurology*. 2021;S0887899421002125.

19. Mortazavi MM, Denning M, Yalcin B et al. The intracranial bridging veins: A comprehensive review of their history, anatomy, histology, pathology, and neurosurgical implications. *Child's Nervous System*. 2013;29(7):1073–8.

20. Cheshire E, Malcolmson R. A systematic autopsy survey of human infant bridging veins. *International Journal of Legal Medicine*. 2018;132:449–61.

21. Case ME. Pathology of fatal abuse. In *Child abuse: Medical diagnosis and management*. 4th ed. A. Laskey, A. Sirotnak , eds. American Academy of Pediatrics, 2020, pp. 765–820.

22. Yamashima T, Friede RL. Why do bridging veins rupture into the virtual subdural space? *Journal of Neurology, Neurosurgery and Psychiatry*. 1984;47(2):121–7.

23. Cohen MC, Scheimberg I. Evidence of occurrence of intradural and subdural hemorrhage in the perinatal and neonatal period in the context of hypoxic ischemic encephalopathy: An observational study from two referral institutions in the United Kingdom. *Pediatric and Developmental Pathology*. 2009;12 (3):169–76.

24. Squier W. The 'shaken baby' syndrome: Pathology and mechanisms. *Acta Neuropathologica*. 2011;122(5):519–42.

25. Till K. Subdural haematoma and effusion in infancy. *BMJ*. 1968;3(5615):400–2.

26. Robinson D, Kreitzer N, Ngwenya LB et al. Diffusion-weighted imaging reveals distinct patterns of cytotoxic edema in patients with subdural hematomas. *Journal of Neurotrauma*. 2021;38(19):2677–85.

27. Squier W, Mack J, Green A, Aziz T. The pathophysiology of brain swelling associated with subdural hemorrhage: The role of the trigeminovascular system. *Child's Nervous System*. 2012;28:2005–15.

28. Muller PJ, Deck JHN. Intraocular and optic nerve sheath hemorrhage in cases of sudden intracranial hypertension. *Journal of Neurosurgery*. 1974;41(2):160–6.

29. Choudhary AK, Servaes S, Slovis TL et al. Consensus statement on abusive head trauma in infants and young children. *Pediatric Radiology*. 2018;48 (8):1048–65.

30. Christian CW, Taylor AA, Hertle RW, Duhaime A-C. Retinal hemorrhages caused by accidental household trauma. *Journal of Pediatrics*. 1999;135(1):125–7.

31. Thiblin I, Andersson J, Wester K, Högberg G, Högberg U. Retinal haemorrhage in infants investigated for suspected maltreatment is strongly correlated with intracranial pathology. *Acta Paediatrica*. 2021:apa.16139.

32. Minns RA, Jones PA, Tandon A et al. Raised intracranial pressure and retinal haemorrhages in childhood encephalopathies. *Developmental Medicine and Child Neurology*. 2017;59(6):597–604.

33. Emerson MV, Jakobs E. Ocular autopsy and histopathologic features of child abuse. *Ophthalmology*. 2007;114:1384–94.

34. Teow Kheng Leong K, Abu Kassim SNA, Sidhu JK et al. Neonatal eye screening for 203 healthy term new-borns using a wide-field digital retinal imaging system. *BMC Ophthalmology*. 2021;21(1):1–10.

35. Caffey J. On the theory and practice of shaking infants: Its potential residual effects of permanent brain damage and mental retardation. *American Journal of Diseases of Children*. 1972;124(2):161.

36. Binenbaum G, Reid JE, Rogers DL et al. Patterns of retinal hemorrhage associated with pediatric cerebral sinovenous thrombosis. *Journal of American Association for Pediatric Ophthalmology and Strabismus*. 2017;21(1):23–7.

37. Mattheij M, Venstermans C, de Veuster I et al. Retinal haemorrhages in a university hospital: Not always abusive head injury. *Acta Neurologica Belgica*. 2017;117 (2):515–22.

38. Mulvihill AO, Jones P, Tandon A, Fleck BW, Minns RA. An inter-observer and intra-observer study of a classification of RetCam images of retinal haemorrhages in children. *British Journal of Ophthalmology*. 2011;95(1):99–104.

39. Recognizing retinal hemorrhage patterns aids in diagnosing abuse [Internet]. https://bit.ly/3Uuts0C.

40. Shaken baby syndrome: Rotational cranial injuries. Technical report. *Pediatrics*. 2001;108(1):206–10.

41. Fuchs S, Barthel MJ, Flannery AM, Christoffel KK. Cervical spine fractures sustained by young children in forward-facing car seats. *Pediatrics*. 1989;84(2):348–54.

42. Winter SCA, Quaghebeur G, Richards PG. Unusual cervical spine injury in a 1 year old. *Injury*. 2003;34(4):316–19.

43. Johnston RA. Paediatric spinal injuries. *Injury*. 2004;35(2):105–6.

44. Brennan LK, Rubin D, Christian CW et al. Neck injuries in young pediatric homicide victims: Clinical article. *Journal of Neurosurgery: Pediatrics*. 2009;3(3):232–9.

45. Molina DK, Clarkson A, Farley KL, Farley NJ. A review of blunt force injury homicides of children aged 0 to 5 years in Bexar County, Texas, from 1988 to 2009. *American Journal of Forensic Medicine and Pathology*. 2012;33(4):344–8.

46. Koumellis P, McConachie NS, Jaspan T. Spinal subdural haematomas in children with non-accidental head injury. *Archives of Disease in Childhood*. 2009;94 (3):216–19.

47. Choudhary AK, Ishak R, Zacharia TT, Dias MS. Imaging of spinal injury in abusive head trauma: A retrospective study. *Pediatric Radiology*. 2014;44 (9):1130–40.

48. Choudhary AK, Bradford RK, Dias MS, Moore GJ, Boal DKB. Spinal subdural hemorrhage in abusive head trauma: A retrospective study. *Radiology*. 2012;262 (1):216–23.

49. Rabbitt AL, Kelly TG, Yan K et al. Characteristics associated with spine injury on magnetic resonance imaging in children evaluated for abusive head trauma. *Pediatric Radiology*. 2020;50(1):83–97.

50. Baerg J, Thirumoorthi A, Vannix R et al. Cervical spine imaging for young children with inflicted trauma: Expanding the injury pattern. *Journal of Pediatric Surgery*. 2017;52(5):816–21.

51. Kadom N, Khademian Z, Vezina G et al. Usefulness of MRI detection of cervical spine and brain injuries in the evaluation of abusive head trauma. *Pediatric Radiology*. 2014;44(7):839–48.

52. Geddes JF. Neuropathology of inflicted head injury in children: II. Microscopic brain injury in infants. *Brain*. 2001;124 (7):1299–1306.

53. Mortazavi MM, Shane Tubbs R, Riech S et al. Anatomy and pathology of the cranial emissary veins: A review with surgical

implications. *Neurosurgery*. 2012;70 (5):1312–19.

54. Ruiz DSM, Gailloud P. The craniocervical venous system in relation to cerebral venous drainage. *American Journal of Neuroradiology*. 2002;23:1500–8.
55. Choudhary A, Dias M. Intracranial venous drainage through spinal veins. *Delaware Medical Journal*. 2014;86(6):181–4.
56. Leestma JE. Forensic aspects of intracranial equilibria. In *Forensic neuropathology*. 2nd ed. JE Leestma, ed. CRC Press, 2009, pp. 386–92.
57. Hadley MN, Sonntag VKH, Rekate HL, Murphy A. The infant whiplash–shake injury syndrome: A clinical and pathological study. *Neurosurgery*. 1989;24 (4):536–40.
58. Rutty GN, Squier WMV, Padfield CJH. Epidural haemorrhage of the cervical spinal cord: A post-mortem artefact? *Neuropathology and Applied Neurobiology*. 2005;31(3):247–57.
59. Kemp AM, Joshi AH, Mann M et al. What are the clinical and radiological characteristics of spinal injuries from physical abuse? A systematic review. *Archives of Disease in Childhood*. 2010;95(5):355–60.
60. Feldman KW, Weinberger E, Milstein JM, Fligner CL. Cervical spine MRI in abused infants. *Child Abuse and Neglect*. 1997;21 (2):199–205.
61. Matshes EW, Evans RM, Pinckard JK. Shaken infants die of neck trauma, not of brain trauma. *Academic Forensic Pathology*. 2011;1(2):82–91.
62. Squier W, Scheimberg I, Smith C. Spinal nerve root β-APP staining in infants is not a reliable indicator of trauma. *Forensic Science International*. 2011;212(1–3): e31–5.
63. Duhaime A-C, Christian CW, Rorke LB, Zimmerman RA. Nonaccidental head injury in infants: The 'shaken-baby syndrome'. *New England Journal of Medicine*. 1998;338(25):1822–9.
64. Adams JH, Graham DI, Murray LS, Scott G. Diffuse axonal injury due to nonmissile head injury in humans: An analysis of 45 cases. *Annals of Neurology*. 1982;12(6):557–63.
65. Case ME, Graham MA, Handy TC, Jentzen JM, Monteleone JA. Position paper on fatal abusive head injuries in infants and young children. *American Journal of Forensic Medicine and Pathology*. 2001;22 (2):112–22.
66. Geddes JF. Neuropathology of inflicted head injury in children: I. Patterns of brain damage. *Brain*. 2001;124(7):1290–8.
67. Oehmichen M, Schleiss D, Pedal I et al. Shaken baby syndrome: Re-examination of diffuse axonal injury as cause of death. *Acta Neuropathology*. 2008;116(3):317–29.
68. Mestre H, Du T, Sweeney AM et al. Cerebrospinal fluid influx drives acute ischemic tissue swelling. *Science*. 2020;367 (6483):eaax7171.
69. Matshes E. Abstract: Retinal and optic nerve sheath hemorrhages are not pathognomonic of abusive head injury. *Annual Conference of American Academy of Forensic Sciences*. 2010.
70. Geddes JF, Tasker RC, Hackshaw AK et al. Dural haemorrhage in non-traumatic infant deaths: Does it explain the bleeding in 'shaken baby syndrome'? Intradural haemorrhage in infants. *Neuropathology and Applied Neurobiology*. 2003;29 (1):14–22.
71. Goodrich JT. Reprint of 'Concerning surgical intervention for the intracranial hemorrhages of the new-born' by Harvey Cushing, M.D. *Child's Nervous System*. 2000;16(8):484–92.
72. Gage J, Gross J, McFarlane J. R v Harris. London: SUPREME COURT OF JUDICATURE COURT OF APPEAL (CRIMINAL DIVISION); 2005. Report No.: [2005] EWCA Crim 1980.
73. Squier W, Austin T, Anslow P, Weller RO. Infant subcortical cystic leucomalacia: A distinct pathological entity resulting from impaired fluid handling. *Early Human Development*. 2011;87(6):421–6.
74. Canedo-Antelo M, Baleato-González S, Mosqueira AJ et al. Radiologic clues to

cerebral venous thrombosis. *RadioGraphics*. 2019;39(6):1611–28.

75. Larsen KB, Barber Z, Squier W. The pathology and aetiology of subcortical clefts in infants. *Forensic Science International*. 2019;296:115–22.

76. Ichord RN, Benedict SL, Chan AK, Kirkham FJ, Nowak-Göttl U. Paediatric cerebral sinovenous thrombosis: Findings of the International Paediatric Stroke Study. *Archives of Disease in Childhood*. 2015;100(2):174–9.

77. Fineschi V, Turillazzi E, Neri M, Pomara C, Riezzo I. Histological age determination of venous thrombosis: A neglected forensic task in fatal pulmonary thrombo-embolism. *Forensic Science International*. 2009;186(1–3):22–8.

78. Wu YW, Hamrick SEG, Miller SP et al. Intraventricular hemorrhage in term neonates caused by sinovenous thrombosis. *Annals of Neurology*. 2003;54(1):123–6.

79. Adamsbaum C, Laurent-Vannier A. Shaken baby syndrome or non-accidental head injury caused by shaking. Update of the guidelines issued by the 2011 hearing commission. Haute Autorité de santé (HAS) and Société française de médecine physique et de réadaptation (SOFMER); 2017.

80. Zahl SM, Mack JA, Rossant C, Squier W, Wester K. Thrombosis is not a marker of bridging vein rupture in infants with alleged abusive head trauma. *Acta Paediatrica*. 2021;110(10):2686–94.

81. Adamsbaum C, Rambaud C. Abusive head trauma: Don't overlook bridging vein thrombosis. *Pediatric Radiology*. 2012;42 (11):1298–1300.

82. Vance BM. Ruptures of surface blood vessels on cerebral hemispheres as a cause of subdural hemorrhage. *Archives of Surgery*. 1950;61:992–1006.

83. Rambaud C. Bridging veins and autopsy findings in abusive head trauma. *Pediatric Radiology*. 2015;45(8):1126–31.

84. Di Maio VJM, Molina K. *DiMaio's forensic pathology*. 3rd ed. CRC Press, 2022. (Practical aspects of criminal and forensic investigations).

85. Arnautović KI, Al-Mefty O, Pait TG, Krisht AF, Husain MM. The suboccipital cavernous sinus. *Journal of Neurosurgery*. 1997;86(2):252–62.

86. Mack J, Squier W, Eastman JT. Anatomy and development of the meninges: Implications for subdural collections and CSF circulation. *Pediatric Radiology*. 2009;39(3):200–10.

87. Dmytriw AA, Song JSA, Yu E, Poon CS. Cerebral venous thrombosis: State of the art diagnosis and management. *Neuroradiology*. 2018;60(7):669–85.

Chapter 4

The Importance of the Correlation between Radiology and Pathology in Shaken Baby Syndrome

Julie Mack and Waney Squier

4.1 Basics of Imaging: What Are Density and Signal Intensity?

Imaging studies of the brain can be broadly divided into two main categories: images made by x-ray (computed tomography (CT)) and magnetic resonance imaging (MRI). The time it takes for images to be produced by CT is much shorter than the time it takes for MRI and CT can often be acquired without sedation of the infant. In addition, CT is much more readily available in the emergency room setting. Therefore, CT is often the first imaging tool used in the evaluation of children who present with neurologic dysfunction.

4.1.1 Computed Tomography Imaging

A CT is a specialised form of x-ray and all of the information gained on CT is based on the relative *density* of the structures imaged. The density of a tissue can be characterised using Hounsfield units (HU). Water is arbitrarily assigned a value of zero HU. Tissues denser than water will have positive values and tissues less dense than water (e.g., fat) will have negative values. The skull bone is much denser than the brain and will be 'white' compared to the brain. The cerebral spinal fluid (CSF), the least dense of the structures imaged around the brain, will look 'black' compared to the brain.

The brain is very vascular, particularly in young children, in whom up to 60% of the cardiac output flows to the growing brain (i.e., between 250 ml and 1,300 ml per minute between the ages of 6 months and 2 years) [1]. Blood inside the vessels cannot be seen as a discrete finding on a CT scan because flowing blood in vessels has a similar relative density to the brain. However, when blood clots, the density of the coagulated protein rises and it is depicted on imaging as white or hyperdense compared to the brain (Figure 4.1). While radiologic imaging can adequately depict the location of the blood, it cannot determine which of the surface vessels leaked the blood nor what provoked the bleeding.

4.1.2 Magnetic Resonance Imaging

Magnetic resonance imaging (MRI) utilises a strong magnetic field, magnetic gradients, and radio waves to generate images of the brain. The resulting images are described in terms of signal *intensity* rather than density. Blood outside of vessels has a unique signal intensity signature depending on the type of imaging sequence employed. Each MRI sequence utilises different radiofrequency pulses and gradients and the combination will produce a particular appearance of the brain and surrounding tissues. For instance, a T2 sequence will produce images where the CSF is high signal or hyperintense (white), whereas a T1 sequence will produce images where the CSF is low signal or hypointense (dark). While a complete review of the physics of MRI and the different sequences employed are outside the scope of this

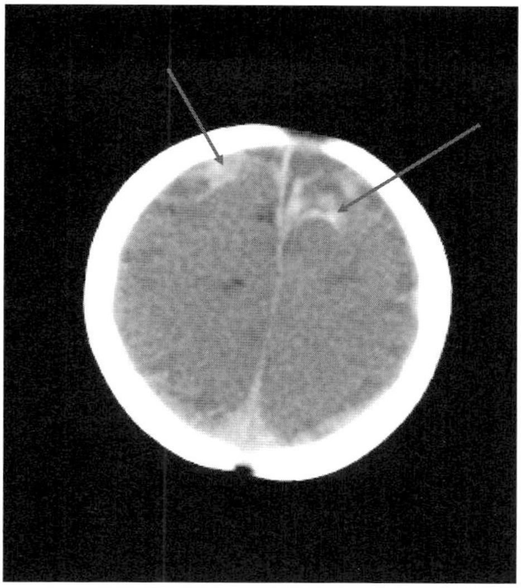

Figure 4.1 Subarachnoid haemorrhage
Image showing clotted blood (arrows) as hyper-dense material inter-digitating into the sulci of the brain, following the contour of the brain surface, confirming the location as within the subarachnoid compartment

chapter, the basic principles of imaging still apply. MRI is capable of imaging alterations of the anatomy with sometimes exquisite detail.

4.1.3 Interpretation of Imaging

When bleeding is identified on imaging, the clinical history plays a role in the analysis of the significance, timing, and potential aetiology of the finding. It is speculative for a radiologist to assert that the findings are due to trauma without corroborating evidence. Imaging findings can give rise to a differential diagnosis (a list of possible causes of the findings) but cannot determine a specific aetiology (e.g., 'shaking' or 'abuse'). The radiographic report should include a range of possible causes for blood or fluid around the brain (e.g., trauma, benign external hydrocephalus (BEH) (see Chapters 5 and 6), infection, vascular malformation, coagulopathy, thrombosis of cortical vessels).

Radiologists need to be careful not to adopt an unverified history when they interpret a study. If the history provided is 'suspected trauma' or 'rule out trauma', the radiologist should not rely on that history or assume there is some clinical or historical evidence of trauma, but should make direct communication with the clinical team, particularly if there is no specific evidence of trauma on the scans. When there is no history of trauma and no clinical evidence of trauma, haemorrhage identified on scans cannot be assumed to be traumatic. One of the worst speculative conclusions is that, if the caretakers do not provide history of a significant trauma and there is bleeding around the brain, then the caretakers are hiding something – because the physicians erroneously are convinced that an unexplained subdural collection can only be caused by trauma. This expectation that a parent or caretaker should be able to explain the neuroimaging does not exist outside the narrow field of child abuse.

When there is bleeding on imaging and the child dies, review of the imaging and correlation with the pathologic findings is a must. What, if any, evidence of trauma is present at pathology? Is the clinical history correct or is it based on the assumption of trauma? How much blood is present on scan? Does pathology confirm the location of the blood, within or outside the dura or within the subarachnoid space? Did the bleeding increase after the scan due to a developing coagulopathy? Can the vessels that were bleeding be identified at pathology? Can the blood be aged? Is it acute/fresh or chronic? Is there parenchymal damage and how has it evolved between imaging and autopsy? All these questions require careful evaluation and review by the pathologist. The radiology in this instance is a guide to the pathologic review. When the imaging shows abnormality in a particular location, that location needs to be carefully evaluated at autopsy with gross pictures and microscopic sections. Any radiological conclusions as to aetiology of the bleeding should be scrutinised for pathologic supportive evidence rather than accepted as a factual finding by the pathologist.

4.2 Subdural Haemorrhage

Unexplained subdural haemorrhage (SDH) found on head imaging represents one of the most common reasons a case is referred to a child abuse team. Bleeding in or around the brain can certainly be due to trauma but trauma should not be the 'default' diagnosis if no other reason is obvious. A detailed investigation of less common causes of subdural bleeding should be undertaken – for example, genetic diseases, inherited or acquired coagulopathies, or infections. If one of these conditions is not found, it is inappropriate to assume a diagnosis of trauma particularly if there is no ancillary evidence of trauma. There are multiple potential sources for bleeding into the subdural compartment and not all require trauma. To understand the significance of SDH, it is essential to understand the anatomy of the membranes (meninges) that surround the brain (see Chapter 3).

Normally, the dura is contiguous with the arachnoid, connected by a tissue layer, the dural border layer, with no subdural space between them. Therefore, SDH must originate within the dura. If the volume of intradural blood or fluid is sufficient, the dural border cell layer will be cleaved and a subdural collection created.

Although it was long believed that bridging vein rupture was the primary cause of dural/subdural haemorrhages, the bridging veins are not the only potential source of dural bleeding. In small-volume haemorrhages, other vessels within the dura are a much more likely source. The small and fragile intrinsic capillaries and venules of the dura are a known source of dural and subdural haemorrhage. These vessels are more numerous in young babies than adults and are most pronounced in the falx, tentorium, parasagittal, and occipital dura, the most common locations of subdural bleeding in infants [2].

The classic explanation of SDH in the context of abuse is that the macroscopic bridging veins extending from the cortex of the brain to the parasagittal dura are ruptured during the act of shaking. Because the bridging veins are relatively large, force is required to rupture them. If SDH exclusively arose from ruptured bridging veins, then trauma may be a reasonable conclusion. However, because they are not the only potential source of haemorrhage into the subdural compartment, it is unsafe to conclude that the presence of SDH indicates that bridging veins are ruptured and therefore significant trauma occurred.

Alternative sources of fluid or haemorrhage include the capillaries that invest the native dura, abnormal capillaries that invest a healing neomembrane, and abnormal vascular structures such as malformations or aneurysms. Sources of bleeding other than large bridging veins are much more likely to be the origin of blood when the volume of bleeding is small, contained, or surrounded by fluid (Figure 4.2).

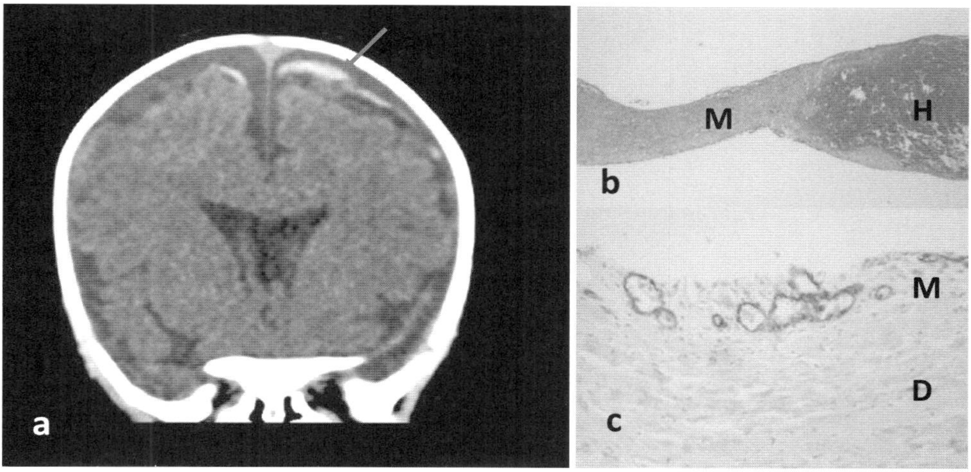

Figure 4.2 Bleeding from a subdural membrane
a CT scan showing bleeding from a neomembrane (arrow) which was confirmed at pathology. The amount of haemorrhage is too small to have originated from bridging vein ruptures. Moreover, the blood is contained and not mixing with the surrounding fluid as would be expected if it represented free bleeding of a ruptured vessel into the subdural compartment.
b Haemorrhage (H, bright pink) from a thin subdural neomembrane (M, pale pink) which has separated from the dura during tissue processing
c An extensive thin membrane (M) adherent to the dura (D). CD 31 stain demonstrates multiple new blood vessels in the membrane as rounded brown profiles. a, b, and c are not the same case. (For the colour version, please refer to the plate section.)

Any disease which may affect the integrity of the vessels within the dura (bleeding diatheses, collagen vascular diseases, etc.) must be considered as potential contributors to an abnormal collection of dural-based blood. In addition, subdural fluid can arise in the context of a previously disrupted subdural compartment (chronic collection), but it can also arise in the context of an acute but non-traumatic event.

4.2.1 Imaging of Subdural Haematoma

Acute SDH on CT is typically identified by high density or white outside the brain that follows the contour of the dura. Acute blood cannot be precisely timed, but when it is hyperdense or white on CT, it is generally considered less than 7–10 days of age.

The dura lines the skull and dural folds dip between the cerebral hemispheres (falx) and between the cerebrum and the cerebellum (tentorium). Therefore, any increased density in these regions is suspect for dural-based haemorrhage. The volume of haemorrhage imaged is important. Larger-volume haemorrhage more often arises from larger-calibre vessels, where small amounts of haemorrhage are more likely the result of bleeding from smaller vessels. Figure 4.3 shows an example of a confirmed single bridging vein rupture in an infant.

Bleeding from smaller vessels rarely produces large volumes of blood, particularly over a short period of time. Bleeding from small vessels in the native dura may be limited to small areas of high density that closely follow the contour of the dura. It may be difficult to differentiate blood within the dura (intradural bleeding) from blood accumulating within and disrupting the border layer between the dura and the arachnoid (subdural) (Figures 4.4, 4.5).

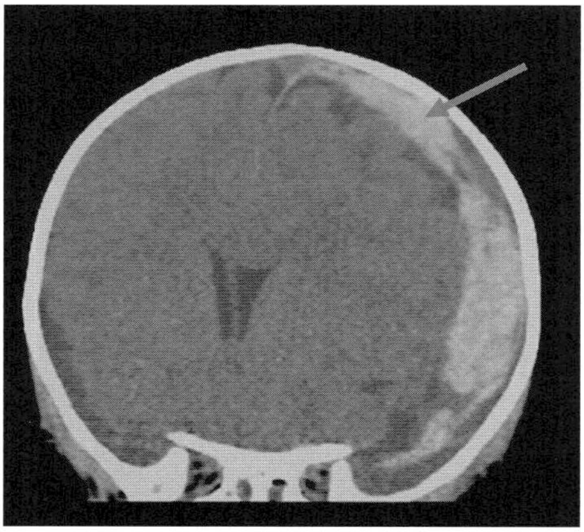

Figure 4.3 Coronal CT of a 7-month-old with confirmed rupture of a single frontal bridging vein. The volume of haemorrhage is large. Acute blood and a ruptured bridging vein were found at surgery.

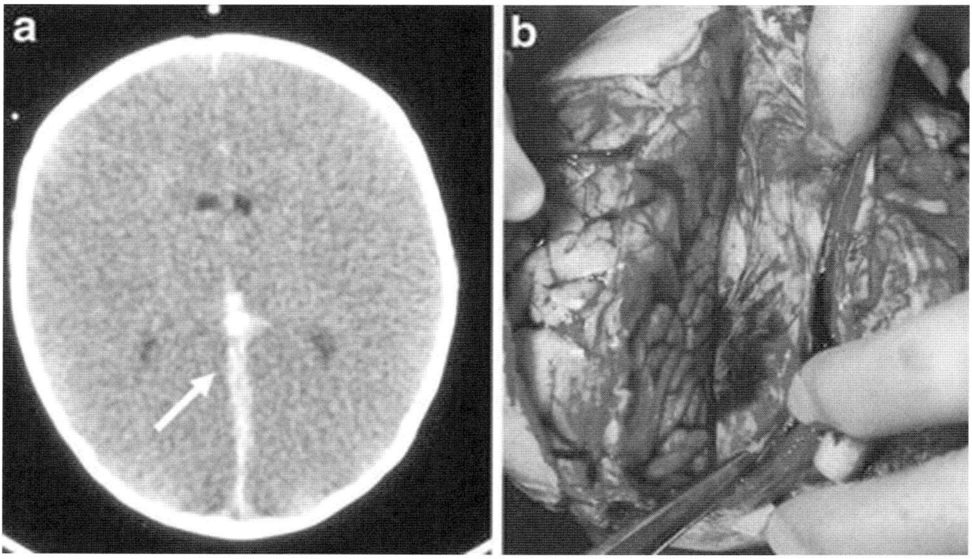

Figure 4.4 Infant 4 months. Sudden death, no trauma.
a CT scan showing thickened, dense falx (arrow) which was reported as SDH
b Autopsy showed the blood to be entirely intradural. There is no SDH (reproduced with permission from Squier W. The "Shaken Baby" syndrome: pathology and mechanisms. Acta Neuropathol (Berl). 2011 Nov;122 (5):519–42.) (For the colour version, please refer to the plate section.)

4.2.2 Subdural Fluid Collections (Chronic Subdural Haemorrhage/ Hygromas/Effusions)

Subdural fluid on CT imaging is a collection that is typically higher in density than CSF, but lower in density than acute blood. The density is due to its proteinaceous or blood-tinged nature. Fluid seen in the subdural compartment may be incorrectly assumed to be evidence of a 'chronic' SDH. While fluid collections can be the result of chronic collection of blood,

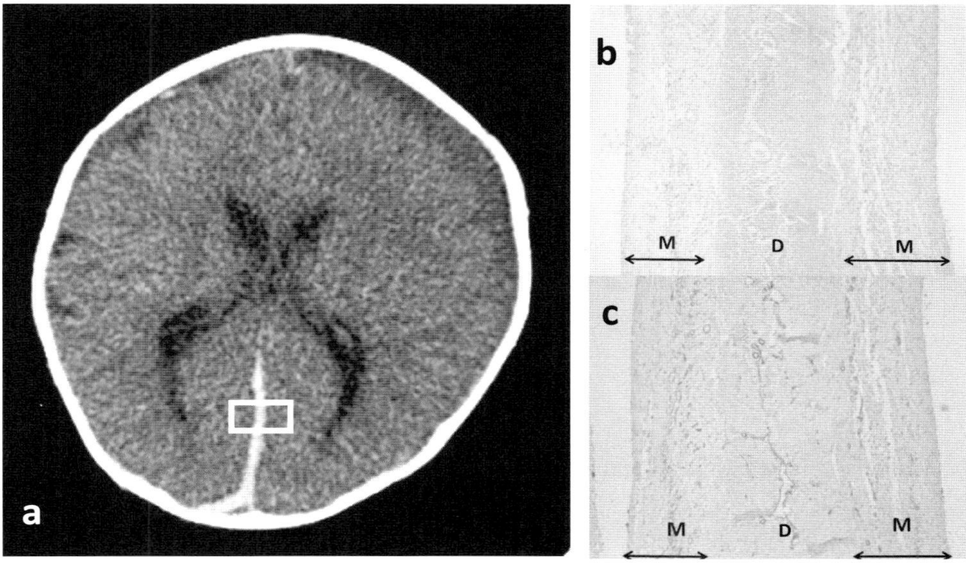

Figure 4.5 Chronic, healing membrane
a CT shows small-volume, hyper-dense (acute) blood following the contour of the falx. The white box represents the area shown in b and c.
b Same case. Sections from the falx showing subdural membrane (M) on each side of the dura (D), more than doubling its thickness (H&E). These could not be distinguished on the scan.
c CD31 stains the newly formed capillary blood vessels brown. (For the colour version, please refer to the plate section.)

proteinaceous subdural fluid may accumulate acutely or slowly over time without antecedent trauma. It is erroneous to presume that an accumulation of proteinaceous or blood-tinged subdural fluid (subdural hygroma) indicates that bridging veins have been ruptured. Ruptured veins would result in significant blood accumulation, not blood-tinged fluid. Proteinaceous subdural fluid is not the result of acute bridging vein rupture and can accumulate without trauma.

When the fluid is similar in density to CSF, it may be difficult to differentiate between excess fluid in the subarachnoid space or subdural fluid on CT imaging. MRI provides a greater degree of tissue contrast and is therefore more sensitive in the depiction of subdural collections.

Fluid collections of more than one density (mixed density) were traditionally thought to reflect a mix of acute and older blood. However, fresh blood may appear to be mixed with fluid when red cells sediment, or when it is mixed with fresh effusions. A chronic process may be confirmed by the presence of membranes or septations. However, when there is no clear radiologic evidence of a neomembrane, the timing and origin of proteinaceous or blood-tinged fluid cannot be determined on imaging.

Subdural effusions are defined as an accumulation of fluid in the subdural compartment (Figure 4.6). They may arise as a delayed finding, days or weeks after minor trauma (post-traumatic or acute-traumatic dural effusions) [3], in association with meningitis [4] or

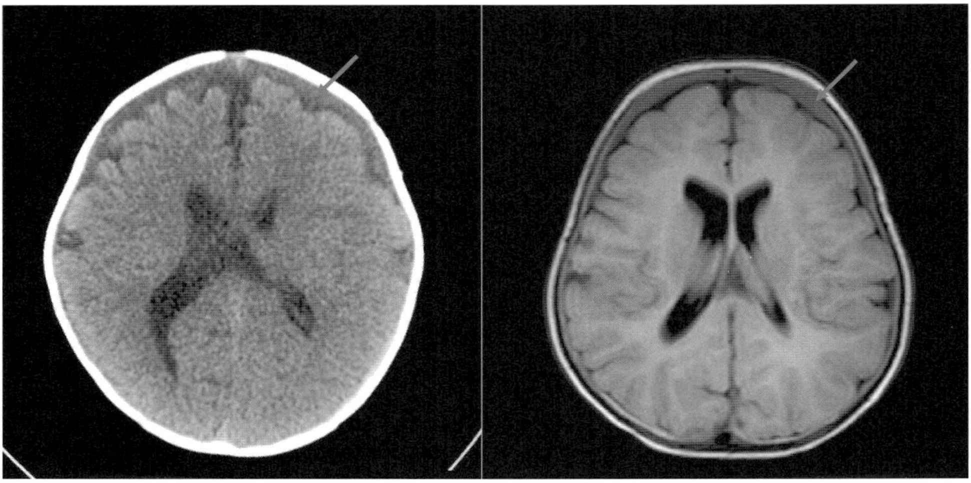

Figure 4.6 Subdural effusion
a CT scan shows fluid in the subdural compartment of slightly higher density than CSF in the ventricles.
b MRI FLAIR sequence of the same case shows proteinaceous fluid in the subdural compartment. The blood-sensitive sequences showed no significant haemorrhage in this collection. The infant was diagnosed with benign subdural collections of infancy (benign external hydrocephalus (BEH)) occurring in the context of an enlarging head circumference.

cerebral venous thrombosis [5]. Subdural fluid collections can arise spontaneously or in association with minor trauma, for instance in the condition known as benign external hydrocephalus (BEH) [6, 7] (see Chapters 5, 6). There may be no clear imaging distinction between subdural effusions and chronic subdural haemorrhagic collections; subdural effusions may be yellow in colour when aspirated (xanthochromic) or haemorrhagic and may evolve into frank subdural hematomas [8, 9].

The source of fluid in effusions is unclear. The meninges communicate with the perivascular space as part of the glymphatic system of the brain [10], which includes transdural efflux pathways. Disruption of the dural-glymphatic pathway may lead to effusions or they may arise by plasma leaking directly from intrinsic dural capillaries and venules, an etiologic mechanism suggested in the development of sterile subdural effusions in association with inflammation and meningitis [11].

4.2.3 The Arachnoid Tear Hypothesis

Some authors suggest that the trauma of shaking tears the arachnoid membrane, allowing transfer of CSF from the subarachnoid space into the dural compartment [12], producing mixed-density fluid collections. These are then interpreted, not as ageing blood, but as 'acute traumatic effusions' occurring immediately before collapse, and used to implicate the person who was last caring for the infant.

This mechanism is untenable for several reasons. Firstly, the arachnoid membrane is a physiologic barrier necessary for normal function of the brain, extremely strong, and unlikely to be torn unless there is a penetrating injury. Secondly, if the arachnoid barrier membrane were damaged, blood accumulating in the dura from bleeding vessels would be expected to flow with the pressure gradient into the large subarachnoid space, rather than

CSF flowing against a pressure gradient into a tissue compartment already congested by extravasated blood.

Support for the arachnoid tear hypothesis has been drawn from a study by Zouros et al. [13], who found that radioisotope injected into the lumbar CSF appeared in drained subdural fluid. There are several problems with this study. Firstly, all the patients studied had undergone percutaneous subdural drain placement, which may have caused iatrogenic injury to the arachnoid membrane. More importantly, the tracer they used is normally transported across the arachnoid barrier layer into the dura so its accumulation within dural collections would be expected as part of normal physiological clearance properties. The suggestion that subdural fluid represents a 'tear' in the arachnoid barrier membrane is not supported by pathology or by surgical examination [14].

4.2.4 'Dating' of Subdural Collections

Head imaging can depict changes in the appearance of blood products as they age. When blood leaves a blood vessel it clots relatively quickly and becomes hyperdense on CT imaging. The blood clot breaks down, becoming thinner and more liquid until it is eventually removed by the lymphatic system and the scavengers of the immune system. The progress of these changes depends on the location, the amount of blood, the presence and amount of any associated fluid, and whether the bleeding is continuing (e.g., in the setting of a coagulopathy). Therefore, the timing of haemorrhage by imaging cannot be precise and is always reported in a range. On CT, the age range for hyperdense blood extends from about 1 hour of age up to 7–10 days in age. MRI, which can depict changes in signal intensity associated with alterations of the haemoglobin molecule, can provide additional information and may serve to slightly narrow the potential age range of the bleeding. However, there is a wide range of overlap and neither CT nor MRI can precisely date the age of the haematoma [15–17]. Subdural fluid, including subdural effusions, cannot be dated on either CT or MRI.

4.3 Brain Swelling

Brain swelling (oedema) is a non-specific response to a range of brain insults, including trauma. The secondary cascades of trauma, including loss of the normal function of the blood–brain barrier, often produce brain swelling, but they are not unique to trauma. Swelling can occur slowly or be rapid in evolution.

On imaging studies, oedema can be broadly divided into two components: cellular (cytotoxic) oedema and extracellular (vasogenic, interstitial) oedema. Cellular oedema, the early response to an insult, involves a shift of fluid from the extracellular to the intracellular compartment with no overall increase of volume of the brain. Extracellular oedema depends on additional fluid drawn in from blood vessels and results in an increase in volume of the brain which can be identified on imaging and increased weight of the brain identified at pathology.

4.3.1 Imaging of Brain Swelling

4.3.1.a Computed Tomography and Oedema

Only oedema that changes the density of the brain is visible on CT. Because water is of lower density than brain tissue, oedema decreases the density of the involved part of the brain. Severe generalised swelling displaces CSF, resulting in reduction or compression of the normal fluid-containing spaces of the brain: the subarachnoid space and the ventricles. Severe swelling also compresses blood vessels, reducing the supply of oxygenated blood and exacerbating tissue hypoxia.

4.3.1.b Magnetic Resonance Imaging and Oedema

MRI is a sensitive tool for imaging cytotoxic oedema. The MRI sequence 'diffusion weighted imaging' (DWI) relies on the normal motion of water molecules (diffusion) within tissue. The degree of tissue cellularity determines the relative impedance (or restriction) of water molecule diffusion between cells. The impedance in specific brain areas can be quantitatively assessed by the apparent diffusion coefficient (ADC).

When cells swell, the motion of extracellular fluid is altered, causing restricted diffusion focally or more diffusely. This is not unique to trauma and can occur in any process that results in cellular swelling. Neither cytotoxic nor extracellular oedema can be dated by imaging.

4.4 Venous Thrombosis

Cortical vein thrombosis with or without sinus thrombosis (collectively cerebral venous thrombosis (CVT)) is increasingly recognised as a cause of stroke and mortality in young babies. Correct diagnosis may be lifesaving because, if thrombosis is not identified or is mistakenly assumed to be the result of trauma, infants will be inadequately treated for a potentially reversible condition.

The majority of infants with CVT present with seizures, focal neurological signs, or decreased level of consciousness [18]. Others have non-specific presentations including lethargy, poor feeding, drowsiness, and vomiting. In many cases there is a predisposing condition such as infection, anaemia, dehydration, thrombophilia, and hypoxic-ischaemic injury. Almost half of infants and children with CVT have middle ear infection which may be missed if not specifically sought on scans and is readily missed at autopsy as the bony sinuses and middle ears are rarely examined. In a small proportion (4%) of cases venous thrombosis follows trauma [18].

4.4.1 Imaging of Venous Thrombosis

4.4.1.a Vessels

Timely neuroimaging is critical to diagnosis. Thrombi causing clinical effects may lyse and no longer be visible if imaging is delayed. Radiologic diagnosis depends on high-quality imaging; standard CT is not sensitive for the depiction of acute or chronic CVT. MRI with contrast venogram has a better sensitivity and should be routinely acquired in cases where the cause of brain dysfunction is uncertain.

The CT findings suggestive of CVT include hyperdensity in the region of the dural sinuses or in the expected locations of cortical veins. There may be delayed enhancement of the vasculature or parenchyma in areas affected by clot. Tortuous or 'corkscrew' collateral vessels that are providing compensatory drainage pathways can be a secondary sign of CVT and should always be sought when reviewing imaging studies. CVT is commonly missed and diagnosis depends on a high index of suspicion. As venous thrombosis is a mimic of SDH [19, 20], accurate diagnosis is vital.

4.4.1.a.1 Varicose Surface Veins

When thrombus obstructs blood flow in a vein, it can become congested, tortuous, stretched, and dilated (varicose) and may form a knotty mass of vessels on the brain surface. This may mimic focal subdural or subarachnoid bleeding [19] (Figure 4.7).

4.4.1.b Parenchymal findings associated with CVT

4.4.1.b.1 Oedema/ Haemorrhage and Cysts

Obstructed or reduced venous blood flow causes localised oedema in the area drained by the involved vessels (Figure 4.8). The superficial veins drain the immediate subcortical white matter which is the watershed of the deep and superficial venous systems. Involvement of deep veins causes damage to the deep tissues of the brain and bleeding into the ventricles. Thrombosis of the superior sagittal sinus causes bilateral parasagittal hemispheric lesions [21]. However, because venous anatomy is variable with extensive collaterals, topographical correlation between the pathology and the site of thrombosis may be poor. Oedema may be transient and reversible or may progress to venous infarction with or without haemorrhage; subcortical cystic lesions can be the end result of a previous venous event (Figure 4.9).

4.4.1.b.2 Meningeal Haemorrhage

Venous obstruction is associated with red blood cell diapedesis – that is, leakage of red blood cells through the vein wall, which on the surface of the brain leads to focal sub-pial or subarachnoid bleeding. In the dura this may lead to intra- or subdural bleeding. However, subdural bleeding or subdural effusions in the setting of CVT may not be directly caused by the thrombosed vessels. Studies using contrast have shown increased dural enhancement in patients with CVT [22]. In these patients, altered flow through the dura, changes in dural vascular permeability, and fluid accumulation due to disruption of the glymphatic pathways may contribute to changes in the appearance of the dura and subdural compartment. In addition, if a chronic subdural collection is present, it may precede CVT or be just a bystander and not directly produced by CVT.

4.4.1.b.3 Sub-pial Haemorrhage

Sub-pial bleeding is an under-recognised feature of venous outflow obstruction and largely ignored in the literature. It can be identified radiologically and macroscopically as a well-defined patch of bleeding beneath the arachnoid membrane, distinguished from subarachnoid bleeding by its cleanly delimited margins, often appearing on scans as a thin crescentic collection at the edge of the crest of a gyrus. It may be associated with subcortical haemorrhage (Figures 4.10, 4.11).

4.4.1.b.4 Intraventricular Haemorrhage

Intraventricular haemorrhage (IVH) is typically seen in very premature babies due to bleeding from the immature germinal matrix. In babies after this premature stage the most common cause of IVH is thrombosis of the deep cerebral veins, seen in a third of neonates with CVT. This diagnosis should be considered in any baby with IVH.

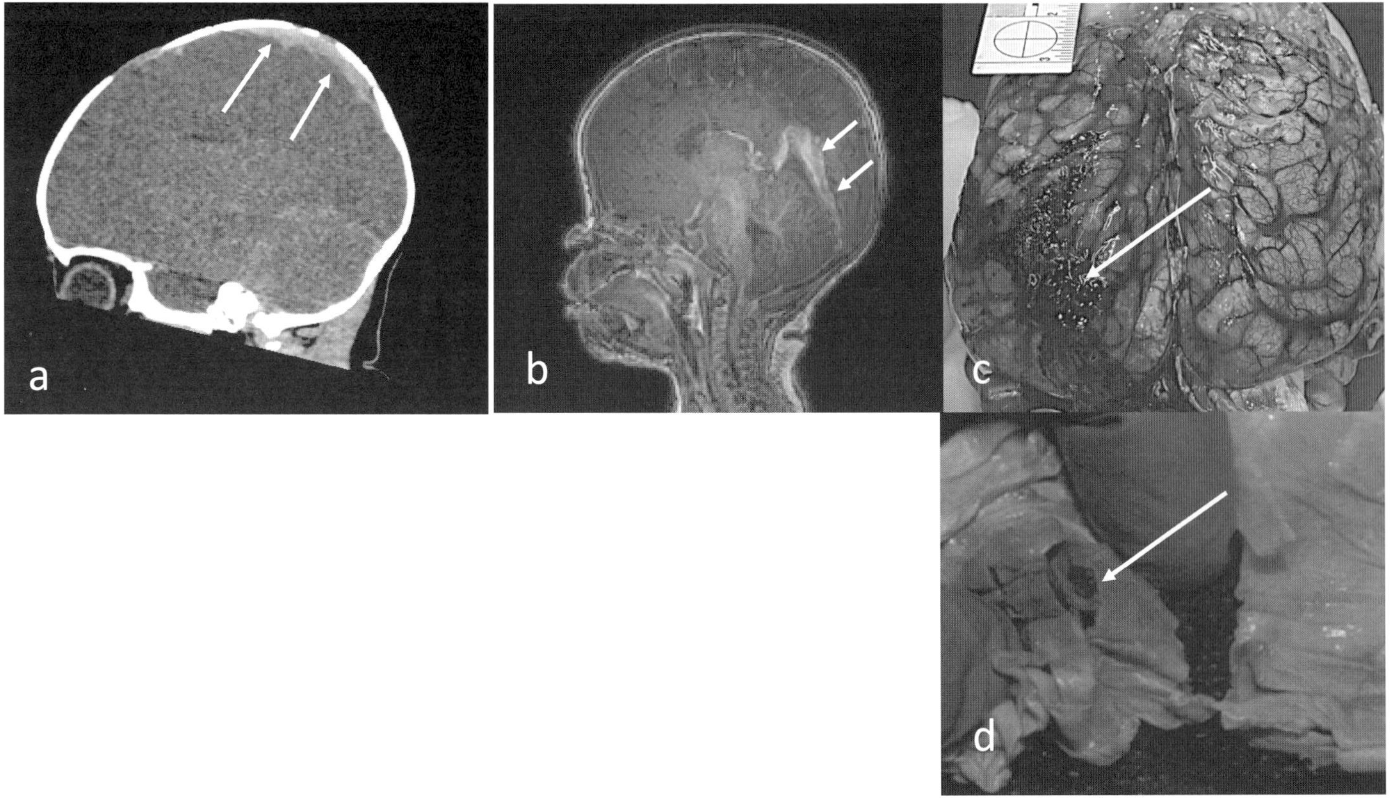

Figure 4.7 CVT in 3-month-old with several days of fever and progressive lethargy
a CT showed extra-axial parasagittal high density (arrows)
b T1-weighted MRI confirmed subacute thrombus ballooning the vein of Galen, straight sinus, and internal cerebral veins. The sagittal sinus also showed subacute thrombus, which was confirmed by pathology.
c Pathologic findings in another patient with confirmed sagittal sinus thrombosis. Dilated, tortuous, and clotted vessels on the surface of the brain were mistaken for SDH on initial CT exam.
d Fixed dura shows the solid clot (white arrow) in the superior sagittal sinus. (For the colour version, please refer to the plate section.)

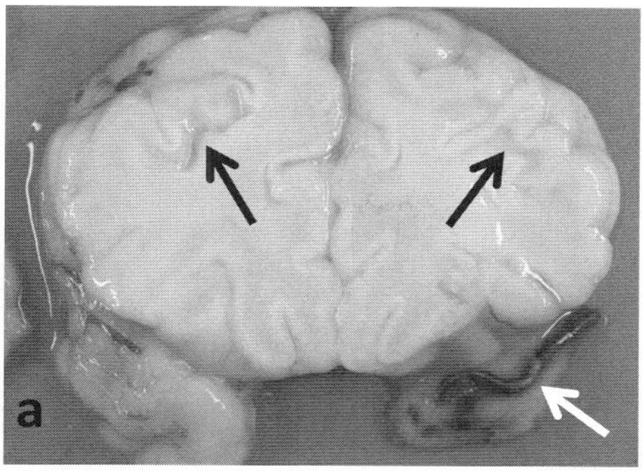

Figure 4.8 Coronal slice of fixed infant brain with thrombosed vein over the right temporal pole (white arrow). There is generalised brain swelling; the subcortical zone is oedematous. Clefts and cysts are developing in the immediate subcortical white matter (black arrows). (For the colour version, please refer to the plate section.)

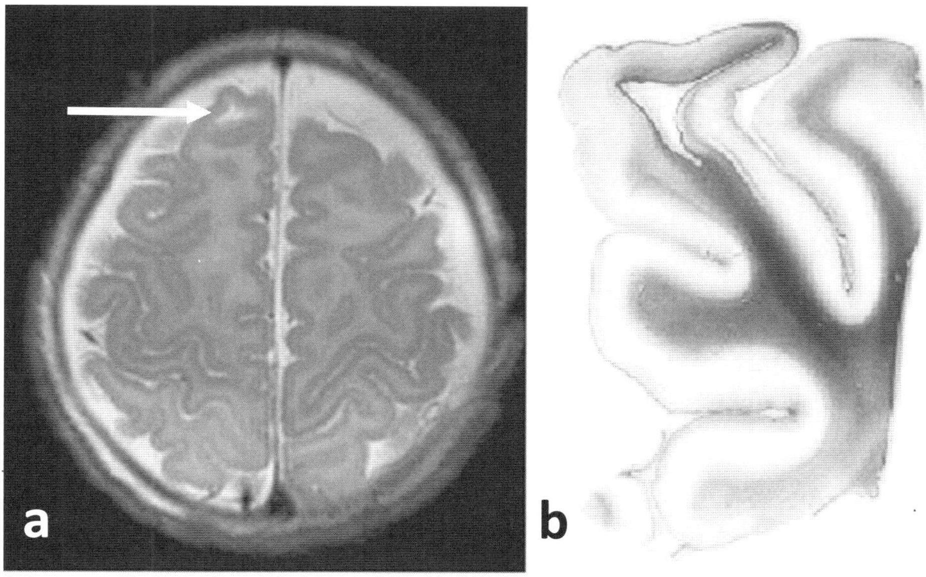

Figure 4.9 a MRI scan showing small cystic lesion beneath intact frontal cortex without evidence of associated swelling or haemorrhage
b Section of frontal lobe from a different case. A 3-month-old baby with bilateral parasagittal subcortical cysts. The section is stained for myelin proteolipid protein (PLP), which stains myelin brown. Note the thinning and aberrant myelination due to scarring of the overlying cortex, indicating the pathology is old. (For the colour version, please refer to the plate section.)

4.4.2 Association of Cerebral Venous Thrombosis with Subdural Haemorrhage

There is no doubt that extra-axial haemorrhage is seen in patients with CVT. In one study of neonates with symptomatic CVT, 46% had subarachnoid and/or subdural bleeding [23], although it should be noted that some may potentially be birth related. Anderst et al. report SDH in 9% of children up to 19 years with CVT. In children less than 2 years of age, SDH

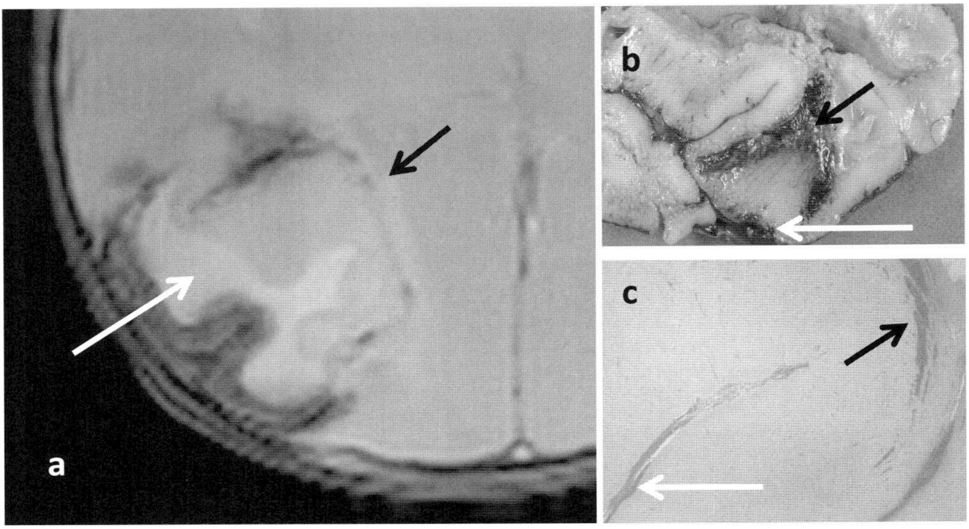

Figure 4.10 Sub-pial haemorrhage with associated subcortical haemorrhage
a MRI scan showing thick sub-pial bleed (white arrow) pushing the cortex away from the meninges. A hypointense linear bleed (black arrow) is seen beneath an apparently intact cortex.
b Fixed brain slice from baby with thrombosis of the sagittal sinus. Note thin sub-pial bleed (white arrow) and thick subcortical bleed (black arrow). The cortex is preserved.
c Section of brain from infant following a recent fall from a high bunk bed. There is a thin fresh sub-pial bleed (white arrow) and thin subcortical bleed (black arrow) following the deep cortical margin. (For the colour version, please refer to the plate section.)

was associated with CVT in 20% [24]. Roach et al. [5] and Canedo et al. [21] describe subdural effusion or hematoma in children with CVT.

Controversy has arisen over whether CVT directly causes SDH. McLean et al. studied a small group of children [25] but there are serious limitations to their study. Only 11 patients were under the age of 1 year and the study was restricted to patients who had undergone contrast enhanced imaging. The patients in their data set who were diagnosed with CVT had no SDH. However, 'SDH' was not one of the search terms used to identify patients with potential CVT. The authors therefore were searching for a correlation between two findings but did not include one of the two findings they were trying to correlate in their search terms. Patients whose imaging study was categorised with SDH as a primary diagnosis would not have been captured in their data set. There was no attempt to retrospectively evaluate those who had SDH to search for missed CVT.

Anderst et al. [24] note an association between CVT and SDH but argue it is not likely causal as those with SDH had predisposing factors for the development of SDH. The fact that SDH and CVT were associated may be because they share common mechanisms; for example, infection, dehydration, and trauma can all promote abnormal coagulation. Anderst et al. also describe a case where SDH preceded CVT [24]. Vaslow [26] suggests that the presence of chronic SDH, an inflammatory condition, is a risk factor for subsequent CVT. Thrombosis is described by pathology in chronic subdural membranes (see Chapter 3, Figure 3.8). CVT may cause alterations in the meningeal vascular flow and interruption of the glymphatic pathways, giving rise to bloody effusions. Trauma can

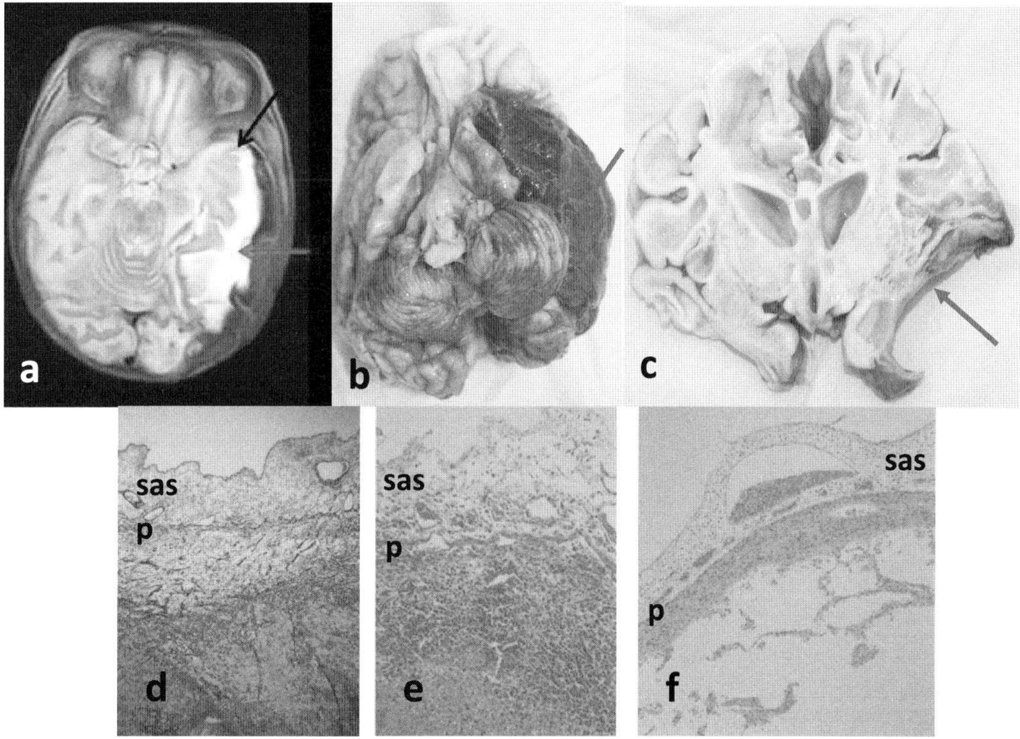

Figure 4.11 Temporal lobe CVT with sub-pial haemorrhage
a Admission brain scan showing right-sided sub-pial collection (gray arrow). The cortex is relatively preserved and the right temporal lobe is pushed towards the midline by the extensive mass effect. Black arrow indicates tip of temporal lobe.
b Baby died three weeks after admission. The image shows the under surface of the fixed brain. The temporal lobe is shrunken and the gyri are not identifiable. The meninges are rust/red in colour due to old sub-pial bleeding.
c Coronal slice through fixed brain. The white matter shows established cerebral hypoxic-ischaemic injury (HII) and is reduced to a mass of clean-walled, non-haemorrhagic, predominantly subcortical cysts. The right temporal lobe has been compressed by sub-pial haemorrhage.
d Reticulin stain for collagen fibres showing the pia (p) and extensive destruction of the superficial cortex. The subarachnoid space is thickened and cellular.
e H&E stained section at higher power showing the pia and superficial cortex, which is necrotic and contains many cells staining brown due to their content of hemosiderin from old blood.
f Cortex distant from the sub-pial bleed showing deeper cortical destruction typical of HII. There was no sub-pial bleeding here and the pial surface is smooth and relatively preserved. (For the colour version, please refer to the plate section.)

give rise to SDH and to CVT, but the trauma need not be severe and symptoms may be delayed.

4.5 Unverified Imaging 'Diagnoses'

The following section discusses a number of entities described in radiological reports of suspected abusive head trauma (AHT). Some have been shown by pathology to be incorrect; others have never been subjected to pathological verification. It is important to recognise that these radiological appearances do not correspond to established pathologies but are speculative.

4.5.1 'Clots' As a Manifestation of Bridging Vein Rupture

In recent years suggestions have been made that radiological observations of focal thrombosis of cortical and bridging veins indicate bridging vein rupture and therefore confirm violent shaking [27, 28]. There is no scientific evidence to support this [29].

Objections to the hypothesis are both physiological and radiological. The pathophysiology of vascular trauma is that loss of vascular integrity will result in immediate bleeding from the injured vessel. The clotting cascade is activated by endothelial damage. However, clotting takes time and a clot would not instantaneously stop an injured vessel from leaking blood. Therefore, if a macroscopic bridging vein were ruptured, it would be surrounded by significant blood and any clot would be obscured by the extravasated blood. This was recognised by the renowned brain surgeon Harvey Cushing in 1905: 'In two of the cases that I have examined I have satisfied myself that such ruptures were present. A positive statement, however, cannot be given even for these cases, since the dissection and exposure, difficult enough under any circumstances, owing to the delicacy of the vessels, is the more so when they are obscured by extravasated blood' [30]. To suggest that imaging can easily identify ruptured macroscopic veins hidden in surrounding haemorrhage ignores both pathophysiology and classical neurosurgical teaching.

Imaging studies promoting this theory do not show macroscopic SDH. Instead, they show small areas of clotted blood surrounded by fluid density on CT or fluid signal intensity on MRI. These tiny areas of clotted blood are described as lollipops [31] or tadpoles [32]. The only reason the clot can be visualised as a discrete entity or in association with a vessel is because it is outlined by fluid and not by extravasated blood. These findings most likely represent thrombosed veins on the background of a chronic SDH or clotted veins surrounded by a subdural effusion. Without pathologic correlation, the tissue changes causing the radiological appearance of lollipops and tadpoles remain unverified.

4.5.2 Diffuse Axonal Injury

Axonal injury results not only from trauma, but also from a range of other insults, including hypoxic ischemic injury. Diffuse axonal injury (DAI) is a pathologic diagnosis which relies on specialised microscopic methods described in Chapter 3. Imaging studies cannot characterise microscopic axonal changes and cannot report 'DAI' as a radiologic diagnosis.

Erroneous extrapolation of adult neuropathology has led to the misconception that small-tissue haemorrhages in infants indicate traumatic axonal injury [33]. In adults, after severe head trauma, parenchymal haemorrhages have been correlated with pathologic evidence of axonal injury. If severe trauma has been documented and typical petechial haemorrhagic changes are noted in the deep white matter in an adult or older child, then a diagnosis of DAI may be appropriate. However, white-matter haemorrhages in an infant cannot be taken to indicate axonal injury and are not a surrogate for DAI. A radiographic report stating that 'findings are consistent with DAI' in an infant is not reliable unless confirmed by pathology.

4.5.3 Non-haemorrhagic Contusions

Contusions are bruises and are haemorrhagic by definition. An MRI report showing focal-restricted diffusion and labelled as non-haemorrhagic contusion ignores the definition of contusion and is meaningless. The radiographic finding is of focal cytotoxic oedema, for which there are other, more common, causes. For instance, focal subcortical swelling is one of the characteristic findings in venous thrombosis [21]. When a radiographic report inappropriately characterises focal cytotoxic oedema as a contusion, trauma is often erroneously presumed. This can lead to significant medical misdiagnosis.

4.5.4 Gliding/Subcortical Contusions

Radiology reports may describe focal haemorrhage in the subcortical zone as 'gliding contusion' or subcortical contusion (Figure 4.10). While haemorrhage within white matter can be seen on radiographic studies, the theory that the cortex 'glides' over the white matter during the act of shaking and creates a cleavage plane of contusions ignores basic anatomy. The cortex contains nerve cells whose densely packed nerve fibres make up the subcortical zone of white matter and anchor the cortex in place (Figure 4.12). The hypothesis that the cortex 'glides' over the white matter is anatomically untenable.

4.5.5 Subcortical 'Tear'

This term is applied to radiological observation of fluid or cystic collections in the subcortical white matter, often referred to as traumatic tears. Review of infant pathology shows that these lesions do not have the typical pathologic signature of trauma [34] but are due to

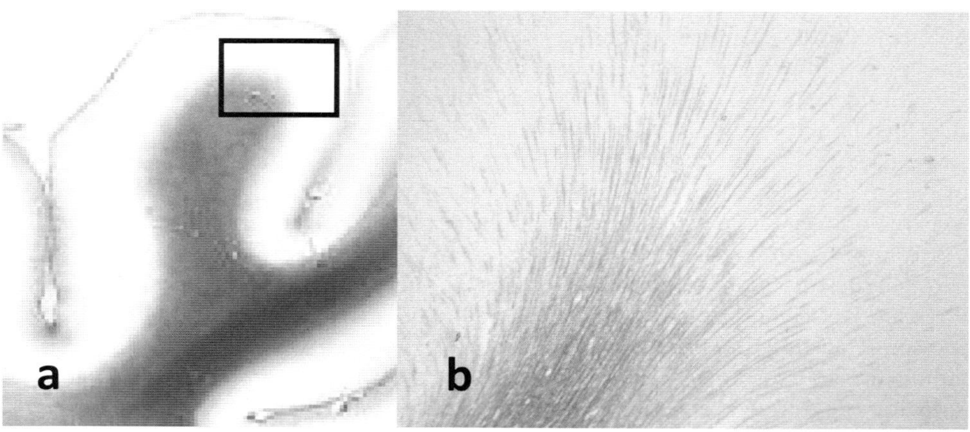

Figure 4.12 Junction of cortex and white matter. PLP myelin stain
a Low-power image showing dense myelinated fibres in the white matter contrasted with the cortex, which is almost devoid of myelin. The area in the box is represented in high power in b.
b Densely packed axons fan out from the white matter into the deep cortex, anchoring it firmly to the underlying white matter. (For the colour version, please refer to the plate section.)

accumulation of fluid following disruption of fluid drainage in this specific zone of the growing brain (Figures 4.8, 4.9).

4.5.6 Spinal Ligamentous Injuries

Spinal 'injuries' are increasingly described in infants with AHT, based on the imaging appearances of the paraspinal soft tissue. The nature of the altered paraspinal signal is unclear. Choudhary et al. [35] describe 'oedema' (based on increased STIR or T2 MRI signal) and assume that the observation is representative of traumatic oedema. However, hyper intensity surrounding (rather than within) ligaments or membranes on an MRI sequence that accentuates fluid does not confirm traumatic damage but may simply represent fluid shift or oedema. The local extensive venous plexuses may contribute to paraspinal oedema in the presence of brain swelling (see Chapter 3).

4.6 Imaging of Spinal Subdural Blood in Abusive Head Trauma

The imaging finding of blood around the spinal cord is assumed by some authors to be a sign of abusive head trauma [36, 37]. This assumption is unjustified. Infant SDH may track and redistribute from the cranial to the spinal compartment and will settle, by gravity, in the dorsal thoracolumbar area, the most dependent area in the supine infant. Choudhary et al. [35] described more than 60% of infant spinal SDH as thoracolumbar and without associated thoracolumbar ligamentous injury. All infants with spinal SDH had a coexisting posterior fossa SDH of similar MRI intensity. Koumellis et al. [37] demonstrated similar findings and, in two cases, anatomic continuity between these bleeds was identified (see Chapter 3). In conclusion, blood in the subdural compartment of the spinal cord can be a natural consequence of gravitational redistribution of intracranial SDH and cannot be regarded as an independent marker of trauma.

4.7 Conclusion

Imaging studies can demonstrate anatomic and physiologic changes in the infant brain in great detail. This chapter provides an overview of the radiologic findings that might be encountered in cases of possible abuse. However, their interpretation must be based on a solid understanding of the correlative pathology. This is standard practice in clinical medicine; no responsible clinician would make a diagnosis of cancer and manage patient care and start treatment on initial radiological evidence alone; confirmation by pathological analysis of the abnormal tissue is routine. This is not possible in the living infant, so we have prepared this chapter to demonstrate examples of radiological and pathological correlation where autopsy confirmation is available.

A physician who is interpreting imaging studies must be keenly aware that signal alteration or change in density may have multiple potential pathologic correlates, and that some imaging findings thought to have a specific meaning have never been verified pathologically. This is particularly relevant in AHT, where the 'diagnosis' cannot be verified as it is not a medical disease that can be confirmed by response to specific treatment. The lack of a feedback loop in cases of suspected abuse means that false positive cases are not identified (see Chapter 10); physicians who make the error of assuming a child has been abused due to the presence of an unexplained SDH are unable to learn from their mistakes. Worse, if findings assumed to represent abuse are repeated in the literature as 'specific' for abuse, mistakes will be propagated. It is only through careful correlation of the radiology with pathology that a complete and accurate differential diagnosis may be reached.

References

1. Wintermark M, Lepori D, Cotting J et al. Brain perfusion in children: Evolution with age assessed by quantitative perfusion computed tomography. *Pediatrics*. 2004;113(6):1642–52.
2. Scheimberg I, Cohen MC, Vazquez REZ et al. Nontraumatic intradural and subdural hemorrhage and hypoxic ischemic encephalopathy in fetuses, infants, and children up to three years of age: Analysis of two audits of 636 cases from two referral centers in the United Kingdom. *Pediatric and Developmental Pathology*. 2013;16(3):149–59.
3. Kumar R, Singhal N, Mahapatra AK. Traumatic subdural effusions in children following minor head injury. *Child's Nervous System*. 2008;24(12):1391–6.
4. Vinchon M, Joriot S, Jissendi-Tchofo P, Dhellemmes P. Postmeningitis subdural fluid collection in infants: Changing pattern and indications for surgery. *Journal of Neurosurgery*. 2006;104(6 Suppl):383–7.
5. Roach ES, Golomb MR, Adams R et al. Management of stroke in infants and children: A scientific statement from a Special Writing Group of the American Heart Association Stroke Council and the Council on Cardiovascular Disease in the Young. *Stroke*. 2008;39(9):2644–91.
6. Hellbusch LC. Benign extracerebral fluid collections in infancy: Clinical presentation and long-term follow-up. *Journal of Neurosurgery: Pediatrics*. 2007;107 (2):119–25.
7. Zahl SM, Egge A, Helseth E, Wester K. Benign external hydrocephalus: A review, with emphasis on management. *Neurosurgery Review*. 2011;34(4):417–32.
8. Caldarelli M, Di Rocco C, Romani R. Surgical treatment of chronic subdural hygromas in infants and children. *Acta Neurochirurgica (Wien)*. 2002;144 (6):581–8.
9. Park CK, Choi KH, Kim MC, Kang JK, Choi CR. Spontaneous evolution of posttraumatic subdural hygroma into chronic subdural haematoma. *Acta Neurochirurgica (Wien)*. 1994;127(1–2):41–7.
10. Klostranec JM, Vucevic D, Bhatia KD et al. Current concepts in intracranial interstitial fluid transport and the glymphatic system: Part I. Anatomy and physiology. *Radiology*. 2021;301(3):502–14.
11. Squier W, Mack J, Green A, Aziz T. The pathophysiology of brain swelling associated with subdural hemorrhage: The role of the trigeminovascular system. *Child's Nervous System*. 2012;28:2005–15.
12. Choudhary AK, Servaes S, Slovis TL et al. Consensus statement on abusive head trauma in infants and young children. *Pediatric Radiology*. 2018;48 (8):1048–65.
13. Zouros A, Bhargava R, Hoskinson M, Aronyk KE. Further characterization of traumatic subdural collections of infancy: Report of five cases. *Journal of Neurosurgery: Pediatrics*. 2004;100 (5):512–18.
14. McConnell AA. Traumatic subdural effusions. *Journal of Neurology, Neurosurgery and Psychiatry*. 1941;4(3–4):237–56.
15. Bradley WG. MR appearance of hemorrhage in the brain. *Radiology*. 1993;189(1):15–26.
16. Sieswerda-Hoogendoorn T, Postema FAM, Verbaan D, Majoie CB, Van Rijn RR. Age determination of subdural hematomas with CT and MRI: A systematic review. *European Journal of Radiology*. 2014;83 (7):1257–68.
17. Vezina G. Assessment of the nature and age of subdural collections in nonaccidental head injury with CT and MRI. *Pediatric Radiology*. 2009;39(6):586–90.

18. Sebire G. Cerebral venous sinus thrombosis in children: Risk factors, presentation, diagnosis and outcome. *Brain*. 2005;128(3):477–89.
19. Bordia R, Le M, Behbahani S. Pitfalls in the diagnosis of subdural hemorrhage: Mimics and uncommon causes. *Journal of Clinical Neuroscience*. 2021;89:71–84.
20. Krasnokutsky MV. Cerebral venous thrombosis: A potential mimic of primary traumatic brain injury in infants. *American Journal of Roentgenology*. 2011;197(3): W503–7.
21. Canedo-Antelo M, Baleato-González S, Mosqueira AJ et al. Radiologic clues to cerebral venous thrombosis. *RadioGraphics*. 2019;39(6):1611–28.
22. Poon CS, Chang J-K, Swarnkar A, Johnson MH, Wasenko J. Radiologic diagnosis of cerebral venous thrombosis: Pictorial review. *American Journal of Roentgenology*. 2007;189(6_supplement): S64–75.
23. Garrido-Barbero M, Arnaez J, Loureiro B et al. The role of Factor V Leiden, Prothrombin G20210A, and MTHFR C677 T mutations in neonatal cerebral sinovenous thrombosis. *Clinical and Applied Thrombosis*. 2019;25:107602961983435.
24. Anderst J, Carpenter S, Frazier T et al. Subdural hemorrhage in a cohort with cerebral sinovenous thrombosis: Application to abusive head trauma. *Child Abuse and Neglect*. 2021;117:105119.
25. McLean LA, Frasier LD, Hedlund GL. Does intracranial venous thrombosis cause subdural hemorrhage in the pediatric population? *American Journal of Neuroradiology*. 2012;33 (7):1281–4.
26. Vaslow DF. Chronic subdural hemorrhage predisposes to development of cerebral venous thrombosis and associated retinal hemorrhages and subdural rebleeds in infants. *Neuroradiology Journal*. 2021;197140092110269.
27. Adamsbaum C, Rambaud C. Abusive head trauma: Don't overlook bridging vein thrombosis. *Pediatric Radiology*. 2012;42 (11):1298–1300.
28. Rambaud C. Bridging veins and autopsy findings in abusive head trauma. *Pediatric Radiology*. 2015;45(8):1126–31.
29. Zahl SM, Mack JA, Rossant C, Squier W, Wester K. Thrombosis is not a marker of bridging vein rupture in infants with alleged abusive head trauma. *Acta Paediatrica*. 2021;110(10):2686–94.
30. Goodrich JT. Reprint of 'Concerning surgical intervention for the intracranial hemorrhages of the new-born' by Harvey Cushing, M.D. *Child's Nervous System*. 2000;16(8):484–92.
31. Choudhary AK, Bradford R, Dias MS, Thamburaj K, Boal DKB. Venous injury in abusive head trauma. *Pediatric Radiology*. 2015;45(12):1803–13.
32. Hahnemann ML, Kinner S, Schweiger B et al. Imaging of bridging vein thrombosis in infants with abusive head trauma: The 'tadpole sign'. *European Radiology*. 2015;25 (2):299–305.
33. Hymel KP, Stoiko MA, Herman BE et al. Head injury depth as an indicator of causes and mechanisms. *Pediatrics*. 2010;125 (4):712–20.
34. Squier W, Austin T, Anslow P, Weller RO. Infant subcortical cystic leucomalacia: A distinct pathological entity resulting from impaired fluid handling. *Early Human Development*. 2011;87(6):421–6.
35. Choudhary AK, Ishak R, Zacharia TT, Dias MS. Imaging of spinal injury in abusive head trauma: A retrospective study. *Pediatric Radiology*. 2014;44 (9):1130–40.
36. Choudhary AK, Bradford RK, Dias MS, Moore GJ, Boal DKB. Spinal subdural hemorrhage in abusive head trauma: A retrospective study. *Radiology*. 2012;262 (1):216–23.
37. Koumellis P, McConachie NS, Jaspan T. Spinal subdural haematomas in children with non-accidental head injury. *Archives of Disease in Childhood*. 2009;94 (3):216–19.

Chapter 5

Shaken Baby Syndrome

Abusive Head Trauma or Just a Type of Hydrocephalus?

Knut Wester and Johan Wikström

Introduction

The First Author's Personal Experience with Shaken Baby Syndrome/ Abusive Head Trauma

I am a retired professor of neurosurgery with some experience in paediatric neurosurgery. Until the age of 74, I believed the diagnoses shaken baby syndrome (SBS) or abusive head trauma (AHT) were based on a sound scientific foundation. At that time, I was by sheer coincidence engaged in a case of alleged violent shaking simply because I had written scientific articles on so-called benign external hydrocephalus (BEH), where cerebrospinal fluid (CSF) accumulates on the outside of the brain. Before that, I had never seen a child with SBS or AHT, possibly because neurosurgeons are rarely or never asked to serve as expert witness in such court cases in Norway.

My first encounter with SBS/AHT was caused by a bright grandmother whose grandson had been removed from his parents by a child protection team and placed in a foster home for 6 months while the police were preparing a case against his father because they suspected SBS/AHT. She had seen the boy's CT and MRI images and was convinced he had BEH, so she contacted me. The boy had a large head and had been sent repeatedly to the regional paediatric department for investigation of possible seizures, but no one there took notice of the large head and he was always sent back home. When he finally fell critically ill, CT and MRI scans were performed and the results were described as typical of SBS/AHT by experts in forensic medicine and paediatrics, despite the fact that the images had the appearance of BEH complicated by bleeding – a rather common complication to BEH, as discussed later in this chapter. Based on a brief report emphasising the BEH diagnosis, the boy was returned to his biological parents 2 days later and the police dropped further investigations.

Had it not been for a second case, I would have thought of this episode as purely incidental and unique. However, a short time later, I was confronted with another infant boy. His father had been sentenced by a lower court to 1.5 years in jail for shaking his son. Once again, the MRI had the appearance of BEH complicated with bleeding [1]. At this point I realised these two cases perhaps were not mere isolated incidents, but more likely reflected a systematic diagnostic error. Since then, I have devoted my scientific work to this possible confusion and am now, based on experience from several countries (Australia, Belgium, Denmark, France, Germany, Norway, and Sweden), quite convinced BEH is very often misdiagnosed as SBS/AHT, thus causing a large proportion of false accusations of SBS/AHT.

The Second Author's Personal Experience with Shaken Baby Syndrome/ Abusive Head Trauma

I am a professor of neuroradiology with almost 30 years of radiological experience and almost 20 years of experience as a neuroradiologist at a university hospital. As a clinical neuroradiologist I have been approached on several occasions by specialists in forensic medicine on my view about cases of alleged AHT. My predominant feeling was at first one of ignorance, since I could not understand how I could confidently ascertain the mechanism of injury from radiological findings. Gradually I have understood there is a lack of solid evidence behind the previously presented theories of ABS/AHT and that this is being acknowledged by an increasing number of colleagues. There is thus a great need for unbiased research on this topic.

The two authors of this chapter realised a combination of their specialties – neuroradiology and neurosurgery – would strengthen their scientific work on this topic. They have therefore worked in collaboration for the past 2 years [2–5]. This chapter is divided into the following sections.

1. Hydrocephalus with emphasis on a special subtype of this condition: benign external hydrocephalus (BEH), also known as benign enlargement of the subarachnoid spaces (BESS).
2. Subdural haematoma: accumulations of blood-containing fluid in the subdural compartment between the dura and the arachnoid membrane.
3. Epilepsy.
4. Retinal haemorrhage (RH): bleeding in the back of the eye.
5. Acute/apparent life-threatening event (ALTE).
6. Abusive head trauma (AHT)/shaken baby syndrome (SBS).

We also try to explain how these conditions and terms can be associated or confused.

5.1 Hydrocephalus

5.1.1 General Comments on Hydrocephalus

Normally, the brain produces CSF in the normal cavities of the brain – the ventricles. Adults produce more than half a litre every 24 hours. Children produce less depending on age and infants produce about 75–100 cc per day. This fluid circulates through the brain into the subarachnoid space on the outside of the brain, to be removed from that space and returned to the bloodstream via fluid transport systems. It is essential that CSF is removed from the intracranial space at the same speed as it is produced. In hydrocephalus, there is a mismatch between production and elimination of CSF: CSF is not filtrated back to the blood vessels at the same speed it is produced. When too much fluid is trapped inside the skull, it will cause increased intracranial pressure (ICP). This increased ICP will cause the skull to grow more rapidly than normal as the skull in infancy is not a rigid case but consists of thin bony plates connected by connective tissue. This abnormal growth is reflected in the routine measurements of the head circumference (HC) performed in infant health clinics in most countries (see Figure 5.1).

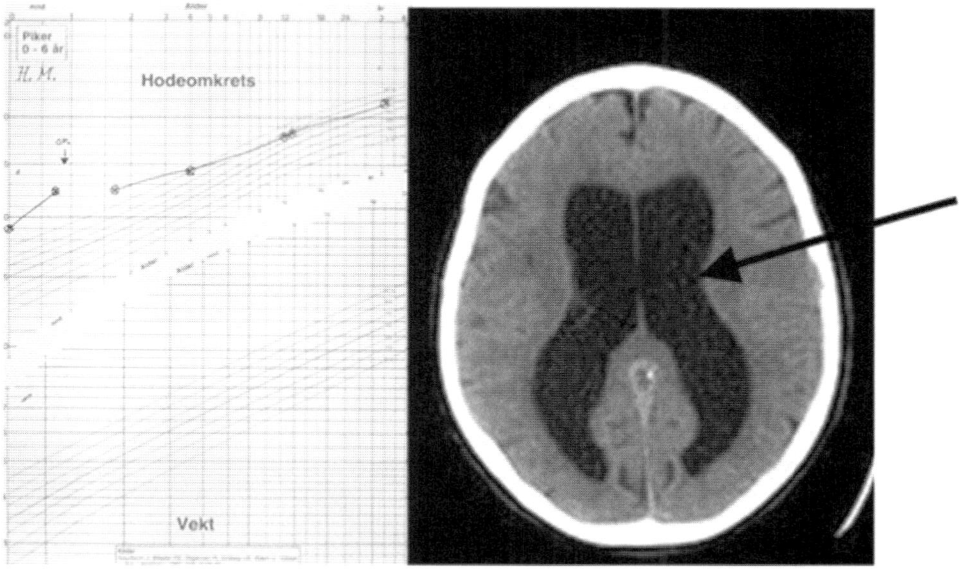

Figure 5.1 'Ordinary' hydrocephalus. Left: head circumference (HC) chart that shows an abnormally rapid (steep) growth. "Hodeomkrets" (HC) starting at birth, and a later normalisation after a neurosurgical procedure (OP = ventriculoperitoneal shunt) allowing permanent drainage of CSF to the abdomen. Right: CT image of a child with 'ordinary' hydrocephalus showing increased CSF (black) in the ventricles of the brain (black arrow). Normal amount of CSF outside the brain, unlike the image of external hydrocephalus (BEH/BESS) (see Figure 5.2) (For the colour version, please refer to the plate section.)

5.1.2 External Hydrocephalus: Epidemiological, Clinical, and Radiological Characteristics

Introduction

This and closely related conditions are known under many aliases: benign/idiopathic external hydrocephalus (BEH), benign familial macrocephaly, benign infantile hydrocephalus, benign subdural collection, benign extra-axial fluid/collection, benign extracerebral fluid collection, benign communicating hydrocephalus, benign enlargement of the subarachnoid spaces (BESS), subarachnoid fluid collection, chronic subdural hygroma, pericerebral fluid collection, idiopathic macrocephaly, chronic subdural haematoma (CSDH), and subdural effusion.

The diagnosis of external hydrocephalus is based on a combination of clinical and radiological characteristics (see Figure 5.2). External refers to the fact that there is accumulated fluid on the outside of the brain. It is a special form of hydrocephalus with a marked male preponderance [6] and an overrepresentation among prematures [7]. The term *benign* has been coined to distinguish it from more aggressive types of hydrocephalus, but this is misleading as it may cause severe brain injury, even death – see later in this chapter. The condition is characterised by increased CSF not only in the ventricles, but also in the subarachnoid compartment between the brain and the skull. This increased fluid causes raised ICP and

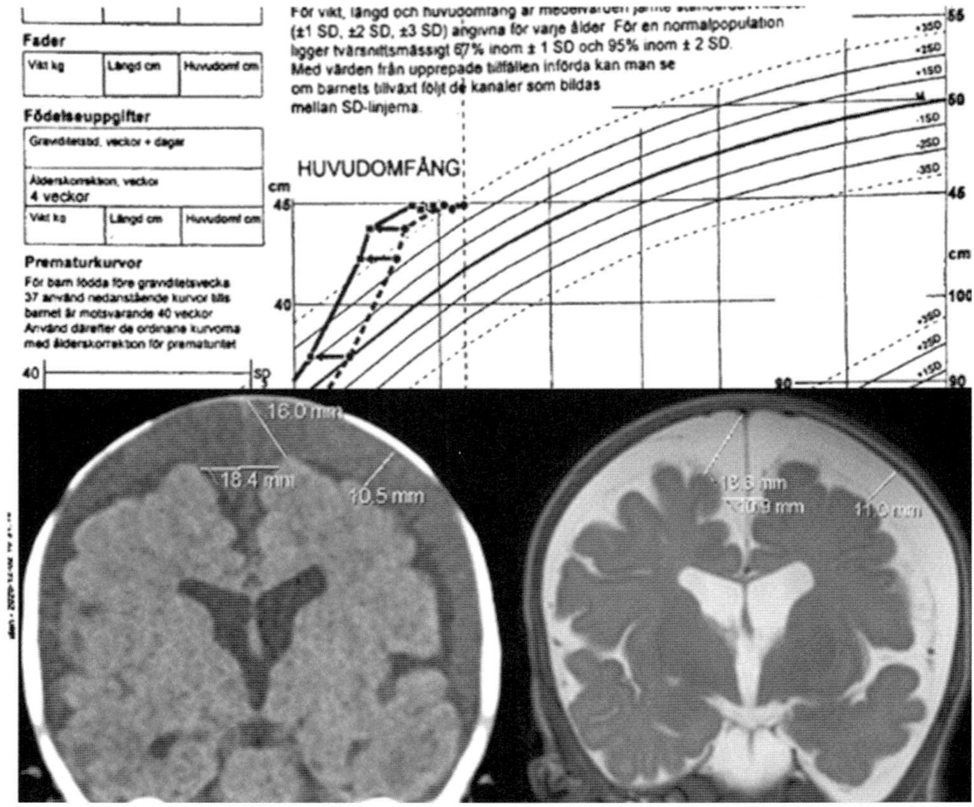

Figure 5.2 Benign external hydrocephalus (BEH). Upper: Swedish head circumference (HC) chart from a prematurely born boy with BEH, showing fast and abnormal HC growth from birth (dashed line) – corrected for prematurity: solid line; Lower: Radiological characteristics. CT and MRI images of the same infant; note the increased CSF is not restricted to the ventricles of the brain; there is also increased fluid in the subdural compartment; which contains blood elements – chronic subdural haematoma (CSDH). Note the small rim of normal CSF between the brain and the subdural fluid – dark on the CT, bright on the MRI. Measurements indicate the inter-hemispheric distance, the sinocortical width, and the craniocortical width. For further radiological details, see Figure 5.7. Reproduced from [4] with permission of *Acta Paediatrica*, John Wiley and Sons through Copyright Clearance Center.

consequently a rapid growth of the head because the ICP forces the thin bony plates of the infant skull to separate from each other (see 'Radiological Signs of Increased Intracranial Pressure' section and Figure 5.8). This increased extracerebral, subarachnoid CSF is known to be a predisposing factor for oozing of blood into the subdural compartment, often referred to as subdural haematoma (SDH) [8]; the amount of blood in the subdural compartment may be quite small and much of the fluid that accumulates in the subdural compartment is proteinaceous rather than frankly bloody. Generally, this oozing of blood and fluid occurs spontaneously – without head trauma [8, 9] (see 'Predisposing Factors for the Development of Subdural Haematomas in Infancy' section and Figure 5.12).

Epidemiology

The only population-based epidemiological study of external hydrocephalus [6] shows a marked male preponderance – 86% of patients are boys. A similar male overrepresentation is found in all larger publications on external hydrocephalus [8, 9]. Prematurity also appears to be highly prevalent among these infants [7]. As shown in Figure 5.3, most infants who develop this condition are born with a close-to-normal HC, but during the first postnatal months the head starts to grow abnormally fast; most of these infants reach HC values compatible with hydrocephalus at the age of 3–6 months. In fact, a later analysis of the same Norwegian infant population revealed the large HC developed before that age, starting between 2 and 3 months (Figure 5.4) [10]. Figure 5.4 shows further detail on the development of increased HC in external hydrocephalus.

Clinical Signs and Findings

External hydrocephalus is characterised by a large and/or rapidly growing head and is often associated with symptoms of delayed development along with symptoms related to elevated ICP, such as sunset gaze (Figure 5.5), tense anterior fontanel, irritability, feeding problems (regurgitating and/or vomiting), and epilepsy (see 'Radiological Signs of Increased Intracranial Pressure' section). When external hydrocephalus is considered to be the cause of SDH, an updated HC chart is of the utmost importance.

Radiological Characteristics

Benign external hydrocephalus is characterised by an increasing amount of CSF in the subarachnoid space during the first weeks/months after birth, in addition to moderately

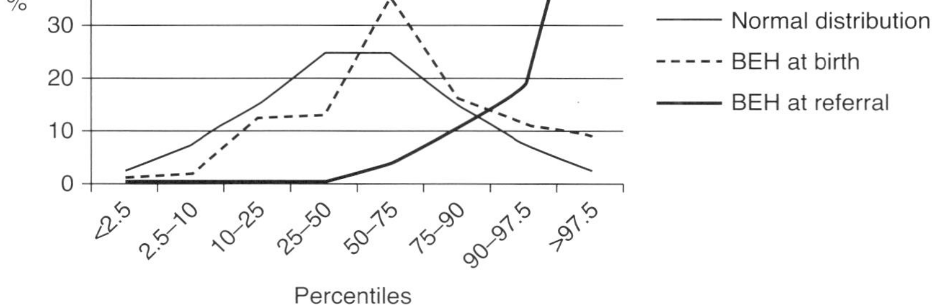

Figure 5.3 This graph shows the abnormal growth of the head circumference (HC) in Norwegian infants who developed external hydrocephalus [6]. The HC of these infants (dashed line) did not deviate much from the normal distribution (thin solid line) at birth; their abnormal increase of HC (arrow) occurred between birth and referral time (mean age 7.3 months). For further details, see Figure 5.4. Reproduced from *Pediatric Neurology* with permission from Elsevier through Copyright Clearance Center.

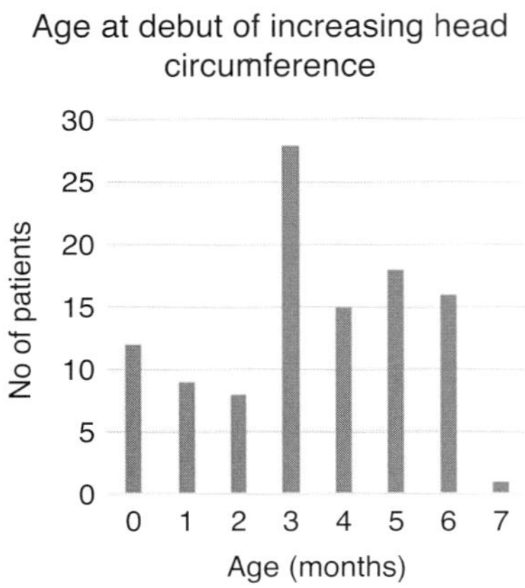

Figure 5.4 The age at which the HC in Norwegian BEH infants becomes abnormally large. In virtually none did routine HC measurements reveal abnormally large heads after the age of 7 months, from [10]. Reproduced from *Pediatric Neurology* with permission from Elsevier through Copyright Clearance Center.

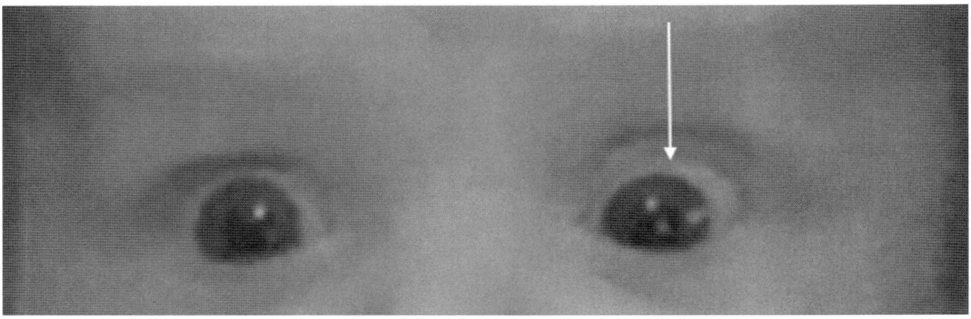

Figure 5.5 'Sunset gaze' resembles a setting sun and indicates increased intracranial pressure (ICP) in a 2-month-old infant. Note the typical rim of white sclera between the upper eyelid and the iris (arrow). (For the colour version, please refer to the plate section.)

increasing CSF in the ventricles of the brain (see Figures 5.6 and 5.7). The first event is usually that the frontal inter-hemispheric distance increases (white horizontal line), followed by an increased subarachnoid layer outside the brain (white double arrow) and finally increased fluid in the ventricles (white arrow) [11].

Intracranial measurements used to characterise external hydrocephalus have been sinocortical width (SCW), craniocortical width (CCW), and inter-hemispheric distance (IHD) (see Figure 5.7). Increase in these intracranial distances has been regarded as characteristic for external hydrocephalus. However, there is no consensus on normal measurements [6] as these depend on the imaging modality and the age of the child; the upper limit of normal CCW has been regarded as ranging from 4 mm to 10 mm [11–15]. The corresponding ranges for SCW are 2 mm to 10 mm and for IHD 6 mm to 8.5 mm. However, there are no validated normal values and the values at which this condition is diagnosed can be variable.

Radiological Signs of Increased Intracranial Pressure

Because the infant skull consists of thin bony plates loosely connected to each other by 'sutures' of connective tissue, increased ICP serves to move the cranial bones apart from

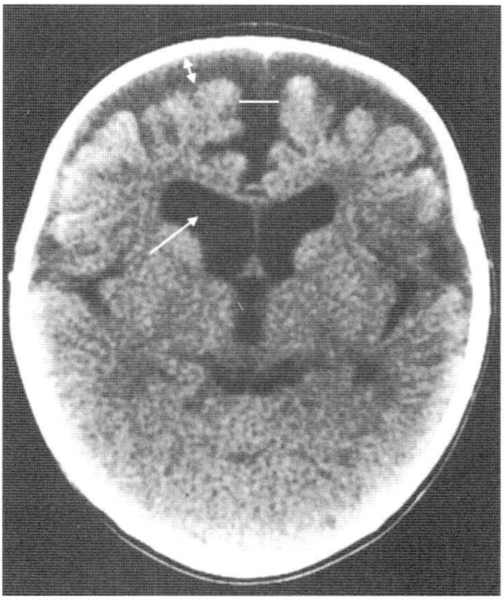

Figure 5.6 Characteristic CT image of BEH taken from [72]. See text and Figure 5.7 for details. The increase of fluid is usually first observed as an increased inter-hemispheric distance (IHD) between the two cerebral frontal lobes (white horizontal line), followed by an increased subarachnoid layer outside of the brain (white double arrow) and finally: increased fluid in the ventricles (white arrow). Reproduced with permission from *American Journal of Neuroradiology*, American Society of Neuroradiology through Copyright Clearance Center.

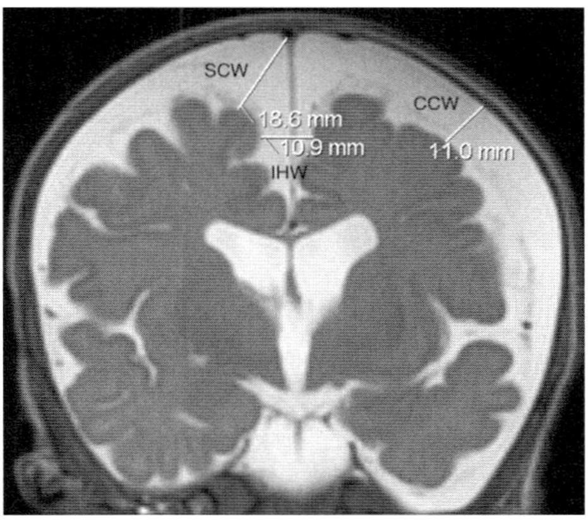

Figure 5.7 Details from Figure 5.2. Intracranial measurements used to characterise external hydrocephalus are sinocortical width (SCW) – 18.6 mm; craniocortical width (CCW) – 11.0 mm; inter-hemispheric distance (IHD) – 10.9 mm. Note the subdural fluid does not compress the ventricles or the convolutions on the brain surface, indicating generally increased ICP with a balance between the intraventricular and the extracerebral pressures. If there were a higher pressure in the subdural fluid, one would expect the brain (and ventricles) to be compressed.

each other. This phenomenon – suture diastasis – can be felt by palpation or seen on a CT (Figure 5.8).

5.2 Subdural Haematoma

The term *subdural haematoma* describes a collection of fluid that contains blood elements (acute or chronic) in the so-called subdural compartment between the arachnoid membrane over the brain surface and the membrane lining the inner aspect of the skull – the 'dura'.

5.2.1 Acute and Chronic Subdural Haematomas

Fresh, acute, and coagulated blood appears white on a CT image and is referred to as an acute subdural haematoma (ASDH). An ASDH is much more dangerous than

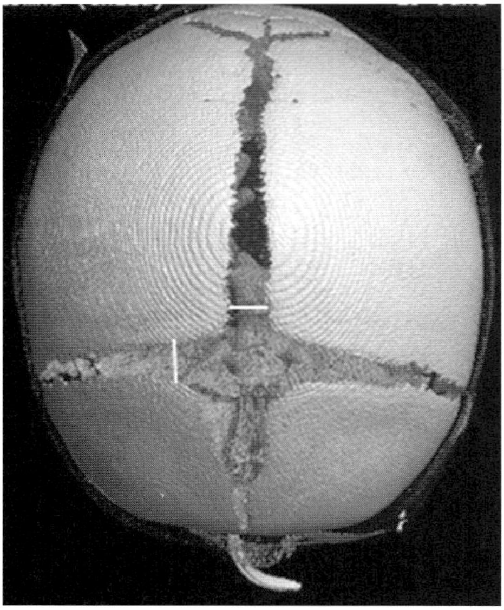

Figure 5.8 Reconstructed CT 3-D image showing suture diastasis (white lines) in infantile external hydrocephalus. Face at lower edge of image (For the colour version, please refer to the plate section.)

a chronic subdural haematoma (CSDH) [5], which develops more slowly (several days or even weeks) by oozing of blood into the subdural compartment. Quite often a CSDH is characterised by old blood elements evenly distributed in the subdural fluid; thus, in a baby positioned in a CT scanner with the nose up, these blood elements will sink by gravity to the posterior portion of the intracranial compartment. The different appearances of ASDH and CSDH are shown in Figure 5.9. As will be apparent from that figure, an ASDH is associated with acute parenchymal swelling (brain oedema); this acute swelling appears to be a more important cause of midline shift than the volume of the ASDH itself.

Acute Subdural Haematoma

Acute SDH appears to be much less common in infants than chronic SDH. Based on striking epidemiological, radiological, and prognostic dissimilarities, a recent article discusses the probability that ASDH and CSDH in fact are two different entities – for example, with a much higher mortality rate in ASDH [5]. Figure 5.10 shows a paediatric ASDH with fast-developing and fatal brain oedema.

Chronic Subdural Haematoma

Figure 5.11 depicts a chronic SDH in an infant with alleged AHT.

Figure 5.12 is an illustration from a textbook chapter on BEH. It shows a widened subarachnoid compartment – typical of BEH – with increased distances (SCW, CCW, IHD) and with stretched, contrast-filled veins extending from the brain surface to the inside of the skull (bridging veins). With increasing subarachnoid fluid, the stretched veins may start to ooze blood into the subdural compartment from where the veins enter the dural membrane on the inside of the skull. This blood will add to the extracerebral fluid and cause additional increase of ICP.

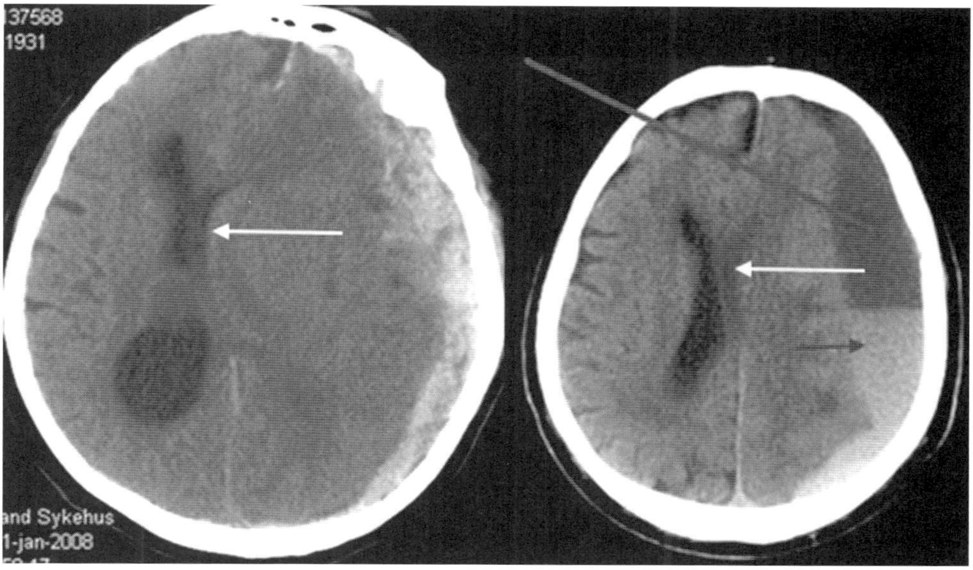

Figure 5.9 SDH in adults. Left: Acute SDH with fresh, partly coagulated blood (light coloured). Right: Chronic SDH with sedimentation of old blood components to the back of the head. Please note that in both types of SDH the brain is squeezed to the opposite side by the haematoma and the ventricle on the side of the haematoma is compressed (white arrows). In a chronic SDH, the chronic blood elements will sink down to the rear of the skull (light colour), leaving the fluid above the blood elements with a darker colour.

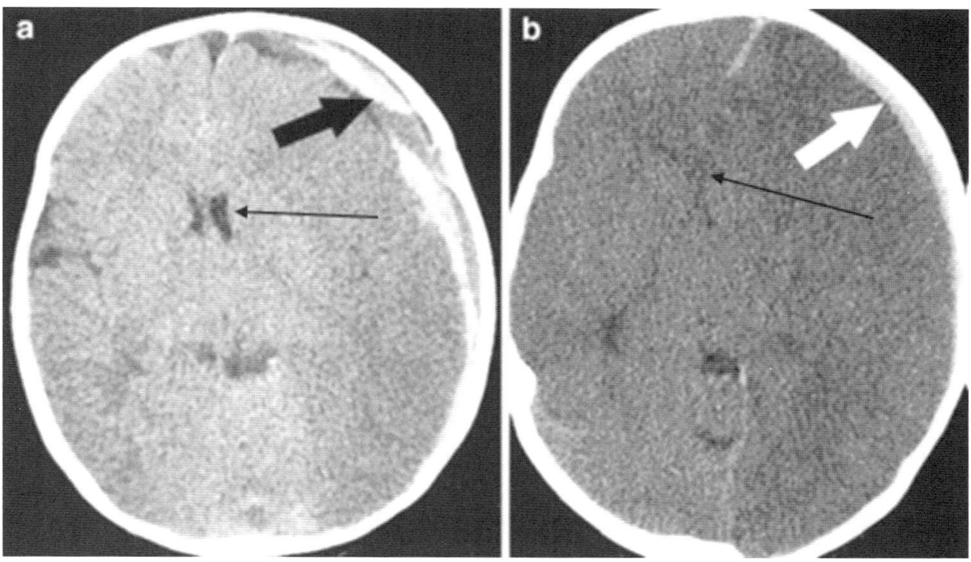

Figure 5.10 A typical ASDH in a small child (thick arrows). Left: shortly after the head injury. Right: 24 hours later. In both images the brain midline is dislocated to the opposite side and the ventricles are compressed (narrow black arrows). Note the marked brain oedema beneath the SDH immediately and then more pronounced after 24 hours (darker grey) in the compressed hemisphere. Figure reproduced from [73] with permission from Springer Nature, Pediatric Radiology through Copyright Clearance Center.

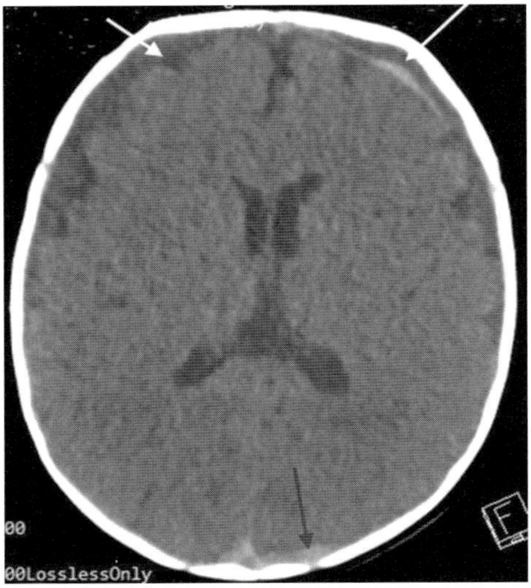

Figure 5.11 CT scan of a 3-month-old infant allegedly subjected to SBS/AHT. Bifrontal CSDH (white arrows), with a small amount of fresh blood over the left frontal lobe (white – on right side of the picture). Dark arrow on a posterior portion of the CSDH, which appears somewhat brighter than the frontal portion due to sedimentation and concentration of blood cells by gravity. Forensic experts diagnosed this case as an acute SDH.

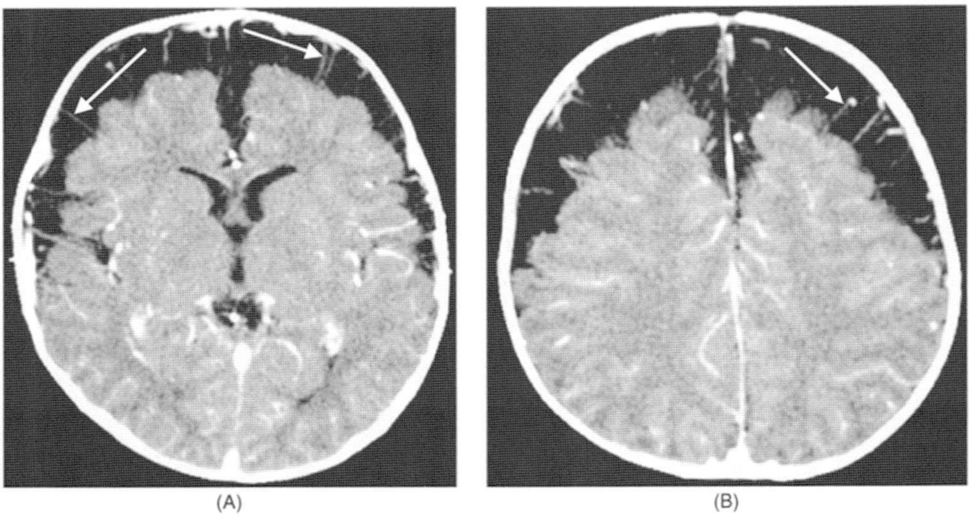

Figure 5.12 Figure from [76], p. 83. In addition to increased extracerebral, subarachnoid fluid with increased distances (SCW, CCW, IHD), these CT scans show stretched, contrast-filled veins (arrows) extending from the brain surface to the inside of the skull (bridging veins). See also text. Republished with permission from Taylor & Francis Group LLC. Permission conveyed through Copyright Clearance Center.

5.2.2 Factors That Predispose to Development of Subdural Haematomas in Infancy

Low Age and Prematurity

In general, infants are markedly more prone to develop SDH in their first 6 months than later in infancy (see Figure 5.13). This fact has been known since at least 1944 [16].

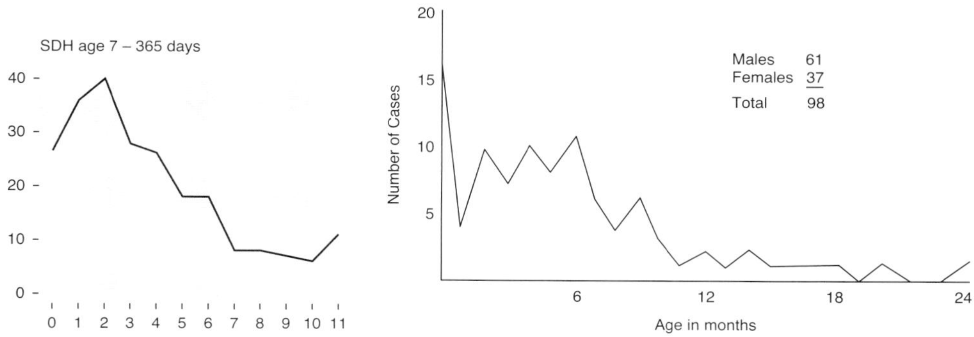

Figure 5.13 Left: Age distribution in a national study comprising Swedish infants with SDH in the period 1997–2014 [17]. Right: Corresponding age distribution in a US cohort from 1944 [74], reproduced with permission from *Journal of Pediatrics*, Elsevier through Copyright Clearance Center. Note very few infants are diagnosed with SDH after the age of 6 months in either population – 70 years apart (infancy: age below 12 months).

Prematurely born children are also more prone to develop SDH than babies born at term [17].

Subdural Haematomas in Newborns

It is now well documented that about half of all newborns have subdural blood collections, more frequently after assisted deliveries and most often after emergency Caesarean procedures [18]. It is assumed these subdural collections will resolve in a few months, but this cannot be concluded from this or other studies as only a fraction (39.1%) of these infants were followed up and in one of them a large chronic SDH had developed at the age of 26 days (see figure 4 in [18]). In this respect, it is important to recognise that re-bleeding may occur into an already existing SDH [19–21].

External Hydrocephalus

External hydrocephalus is a well-documented predisposing factor for SDH, as shown in many articles; only a few are referred to here [8, 9, 22–35]. In fact, a causal relationship between these two conditions has been proposed – that the birth-related small rim of SDH blocks the normal 'escape' routes for the CSF and thus causes an extracerebral fluid accumulation [36]. Figure 5.14 shows a spontaneous SDH occurring between 6 and 12 months of age in an infant with BEH [25].

Based on the vast, existing literature, it appears clear that external hydrocephalus represents a definite risk of SDH in infancy. Such an SDH is most often old (chronic) or with a mixture of old and freshly coagulated blood (acute on chronic) (see Figure 5.14) [5].

Gender

There is a marked male preponderance in nearly all articles on SDH in infancy, with close to twice as many boys as girls [17, 37]. As mentioned, the only population-based study on external hydrocephalus also shows a marked male overrepresentation (86%) [6] and early age of onset [10]. A similar age and gender distribution can be found in most larger articles on AHT/SBS (e.g., [38–40]). Pooled together, the infants in these publications had a male preponderance of 70% and a mean age of 4 months.

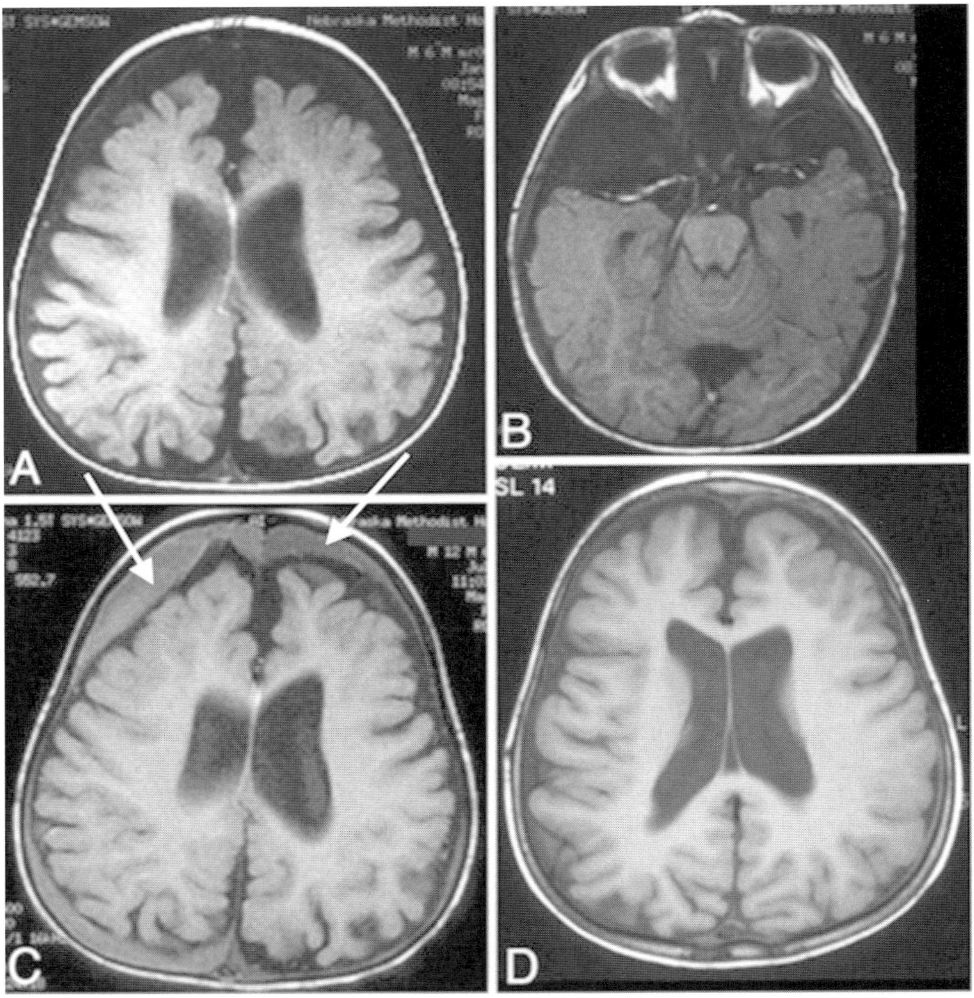

Figure 5.14 Development of an SDH in an infant with external hydrocephalus. Illustration from [25] reproduced from *Journal of Neurosurgery* with permission from American Association of Neurological Surgeons. Image A: MRI without signs of SDH with characteristic radiological features for BEH: wide frontal inter-hemispheric distance, wide subarachnoid fluid space, and enlarged ventricles. Image B: MRI at the same time as image A closer to the skull base. Image C: At 12 months of age large, spontaneously occurring subdural haematomas of different ages can be seen overlying both cerebral hemispheres (arrows). Note absence of compression of the brain surface, indicating this is not acute subdural haematoma caused by a trauma – accidental or by abuse. Image D: spontaneous recovery.

Similarities between External Hydrocephalus, Subdural Haematoma, and Shaken Baby Syndrome/Acute Head Trauma

There are very striking epidemiological similarities between external hydrocephalus, SDH, and AHT/SBS in infancy regarding gender and age. It is our experience that external hydrocephalus complicated by an SDH can be – and has been – misdiagnosed as AHT/SBS within Scandinavian judicial systems [1, 3]. Based on our international experience, we are of the opinion this may be the case in other regions of the world as well. There is also a high degree of similarity between neuroimages published as typical examples of AHT/SBS and those published as examples of external hydrocephalus complicated by SDH (see Figure 5.15).

Having discovered that apparently similar images had been published in international articles as typical examples of AHT/SBS and BEH complicated by SDH or subdural hygroma, we went through the relevant literature on AHT/SBS published in the period 2008–21 together with a colleague who is trained in neuroradiology. We found 63 articles with a total of 172 illustrations that claimed to show AHT/SBS and that were of sufficient quality to allow classification. Of these, radiological findings suggesting BEH were detected in 59 (34.1%), whereas only 24 (14.1%) were compatible with what one would expect to find after an *acute traumatic* event: an acute SDH (ASDH), with an appearance like that shown in Figures 5.9 and 5.10. For further details of this review, see Chapter 6.

The different age distributions between the ASDH-like images and those resembling BEH were striking. The BEH-like images nearly all came from very young infants, whereas the children with ASDH-like images were evenly distributed throughout an age range of 0–48 months (see Figure 5.16).

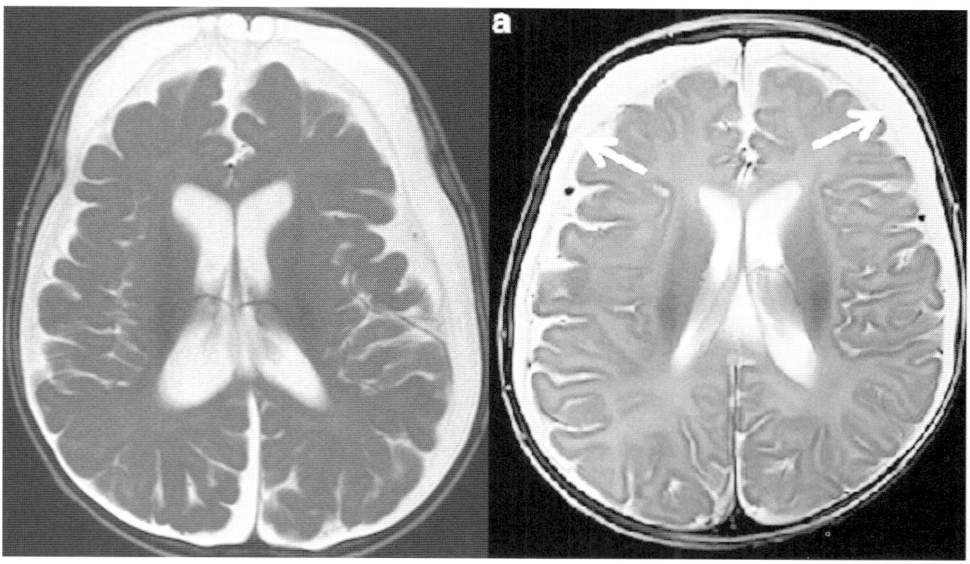

Figure 5.15 Examples of the confusion regarding the radiological diagnosis of SBS/AHT. Left: MRI described as showing 'spontaneous SDH in [an] infant' associated with external hydrocephalus. Reproduced from [35] with permission from *Child's Nervous System*. Right: MRI described as strongly suggesting child abuse (AHT). Reproduced from [75] with permission from *Pediatric Radiology*, Springer Nature through Copyright Clearance Center. Arrows delineate the border between the normal subarachnoid brain fluid (CSF) overlying the brain surface and the outer (whiter) subdural fluid collection with blood components. Note that the subdural fluid in neither case compresses the cortical surface, the subarachnoid space or the fluid producing cavities – the slightly enlarged ventricles. Radiologically, these images appear to share the same features.

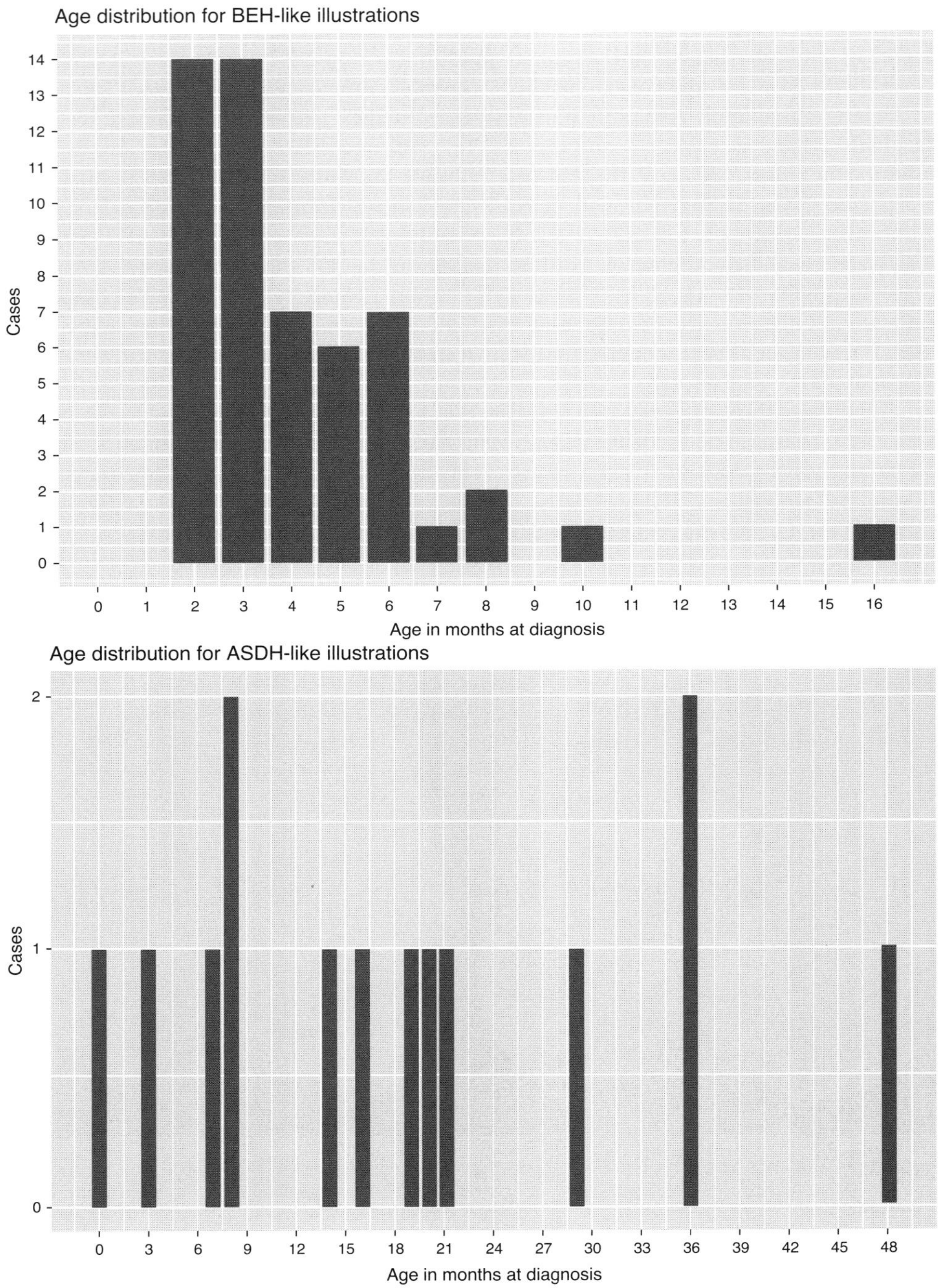

Figure 5.16 Age distribution of children diagnosed as AHT/SBS in the world literature during the period 2008–18. Upper graph: children with BEH-like images. Note the low age and hardly any older than 6 months. Lower graph: children with ASDH-like images distributed throughout the age range. Note that the X axes (ages) are different – the age range on the lower graph is 0–48 months.

5.3 Epilepsy

Epilepsy is not a disease but a symptom. Brain cells communicate by exchanging controlled bioelectric signals. Many intracranial pathological conditions, such as increased ICP, tumours, failing blood supply to the brain, intracranial or intracerebral bleeding, and brain infarctions, can disturb the finely tuned rhythm of these bioelectric signals, resulting in a massive discharge of uncontrolled impulses. Epileptic seizures (fits) can manifest themselves in different ways; most often they cause loss of consciousness, rhythmic convulsions, and/or a temporary stiffness followed by limpness. Epileptic seizures are common in infants with external hydrocephalus, often as the first dramatic symptom, especially in infants with external hydrocephalus complicated by SDH [8, 9, 23, 25, 27, 32, 41–46].

5.4 Retinal Haemorrhage

Retinal haemorrhage (RH) has been claimed as a significant, pathognomonic, and indeed nearly imperative finding in AHT/SBS [40, 47]. Bilateral, extensive bleeding in several retinal layers has been regarded as a key feature of AHT [48–55]. However, in truth bilateral RH is not specific or pathognomonic for AHT/SBS. It has been known for more than a century that increased ICP can cause RH; the increased ICP is mediated by the sheath around the optic nerve to the inside of the eye bulb and can thus cause haemorrhage there – a phenomenon referred to as Terson's syndrome [56]. The optic nerve sheath in infants is very short – only a few millimetres – which makes this pressure mediation easier. Retinal haemorrhage can also be found in infants in situations unrelated to abuse – for example, in a large number of healthy newborns [57–59], in infants with 'macrocephaly'/BEH [32, 60], after 'high-risk' deliveries [61], following ALTE (see later in this chapter) with dysphagic choking [62], and after cardiopulmonary resuscitation [63–65]. Retinal haemorrhage has also been documented in premature infants. Contrary to the rapid resolution of the bleeding one usually sees in most newborns, the bleeding in preterms tend to be longer-lasting [66]. An example of large RH in ALTE can be seen in Figure 5.17. The correlation between

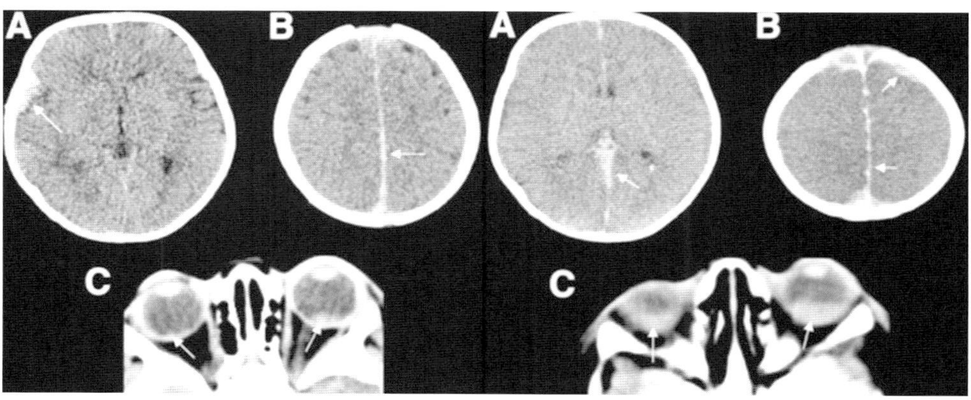

Figure 5.17 Retinal haemorrhage (RH) in a 4.5-month-old male infant found 'choking and blue' with a bulging fontanel. Left: 1.5 hours after the acute event. Right: 12 hours after the acute event. RHs are shown in the posterior parts of the eye bulbs, see lower part (C) of each image. White arrows are pointing to the bilateral RHs, which increase dramatically in size from 1.5 to 12 hours. Reproduced from [62] with permission from *Seminars in Pediatric Neurology*, Elsevier through Copyright Clearance Center.

increased ICP (due to medical conditions) and RH in children (aged 3–17 years) has been demonstrated [67].

A recent study of allegedly shaken babies shows RH was found only in infants who also had intracranial pathology [68]. This study indicates RH is *not* caused by traction forces between the retina and vitreous body acting directly on retinal vessels, but they more likely are the result of increased ICP – Terson's syndrome [56].

5.5 Acute/Apparent Life-Threatening Event

An acute/apparent life-threatening event has been defined as 'an episode that is frightening to the observer and that is characterised by some combination of apnoea (central or occasionally obstructive), colour change (usually cyanotic or pallid), marked change in muscle tone, choking or gagging' [69]. The condition is not uncommon and usually has no serious consequences. However, there are exceptions as fatal outcomes also have been reported [62, 70]. Epilepsy has been reported as frequently as 25% in infants with ALTE [71].

5.6 Abusive Head Trauma/Shaken Baby Syndrome

Abusive head trauma and shaken baby syndrome are *not* valid medical diagnoses. These terms have been used synonymously and indeed they have been used both as a medical diagnosis and as a description of an assumed criminal act, namely intentional violent shaking or physical child abuse including head impact.

More than 1,000 articles have been published internationally that claim to report findings in infants subjected to AHT. The lack of objectively based *observations* of this assumed violence is, however, striking; most AHT/SBS diagnoses are based on assumptions made by child protection teams on the basis of what these teams believe is solid evidence of violence (see [47]: 'evaluated by the hospital's child abuse evaluation team'). One problem with this assumption is that these same medical and radiological findings can be present in several other medical – nonviolent – conditions.

Violent shaking has in fact extremely rarely been observed. When it *has* been observed, the victims who were subjected to shaking apparently did not have the typical findings believed to be associated with shaking [2]. Nevertheless, this alleged shaking or abusive violence, and thus also the criminal act behind it, has been 'diagnosed' based on certain clinical and/or radiological findings – the *triad.*

Due to the lack of *observation* of the criminal act or other *objective* proof, the 'diagnosis' of the criminal act is in fact based on medical findings in the baby *after* the criminal event has allegedly taken place; findings the proponents of the triad claim to be certain or close-to-certain proofs of abuse. In other words, the triad or one of its three components – SDH, RH, and signs/symptoms of brain damage (encephalopathy) – has been widely regarded as solid proof of violent child abuse.

A final note from the first author: prior to my involvement – at a relatively advanced age – in AHT/SBS cases, I was convinced this was a scientifically solid diagnosis that could be used to prove guilt 'beyond reasonable doubt' in criminal cases. Later, however, I discovered this was false and that the diagnosis was based on assumptions only. After having thoroughly read the relevant literature, including all the major articles concerning AHT/SBS, this diagnosis has struck me as being based on very *weak scientific documentation*. The main reason for this weakness is that nearly all published studies are based on circular reasoning, which in most cases invalidates any conclusions these studies propose.

References

1. Wester K. Two infant boys misdiagnosed as 'shaken baby' and their twin sisters: A cautionary tale. *Pediatric Neurology*. 2019;97:3–11.
2. Thiblin I, Andersson J, Wester K et al. Medical findings and symptoms in infants exposed to witnessed or admitted abusive shaking: A nationwide registry study. *PLoS One*. 2020;15(10):e0240182.
3. Wester K, Stridbeck U, Syse A, Wikstrom J. Re-evaluation of medical findings in alleged shaken baby syndrome and abusive head trauma in Norwegian courts fails to support abuse diagnoses. *Acta Paediatrica*. 2022;111(4):779–92.
4. Wester K, Wikström J, Lynøe N, Eriksson A. Unsubstantiated belief in the diagnostic accuracy of the triad of abusive head trauma may lead to incorrect diagnoses of alleged abuse cases. *Acta Paediatrica*. 2022;111(4):809–11.
5. Andersson J, Wikstrom J, Hogberg U, Wester K, Thiblin I. External hydrocephalus as a cause of infant subdural hematoma: Epidemiological and radiological investigations of infants suspected of being abused. *Pediatric Neurology*. 2021;126:26–34.
6. Wiig US, Zahl SM, Egge A, Helseth E, Wester K. Epidemiology of benign external hydrocephalus in Norway: A population-based study. *Pediatric Neurology*. 2017;73:36–41.
7. Yew AY, Maher CO, Muraszko KM, Garton HJ. Long-term health status in benign external hydrocephalus. *Pediatric Neurosurgery*. 2011;47(1):1–6.
8. Lee HC, Chong S, Lee JY et al. Benign extracerebral fluid collection complicated by subdural hematoma and fluid collection: Clinical characteristics and management. *Child's Nervous System*. 2018;34(2):235–45.
9. McNeely PD, Atkinson JD, Saigal G, O'Gorman AM, Farmer JP. Subdural hematomas in infants with benign enlargement of the subarachnoid spaces are not pathognomonic for child abuse. *American Journal of Neuroradiology*. 2006;27(8):1725–8.
10. Zahl SM, Egge A, Helseth E, Wester K. Clinical, radiological, and demographic details of benign external hydrocephalus: A population-based study. *Pediatric Neurology*. 2019;96:53–7.
11. Alvarez LA, Maytal J, Shinnar S. Idiopathic external hydrocephalus: Natural history and relationship to benign familial macrocephaly. *Pediatrics*. 1986;77(6):901–7.
12. Fessell DP, Frankel DA, Wolfson WP. Sonography of extraaxial fluid in neurologically normal infants with head circumference greater than or equal to the 95th percentile for age. *Journal of Ultrasound Medicine*. 2000;19(7):443–7.
13. Fukuyama Y, Miyao M, Ishizu T, Maruyama H. Developmental changes in normal cranial measurements by computed-tomography. *Developmental Medicine and Child Neurology*. 1979;21(4):425–32.
14. Libicher M, Troger J. Us measurement of the subarachnoid space in infants: Normal values. *Radiology*. 1992;184(3):749–51.
15. Marino MA, Morabito R, Vinci S et al. Benign external hydrocephalus in infants. A single centre experience and literature review. *Neuroradiology Journal*. 2014;27(2):245–50.
16. Ingraham F, Matson D. Subdural hematoma in infancy. *Journal of Pediatrics*. 1944;24(1):1–37.
17. Hogberg U, Andersson J, Squier et al. Epidemiology of subdural haemorrhage during infancy: A population-based register study. *PLoS One*. 2018;13(10):1–17.
18. Rooks VJ, Eaton JP, Ruess L et al. Prevalence and evolution of intracranial hemorrhage in asymptomatic term infants.

American Journal of Neuroradiology. 2008;29(6):1082–9.

19. Ito H, Yamamoto S, Komai T, Mizukoshi H. Role of local hyperfibrinolysis in etiology of chronic subdural hematoma. *Journal of Neurosurgery*. 1976;45(1):26–31.
20. Kawakami Y, Chikama M, Tamiya T, Shimamura Y. Coagulation and fibrinolysis in chronic subdural hematoma. *Neurosurgery*. 1989;25(1):25–9.
21. Murakami H, Hirose Y, Sagoh M et al. Why do chronic subdural hematomas continue to grow slowly and not coagulate? Role of thrombomodulin in the mechanism. *Journal of Neurosurgery*. 2002;96 (5):877–84.
22. Azais M, Echenne B. Idiopathic subarachnoid space enlargement (benign external hydrocephalus) in infants. *Annales de pediatrie*. 1992;39(9):550–8.
23. Ghosh PS, Ghosh D. Subdural hematoma in infants without accidental or nonaccidental injury: Benign external hydrocephalus, a risk factor. *Clinical Pediatrics*. 2011;50(10):897–903.
24. Gout A, Gautier I, Bellaiche M et al. Idiopathic subarachnoid space enlargement in infancy: Simple anatomic variant or hemorrhagic risk factor? *Archives de pediatrie*. 1997;4(10):983–7.
25. Hellbusch LC. Benign extracerebral fluid collections in infancy: Clinical presentation and long-term follow-up. *Journal of Neurosurgery*. 2007;107(2 Suppl):119–25.
26. Kapila A, Trice J, Spies WG, Siegel BA, Gado MH. Enlarged cerebrospinal fluid spaces in infants with subdural hematomas. *Radiology*. 1982;142 (3):669–72.
27. Laubscher B, Deonna T, Uske A, Van MG. Primitive megalocephaly in children: Natural history, medium term prognosis with special reference to external hydrocephalus. *European Journal of Pediatrics*. 1990;149(7):502–7.
28. McKeag H, Christian CW, Rubin D et al. Subdural hemorrhage in pediatric patients with enlargement of the subarachnoid spaces Clinical article. *Journal of Neurosurgery: Pediatrics*. 2013;11 (4):438–44.
29. Miller D, Barnes P, Miller M. The significance of macrocephaly or enlarging head circumference in infants with the triad further evidence of mimics of shaken baby syndrome. *American Journal of Forensic Medical Pathology*. 2015;36 (2):111–20.
30. Mori K, Sakamoto T, Nishimura K, Fujiwara K. Subarachnoid fluid collection in infants complicated by subdural-hematoma. *Child's Nervous System*. 1993;9(5):282–4.
31. Papasian NC, Frim DM. A theoretical model of benign external hydrocephalus that predicts a predisposition towards extra-axial hemorrhage after minor head trauma. *Pediatric Neurosurgery*. 2000;33 (4):188–93.
32. Piatt JH, Jr. A pitfall in the diagnosis of child abuse: External hydrocephalus, subdural hematoma, and retinal hemorrhages. *Neurosurgery Focus*. 1999;7 (4):e4.
33. Ravid S, Maytal J. External hydrocephalus: A probable cause for subdural hematoma in infancy. *Pediatric Neurology*. 2003;28 (2):139–41.
34. Tucker J, Choudhary AK, Piatt J. Macrocephaly in infancy: Benign enlargement of the subarachnoid spaces and subdural collections. *Journal of Neurosurgery: Pediatrics*. 2016;18(1):16–20.
35. Vinchon M, Delestret I, DeFoort-Dhellemmes S, Desurmont M, Noule N. Subdural hematoma in infants: can it occur spontaneously? Data from a prospective series and critical review of the literature. *Child's Nervous System*. 2010;26 (9):1195–1205.
36. Zahl SM, Wester K, Gabaeff S. Examining perinatal subdural haematoma as an aetiology of extra-axial hygroma and chronic subdural haematoma. *Acta Paediatrica*. 2020;109(4):659–66.
37. Ingraham FD, Matson, D. D. Subdural hematoma in infancy. *Journal of Pediatrics*. 1944;24(1):1–37.

38. Adamsbaum C, Grabar S, Mejean N, Rey-Salmon C. Abusive head trauma: Judicial admissions highlight violent and repetitive shaking. *Pediatrics*. 2010;126(3):546–55.

39. Hobbs C, Childs AM, Wynne J, Livingston J, Seal A. Subdural haematoma and effusion in infancy: An epidemiological study. *Archives of Disease in Childhood*. 2005;90(9):952–5.

40. Vinchon M, de Foort-Dhellemmes S, Desurmont M, Delestret I. Confessed abuse versus witnessed accidents in infants: Comparison of clinical, radiological, and ophthalmological data in corroborated cases. *Child's Nervous System*. 2010;26 (5):637–45.

41. Alper G, Ekinci G, Yilmaz Y et al. Magnetic resonance imaging characteristics of benign macrocephaly in children. *Journal of Child Neurology*. 1999;14(10):678–82.

42. Govaert P, Oostra A, Matthys D, Vanhaesebrouck P, Leroy J. How idiopathic is idiopathic external hydrocephalus? *Developmental Medicine and Child Neurology*. 1991;33(3):274–6.

43. Miller M, Ward T, Stolfi A, Ayoub D. Overrepresentation of multiple birth pregnancies in young infants with four metabolic bone disorders: Further evidence that fetal bone loading is a critical determinant of fetal and young infant bone strength. *Osteoporosis International*. 2014;25(7):1861–73.

44. Nogueira GJ, Zaglul HF. Hypodense extracerebral images on computed-tomography in children: External hydrocephalus. A misnomer. *Child's Nervous System*. 1991;7(6):336–41.

45. Roshan K, Elizabeth C, Chacko A et al. External hydrocephalus: A report of 16 cases from Oman. *Journal of Tropical Pediatrics*. 1998;44(3):153–6.

46. Sahar A. Pseudohydrocephalus: Megalocephaly, increased intracranial pressure and widened subarachnoid space. *Neuropadiatrie*. 1978;9(2):131–9.

47. Binenbaum G, Mirza-George N, Christian CW, Forbes BJ. Odds of abuse associated with retinal hemorrhages in children suspected of child abuse. *Journal of the American Association for Pediatric Ophthalmology*. 2009;13(3):268–72.

48. Binenbaum G, Forbes BJ. The eye in child abuse: Key points on retinal hemorrhages and abusive head trauma. *Pediatric Radiology*. 2014;44 Suppl 4:S571–S577.

49. Levin AV. Retinal hemorrhage in abusive head trauma. *Pediatrics*. 2010;126 (5):961–70.

50. Maguire S, Pickerd N, Farewell D et al. Which clinical features distinguish inflicted from non-inflicted brain injury? A systematic review. *Archives of Disease in Childhood*. 2009;94(11):860–7.

51. Maguire SA, Lumb RC, Kemp AM et al. A systematic review of the differential diagnosis of retinal haemorrhages in children with clinical features associated with child abuse. *Child Abuse Review*. 2013;22(1):29–43.

52. Maguire SA, Watts PO, Shaw AD et al. Retinal haemorrhages and related findings in abusive and non-abusive head trauma: A systematic review. *Eye*. 2013;27 (1):28–36.

53. Morad Y, Wygnansky-Jaffe T, Levin AV. Retinal haemorrhage in abusive head trauma. *Clinical and Experimental Ophthalmology*. 2010;38(5):514–20.

54. Parulekar MV, Elston JS. The evidence base for retinal haemorrhages in shaken baby syndrome. *Developmental Medicine and Child Neurology*. 2008;50 (10):793–4.

55. Pierre-Kahn V, Roche O, Dureau P et al. Ophthalmologic findings in suspected child abuse victims with subdural hematomas. *Ophthalmology*. 2003;110 (9):1718–23.

56. de Terson A. L' hemorrhagie dans le corps vitre au cours de l'hemorrhagie cerebrale. *Clinical Ophthalmology*. 1900;6:309–12.

57. Li LH, Li N, Zhao JY et al. Findings of perinatal ocular examination performed on 3573, healthy full-term newborns. *British Journal of Ophthalmology*. 2013;97 (5):588–91.

58. Nemivant K, Bhalerao A. Retinal haemorrhages in the newborn. *Journal of*

Evolution of Medical and Dental Sciences. 2015;4(46):8028–40.

59. Vinekar A, Govindaraj I, Jayadev C et al. Universal ocular screening of 1021 term infants using wide-field digital imaging in a single public hospital in India: A pilot study. *Acta Ophthalmology.* 2015;93(5): E372–E6.
60. Scheller J. Infantile retinal haemorrhages in the absence of brain and bodily injury. *Acta Paediatrica.* 2017;106(12):1902–4.
61. Pu QL, Li P, Jiang HQ et al. Factors related to retinal haemorrhage in infants born at high risk. *Acta Ophthalmology.* 2017;95(6): E477–E80.
62. Barnes PD, Galaznik J, Gardner H, Shuman M. Infant acute life-threatening event: Dysphagic choking versus nonaccidental injury. *Seminars in Pediatric Neurology.* 2010;17(1):7–11.
63. Kramer K, Goldstein B. Retinal hemorrhages following cardiopulmonary resuscitation. *Clinical Pediatrics.* 1993;32 (6):366–8.
64. Pham H, Enzenauer RW, Elder JE, Levin AV. Retinal hemorrhage after cardiopulmonary resuscitation with chest compressions. *American Journal of Forensic and Medical Pathology.* 2013;34 (2):122–4.
65. Polito A, Eong KGA, Repka MX, Pieramici DJ. Bilateral retinal hemorrhages in a preterm infant with retinopathy at prematurity immediately following cardiopulmonary resuscitation. *Archives of Ophthalmology (Chicago).* 2001;119 (6):913–14.
66. Fledelius HC. Retinal haemorrhages in premature infants: A pathogenetic alternative diagnosis to child abuse. *Acta Ophthalmologica Scandinavica.* 2005;83 (4):424–7.
67. Binenbaum G, Rogers DL, Forbes BJ et al. Patterns of retinal hemorrhage associated with increased intracranial pressure in children. *Pediatrics.* 2013;132(2):e430–e434.
68. Thiblin I, Andersson J, Wester K, Hogberg G, Hogberg U. Retinal haemorrhage in infants investigated for suspected maltreatment is strongly correlated with intracranial pathology. *Acta Paediatrica.* 2022;111(4):808–8.
69. Davies F, Gupta R. Apparent life threatening events in infants presenting to an emergency department. *Emergency Medicine Journal.* 2002;19(1):11–16.
70. Meert K, Telford R, Holubkov R et al. Exploring the safety and efficacy of targeted temperature management amongst infants with out-of-hospital cardiac arrest due to apparent life threatening events. *Resuscitation.* 2016;109:40–8.
71. Gray C, Davies F, Molyneux E. Apparent life-threatening events presenting to a pediatric emergency department. *Pediatric Emergency Care.* 1999;15 (3):195–9.
72. Maytal J, Alvarez LA, Elkin CM, Shinnar S. External hydrocephalus: Radiologic spectrum and differentiation from cerebral atrophy. *American Journal of Roentgenology.* 1987;148(6):1223–30.
73. Fernando S, Obaldo RE, Walsh IR, Lowe LH. Neuroimaging of nonaccidental head trauma: Pitfalls and controversies. *Pediatric Radiology.* 2008;38(8):827–38.
74. Ingraham FD, Matson DD. Subdural hematoma in infancy. *Journal of Pediatrics.* 1944;24(1):1–37.
75. Flom L, Fromkin J, Panigrahy A, Tyler-Kabara E, Berger RP. Development of a screening MRI for infants at risk for abusive head trauma. *Pediatric Radiology.* 2016;46(4):519–26.
76. Raybaud C, Greenberg G. Imaging (normal and abnormal). In *Cerebrospinal fluid disorders.* C Malluci, S Sgouros, eds., 2010, CRC Press, Taylor & Francis, chapter 3.

Chapter 6

Shaken Baby Syndrome or Benign External Hydrocephalus

How Is Abusive Head Trauma Depicted in the Scientific Literature?

Knut Wester, Johan Wikström, and Joseph Scheller

6.1 Introduction

Over the past decades, numerous articles have been published that deal with abusive head injuries in children, mostly in infants. Such traumas have been given a variety of names, most of which imply intent, such as 'shaken baby syndrome' (SBS), 'abusive head trauma/injury' (AHT), 'non-accidental head/brain trauma/injury', and 'inflicted' or even 'intentional injuries'.

Upon reading the relevant literature, the present authors were struck by three facts; first, the lack of solid evidence for the current assumption that the triad of subdural haematoma (SDH), retinal haemorrhages (RH), and encephalopathy could be regarded as pathognomonic for SBS, almost taken as a proof of violent shaking [1–3]. Second, an equally adamant group suggests there is no such thing as a triad. Third, puzzling neuroimaging evidence has been presented as typical for SBS. After having worked with benign external hydrocephalus (BEH) both clinically and scientifically for some years, we were surprised to find that neuroimaging presented as typical for AHT/SBS often also seemed to fit the radiological criteria for external hydrocephalus, described by Dandy back in 1946 [4] and defined radiologically more accurately by Alvarez et al. and Maytal et al. more than three decades ago [5, 6].

As a matter of fact, two almost identical MRI axial images have been presented in the following way: 'Abnormal screening head MRI sequences in a 2-month-old boy with abusive head trauma' (Flom et al.'s figure 6.3a in [3]) and as 'macrocrania, raised ICP' and 'preexisting idiopathic macrocrania (+3 SD), without other past medical history, who presented with a 10-day duration syndrome of raised intracranial pressure with increased head circumference' (Vinchon et al.'s figure 6.2 in [7]). See Figure 6.1 for comparison of these two illustrations; see also a similar scan in Wittschieber et al.'s figure 6.3 B [8], described as strongly suggestive of child abuse (AHT).

Benign external hydrocephalus is regarded as a subtype of hydrocephalus that develops during infancy with a rapid increase of the head circumference (HC) during the first months of life, in most cases from almost normal values at birth [9–11]. According to Alvarez et al. and Maytal et al., the condition is characterised by three separate neuroimaging features: enlarged subarachnoid spaces, especially overlying the frontal lobes; normal – or most often – moderately enlarged ventricles; and a characteristic widening of the frontal inter-hemispheric fissure [5, 6].

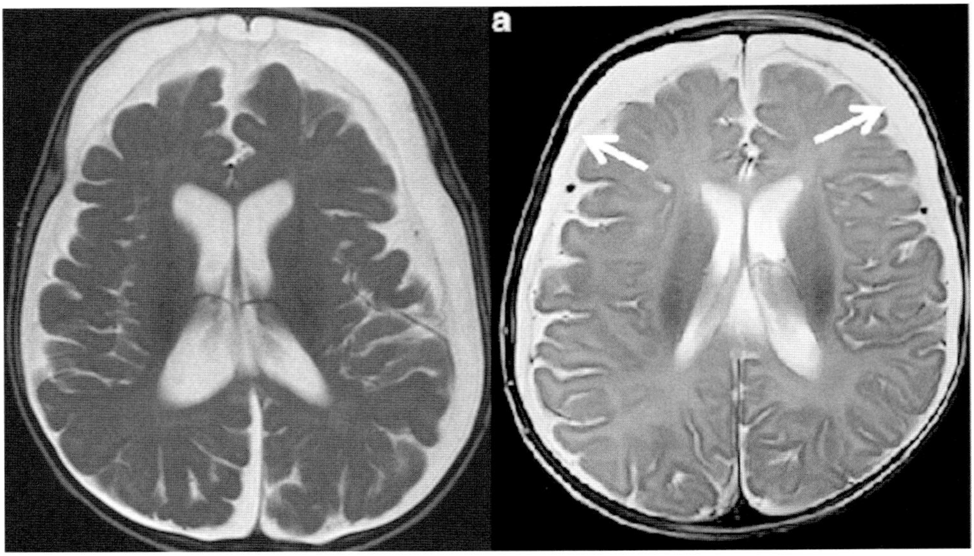

Figure 6.1 MRIs presented as a complication to external hydrocephalus (left) [7] and as typical of child abuse [3] (right). Please note the subdural fluid, which appears a little whiter than the greyish CSF closer to cortex, does not compress the cortical convolutions or the ventricles and there is no midline shift. White arrows are pointing to the arachnoid. Both illustrations are reproduced with the kind permission of the publishers of *Child's Nervous System* and *Pediatric Radiology*, respectively.

Other terms have been used to describe the presence of an excess of cerebrospinal fluid (CSF) around the brain – for example, 'benign enlargement of the subarachnoid spaces' (BESS) [12, 13] and 'macrocephaly' [14, 15]. For details see Chapter 5. For the sake of specificity, this condition will be referred to as BEH in this chapter.

Other infants have an excess of fluid between the brain and skull that is outside the arachnoid membrane. This condition too has been given multiple names, including 'subdural hygroma' [16], 'subdural effusion' [17], and 'benign subdural collections' [18]. Again, for specificity's sake, we will use the term 'subdural hygroma'.

Some of the names suggest these conditions are benign; in most cases that may be true, but even in children with a seemingly benign course, the conditions may leave some imprint, including cognitive problems [19]. However, other reports indicate considerably more serious consequences such as marked dyscognition [20], epilepsy [12, 21–25], and, above all, subdural haematomas (SDH), as described by many authors [7, 12, 21–33]. It is well known that BEH and subdural hygromas predispose to SDH.

The subarachnoid space enlargement in BEH and subdural hygromas seem to gradually decrease and disappear as the infant grows older [6, 20, 34, 35]. Ventricular dilatation of varying magnitude has been described in many infants with BEH [6, 20, 23, 35–43]; most of the reports conclude these infants also have enlarged ventricles. One article indicates that approximately 80% of the infants had enlarged ventricles [11]. The frontal portion of the inter-hemispheric fissure appears to be the first subarachnoid compartment to enlarge, followed by the fluid space over the frontal convexities; ventricular dilation seems to appear later [6]. For an extensive review of the condition, see Zahl et al. [9].

In most cases of suspected AHT, it is the person who cared for the infant when the baby became critically ill who is assumed to have shaken the baby and is consequently accused because it is assumed that the shaking took place close to the time of the acute worsening of the clinical condition As the neuroimaging often is performed shortly after the acute worsening, one would expect these early CT and/or MRI scans to show features compatible with an acute intracranial traumatic haemorrhagic event such as an acute subdural haematoma (ASDH), and that this haematoma had caused a compression of the ipsilateral brain and ventricle with a midline shift when unilateral, and compression of both hemispheres and lateral ventricles if bilateral, as one usually sees in ASDHs.

In this chapter, we try to find out how SDH, assumed to be caused by SBS/AHT, has been presented radiologically in the relevant literature. More precisely, we wanted to see if the illustrations looked like a 'classical' ASDH with or without brain contusions or, conversely, how often the presented images showed radiological signs compatible with BEH.

6.2 Material and Methods

This chapter is based on a review of relevant articles that present neuroimaging illustrations of what is claimed to be the result of violent shaking or AHT. The review was performed by the authors, who are specialists in neuro-medicine: a neurosurgeon experienced in paediatric neurosurgery, a paediatric neurologist licensed in interpretation of neuroimaging, and a specialist in neuroradiology. CT or MRI scans showing signs of impact such as localised bruises, swelling of the head, or cranial fractures were not included as the main object of this study was to find out how brain injuries caused by alleged shaking alone is depicted in the literature.

The search was limited to articles that may give an updated view on the topic; only articles published after January 2008 were therefore included in the survey. Besides this limitation in time, the only inclusion criteria were that the publications had been written in English or German and that they contained neuroimaging examples of SDH associated with or caused by violent shaking. In the literature search (Web of Science), the following words and combinations were used: (subdural OR intracerebral OR intracranial OR subarachnoi* OR head OR brain) AND (haematoma OR bleeding OR hygroma OR injur* OR traum*) AND (chil* OR infan* OR kid OR bab*) AND (abusive OR nonaccidental OR inflict* OR shaken) AND (CT OR MRI OR imag*).

Cases were assigned to one of four categories: (1) BEH, (2) possible BEH (3) no evidence of BEH or expansive ASDH or inconclusive, or (4) expansive ASDH. When looking for cases that could be BEH, the features described as typical for external hydrocephalus were emphasised: 'prominent widened subarachnoid space frontally', 'enlarged interhemispheric fissure', and 'mild ventricular enlargement' [6]. In addition, a preserved subarachnoid space despite an overlying SDH was regarded as indicative of BEH. Cases with signs of BEH but that were difficult to interpret – for instance, because the ventricles were not visualised – were regarded as possible BEH. Criteria for an expansive ASDH were an SDH with higher attenuation than adjacent parenchyma that caused compression of adjacent gyri or a midline shift. Only illustrations showing the results of first obtained scanning were included; late scans and inconclusive scans that did not allow a precise assessment were not. All authors reviewed all the illustrations independently, after which a decision on the classification of each illustration was reached. The neuroradiologist had the final say in this decision.

6.3 Results

A total of 63 articles with 172 illustrations of alleged abuse were identified, 59 through the Web of Science search, and 4 through manual search in the references found in the literature search [2, 3, 8, 44–103]. Many of the illustrations did not allow a definite conclusion.

A detailed description of the survey is presented in Table 6.1. A substantial proportion (59/172 (34.3%)) of the illustrations that were presented as evidence or examples of child abuse seemed to us compatible with a BEH condition ('BEH-like') complicated with a hygroma/chronic subdural haematoma (CSDH) with or without acute blood elements, whereas findings compatible with an expansive ASDH ('ASDH-like') were found in only 24/170 (14.0%). Another 32 images (18.6%) raised a weaker suspicion of BEH and findings not compatible with either BEH or ASDH or inconclusive images were found in 57 illustrations (33.1%). Information about gender and age was not available for all children, but, where this information was given, males were overrepresented in all groups: 78 males (71.6%) and 31 females (28.8%). Mean age was 4.2 months in the BEH group and 17.6 months in the ASDH group; for details see later in this chapter. An acute SDH is shown in Figure 6.2.

The BEH-like illustrations shared more or less the features described by Alvarez et al. and Maytal et al. as typical for external hydrocephalus [6] (see Figure 6.3). Fifteen of these BEH-like illustrations are shown in Figure 6.4.

For the BEH-like group, the widened subarachnoid and subdural spaces appeared bilaterally and there was no midline shift, not even in cases with a predominant unilateral chronic or subacute haematoma. Most often the subdural effusions seemed to contain subacute or chronic blood rather than acute, as can be seen in CSDH. In some of the illustrations, acute coagulated blood clots could be seen in the subdural effusions, then, however, only as minor proportions of the total subdural fluid volume. Even in cases with thick CSDHs, there still appeared to be a rim of CSF between the haematoma and the cortical surface, and the CSDH had not compressed the cortical surface or the lateral ventricles that remained normal or slightly enlarged as is the case in BEH. On the other hand, the 24 illustrations that seemed compatible with an ASDH all exhibited ipsilateral cortical and/or ventricular compression and a midline shift with compression also of the contralateral subarachnoid space, as one would expect in a unilateral ASDH, or bilateral compression of the cortices and ventricles as expected in bilateral ASDH.

Age

In the BEH-like group, age was indicated for 46 patients; the mean age in these infants was 4.2 months (median 4 months). Only 3 were older than 6 months; the remaining 43 were ≤ 6 months (Figure 6.5). Age was given for a total of 35 gender-specified children (21 boys and 14 girls). The mean age in boys and girls was 4.1 months and 4.4 months, respectively. In the ASDH-like group, age was given for 21 children. The mean age in this group was four times higher than in the BEH group –17.6 months with a median of 16 months (Figure 6.5).

Gender

Gender was given for 37 children in the BEH-like group: 23 boys (62.1%) and 14 girls (37.8%). In the much smaller ASDH-like group, gender was indicated for only 16 children: 13 boys (81.3%) and 3 girls (18.8%). Seven of the boys in the ASDH group were older than 12 months (mean age 30 months). In the 'possible BEH-like group', there were 14 boys (70%) and 6 girls (30%).

Table 6.1 Overview of the included illustrations, authors, publications, figure/case numbers, sex, and age (in months)

No.	Author, year [reference]	BEH-like illustration	Possible BEH-like	Undetermined	ASDH-like illustration	Comments
1.	Rolfes 2018 [87]		**Fig. 6 C/D/H** Male 2 **Fig. 9** 3			
2.	Elliott 2017 [55]			**Case 2–4** Male 18 Male 6 Female 19	**Fig 1 case 1** Male 16	
3.	Vinchon 2017 [99]		**Fig. 6** Male 3	**Fig. 3** Male 2		
4.	Kralik 2017 [72]	**Fig. 3** Female 3				
5.	Kralik 2017 [73]	**Fig. 1** Infant 4				Gender not given
6.	Pfeifer 2017 [83]	**Fig. 7**				No patient information given
7.	Knox 2016 [71]	**Fig. 3** Female 8				
8.	Flom 2016 [3]	**Fig. 3** Male 2		**Fig. 2** Male 2.5		

Table 6.1 (cont.)

No.	Author, year [reference]	BEH-like illustration	Possible BEH-like	Undetermined	ASDH-like illustration	Comments
9.	Girard 2016 [62]	**Fig. 12** Female 3		**Fig. 5/9** Male 1.5 **Fig. 8** Male 3 **Fig.11** Female 4	**Fig. 7** Male 4 years	
10.	Reith 2016 [86]	**Fig. 1** Infant of unspec. age **Fig. 2** Infant 3 **Fig. 3** Infant 2.5 **Fig. 4** Infant 2 **Fig. 5** Female 2.5				Gender not given for figs. 1–3 Age not given for fig. 1
11.	Shekdar 2016 [90]	**Fig. 4** No info	**Fig. 7** No info **Fig. 6** No info	**Fig. 5** No info		
12.	Choudhary 2015 [112]	**Fig. 6** Male 2 **Fig. 7** Male 3	**Fig. 4** Male 7 **Fig 5** Female 5			

13.	Langford 2015 [74]			**Fig. 3** Infant 3 weeks **Fig. 4** Infant 2	**Fig. 1** Infant 16	No detailed patient information given
14.	Feldman 2015 [57]	**Fig. 2** Male 2	**Fig. 1** Female 1 **Fig. 3** Male 10			
15.	Hahnemann 2015 [66]		**Fig. 1** No info **Fig. 2** No info			
16.	Hsieh 2015 [68]	**Fig. 4A** Male 4 **Fig. 4B** Female 4	**Fig. 5B** Female 9	**Fig. 5A** Male 10 **Fig. 10** Male 2 weeks	**Fig. 3B** Male 11	
17.	Nishimoto 2015 [76]		**Fig. 4 Case 1** Female 2			
18.	Wittschieber2015 [8]	**Fig. 1** Male 2 **Fig. 3** Female 5				
19.	Yilmaz 2015 [100]	**Fig. 1 Case 1** Female 2 **Fig. 2 Case 2** Male 6				

Table 6.1 (cont.)

No.	Author, year [reference]	BEH-like illustration	Possible BEH-like	Undetermined	ASDH-like illustration	Comments
20.	Adamsbaum 2014 [46]	**Fig. 4** Female 6 **Fig. 6** Male 6 **Fig. 7** Female 2 **Fig. 10** Male 6		**Fig. 8** Female 5 **Fig. 2** Male 1.5 **Fig. 5** Male 3	**Fig. 1** Male 8 **Fig. 9** Male 3	
21.	Kadom 2014 [70]		**Fig. 8** Male 14	**Fig. 4** Male 4	**Fig. 9** Male 3 years	
22.	Vásquez 2014 [96]	**Fig. 1** Female 3 **Fig. 6** Male 6 **Fig. 10** Male 3		**Fig. 11** Male 7 weeks **Fig. 9** Male 5		
23.	Greiner 2013 [63]	**Fig. 1 Case 3** Female 8 **Fig. 2 Case 4** Male 3				
24.	Caylan 2013 [54]	**Fig. 3 Case 3** Male 3		**Fig. 1** **Case 1** Female 3		
25.	Binenbaum 2013 [51]	**Fig. 1A** Infant 4				

26.	Sieswerda-Hoogendoorn 2012 [113]			**Fig. 6** Female 24	**Fig. 5** Male 3years	
27.	Tysiak 2012 [94]	**Fig. 2** Infant 5				Gender not given
28.	Van Rijn 2011 [95]		**Fig. 7** Male 1.5	**Fig. 8** Female 2	**Fig. 6** Female 29	
29.	Rajaram 2011 [85]	**Fig. 3** Infant 6 **Fig. 8** No info		**Fig. 4** Infant 3 **Fig. 6** Infant 3		Gender not given
30.	Erfurt 2011 [56]	**Fig. 16**		**Fig. 13**		No patient information given
31.	Barnes 2011 [48]	**Fig. 4** Infant 6 **Fig. 15** Infant 5		**Fig. 2** Infant 5 weeks **Fig. 7** Infant 28 **Fig. 8** Infant 14	**Fig. 3** Infant 8 **Fig. 6** Infant 21 **Fig. 9** Infant 20 **Fig. 11** Female 9 **Fig. 16** Infant 16	
32.	Ashwal 2010 [47]		**Fig. 1b** Male 5 **Fig. 2** Female 3	**Fig. 1a** Male 2 **Fig. 5** Infant 7		

Table 6.1 (cont.)

No.	Author, year [reference]	BEH-like illustration	Possible BEH-like	Undetermined	ASDH-like illustration	Comments
33.	Adamsbaum 2010 [44]	**Fig. 1** Infant 5		**Fig. 2** Infant 6 **Fig. 3** Infant 6		No gender information given
34.	Adamsbaum 2010b [45]	**Fig. 4** Male 5		**Fig. 5** No info		
35.	Foerster 2009 [59]		**'Figure'** No info			
36.	Hedlund 2009 [67]	**Fig. 4** **Figs. 6, 7**	**Fig. 3** **Fig. 5** **Fig. 9**	**Fig. 1**		No patient information given
37	Matschke 2009 [75]	**Fig. 2A** Male	**Fig. 2B** Male			
38.	Vezina 2009 [97]		**Fig. 3b/c**	**Fig. 1** No info **Fig. 2** Infant 4		No detailed patient information given
39.	Fernando 2008 [58]			**Fig. 7** Male 12 **Fig. 18** Male 5 **Fig. 1** Male 5	**Fig. 10** Male 14	

40.	Stöver 2008 [92]		**Fig. 9** Infant 3	**Fig. 8** No info		
41.	Beez 2018 [49]			**Fig. 1** Male 2		
42.	Berger 2020 [50]	**Fig. 1** Male 2.4				
43.	Boehnke 2018 [53]	**Fig. 2** Male 5				
44.	Gencturk 2019 [61]	**Fig. 4** Female 4			**Fig. 5** Male 41	
45.	Gunda 2019 [64]	**Fig. 6** Male 4 **Fig. 7** Male 12	**Fig. 5** Male 9 **Fig. 8/10** Male 10 w			
46.	Haas-Lude 2019 [65]	**Case 2** Female 5		**Case 1** Male 4		
47.	O´Brien 2018 [78]	**Fig. 29** **Fig. 26**		**Fig. 25**	**Fig. 30** **Fig. 27** **Fig. 31**	Age and gender not reported
48.	Orru 2018 [80]	**Fig. 1B/C** Female 6				
49.	Orru 2018 [81] (J Neuroimaging)			**Fig. 1** Male 3 **Fig. 2** Male 4		

Table 6.1 (cont.)

No.	Author, year [reference]	BEH-like illustration	Possible BEH-like	Undetermined	ASDH-like illustration	Comments
50.	Palmer 2019 [82]	**Figs. 2, 3**				Age and gender not reported
51.	Ronning 2018 [88]		**Fig. 1/2** Male 5			
52.	Saigal 2018 [89]			**Fig. 14** 2 years		
53.	Takeda 2020 [93]				**Fig. 1** Male 5	
54.	Blumfield 2020 [52]			**Fig. 3** Male 9 weeks **Fig. 5 c** Male 4	**Fig. 2** Male 7	
55.	Cartocci 2021 [60]			**Fig. 4** Infant		Age and gender not reported
56.	Hung 2020 [69]			**Fig. 1 c, d** Female 12		
57.	Oates 2020 [77]			**Fig. 2a** Male 2 **Fig. 6** Male 1		
58.	Orman 2020 [79]		**Fig. 7** Female 2			

59.	Porto 2021 [84]		**Fig. 1** Infant 5	**Fig. 2** 2 years		Gender not reported. Fig. 2 acute or subacute?
60.	Vilanilam 2021 [98]	**Fig. 2** Male 4	**Fig. 1** Male 5 **Fig. 3** Male 5			
61.	Wittschieber 2019 [101]	**Fig. 1c** Male 4 **Fig. 1d** Male 3	**Fig. 1i** Male 4	**Fig. 1b** Male 2 **Fig. 1f** Female 4 **Fig. 1g** Male 7	**Fig. 1a** Male 2 **Fig. 1e** Male 19	
62.	Wittschieber 2021 [102]			**Fig. 1** Male 2		
63.	Wright 2019 [103]	**Fig 2a** Male 3			**Fig. 1** Female 4	Fig. 2 had also enlarged head (+2.26 z-score)
	Total (males/females)	59 (23/14)	32 (14/6)	57 (28/8)	24 (13/3)	

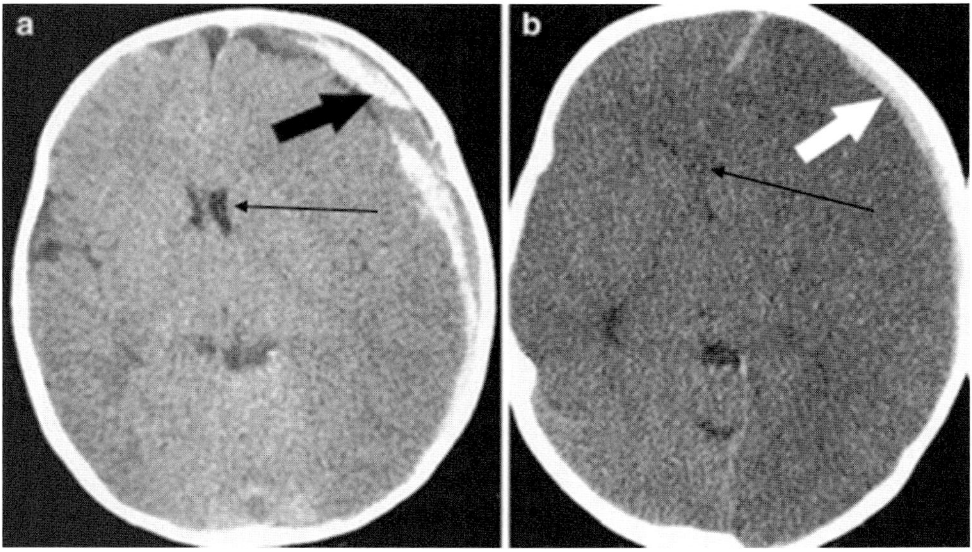

Figure 6.2 A typical ASDH in a small child (thick arrows). Left: shortly after the head injury. Right: 24 hours later. In both images the brain midline is dislocated to the opposite side and the ventricles are compressed (narrow black arrows). Note the marked brain oedema beneath the SDH immediately and then more pronounced after 24 hours (darker grey) in the compressed hemisphere. Figure reproduced from [74] with permission from Springer Nature, *Pediatric Radiology* through Copyright Clearance Center.

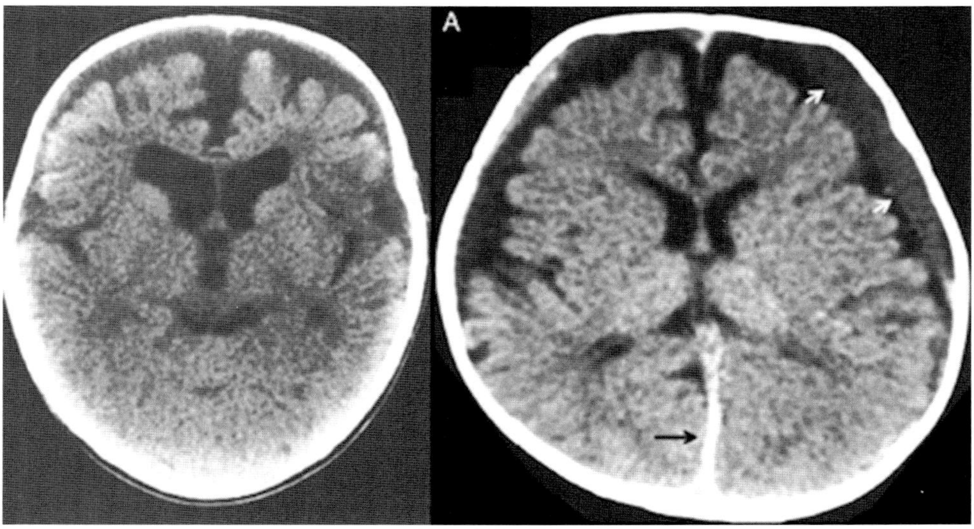

Figure 6.3 CT scans presented as typical for external hydrocephalus (left) [6] and child abuse (right) [46], respectively. Please note the widened frontal inter-hemispheric fissure (regarded as typical for external hydrocephalus) in both scans. Please also note the subdural haematoma/hygroma over the left hemisphere (white arrows) in the alleged abuse case does not compress the cortical surface or the ipsilateral ventricle, nor does it cause a midline shift. Both illustrations are reproduced with the kind permission of the publishers of *American Journal of Neuroradiology* and *Pediatric Radiology*, respectively.

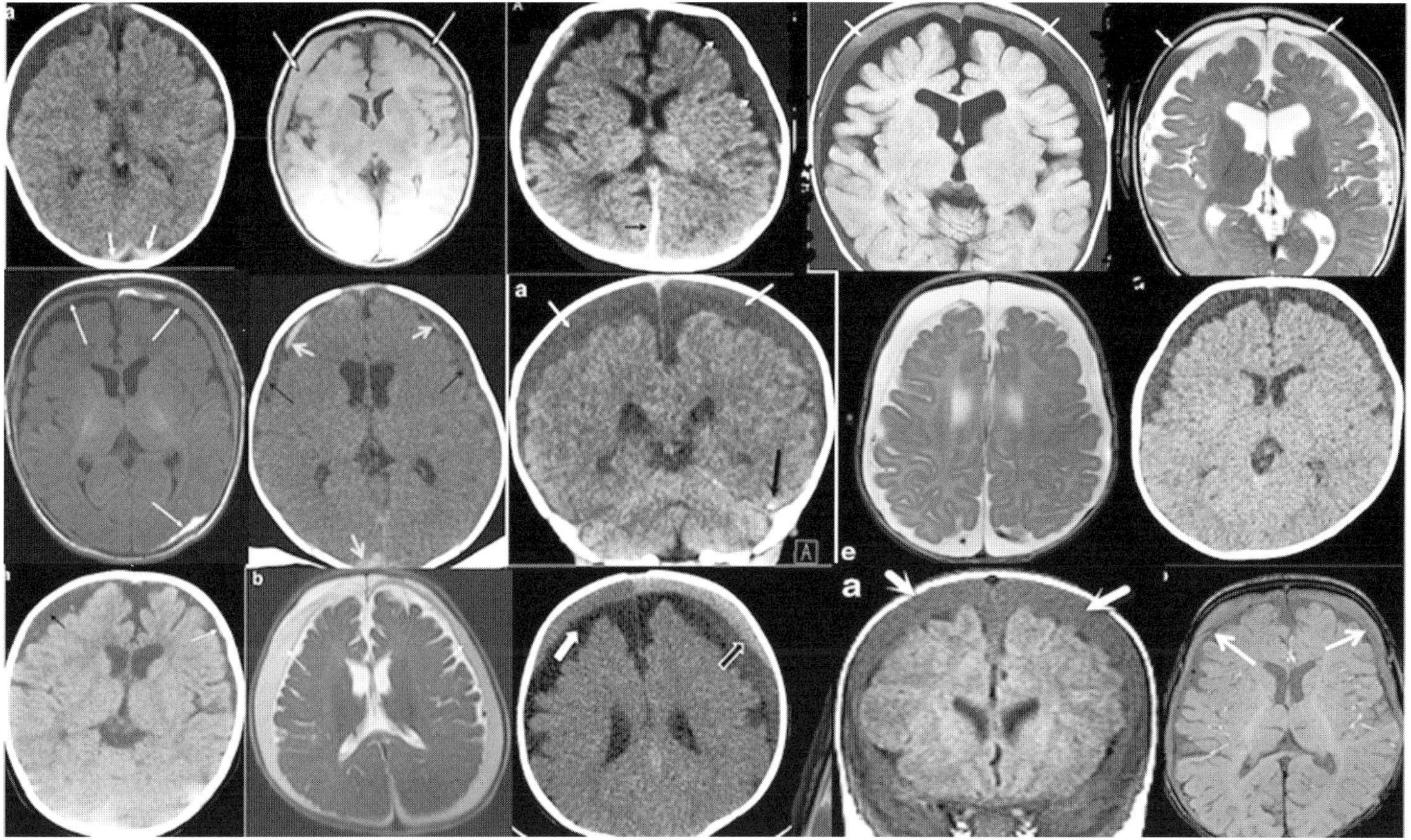

Figure 6.4 Examples of some of the BEH-like illustrations, numbered according to case numbers (#) given in Table 1 and presented from left to right. Bottom row:#4 Figs. 1 and 3, #6 Fig. 7,#12 Fig. 6,#8 Fig. 3. Middle row:#30 Fig. 16,#11 Fig. 4,#12 Fig. 7a,#19 Fig. 1,#20 Fig. 4. Upper row:#22 Fig 10,#24 Fig. 3,#33 Fig. 1,#36 Fig. 7,#36 Fig. 4

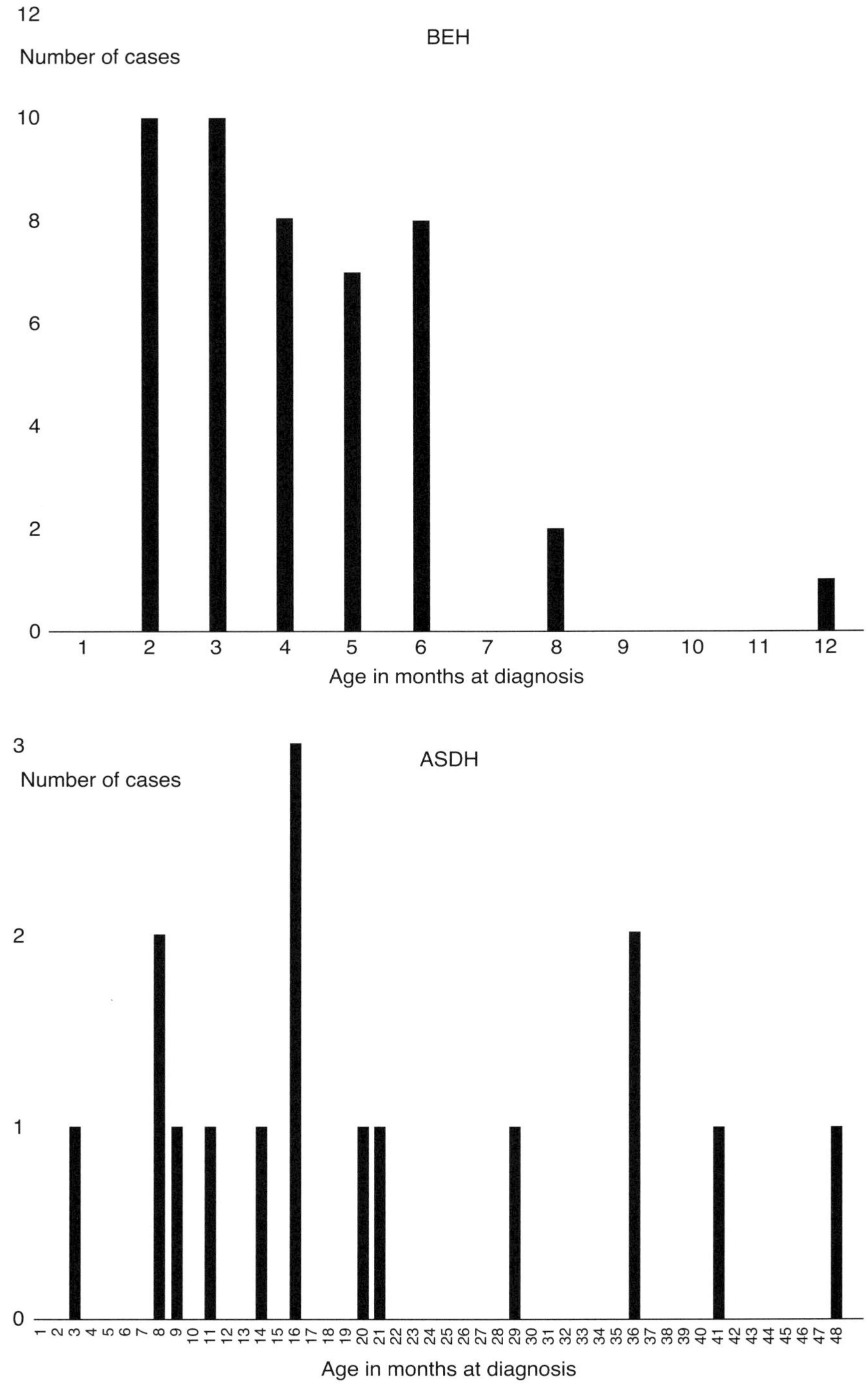

Figure 6.5 Age distribution for BEH-like (upper) and ASDH-like illustrations (lower). Please note the age intervals on the X-axes are different; the age axes cover ages from 0 to 12 months (BEH – upper) and from 0 to 48 months (ASDH – lower).

6.4 Discussion

The findings in the present literature survey, which emphasises how SDH following alleged child abuse has been depicted in the literature, are indeed surprising. Contrary to what one might expect, many illustrations appeared to lack the features one would expect in a haematoma caused by some *acute* external trauma. Above all, acute, coagulated blood was not prevailing in these illustrations; on the contrary, the subdural, extracerebral fluid seemed more compatible with a hygroma or CSDH, sometimes with small amounts of coagulated blood. Moreover, the subdural fluid collections did not appear to compress the cortical surface or the lateral ventricles, which mostly seemed to be of normal size or slightly enlarged, as is often seen in BEH, neither did they cause midline shift, not even in large, predominantly unilateral fluid collections. In short, this group of illustrations looked more like external hydrocephalus complicated by subdural bleeding. A large series of publications has confirmed this predisposition for SDH in BEH infants [7, 12, 21, 22, 24, 25, 27, 28, 30, 33, 41, 104, 105]. Especially the large series of infants published by Lee et al. demonstrates this predisposition for SDH in 'macrocephaly'; their figures 6.1 through 6.4 are confusingly like the ones presented as examples of SBS or abusive head injury in the publications included in the present survey [106]. This predisposition has been suggested to represent a pitfall in the diagnosis of abusive head trauma [12, 24, 25, 43, 107, 108].

Fewer of the illustrations had features that seemed more compatible with a 'classical' ASDH, containing mostly acute, coagulated blood. When unilateral, the ASDH was seen to compress the ipsilateral cortical surface and lateral ventricle, in addition to causing a midline shift. When the ASDH was bilateral, both cortices and lateral ventricles were compressed.

The CT scans shown in Adamsbaum et al. [44] (their figure 1) show almost exactly the same features as Maytal et al.'s [6] figure 1: a prominent widened subarachnoid space frontally, an enlarged frontal inter-hemispheric fissure, and normal or mildly enlarged ventricles. Except for what appears to be a large left-sided chronic SDH/fluid collection that does not cause midline shift, compression of the ipsilateral or contralateral cortical surfaces, or compression of the ipsilateral ventricle, the Adamsbaum figure bears a striking resemblance to the figure Maytal et al. presented decades ago as typical for external hydrocephalus (see Figure 6.2 in the present chapter for comparison). Similarly, if one compares the MRI scans presented in Vinchon et al.'s figure 2 [7] and Flom et al.'s figure 3 [3] presented as compatible with a haemorrhagic complication to external hydrocephalus and abuse, respectively, it is difficult to see the large differences (Figure 6.1).

It was a rather unexpected finding in this study that such a large fraction of neuroimaging illustrations of alleged SBS appeared more compatible with a BEH complicated by a CSDH than with an ASDH. This striking similarity makes one wonder whether a BEH complicated by an SDH in certain cases has been misdiagnosed as caused by abuse. A series of articles has discussed or even demonstrated the possibility of misdiagnosing a BEH-related SDH as SBS/AHT [12, 24, 25, 107, 109–111].

Another thought-provoking similarity between the BEH-like illustrations presented here and BEH is the marked male preponderance. The male preponderance for BEH is well known and has been described in a series of publications [11, 20, 23]. Similarly thought-provoking are the marked differences in age distribution between the two groups of neuroimaging illustrations. Why should BEH-like illustrations be found only for infants – and mostly during the first 6 months of life – and the ASDH-like scans be distributed over a much larger age span? Most infants who develop BEH seem to be born with normal head circumference, which then starts to increase abnormally fast during the first months of life [10, 11]. The infants with the BEH-like illustrations reported in this chapter were with three exceptions 6 months or younger. The majority were 4 months or younger, thus matching what is known about BEH with or without subdural haematomas or hygromas [10, 11, 20, 106].

The similarities in radiological appearance, age, and gender distribution between these two groups of infants – BEH and alleged SBS/AHT – raise a crucial question: are all of these allegedly shaken babies really shaken babies?

In criminal cases that involve violence and bodily harm, guilt must be proven beyond reasonable doubt in most civilised countries. The striking similarities between illustrations that are claimed to be typical of abuse and external hydrocephalus render it difficult from a medical point of view to rule out any such reasonable doubt.

A weakness of this study is of course that the present authors had limited access to clinical information or the complete series of neuroimaging documentation. On the other hand, the included illustrations were picked by the authors of the included articles to depict SBS/AHT – without any reservations. Our idea was to present what is published as examples of SBS and how we perceived these illustrations.

In conclusion, about one third of the illustrations that claimed to portray AHT/SBS in the reviewed literature seemed more compatible with BEH complicated with a chronic SDH than with an acutely inflicted injury. If our findings reflect a similar wrongful diagnostic workup in criminal court cases, it is indeed frightening.

References

1. Duhaime AC, Alario AJ, Lewander WJ et al. Head injury in very young children: Mechanisms, injury types, and ophthalmologic findings in 100 hospitalized patients younger than 2 years of age. *Pediatrics*. 1992;90(2):179–85.
2. Choudhary AK, Servaes S, Slovis TL et al. Consensus statement on abusive head trauma in infants and young children. *Pediatric Radiology*. 2018;48(8):1048–65.
3. Flom L, Fromkin J, Panigrahy A, Tyler-Kabara E, Berger RP. Development of a screening MRI for infants at risk for abusive head trauma. *Pediatric Radiology*. 2016;46 (4):519–26.
4. Dandy WE. Treatment of an unusual subdural hydroma (external hydrocephalus). *Archives of Surgery (Chicago)*. 1946;52(4):421–8.
5. Alvarez LA, Maytal J, Shinnar S. Idiopathic external hydrocephalus: Natural history and relationship to benign familial macrocephaly. *Pediatrics*. 1986;77(6):901–7.
6. Maytal J, Alvarez LA, Elkin CM, Shinnar S. External hydrocephalus: Radiologic spectrum and differentiation from cerebral atrophy. *American Journal of Roentgenology*. 1987;148(6):1223–30.
7. Vinchon M. Subdural hematoma in infants: Can it occur spontaneously? Data from a prospective series and critical review of the literature by Vinchon et al. Reply. *Child's Nervous System*. 2010;26(11):1195–1205.
8. Wittschieber D, Karger B, Niederstadt T, Pfeiffer H, Hahnemann ML. Subdural hygromas in abusive head trauma: Pathogenesis, diagnosis, and forensic implications. *American Journal of Neuroradiology*. 2015;36(3):432–9.
9. Zahl SM, Egge A, Helseth E, Wester K. Benign external hydrocephalus: A review, with emphasis on management. *Neurosurgery Review*. 2011;34(4):417–32.
10. Zahl SM, Egge A, Helseth E, Wester K. Clinical, radiological, and demographic details of benign external hydrocephalus: A

population-based study. *Pediatric Neurology*. 2019;96:53–7.

11. Wiig US, Zahl SM, Egge A, Helseth E, Wester K. Epidemiology of benign external hydrocephalus in Norway: A population-based study. *Pediatric Neurology*. 2017;73:36–41.
12. McNeely PD, Atkinson JD, Saigal G, O'Gorman AM, Farmer JP. Subdural hematomas in infants with benign enlargement of the subarachnoid spaces are not pathognomonic for child abuse. *American Journal of Neuroradiology*. 2006;27(8):1725–8.
13. Ment LR, Duncan CC, Geehr R. Benign enlargement of the subarachnoid spaces in the infant. *Journal of Neurosurgery*. 1981;54 (4):504–8.
14. Korbin MA. Macrocephaly: Report of case verified by ventriculography and autopsy. *Bulletin of the Los Angeles Neurological Society*. 1954;19(3):178–85.
15. Riley HD, Smith WR. Macrocephaly, pseudopapilledema and multiple hemangiomata: A previously undescribed heredofamilial syndrome. *Pediatrics*. 1960;26(2):293–300.
16. Dickinson EH, Pastor BH. 2 cases of acute subdural hygroma simulating massive intracranial hemorrhage. *Journal of Neurosurgery*. 1948;5(1):98–101.
17. Kumar R, Singhal N, Mahapatra AK. Traumatic subdural effusions in children following minor head injury. *Child's Nervous System*. 2008;24(12):1391–6.
18. Robertson WC Jr., Chun RW, Orrison WW, Sackett JF. Benign subdural collections of infancy. *Journal of Pediatrics*. 1979;94(3):382–6.
19. Mikkelsen R, Rodevand LN, Wiig US, et al. Neurocognitive and psychosocial function in children with benign external hydrocephalus (BEH): A long-term follow-up study. *Child's Nervous System*. 2017;33 (1):91–9.
20. Muenchberger H, Assaad N, Joy P, Brunsdon R, Shores EA. Idiopathic macrocephaly in the infant: Long-term neurological and neuropsychological outcome. *Child's Nervous System*. 2006;22 (10):1242–8.
21. Ghosh PS, Ghosh D. Subdural hematoma in infants without accidental or nonaccidental injury: Benign external hydrocephalus, a risk factor. *Clinical Pediatrics*. 2011;50(10):897–903.
22. Hellbusch LC. Benign extracerebral fluid collections in infancy: Clinical presentation and long-term follow-up. *Journal of Neurosurgery*. 2007;107(2 Suppl):119–25.
23. Laubscher B, Deonna T, Uske A, Van MG. Primitive megalencephaly in children: Natural history, medium term prognosis with special reference to external hydrocephalus. *European Journal of Pediatrics*. 1990;149(7):502–7.
24. Miller D, Barnes P, Miller M. The significance of macrocephaly or enlarging head circumference in infants with the triad: Further evidence of mimics of shaken baby syndrome. *American Journal of Forensic Medicine and Pathology*. 2015;36 (2):111–20.
25. Piatt JH Jr. A pitfall in the diagnosis of child abuse: External hydrocephalus, subdural hematoma, and retinal hemorrhages. *Neurosurgery in Focus*. 1999;7(4):e4.
26. Azais M, Echenne B. Idiopathic subarachnoid space enlargement (benign external hydrocephalus) in infants. *Annales de pediatrie*. 1992;39(9):550–8.
27. Gout A, Gautier I, Bellaiche M et al. Idiopathic subarachnoid space enlargement in infancy: Simple anatomic variant or hemorrhagic risk factor? *Archives de pediatrie*. 1997;4(10):983–7.
28. Kapila A, Trice J, Spies WG, Siegel BA, Gado MH. Enlarged cerebrospinal fluid spaces in infants with subdural hematomas. *Radiology*. 1982;142 (3):669–72.
29. McKeag H, Christian CW, Rubin D et al. Subdural hemorrhage in pediatric patients with enlargement of the subarachnoid spaces: Clinical article. *Journal of Neurosurgery: Pediatric*. 2013;11 (4):438–44.

30. Mori K, Sakamoto T, Nishimura K, Fujiwara K. Subarachnoid fluid collection in infants complicated by subdural hematoma. *Child's Nervous System*. 1993;9 (5):282–4.

31. Papasian NC, Frim DM. A theoretical model of benign external hydrocephalus that predicts a predisposition towards extra-axial hemorrhage after minor head trauma. *Pediatric Neurosurgery*. 2000;33 (4):188–93.

32. Pittman T. Significance of a subdural hematoma in a child with external hydrocephalus. *Pediatric Neurosurgery*. 2003;39(2):57–9.

33. Ravid S, Maytal J. External hydrocephalus: A probable cause for subdural hematoma in infancy. *Pediatric Neurology*. 2003;28 (2):139–41.

34. Caldarelli M, Di Rocco C, Romani R. Surgical treatment of chronic subdural hygromas in infants and children. *Acta Neurochirurgica*. 2002;144(6):581–8.

35. Kumar R. External hydrocephalus in small children. *Child's Nervous System*. 2006;22 (10):1237–41.

36. Alper G, Ekinci G, Yilmaz Y et al. Magnetic resonance imaging characteristics of benign macrocephaly in children. *Journal of Child Neurology*. 1999;14(10):678–82.

37. Barlow CF. CSF dynamics in hydrocephalus: With special attention to external hydrocephalus. *Brain Development*. 1984;6(2):119–27.

38. Carolan PL, Mclaurin RL, Towbin RB, Towbin JA, Egelhoff JC. Benign extraaxial collections of infancy. *Pediatric Neuroscience*. 1986;12(3):140–4.

39. Castro-Gago M, Perez-Gomez C, Novo-Rodriguez MI et al. [Benign idiopathic external hydrocephalus (benign subdural collection) in 39 children: Its natural history and relation to familial macrocephaly]. *Review of Neurology*. 2005;40(9):513–17.

40. Gherpelli JL, Scaramuzzi V, Manreza ML, Diament AJ. Follow-up study of macrocephalic children with enlargement of the subarachnoid space. *Arquivos neuropsiquiatria*. 1992;50(2):156–62.

41. Medina LS, Frawley K, Zurakowski D et al. Children with macrocrania: Clinical and imaging predictors of disorders requiring surgery. *American Journal of Neuroradiology*. 2001;22(3):564–70.

42. Prassopoulos P, Cavouras D, Golfinopoulos S, Nezi M. The size of the intraventricular and extraventricular cerebrospinal fluid compartments in children with idiopathic benign widening of the frontal subarachnoid space. *Neuroradiology*. 1995;37(5):418–21.

43. Robertson WC Jr, Gomez MR. External hydrocephalus: Early finding in congenital communicating hydrocephalus. *Archives of Neurology*. 1978;35(8):541–4.

44. Adamsbaum C, Grabar S, Mejean N, Rey-Salmon C. Abusive head trauma: Judicial admissions highlight violent and repetitive shaking. *Pediatrics*. 2010;126 (3):546–55.

45. Adamsbaum C, Mejean N, Merzoug V, Rey-Salmon C. How to explore and report children with suspected non-accidental trauma. *Pediatric Radiology*. 2010;40 (6):932–8.

46. Adamsbaum C, Morel B, Ducot B, Antoni G, Rey-Salmon C. Dating the abusive head trauma episode and perpetrator statements: Key points for imaging. *Pediatric Radiology*. 2014;44:578–88.

47. Ashwal S, Wycliffe ND, Holshouser BA. Advanced neuroimaging in children with nonaccidental trauma. *Developments in Neuroscience (Basel)*. 2010;32(5–6):343–60.

48. Barnes PD. Imaging of nonaccidental injury and the mimics: Issues and controversies in the era of evidence-based medicine. *Radiologic Clinics of North America*. 2011;49(1):205–29.

49. Beez T, Schmitz AK, Steiger HJ, Munoz-Bendix C. Endoscopic lavage of extensive chronic subdural hematoma in an infant after abusive head trauma: Adaptation of a technique from ventricular neuroendoscopy. *Cureus*. 2018;10(3):1–6. https://doi.org/10.7759/cureus.2258.

50. Berger RP, Furtado AD, Flom LL, Fromkin JB, Panigrahy A. Implementation of a brain injury screen MRI for infants at risk for abusive head trauma. *Pediatric Radiology*. 2020;50(1):75–82.

51. Binenbaum G, Christian CW, Ichord RN et al. Retinal hemorrhage and brain injury patterns on diffusion-weighted magnetic resonance imaging in children with head trauma. *Journal of the American Association for Pediatric Ophthalmology*. 2013;17(6):603–8.

52. Blumfield E. Pearls and pitfalls in imaging of abusive head trauma. *Seminars in Ultrasound, CT and MRI*. 2020;41 (5):411–20.

53. Boehnke M, Mirsky D, Stence N et al. Occult head injury is common in children with concern for physical abuse. *Pediatric Radiology*. 2018;48(8):1123–9.

54. Caylan ND, Yilmaz G, Oral R, Karacan CD, Zorlu P. Abusive head trauma: Report of 3 cases. *Turkish Journal of Trauma and Emergency Surgery*. 2013;19(3):261–6.

55. Elliott CA, Ramaswamy V, Jacob FD, Sankar T, Mehta V. Early diffusion restriction of white matter in infants with small subdural hematomas is associated with delayed atrophy. *Child's Nervous System*. 2017;33(2):289–95.

56. Erfurt C, Hahn G, Roesner D, Schmidt U. Pediatric radiological diagnostic procedures in cases of suspected child abuse. *Forensic Science and Medical Pathology*. 2011;7(1):65–74.

57. Feldman KW, Sugar NF, Browd SR. Initial clinical presentation of children with acute and chronic versus acute subdural hemorrhage resulting from abusive head trauma. *Journal of Neurosurgery: Pediatric*. 2015;16(2):177–85.

58. Fernando S, Obaldo RE, Walsh IR, Lowe LH. Neuroimaging of nonaccidental head trauma: Pitfalls and controversies. *Pediatric Radiology*. 2008;38(8):827–38.

59. Foerster BR, Petrou M, Lin D, et al. Neuroimaging evaluation of non-accidental head trauma with correlation to clinical outcomes: A review of 57 cases. *Journal of Pediatrics*. 2009;154(4):573–7.

60. Cartocci G, Fineschi V, Padovano M et al. Shaken baby syndrome: Magnetic resonance imaging features in abusive head trauma. *Brain Science*. 2021;11(2):1–16.

61. Gencturk M, Tore HG, Nascene DR et al. Various cranial and orbital imaging findings in pediatric abusive and non-abusive head trauma, and relation to outcomes. *Clinical Neuroradiology*. 2019;29 (2):253–61.

62. Girard N, Brunel H, Dory-Lautrec P, Chabrol B. Neuroimaging differential diagnoses to abusive head trauma. *Pediatric Radiology*. 2016;46(5):603–14.

63. Greiner MV, Richards TJ, Care MM, Leach JL. Prevalence of subdural collections in children with macrocrania. *American Journal of Neuroradiology*. 2013;34 (12):2373–8.

64. Gunda D, Cornwell BO, Dahmoush HM, Jazbeh S, Alleman AM. Pediatric central nervous system imaging of nonaccidental trauma: Beyond subdural hematomas. *Radiographics*. 2019;39(1):213–28.

65. Haas-Lude K, Roulet-Perez E, Dobler-Neumann M et al. Cerebellar lesions in pediatric abusive head trauma. *European Journal of Paediatric Neurology*. 2019;23 (4):604–8.

66. Hahnemann ML, Kinner S, Schweiger B et al. Imaging of bridging vein thrombosis in infants with abusive head trauma: The 'tadpole sign'. *European Radiology*. 2015;25 (2):299–305.

67. Hedlund GL, Frasier LD. Neuroimaging of abusive head trauma. *Forensic Science and Medical Pathology*. 2009;5(4):280–90.

68. Hsieh KLC, Zimmerman RA, Kao HW, Chen CY. Revisiting neuroimaging of abusive head trauma in infants and young children. *American Journal of Roentgenology*. 2015;204(5):944–52.

69. Hung KL. Pediatric abusive head trauma. *Biomedical Journal*. 2020;43(3):240–50.

70. Kadom N, Khademian Z, Vezina G et al. Usefulness of MRI detection of cervical spine and brain injuries in the evaluation of abusive head trauma. *Pediatric Radiology*. 2014;44(7):839–48.

71. Knox B, Rorke-Adams LB, Luyet FM. Subdural hematoma rebleeding in relation to abusive head trauma. *Journal of Family Violence*. 2016;31(7):815–21.

72. Kralik SF, Finke W, Wu IC et al. Radiologic head CT interpretation errors in pediatric abusive and non-abusive head trauma patients. *Pediatric Radiology*. 2017;47 (8):942–51.

73. Kralik SF, Yasrebi M, Supakul N et al. Diagnostic performance of ultrafast brain MRI for evaluation of abusive head trauma. *American Journal of Neuroradiology*. 2017;38(4):807–13.

74. Langford S, Panigrahy A, Narayanan S et al. Multiplanar reconstructed CT images increased depiction of intracranial hemorrhages in pediatric head trauma. *Neuroradiology*. 2015;57(12):1263–8.

75. Matschke J, Voss J, Obi N et al. Nonaccidental head injury is the most common cause of subdural bleeding in infants < 1 year of age. *Pediatrics*. 2009;124 (6):1587–94.

76. Nishimoto H. Recent progress and future issues in the management of abusive head trauma. *Neurologia Medico-chirurgica*. 2015;55(4):296–304.

77. Oates AJ, Sidpra J, Mankad K. Parenchymal brain injuries in abusive head trauma. *Pediatric Radiology*. 2021;51 (6):898–910.

78. O'Brien WT, Care MM, Leach JL. Pediatric emergencies: Imaging of pediatric head trauma. *Seminars in Ultrasound, CT and MRI*. 2018;39(5):495–514.

79. Orman G, Kralik SF, Meoded A et al. MRI findings in pediatric abusive head trauma: A review. *Journal of Neuroimaging*. 2020;30 (1):15–27.

80. Orru E, Calloni SF, Tekes A, Huisman TAGM, Soares BP. The child with macrocephaly: Differential diagnosis and neuroimaging findings. *American Journal of Roentgenology*. 2018;210 (4):848–59.

81. Orru' E, Huisman TAGM, Izbudak I. Prevalence, patterns, and clinical relevance of hypoxic-ischemic injuries in children exposed to abusive head trauma. *Journal of Neuroimaging*. 2018;28(6):608–14.

82. Palmer AW, Albert GW. Minicraniotomy with a subgaleal pocket for the treatment of subdural fluid collections in infants. *Journal of Neurosurgery: Pediatrics*. 2019;23 (4):480–5.

83. Pfeifer CM, Hammer MR, Mangona KL, Booth TN. Non-accidental trauma: The role of radiology. *Emergency Radiology*. 2017;24(2):207–13.

84. Porto L, Bartels MB, Zwaschka J et al. Abusive head trauma: Experience improves diagnosis. *Neuroradiology*. 2020;63 (3):417–30.

85. Rajaram S, Batty R, Rittey CDC, Griffiths PD, Connolly DJA. Neuroimaging in non-accidental head injury in children: An important element of assessment. *Postgraduate Medical Journal*. 2011;87 (1027):355–61.

86. Reith W, Yilmaz U, Kraus C. Shaken baby syndrome. *Radiologe*. 2016;56 (5):424–31.

87. Rolfes MC, Guerin JB, Brucker J, Kalina P. Pediatric abusive head trauma: Review of standard imaging evaluation and typical findings. *Journal of Pediatric Neurology*. 2018;16(2):39–55.

88. Ronning MM, Carolan PL, Cutler GJ, Patterson RJ. Parasagittal vertex clots on head CT in infants with subdural hemorrhage as a predictor for abusive head trauma. *Pediatric Radiology*. 2018;48 (13):1915–23.

89. Saigal G, Ezuddin NS, de la Vega G. Neurologic emergencies in pediatric patients including accidental and nonaccidental trauma. *Neuroimaging Clinics of North America*. 2018;28 (3):453–70.

90. Shekdar K. Imaging of abusive trauma. *Indian Journal of Pediatrics*. 2016;83 (6):578–88.

91. Sieswerda-Hoogendoorn T, Boos S, Spivack B, Bilo RAC, Van Rijn RR. Educational paper. Abusive head trauma part II: Radiological aspects. *European Journal of Pediatrics*. 2012;171(4):617–23.

92. Stöver B. Bildgebende Diagnostik der Kindesmisshandlung. *Monatsschrift Kinderheilkde*. 2008;156:385–98.

93. Takeda R, Kobayashi S, Kamioka N et al. Post-traumatic stress syndrome due to abusive head trauma in two infants with different brain imaging findings. *Tohoku Journal of Experimental Medicine*. 2020;250(3):167–71.

94. Tysiak EWN, Petersen D, Gottschalk S et al. Progression of chronic subdural haematomas in an infant boy after abusive head trauma. *European Journal of Paediatric Neurology*. 2012;16(6):736–9.

95. Van Rijn RR, Spevak MR. Imaging of neonatal child abuse with an emphasis on abusive head trauma. *Magnetic Resonance Imaging Clinics of North America*. 2011;19 (4):791–812, viii.

96. Vazquez E, Delgado I, Sanchez-Montanez A et al. Imaging abusive head trauma: Why use both computed tomography and magnetic resonance imaging? *Pediatric Radiology*. 2014;44:589–603.

97. Vezina G. Assessment of the nature and age of subdural collections in nonaccidental head injury with CT and MRI. *Pediatric Radiology*. 2009;39 (6):586–90.

98. Vilanilam GK, Jayappa S, Desai S et al. Venous injury in pediatric abusive head trauma: A pictorial review. *Pediatric Radiology*. 2021;51(6):918–26.

99. Vinchon M. Shaken baby syndrome: What certainty do we have? *Child's Nervous System*. 2017;33(10):1727–33.

100. Yilmaz U, Korner H, Meyer S, Reith W. Multifocal signal loss at bridging veins on susceptibility-weighted imaging in abusive head trauma. *Clinical Neuroradiology*. 2015;25(2):181–5.

101. Wittschieber D, Karger B, Pfeiffer H, Hahnemann ML. Understanding subdural collections in pediatric abusive head trauma. *American Journal of Neuroradiology*. 2019;40(3):388–95.

102. Wittschieber D, Muggenthaler H, Mall G, Mentzel HJ. [Bridging vein injuries in shaken baby syndrome: Forensic-radiological meta-analysis with special focus on the tadpole sign]. *Radiologe*. 2021;61(1):71–9.

103. Wright JN, Feyma TJ, Ishak GE et al. Subdural hemorrhage rebleeding in abused children: Frequency, associations and clinical presentation. *Pediatric Radiology*. 2019;49(13):1762–72.

104. Mori K, Yamamoto T, Horinaka N, Maeda M. Arachnoid cyst is a risk factor for chronic subdural hematoma in juveniles: Twelve cases of chronic subdural hematoma associated with arachnoid cyst. *Journal of Neurotrauma*. 2002;19(9):1017–27.

105. Tucker J, Choudhary AK, Piatt J. Macrocephaly in infancy: Benign enlargement of the subarachnoid spaces and subdural collections. *Journal of Neurosurgery: Pediatrics*. 2016;18 (1):16–20.

106. Lee HC, Chong S, Lee JY et al. Benign extracerebral fluid collection complicated by subdural hematoma and fluid collection: Clinical characteristics and management. *Child's Nervous System*. 2018;34(2):235–45.

107. Wester K. Two infant boys misdiagnosed as 'shaken baby' and their twin sisters: A cautionary tale. *Pediatric Neurology*. 2019;97:3–11.

108. Wester K, Wikström J, Lynøe N, Eriksson A. Unsubstantiated belief in the diagnostic accuracy of the triad of abusive head trauma may lead to incorrect diagnoses of alleged abuse cases. *Acta Paediatrica*. 2022;111(4):809–11.

109. Miller R, Miller M. Overrepresentation of males in traumatic brain injury of infancy and in infants with macrocephaly: Further evidence that questions the existence of shaken baby syndrome. *American Journal of Forensic Medicine and Pathology*. 2010;31 (2):165–73.

110. Piatt JH. Monozygotic twins discordant for external hydrocephalus. *Pediatric Neurosurgery*. 2001;35(4):211–15.

111. Wester K, Stridbeck U, Syse A, Wikstrom J. Re-evaluation of medical findings in

alleged shaken baby syndrome and abusive head trauma in Norwegian courts fails to support abuse diagnoses. *Acta Paediatrica*. 2021;111 (4):779–92.

112. Choudhary AK, Bradford R, Dias MS, Thamburaj K, Boal DKB. Venous injury in abusive head trauma. *Pediatric Radiology*. 2015;45(12):1803–13.

113. Sieswerda-Hoogendoorn T, Boos S, Spivack B, Bilo RAC, Van Rijn RR. Educational paper. Abusive head trauma part I: Clinical aspects. *European Journal of Pediatrics*. 2012;171(3):415–23.

Chapter 7 Are Some Cases of Sudden Infant Death Syndrome Incorrectly Diagnosed as Shaken Baby Syndrome?

Marta Cohen

7.1 Sudden Infant Death

7.1.1 Definition

Sudden infant death syndrome (SIDS) is 'the sudden death of an infant under 1 year of age which remains unexplained after a thorough case investigation, including performance of a complete autopsy, examination of the death scene, and review of the clinical history' [1]. This definition, coined by the National Institute of Child Health and Human Development three decades ago, remains valid. Characteristically, sudden infant death occurs in a seemingly healthy infant typically associated with a sleep period – either during sleep itself or during one of the many spontaneous arousals that occur from sleep.

Importantly, SIDS is characterised by a 'negative' post-mortem, and it is therefore a 'default' diagnosis. In 1994, Filiano and Kinney [2] proposed the 'triple risk' hypothesis: SIDS results from the intersection of three overlapping factors: (1) a vulnerable infant, (2) a critical developmental period, and (3) an exogenous stressor. In other words, SIDS is the result of the combination of a baby who is vulnerable due to its genetic constitution, of a particular developmental age (2 to 6 months), who is exposed to risk factors. Similarly, Kahn [3] describes SIDS as the result of multifactorial situations, associating inadequate cardiac, breathing, autonomic, and/or arousal controls and comprising three main groups of causes: maturational processes, medical conditions, and environmental factors. These three conditions, either independently or in combination, may lead to the same common final pathway: a decreased propensity to arouse from sleep and an increase in sympathovagal balance of the heart rate.

7.1.2 Risk Factors and Epidemiological Features of Sudden Infant Death Syndrome

Rates of SIDS declined considerably from 130.3 deaths per 100,000 live births in 1990 to 33.3 deaths per 100,000 live births in 2019 [4]. Similarly, although the incidence was initially reported to be higher during the cold months (autumn and winter) than in the spring and summer across several high-income countries, this seasonal difference appears to have reduced, with a similar distribution of SIDS throughout the year [5]. A crucial point in the decline of SIDS deaths was the implementation of the 'back to sleep' campaign in the late 1980s and early 1990s. The success of the campaign, which advised parents to put babies to sleep on their back and avoid prone or side sleeping positions, decreased the incidence of

SIDS in many countries. In the United Kingdom, the number of SIDS deaths was reduced by up to 40% within the first year of the campaign [6], while in the United States there was a 41% decrease from 1.30 deaths per 1,000 live births in 1989–91 to 0.77 per 1,000 live births in 1995–8 [5, 7].

Risk factors for SIDS include male sex, prematurity, low birth weight, prone sleeping position, smoking, young parents, and low socioeconomic status [4, 5, 8]. Approximately 80% of SIDS deaths occurred before the age of 4 months with a peak between 2 and 3 months of age [5]. Moreover, a study from Ireland documented that 83% of SIDS cases were below 6 months of age [9].

Male sex is considered a risk factor for SIDS, and a study from the United States showed an incidence of 0.45 SIDS deaths per 1,000 live births for males and 0.38 for females [10]. The causative mechanisms behind the sex difference in the incidence of SIDS remain unknown. However, research has shown increased apoptosis in the brainstem of SIDS infants, which is affected by age and gender, and by clinical risk factors such as sleep position and cigarette smoke exposure [11]. Machaalani et al. [11] revealed that neuronal cell death in specific areas of the brainstem was increased in SIDS compared with non-SIDS cases. They also demonstrated a statistically significant difference for male SIDS compared to male non-SIDS ($p = 0.04$) in neuronal cell necrosis, specifically in the arcuate nuclei in the brainstem, which plays an important role in regulation of respiration in response to increasing levels of carbon dioxide [12]. Of relevance, despite a major decrease in the incidence of SIDS, the sex difference has remained unaltered. This gives support to the hypothesis that sex differences in brain structure and function may influence arousal during sleep.

Preterm birth (< 37 weeks' gestation) is a known risk factor for SIDS, with a decline of the incidence of SIDS as gestational age at birth increases [5, 13]. Malloy et al. [14] demonstrated that SIDS was 2.6, 2.7, and 1.9 times more likely when the infant was born at 24–28, 29–32, and 33–36 weeks' gestation compared to full term. These authors also remarked on the fact that, despite the significant drop in the incidence of SIDS since 1987, the risk for SIDS among preterm infants remains elevated.

Young parents and low socioeconomic status (SES) are well-known risk factors for SIDS. A study of infants born to Kentucky residents in the 1990s identified adjusted relative risks for SIDS as maternal age under 20 (1. 73, $p \leq 0.08$), maternal cigarette use (1.92 for one pack per day, $p < 0.01$), Caesarean delivery (both emergency and elective) (2.09, $p \leq 0.01$), and premature birth (1. 76, $p \leq 0.08$) [15]. The link between low SES and SIDS was also demonstrated in a systematic review of observational studies, which reported the significant association of SES with sudden unexpected death in infancy [16].[1]

This review also showed the increasing risk of infant death with greater exposure to adverse social circumstances. Low SES correlates with lower educational achievements, poor health, and poverty [17]. Moreover, lower SES has been linked to a variety of negative health outcomes at birth and throughout the life span, such as higher infant mortality. In the United States, babies born to white mothers have an expected mortality rate of 5.35 per 1,000 births. In comparison, babies born to black mothers have a mortality rate of 12.35 per 1,000 births [18, 19]. In SIDS, infants frequently have history of a recent 'cold' and a study

[1] Sudden unexpected death in infancy (SUDI) is a term some authors use to describe SIDS. Others use SUDI to define a child who dies suddenly and unexpectedly, although a cause of death may be found at post mortem.

found that 41.2% of these cases had a potentially pathogenic organism identified with bacteriology or virology (20).

Delayed Sudden Infant Death Syndrome

Although SIDS cases are usually found dead in the early hours of the morning, in a small percentage of cases advanced resuscitation may be successful and these infants may die later (delayed SIDS) [21]. In these circumstances, there is an overlap between findings most frequently found in SIDS (such as thymic petechiae and pulmonary haemorrhage) and those secondary to hypoxic ischaemic injury to vital organs (including the central nervous system). Notably, a percentage of delayed SIDS cases had subdural bleeding (4%), intradural haemorrhage (12%), subgaleal haemorrhage (7%), subarachnoid haemorrhage (7%), brain haemorrhage (42%), brain oedema (cerebellar herniation, 10%), spinal haemorrhage (10%), and/or retinal haemorrhages (18%). In this group, there was also a higher incidence of male sex (79% males vs. 21% females). In Krous et al.'s study [21], all delayed SIDS cases occurred during the daytime, while most non-delayed SIDS cases were discovered between 00.00 and 07.59 hours. As expected, histopathological studies of the brain of those cases with delayed SIDS showed – as a function of survival interval – parenchymal infarction, neuronal necrosis, gliosis, as well as pulmonary haemorrhage, aspiration of gastric contents, and/or acute bronchopneumonia.

Infants who are victims of delayed SIDS were significantly more often in day-care or other locations compared to infants dying during the late evening and early morning hours, when they are more likely to be in their own homes. In addition to delayed SIDS, the sudden death of an infant while awake at the onset of their terminal events is associated with entirely similar demographic and pathologic profiles to those cases of SIDS discovered between 00.00 and 07.59 hours [22]. As Krous et al. rightly pointed out, altered responses to severe hypotension, bradycardia, and apnoea perhaps elicited by aspiration and mediated by cerebellar and vestibular structures may be involved in the pathogenesis of these deaths [22].

Acute Life-Threatening Event/ Brief Resolved Unexplained Event

The so-called acute life-threatening event (ALTE) currently known as brief resolved unexplained event (BRUE) shares with delayed SIDS the timing of the collapse, as both groups are more likely to be found in distress during the daytime [22, 23].

Gastro-oesophageal Reflux and Aspiration

Young infants are prone to a variety of conditions that result in transient but severe episodes of hypoxemia and/or ischemia. This can result in prolonged apnoeic spells. In most cases, cardiovascular and neural recovery occur rapidly and spontaneously after the onset of swallowing, arousal, and expiratory reflexes that re-oxygenate the body. This mode of spontaneous recovery has been termed 'autoresuscitation' – a brainstem response to hypoxia that initiates gasping respirations, leading to spontaneous recovery – and is said to allow mammals to survive transient episodes of hypoxia. Under normal circumstances, stimulation of the pharynx by fluid initiates mechanisms that protect the airway from fluid entry. If these mechanisms are depressed or interfered with, fluid reaching the larynx and stimulate the laryngeal chemoreflex with possible fatal consequences [24, 25]. Activation of the laryngeal chemoreflex by the presence of fluid in the pharynx can also result in the failure of autoresuscitation.

Aspiration of gastric acid has been identified as a possible risk factor for SIDS [24]. However, the fact that gastric contents are seen in the lungs in 20–40% of SIDS autopsies [26–28], and it is possible that this occurs during cardio-pulmonary resuscitation, makes this finding less or not relevant as a cause of death in SIDS. Histological evidence of gastro-oesophageal reflux (GOR) has been demonstrated at post mortem in cases of SIDS [28]. In one of the cases described by Al-Adnani et al., gastric contents were present in the lungs, surrounded by oedema and haemorrhage, in keeping with asphyxia involved in the mechanism of death [28]. Gastro-oesophageal reflux itself does not appear to be a direct cause of death but is likely linked to sudden death through a choking episode or cardiorespiratory events initiated to prevent gastric contents being aspirated into the airways and lungs [25, 26]. Similarly, in a prospective study conducted in the United Kingdom, 26% of infants who presented with BRUE were diagnosed with GOR [29].

7.2 Shaken Baby Syndrome

7.2.1 Definition

Shaken baby syndrome – also known as abusive head trauma, shaken impact syndrome, inflicted head injury, or whiplash shake syndrome – is usually defined as a serious brain injury resulting from forcefully shaking an infant or toddler [30, 31]. The diagnosis has conventionally been based on three findings – referred to collectively as the triad – namely subdural haematoma (SDH), retinal haemorrhages (RH), and various forms of brain symptoms (encephalopathy) [32].

In the United Kingdom, the Crown Prosecution Service's legal guidance to those cases presenting with the triad states very clearly its approach to these cases as 'Non- Accidental Head Injury Cases (NAHI, formerly referred to as Shaken Baby Syndrome [SBS])' [33]. The Crown Prosecution Service discourages the use of the term *shaken baby syndrome* as it has emotive connotations and, more importantly, it does not adequately describe the range of causes of head injuries. The Crown Prosecution Service's guidelines appear extremely simplistic in the explanation of the physio-pathological mechanisms leading to these features as 'thought to be the shaking of the infant, with or without impact on a solid surface. This moves the brain within the skull, damaging the brain and shearing the bridging veins between the dura and the arachnoid and sometimes causing retinal haemorrhages. Nevertheless, despite medical uncertainty surrounding the mechanism, the triad of injuries is a strong medical pointer to the infliction of NAHI'. It also noted that 'Cases which involve the triad must be approached with caution' and 'In a case where a child dies (or suffers serious injury) . . . it is rare that a charge of homicide (or attempted murder or assault) could be sustained where the only evidence available is the triad of pathological features. Such evidence is rarely conclusive of NAHI and prosecutors should look for other, supporting evidence.'

7.2.2 Risk Factors and Epidemiological Features of Shaken Baby Syndrome

A British survey retrospectively reviewed cases of SDH and effusion during a 12-month period in infants and children up to 2 years of age. The cases – reported by paediatricians, neurosurgeons, and paediatric and forensic pathologists – identified a total of 186 infants

(121 boys, 65 girls) [34]. One hundred and six infants allegedly suffered NAHI, 7 accidental head injuries, 26 a perinatal cause, 7 a non-traumatic medical condition, and 23 meningitis. In 17 the cause was undetermined.

A recent population-based study from Sweden showed the incidence of SDH was 16.5 per 100,000 infants [35]. Of the 251 SDH identified, 139 were traumatic in origin while 112 were non-traumatic. The median age was found to be 2.5 months, although when only those whose age was more than 1 week were considered, the median age was 3.5 months. In this latter group, the presence of acute non-traumatic SDH was associated with multiple birth, preterm birth, perinatal complications, and small-for-gestational age. As in SIDS, male sex was overrepresented, with a significant difference in the incidence in males (64.7%) compared with females (35.3%) ($p < 0.001$).

7.2.3 Shared Epidemiological Features between Sudden Infant Death Syndrome and Shaken Baby Syndrome

Infants who develop the triad of SDH, RH, and encephalopathy share many epidemiological features with infants whose death is attributed to SIDS: age, male sex, higher incidence of prematurity, small for gestational age, young mothers, multiple births, high parity, low SES, smoking during pregnancy, and minor respiratory infections [4–21, 35–41].[2] See Figure 7.1.

7.3 Is There a Common Final Pathway for Infants Dying of Sudden Infant Death Syndrome and for Those Presenting with the Triad of Subdural Haematoma, Retinal Haematoma, and Encephalopathy?

The data sets were analysed of eight studies of sudden and unexpected deaths of infants in which no cause of death could be found (SIDS) or in which a possible cause could be found – 'Accidental Suffocation and Strangulation in Bed', 'Anoxic Encephalopathy', 'Unknown', or 'Explained Sudden Unexpected Death in Infancy'. The authors [42] interpreted that in all these cases sudden death was a consequence of a common process as yet undetermined, brought about by genetic and physiological susceptibility interacting with environmental risk factors and other disease states.

A common final pathway to SIDS is believed to involve immature cardiorespiratory autonomic control together with a failure of arousal responsiveness from sleep [43]. See Figure 7.1. This pathway might subsequently be involved in the development of hypoxia. Abnormal and reduced number of spontaneous arousal episodes have been confirmed in infants who subsequently died of SIDS [3, 15, 44]. The increased risk of SIDS appears to be related to abnormalities in serotoninergic and glutamatergic brainstem neurons involved in automatic breathing during sleep. These chemoreceptive neurons respond to changes in oxygen, carbon dioxide, and pH in the blood and cerebrospinal fluid [45]. The relevance of each particular receptor may vary among infants who die of SIDS, and possibly no single receptor defect is solely responsible for the vulnerability that leads to the sudden death [46].

[2] It is increasingly clear that chronic enlargement of the extra-axial spaces is another group sharing similar demographic features. This condition is described in Chapter 5.

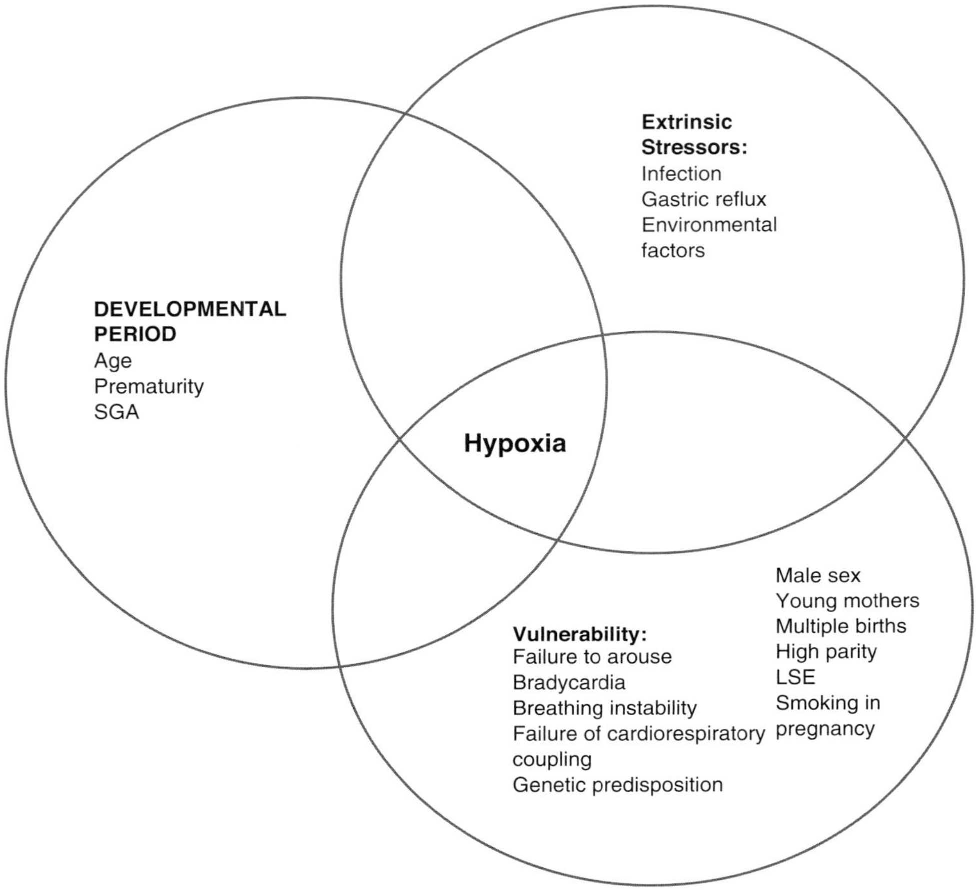

Figure 7.1 Proposed triple-risk model sharing features of vulnerability, external stressors, and development between SIDS and so-called SBS
SGA: Small for gestational age; LSE: Low socioeconomic status

The release of nucleated red blood cell precursors (also known as erythroblasts) into the peripheral blood has been described in cases with a probable hypoxic mode of death [47]. A previous study from our centre [48] identified that higher levels of nucleated red blood cells (nRBCs) were associated with intra-alveolar haemorrhage in the lungs and intradural haemorrhages (IDH) (specifically falx cerebri and tentorium cerebelli) in infants dying with SIDS, SUDI, or causes of deaths associated with a known hypoxic mode of death (i.e., hanging, cardiac malformation, diazepam intoxication). This association strongly suggests that – in all of these cases – hypoxia is a common factor leading to these phenomena, presumably as a result of agonal breathing during hypoxia causing micro ruptures of the vessels in key locations (dura mater and lungs). Interestingly, the occurrence of haemorrhages in the dura was seen in more than two-thirds of cases and was associated with higher values of nRBCs; this was more common in younger infants. The release of nRBCs into the peripheral blood was a significant feature.

The association of hypoxia-IDH-SDH in young infants dying of natural causes has been confirmed using magnetic resonance imaging (MRI) with T2 weighted images to examine the central nervous system at autopsy [49]. In this study, SDH was associated with diffuse IDH and it was also frequently associated with hypoxia. The link between hypoxia-IDH-SDH was further established with two other post-mortem studies [50, 51], which demonstrated that the presence of thin-film bilateral SDH is associated with hypoxic ischaemic encephalopathy ($p < 0.0001$), that these are more common in autopsies of infants under 1 month corrected age and that, although less frequent, they can also be found in children between 1 month and 3 years of age in the absence of trauma.

Of relevance, *none* of the SIDS/SUDI cases had been resuscitated in two of these studies [49, 50]. Yet another of the studies [53] showed that, in those cases in which there was evidence of successful but short-lived cardio-pulmonary resuscitation (CPR), a total of 29% had macroscopic IDH and 46% also had SDH. This percentage was very similar to the babies with established hypoxia and was independent of age. When the analysis was restricted to babies with successful CPR, 73% of them had either as macro IDH or SDH or both ($P < 0.01$). The study [51] also showed SDH was significantly associated with IDH and hypoxic ischaemic encephalopathy (HIE), strongly suggesting IDHs can lead to SDHs. The reason for this is that bleeding from the capillaries and small venules within the dura itself increases with hypoxia, dissecting the thin connective tissue of the dura, eventually leaking out of the tissue itself. The presence of IDH at early stages of hypoxia is consistent with findings in asphyxial deaths in infants, who also develop interstitial bleeding in the lungs, kidneys, and other organs.

Therefore, it is reasonable to consider that, if an infant collapses while awake and is successfully resuscitated (even if short-lived), the ongoing hypoxia can trigger intradural and subdural haemorrhages [22, 23]. The development of raised intracranial pressure, encephalopathy (swollen brain), and RH in the context of hypoxia is discussed in Chapter 3.

References

1. Willinger M, James LS, Catz C. Defining the sudden infant death syndrome (SIDS): Deliberations of an expert panel convened by the National Institute of Child Health and Human Development. *Pediatric Pathology*. 1991;11(5):677–84.
2. Filiano JJ, Kinney HC. A perspective on neuropathologic findings in victims of the sudden infant death syndrome: The triple-risk model. *Biology of the Neonate*. 1994;65:194–7.
3. Kahn A, Sawaguchib T, Sawaguchib A et al. Sudden infant deaths: From epidemiology to physiology. *Forensic Science International*. 2002;130S:S8–S20.
4. Byard RW, Krous HF. Sudden infant death syndrome: Overview and update. *Pediatric Developmental Pathology*. 2003;6:112–27.
5. Shapiro-Mendoza CK, Parks S, Lambert AE et al. The epidemiology of sudden infant death syndrome and sudden unexpected infant deaths: Diagnostic shift and other temporal changes. In *SIDS sudden infant and early childhood death: The past, the present and the future*. JR Duncan, RW Byard, eds. University of Adelaide Press, 2018, chapter 13. www.ncbi.nlm.nih.gov/books/NBK513373.
6. Her Majesty's Stationery Office. *Report of the Chief Medical Officer's Expert Group on the Sleeping Position of Infants and Cot Death*. Her Majesty's Stationery Office, 1993
7. www.cdc.gov/sids/data.htm.
8. Shapiro-Mendoza CK, Tomashek KM, Anderson RN, Wingo J. Recent national trends in sudden, unexpected infant deaths: More evidence supporting a change in

classification or reporting. *American Journal of Epidemiology*. 2006;163(8):762–9.

9. Mehanni M, Cullen A, Kiberd B et al. The current epidemiology of SIDS in Ireland. *Irish Medical Journal*. 2000;93(9):264–8.
10. Heron M. Deaths: Leading causes for 2014. National vital statistics reports from the Centers for Disease Control and Prevention, National Center for Health Statistics, National Vital Statistics System. *National Vital Statistics Reports*. 2016;65(5):1–96.
11. Machaalani R, Waters KA. Neuronal cell death in the sudden infant death syndrome brainstem and associations with risk factors. *Brain*. 2008;131(Pt 1):218–28.
12. Stonebridge R, Taliano RJ, Velilla TD, Anthony DC. Hypertrophy of the anterior external arcuate fasciculus: A rare variant with implications for the development of the arcuate nucleus. *Front Neuroanatomy*. 2020;14:595500.
13. Matthews TJ, MacDorman MF, Thoma ME. Infant mortality statistics from the 2013 period linked birth/infant death data set. *National Vital Statistics Report*. 2015;64(9):1–30.
14. Malloy MH. Prematurity and sudden infant death syndrome: United States 2005–2007. *Journal of Perinatology*. 2013;33(6):470–5.
15. Sanghavi DM. Epidemiology of sudden infant death syndrome (SIDS) for Kentucky infants born in 1990: Maternal, prenatal, and perinatal risk factors. *Journal of the Kentucky Medical Association*. 1995;93(7):286–90.
16. Spencer N, Logan S. Sudden unexpected death in infancy and socioeconomic status: A systematic review. *Journal of Epidemiology and Community Health*. 2004;58(5):366–73.
17. www.apa.org/pi/ses/resources/publications/children-families.
18. Haider, S. J. Racial and ethnic infant mortality gaps and socioeconomic status. *Focus*. 2014;31:18–20.
19. Elder TE, Goddeeris JH, Haider SJ. Racial and ethnic infant mortality gaps and the role of socio-economic status. *Labour Economics*. 2016;43:42–54.
20. Prtak L, Al-Adnani M, Fenton P et al. Contribution of bacteriology and virology in sudden unexpected death in infancy. *Archive of Diseases in Childhood*. 2010;95 (5):371–6.
21. Krous HF, Haas EA, Chadwick AE et al. Delayed death in sudden infant death syndrome: A San Diego SIDS/SUDC Research Project 15-year population-based report. *Forensic Science International*. 2008;176(2–3):209–16.
22. Krous HF, Chadwick AE, Haas E et al. Sudden infant death while awake. *Forensic Science, Medicine and Pathology*. 2008;4 (1):40–6.
23. Kahn A, Blum D, Hennart P et al. A critical comparison of the history of sudden-death infants and infants hospitalised for near-miss for SIDS. *European Journal of Pediatrics*. 1984;143(2):103–7.
24. Page M, Jeffrey H. The role of gastro-oesophageal reflux in the aetiology of SIDS. *Early Human Development*. 2000;59:127–49.
25. Thach BT. Sudden infant death syndrome: Can gastroesophageal reflux cause sudden infant death? *American Journal of Medicine*. 2000;108:S144–S148.
26. Krous HF, Masoumi H, Haas EA et al. Aspiration of gastric contents in sudden infant death syndrome without cardiopulmonary resuscitation. *Journal of Pediatrics*. 2007;150:241–6.
27. Alex N, Thompson JMD, Becroft DMO, Mitchell EA. Pulmonary aspiration of gastric contents and the sudden infant death syndrome. *Journal of Paediatrics and Child Health*. 2005;41:428–31.
28. Al-Adnani M, Cohen MC, Scheimberg I. Gastroesophageal reflux disease and sudden infant death: Mechanisms behind an under-recognized association. *Pediatric Development and Pathology*. 2011;14(1):53–6.
29. Davies F, Gupta R. Apparent life threatening events in infants presenting to an emergency department. *Emergency Medicine Journal*. 2002;19:11–16.

30. https://bit.ly/3V83gdp.
31. https://mayocl.in/3SW5zhM.
32. Elinder G, Eriksson A, Hallberg B et al. Traumatic shaking: The role of the triad in medical investigations of suspected traumatic shaking. *Acta Paediatrica*. 2018;107:3–23.
33. https://bit.ly/3fIYdQJ.
34. Hobbs C, Childs AM, Wynne J et al. Subdural haematoma and effusion in infancy: An epidemiological study. *Archive of Diseases in Childhood*. 2005;90(9):952–5.
35. Högberg U, Andersson J, Squier W et al. Epidemiology of subdural haemorrhage during infancy: A population-based register study. *PLoS One*. 2018;13(10): e0206340.
36. Squier W, Mack J, Jansen AC. Infants dying suddenly and unexpectedly share demographic features with infants who die with retinal and dural bleeding: A review of neural mechanisms. *Developmental Medicine and Child Neurology*. 2016;58 (12):1223–34.
37. Duhaime AC, Christian CW, Rorke LB, Zimmerman RA. Nonaccidental head injury in infants: The 'shaken baby syndrome'. *New England Journal of Medicine*. 1998;338:1822–9.
38. Gerber P, Coffman K. Nonaccidental head trauma in infants. *Child's Nervous System* 2007;23:499–507.
39. Keenan HT, Runyan DK, Marshall SW et al. A population-based study of inflicted traumatic brain injury in young children. *JAMA*. 2003;290:621–6.
40. Oehmichen M, Schleiss D, Pedal I et al. Shaken baby syndrome: Re-examination of diffuse axonal injury as cause of death. *Acta Neuropathologica*. 2008;116:317–29.
41. Blair PS, Sidebotham P, Evason-Coombe C et al. Hazardous cosleeping environments and risk factors amenable to change: Case-control study of SIDS in south west England. *BMJ*.2009;13(339):b3666.
42. Mage D, Donner E, Vennemann M et al. All sudden unexplained infant respiratory deaths may result from the same underlying mechanism. *Scandinavian Journal of Forensic Science*. 2012;18(1):1–9.
43. Moon RY, Horne RSC, Hauck FR. Sudden infant death syndrome. *Lancet*. 2007;370:1578–87.
44. Kato I, Franco P, Groswasser J et al. Incomplete arousal processes in infants who were victims of sudden death. *American Journal of Respiratory and Critical Care Medicine*. 2003;168:1298–1303.
45. Benarroch EE. Brainstem respiratory chemosensitivity. New insights and clinical implications. *Neurology*. 2007:2140–3.
46. Leiter JC, Böhm I. Mechanisms of pathogenesis in the sudden infant death syndrome. *Respiratory Physiology and Neurobiology*. 2007;159:127–38.
47. Naeye RL. Sudden death in infants. In *Potter's pathology of the fetus, infant and child*, vol. 1. E Gilbert-Barness, ed. Elsevier, 2007, pp. 857–69.
48. Cohen MC, Yong CY, Evans C et al. Release of erythroblasts to the peripheral blood suggests higher exposure to hypoxia in cases of SIDS with co-sleeping compared to SIDS non-co-sleeping. *Forensic Science International*. 2010;197(1–3):54–8.
49. Cohen MC, Sprigg A, Whitby EH. Subdural hemorrhage, intradural hemorrhage and hypoxia in the pediatric and perinatal post mortem: Are they related? An observational study combining the use of post mortem pathology and magnetic resonance imaging. *Forensic Science International*. 2010;200(1–3):100–7.
50. Cohen MC, Scheimberg I. Evidence of occurrence of intradural and subdural hemorrhage in the perinatal and neonatal period in the context of hypoxic ischemic encephalopathy. An observational study from two referral institutions in the United Kingdom. *Pediatric Development Pathology*. 2009;12:169–76.
51. Scheimberg I, Cohen MC, Zapata Vazquez RE et al. Nontraumatic intradural and subdural hemorrhage and hypoxic ischemic encephalopathy in fetuses, infants, and children up to three years of age: Analysis of two audits of 636 cases from two referral centers in the United Kingdom. *Pediatric Developmental Pathology*. 2013;16(3):149–59.

Chapter 8

Abusive Head Trauma
The Importance of Predisposing Factors

Bernard Echenne

Subdural haematomas (SDH) in infants: are they always the consequence of abusive or inflicted head trauma? For a neuropaediatric clinician, pathologies involving infants are always related to several, often many, aetiologies and mechanisms. Nowadays, especially in France since the 2011 diagnosis guidelines published by the national health agency, the Haute Autorité de Santé (HAS) (see Chapter 22), when SDH is diagnosed in young babies, only one diagnosis is ever evoked: inflicted head trauma, a wilful aggression. It is always an extrinsic, traumatic, inflicted, mechanism: abusive head trauma (AHT). Nothing is usually said about the responsibility of intrinsic factors, nothing either about the existence of one or more predisposing or risk factors.

We believe these factors do exist and they are most often ignored or misdiagnosed. However, when they are present, they can lead to spontaneous bleeding into the subdural space, or they can represent an additional risk factor after another event such as a short fall. In this chapter, we highlight some of these risk factors.

8.1 Immature Venous Plexus

The first risk factor is the set of anatomical particularities specific to very young infants in whom the venous drainage originates from the prenatal circulation (see Chapter 3). The veins have a plexiform appearance. They are larger and more numerous in young infants than in older children. These venous lakes predominate at the posterior level of the falx and at the cerebellar tentorium level. In contrast to other areas of the body, the cerebral venous system of the brain shows much more morphological variability than the arterial system.

Throughout foetal and early postnatal development, the venous system is continuously rebuilt in a process of integrative development as a result of morphological changes occurring in the skull base and cerebral vesicles [38]. These abundant venous plexuses become shorter and less numerous in the years after birth [3, 20, 26]. Cerebral angiography shows intradural venous plexuses in 20% of infants, compared with 1% of adults [20]. In AHT, bleeding often predominates at the falx and tentorium level. That is not surprising according to the normal venous anatomy during the first months of life. On the other hand, the meningeal membranes in young babies are thin and fragile. This immaturity is one of the factors that explain why SDH occurs in 87% of cases in infants younger than 6 months [23].

8.2 Intradural Haemorrhage

It is now understood that subdural haemorrhage originates within the dura. Although the bridging veins may sometimes be the source of haemorrhage, the bleeding starts within the dura. If the volume of intradural blood is large enough, the dural border cell layer between the dura and arachnoid will be cleaved and a 'subdural' haematoma will appear (see Chapter 3).

The number of the bridging veins and smaller veins draining the blood from the brain to the sinus or to the venous plexus close to the sinus is much higher than previously supposed: the mean number of veins is 54.1 and the largest number is 94, according to the studies of Cheshire et al., with great individual variations [8]. The mean diameter of the bridging veins in this study is 0.93 mm, with measurements ranging from 0.05 to 3.07 mm. These data demonstrate that some veins are extremely small and delicate.

One can also observe that some bridging veins are too large to rupture when subject to the forces associated with AHT. Using optical coherence tomography, the same group has shown that the approximate median diameters of blood vessels entering anterior and posterior segments of the superior sagittal sinus were 110 μm (70–670 μm) and 125 μm (70–740 μm), respectively [7].

These studies also demonstrate that imaging modalities such as magnetic resonance imaging (MRI) and computed tomography do not have the resolution capabilities to image small blood vessels. The importance of these small vessels within the dura cannot be overstated, as they are in many cases the source of bleeding and consequently, responsible for SDH [9]. The vein–dura junction can be more or less weak and fragile, with a length within the dura that can be up to 1 mm.

8.3 Perinatal Subdural Haemorrhage

The third predisposing factor relates to the macro or micro haemorrhages which occur within the meningeal membranes during delivery. Such haemorrhages have represented a very important underdiagnosed factor so far. Incidental intracranial haemorrhages are common findings in neonatal cerebral MRI, as are retinal and optic nerve haemorrhages [4], which can still be present at 58 days in a child born by vacuum delivery [24]. They are observed in children with normal examination, without any abnormal neurological sign. This is not surprising given the remarkable moulding and deformation of the foetal head in the birth canal [1]. Vacuum-assisted delivery is found to be another supplementary risk factor. The relevance of birth-related intracranial haemorrhages is still partially unclear, as are their consequences [29]. The early development of a chronic subdural collection, hygroma, or hygro-haematoma could be the consequence of these deliveries [51].

The estimated prevalence of intracranial haemorrhages in term asymptomatic healthy newborn populations deviates greatly, from 6.9% to 46% [29, 31, 39, 49]. One study reported a high prevalence of supra-tentorial haemorrhages [39], but they were infra-tentorial in the others [31, 43, 49]. These haemorrhages may be responsible for the early constitution of a chronic subdural collection, as shown by one of the 18 newborns and infants followed up to 5 weeks by Rooks et al. [39].

The variations in estimations between the studies could be partly explained by differences in infant ages at time of scanning, as the highest prevalence was detected when imaging was performed during the first 72 hours post partum, with a higher prevalence of SDH [29]. It remains elusive whether the location of the haemorrhages could play a role in possible consequences.

Most of these haemorrhages spontaneously disappear during the first weeks of life. But how many are followed by the constitution of a chronic hygroma or a marked expansion of the subarachnoid space? Up to now, no large systematic study which could answer this question has been carried out using ultrasound or MRI during the first 6 months of life in young infants.

8.4 Cephalhaematomas

There is another open question: what could be the role of soft tissue swelling/cephalhaematoma linked to traumatic delivery since the coexistence of subdural effusion and cephalhaematoma seems frequent but underdiagnosed [14, 39]?

8.5 Prematurity and Low Birth Weight

Other important risk factors are prematurity and low birth weight. Prematurity is considered a predisposing factor of AHT. However, there is no explanation for this. On the other hand, premature infants constantly present a larger subarachnoid space than term babies, and they also have immature meningeal membranes, immature venous distribution, and a brittleness of these tissues which also applies to the retina and the retinal vessels. They may also present with hyperparathyroidism secondary to their mineral deficiency (in 15% of cases [34] leading to a higher risk of bone fractures, especially ribs and metaphyseal fractures [6, 15]).

Premature infants have a higher risk of intradural and subdural bleeding than term infants. This is more likely related to intrinsic factors rather than unproven abuse. A recently published paper underlines the fact that perinatal intradural bleeding may lead to the constitution of chronic subdural and/or large subarachnoid collections, which constitute a predisposing factor for further bleeding [52].

8.6 Benign External Hydrocephalus

The most important risk factor is the expansion of the subarachnoid space, also called benign external hydrocephalus (BEH), in some young infants (see Chapters 5 and 6). This anatomical situation is most often neglected – and not described – by radiologists, since the publications of Paul Kleinman in the 1980s and 1990s. This author considered this situation absolutely and undoubtedly physiologic and irrelevant to the pathophysiology of SDH, even in preterm infants. But it is certainly not physiologic when an expansion of this space leads to a rapid increase of the head circumference, above the 98th percentile, reaching more than 5–10 mm of depth in the frontal area.

An important risk of bleeding results from this situation, with stretching of the bridging veins at the most fragile level of their course, in the dura itself, or by decrease of the output into the venous intradural microvasculature. More than 30 publications in the literature report the occurrence of bleeding in cases of BEH or subdural chronic collections [13]. This situation fortunately remains rare, but its current incidence has yet to be demonstrated. We describe here a case report which demonstrates that this question is still relevant:

> Case report: PN, male. Second uneventful pregnancy, except for an increase of the fetal head circumference observed on US survey, linked to a pericerebral hypo-echogenic collection, with then regular growth always above the 97th percentile [see Figures 8.1 and 8.2]. Normal delivery. Neonatal head circumference 38.5 cm (> 97th centile). Normal psychomotor development except for a slight motor retardation with hypotonia. He never convulsed.

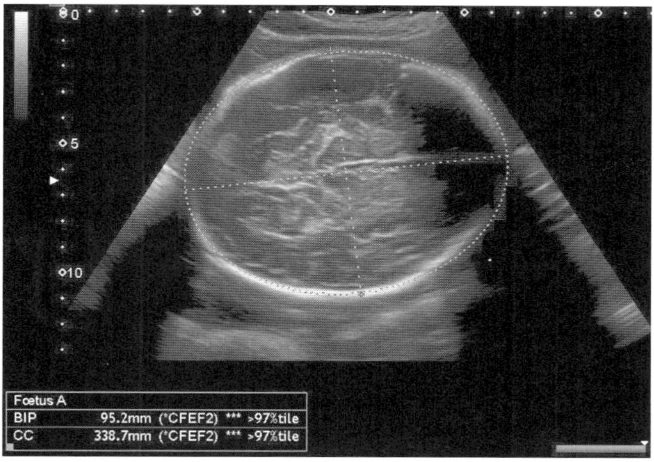

Figure 8.1 Antenatal ultrasound examination performed 3 weeks before delivery: large hypoechogenic cerebrospinal fluid (CSF) collection predominating at the frontal level

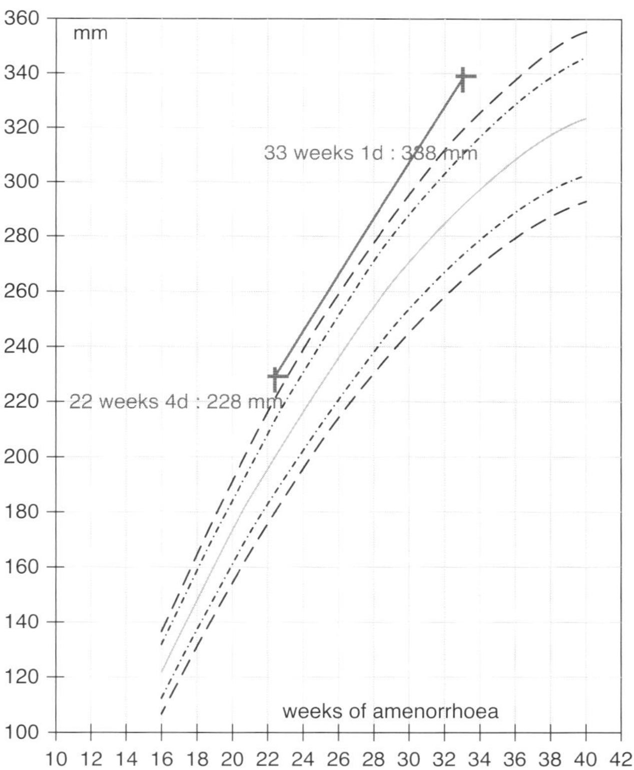

Figure 8.2 Antenatal head circumference curve

His head growth was always above the 97th centile. He never had episodes of marked discomfort.

At 9 months, a short fall from a changing table occurred (about 2/3 inches) with frontal impact. Fifteen minutes later, brief loss of consciousness with hypotonia lasting

15 minutes, with rapid recovery (corresponding to a so-called brief resolved unexplained event (BRUE)).

Despite the clinical normalisation, the parents immediately went to the hospital emergency reception (about 20 minutes later). The neurologic examination was normal. The head circumference was 48 cm (for an age of 9 months, that corresponds to a macrocrania above the 98th centile).

A CT scan was performed which showed a left SDH. The MRI 24 h later confirmed this diagnosis. It showed a bilateral subarachnoidal collection, associated with a bilateral subdural collection with a heterogeneous content: areas of slightly increased signal, of different ages, with a limited left bleed in the subdural space interpreted as an acute subdural hematoma [see Figures 8.3 and 8.4].

Fortunately, the evolution was favorable, with complete normalisation, except for a macrocrania. The diagnosis in this university hospital was: AHT (denied by the parents).

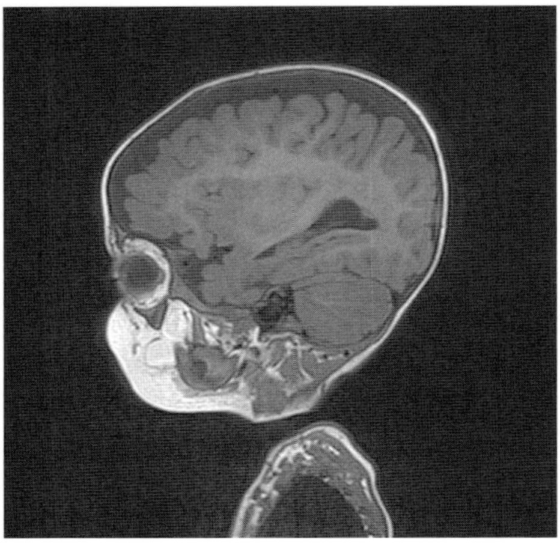

Figure 8.3 MRI T1: images obtained at 9 months of age, 24 hours after a short fall from a changing table: CSF intensity, slightly heterogeneous, pericerebral collection.

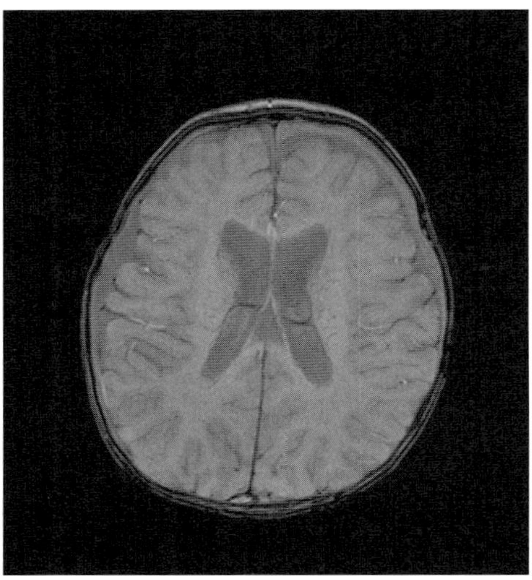

Figure 8.4 MRI SWI: left subdural collections with different signal intensity consistent with spontaneous bleeding

We believe this boy had early, prenatal development of a marked subarachnoid collection (probably of cerebrospinal fluid (CSF)), with constitution of chronic subdural collection and hemato-hygroma linked to recurrent limited asymptomatic micro bleeds, and, finally, limited acute subdural haemorrhage, secondary to a short fall, in an infant presenting anatomical predisposing factors.

Chronic subdural collection or pericerebral collections diagnosed with ultrasound examination in utero have been reported in a few cases [16]. To our knowledge, however, no systematic survey has been performed up to now in order to study the characteristics and evolution of such cases. Of note is that, according to the surprising assertions of a recently published paper by Laurent-Vannier et al., this case could correspond to the first in utero diagnosed shaken baby or prenatal shaken foetus [30].

8.7 Pericerebral Collections

It has been widely claimed in the medical literature that multiple SDH over the convexities, inter-hemispheric haemorrhages, posterior fossa SDH, and even hypoxic-ischemic injury and cerebral oedema are 'significantly' associated with AHT [27]. It has also been claimed that chronic SDH could be specific for AHT [25, 30].

All of these simplistic assertions result from circular reasoning. Nothing is said, particularly in France, about the different factors acting on the physiopathology and development of the pericerebral membranes, nor about the different mechanisms leading to the constitution of subacute or chronic pericerebral collections, as demonstrated by Tucker et al. [47]. It is unfortunate that scientists are embracing a restricted point of view according to which AHT is the only possible cause of SDH, with no consideration of risk factors.

8.8 Genetic Predisposing Factors

The existence of underlying genetic predisposing factors is typically not discussed in cases of so-called AHT. Nevertheless, many publications support the existence of genetic factors as risk factors for subdural bleedings.

The male predominance in SDH, as in AHT, is constantly mentioned in the literature, with a male:female ratio of about 2:1 or more in all reported series. This cannot be coincidental. A controversy has been recently introduced by O'Meara [25]. The references suggesting females may be equally represented concern older infants [33] on only 13 AHT patients [12]. Such references should be considered with great caution given the small number of cases.

The familial occurrence, including in twins, of an abnormal expansion of the subarachnoid spaces associated with subdural effusions and/or haematomas has been reported in several publications, suggesting genetic factors are involved in these cases, factors which remain unknown up to now [2, 13, 48, 50]. The occurrence of subdural or intradural bleeding is a rare complication in well-known genetic diseases such as haemophilia, Menkes disease, glutaric aciduria type I, coagulopathies, anticoagulant protein (antithrombin III, protein C, protein S) deficiencies or anti-phospholipid and anti-cardiolipin antibodies [41].

Spontaneous intradural bleeding may occur in some forms of Ehlers-Danlos disease and osteogenesis imperfecta, giving some proof that internal predisposing factors could favour or even provoke subdural bleeding [42]. However, nothing is described about the responsibility of gene dysfunction involved in collagen synthesis in these cases.

For a long time, we have known that intracranial haemorrhages and retinal haemorrhages have been documented either spontaneously, or after minor trauma in children with types I, II, III osteogenesis imperfecta [11, 18, 21, 40, 46]. We actually know about 19 genes involved in collagen synthesis [32]. Collagen is the main component of the meningeal membranes. The occurrence of SDH has been reported in collagen III, I, IV, and V diseases [35, 45]. However, up to now, no systematic molecular biologic study of the *COL5A1*, *COL3A1*, *COL4A1*, *COL4A2*, *COL1A1*, and *COL1A2* genes has ever been performed in cases of SDH occurring in young infants [44].

As far as bone-associated fractures are concerned, we should emphasise the importance of also investigating in these cases phosphocalcic metabolism and the levels of vitamins D and C in the baby and in the mother as well [36, 42, 44]. We can say the same in cases of cerebral thrombophlebitis associated with SDH: *G1691A* (Leiden factor), *G20210A* (factor 11), and *MTHFRC577 T* gene mutations are rarely studied [19].

8.9 Cerebral Venous Sinus Thrombosis

The responsibility, in rare cases of SDH, of a cerebral venous sinus thrombosis (CVST) needs to be highlighted (see Chapters 3 and 4). According to the seventh AHT Hershey conference, CVST could be secondary to an abusive trauma. That is a new dogma, as it has been previously demonstrated that CVST could be responsible for SDH. An MRI has to be performed less than 72 hours after presentation, and if possible within 48 hours. Parenchymal haemorrhages are observed in 30–35% of these cases, typically in the cortex and extending subcortically with gyral enhancement, tentorial and leptomeningeal enhancement, and SDH or subarachnoid haemorrhage [5, 37].

Moreover, thrombus within the inferior sagittal venous sinus may be occasionally misinterpreted as acute intradural haemorrhages, as shown by Hedlund [22], even if a study of 36 cases of CVST published by McLean et al. [53] didn't show any case of SDH. As suggested by Galaznik [17], CVST may be mistaken for AHT, even if subarachnoid haemorrhages and SDH are rarely associated with CVST [41].

8.10 Sudden Infant Death Syndrome

Finally, an important question remains without response: are there any relationships between AHT and sudden infant death syndrome (SIDS) (see Chapter 7)? Sudden infant death populations are predominantly male with an overrepresentation of prematurely born infants and low birth weight babies [28]. Sudden infant death and SDH occur at the same age. The clinical manifestations of SIDS are very often observed after a nap, with the same apparent life-threatening events revealing the SDH as observed in cases of near or delayed death in SIDS. In these delayed deaths, intradural hemorrhage, SDH, and subarachnoid hemorrhage have been observed in respectively 12%, 4%, and 7% of cases [28]. Of course, most SIDS are the result of a respiratory arrest linked to receptors, genes, and/or regions dysfunction in the brainstem, the limbic system, and the inner ear [10]. Nevertheless, this hypothesis needs to be investigated.

8.11 Conclusion

In conclusion, the risk factors, directly related to the young age of the infant, are too rarely investigated in cases of SDH occurring in young infants. How can we presume only external factors, always inflicted or traumatic, could be involved in all diagnosed cases? Our knowledge about the biochemical and genetic mechanisms regulating the membranes' development and pathology during the first months of life remains incomplete.

We are still functioning in the same manner as we functioned 40 years ago. Although radiological technology has improved, imaging shows images rather than the biochemical characteristics of the fluid collections or the mechanism of constitution of the observed anomalies. It gives no information about the histopathology of these lesions or about the underlying biochemical dysfunctions (see Chapter 3). Half a century ago, we talked about 'idiopathic' SDH in infancy. We are not sure this statement has been greatly modified with time.

References

1. Ami O Maran JC, Gabor P et al. Three dimensional magnetic resonance imaging of fetal head molding and brain shape during the second stage of labor. *PLoS One*. 2019. https://doi.org/10.1371/journal.pone.0215721.
2. Azais M, Echenne B. Epanchements péricérébraux idiopathiques (hydrocéphalie externe) du nourrisson. *Annales de Pédiatrie*. 1992;39:550–8.
3. Browder J, Kaplan HA, Krieger AJ. Veinous lakes in the suboccipital dura matter and falx cerebelli in infants: Surgical significance. *Surgical Neurology*. 1975;4:53–5.
4. Callaway NF, Ludwig CA, Blumenkranz MS et al. Retinal and optic nerve hemorrhages in the newborn infant. *Ophthalmology*. 2016;123(5):1043–52.
5. Canedo Antelo M, Baleato-González S, Mosqueira AJ et al. Radiologic clues to cerebral venous thrombosis. *RadioGraphics*. 2019;39:1611–28.
6. Chen W, Yang C, Chen H, Zhang B. Risk factor analysis and prevention of metabolic bone disease of prematurity. *Medicine*. 2018;97:e12861.
7. Cheshire EC, Malcomson RDG, Joseph S et al. Post-mortem imaging of the infant and perinatal dura matter and superior sagittal sinus using optical coherence tomography. *International Journal of Legal Medicine*. 2017;131:1377–83.
8. Cheshire EC, Malcomson RDG, Sun P et al. A systematic autopsy survey of human infant bridging veins. *International Journal of Legal Medicine*. 2018;132:449–61.
9. Cohen MC, Scheimberg I. Histology of the dural membrane supports the theoretical considerations of its role in the pathophysiology of subdural collections in non-traumatic circumstances. *Pediatric Radiology*. 2009;39:880–1.
10. Cohen MC, Scheimberg I, Beckwith J, Hauck F (eds.). *Investigation of sudden infant death syndrome*. Cambridge University Press, 2019. https://doi.org/10.1017/9781108186001.
11. Cole WG, Lam TP Arachnoid cyst and chronic subdural hematoma in a child with osteogenesis imperfecta type III resulting from the substitution of glycine 1006 by alanine in the pro alpha 2 chain of type I procollagen. *Journal of Medical Genetics*. 1996;33:193–6.
12. Diaz-Olavarrieta C, García-Piña CA, Loredo-Abdala A et al. AHT at a tertiary care children's hospital in Mexico City: A preliminary study. *Child Abuse and Neglect*. 2011;35:915–23.
13. Echenne B. Expansion de l'espace sous-arachnoidien: du physiologique au pathologique. In *Le syndrome du bébé secoué*. B Echenne, A Couture, G Sebire, eds. Sauramps, 2020, pp. 25–47.
14. Echenne B. Notions de terrain et de facteur inhérents à l'enfant lui-même. In *Le syndrome du bébé secoué*. B Echenne, A Couture, G Sébire, eds. Sauramps, 2020, pp. 219–38.
15. Figueras-Aloy J, Álvarez-Domínguez E, Pérez-Fernández JM et al. Metabolic bone disease and bone mineral density in very preterm infants. *Journal of Pediatrics*. 2014;164:499–504.

16. Galaznik JG. A case for an utero etiology of chronic SDH/effusions of infancy. *Journal of Perinatology*. 2011;31:320–2.

17. Galaznik JG. Cerebral sinovenous thrombosis is a valid mimic of AHT. *Pediatrics*. 2013;131:e1357–e1373.

18. Ganesh A, Jenny C, Geyer J, Shouldice M, Levin AV. Retinal hemorrhages in type I osteogenesis imperfecta after minor trauma. *Ophthalmology*. 2004;111:1428–31.

19. Garrido Barbero M, Arnaez J, Loureiro B et al. The role of factor Leiden, prothrombin G20210A, and MTHFR C677 T mutations in neonatal cerebral sinovenous thrombosis. *Clinical and Applied Thrombosis/Hemostasis*. 2019;25:1–6.

20. Gooding CA, Price DC, Newton TH. Experimental studies of falx and tentorial opacification during cerebral angiography. *Radiology*. 1972;103:77–82.

21. Groninger A, Schaper J, Messing-Juenger M, Mayatepek E, Rosenbaum T. Subdural hematoma as clinical presentation of osteogenesis imperfecta. *Pediatric Neurology*. 2005;32:140–2.

22. Hedlund GL. Cerebral sinovenous thrombosis in pediatric practice. *Pediatric Radiology*. 2013;43:173–88.

23. Högberg U, Andersson J, Squier W et al. Epidemiology of subdural haemorrhage during infancy: A population-based register study. *PLoS One*. 2018;13(10): e0206340.

24. Hughes LA, May K, Talbot JF, Parsons MA. Incidence, distribution, and duration of birth-related hemorrhages: A prospective study. *Journal of the American Association for Pediatric Ophthalmology*. 2006;10:102–6.

25. Iqbal O'Meara AM, Sequeira J, Ferguson NM. Advances and future directions of diagnosis and management of pediatric abusive head trauma: A revue of literature. *Frontiers in Neurology*. 2020;11:1–12.

26. Kaplan HA, Browder J, Krieger AJ. Venous channels within the intracranial dural partitions. *Radiology*. 1975;115:641–5.

27. Kemp AM, Jaspan T, Griffiths J et al. Neuroimaging: What neuroradiological features distinguish abusive from non-abusive head trauma? A systematic review. *Archives of Disease in Childhood*. 2011;96:1103–12.

28. Krous HF, Haas EA, Chadwick A et al. Delayed death in sudden infant death syndrome: A San Diego SIDS/SUDC research project 15-year population-based report. *Forensic Science International*. 2008;176:209–16.

29. Kumpulainen V, Lehtola SJ, Tuulari JJ et al. Prevalence and risk factors of incidental findings in brain MRIs of healthy neonates: The FinnBrain Birth Cohort Study. *Frontiers in Neurology*. 2019;10:1347. https://doi.org/10.3389/fneur.2019.01347.

30. Laurent Vannier A, Bernard JY, Chevignard M. High frequency of previous abuse and missed diagnoses prior to abusive head trauma: A consecutive case series of 100 forensic examinations. *Child Abuse Review*. 2020. https://doi.org/10.1002/car.2638.

31. Looney CB, Smith JK, Merck LH et al. Intracranial hemorrhage in asymptomatic neonates: Prevalence on MR images and relationship to obstetric and neonatal risk factors. *Radiology*. 2007;242:535–41.

32. Mäkitie RE, Constantini A, Kämpe A, Alm J, Mäkitie O. New insights into monogenic causes of osteoporosis. *Frontiers in Endocrinology*. 2019;10:1–15.

33. Miller Ferguson M, Sarnaik A, Miles D et al. AHT and mortality: An analysis from an international comparative effectiveness study of children with severe traumatic brain injury. *Critical Care Medicine*. 2017;45:1398–1407.

34. Mitchell SM, Rogers SP, Hicks PD et al. High frequency of elevated alkaline phosphatise activity and rickets exist in extremely low birth weight infants despite current nutritional support. *BMC Pediatrics*. 2009;9:47.

35. Ortiz Remacha PP, Candia J, Conde M. Recurrent subdural hemorrhages: The form of presentation of a type IV

Ehlers–Danlos syndrome. *Revista Clínica Española*. 2000;200:181–2.

36. Paterson CR, Paterson EC. Maternal vitamin deficiencies causing bone disorders and fractures in infants. *Medical Research Archives*. 2019;10:1–13.
37. Poon CS, Chang JK, Swarnkar A, Johnson MH, Wasenko J. Radiologic diagnosis of cerebral venous thrombosis: Pictorial review. *American Journal of Roentgenology*. 2007;189(6 suppl):s64–s75.
38. Raybaud C. Normal and abnormal embryology and development of the intracranial vascular system. *Neurosurgical Clinics of North America*. 2010;21:399–426.
39. Rooks VJ, Eaton JP, Ruess L et al. Prevalence and evolution of intracranial hemorrhage in asymptomatic term infants. *American Journal of Neuroradiology*. 2008;29:1082–9.
40. Sasaki-Adams D, Kulkarni A, Rutka J et al. Neurosurgical implications of osteogenesis imperfecta in children: Report of 4 cases. *Journal of Neurosurgery: Pediatrics*. 2008;1:229–36.
41. Saposnik G, Barinagarrementeria F, Brown RD et al. Diagnosis and management of cerebral venous thrombosis. *Stroke*. 2011;42:1158–92.
42. Singh Kocher M, Dichtel L. Osteogenesis imperfecta misdiagnosed as child abuse. *Journal of Pediatric Orthopaedics B*. 2011;20:440–3.
43. Sirgiovanni I, Avignone S, Groppo M et al. Intracranial hemorrhage: An incidental finding at magnetic resonance imaging in a cohort of late preterm and term infants. *Pediatric Radiology*. 2014;44:289–96.
44. Sturtz F, Echenne B. Les notions de terrain et de facteur favorisants: Maladies génétiques. In *Le syndrome du bébé secoué*. B Echenne, A Couture, G Sebire, eds. Sauramps, 2020, pp. 241–55.
45. Tosun A, Kurtgoz S, Dursun S, Bozkurt G. A case of Ehlers–Danlos syndrome type VI A with novel *PLOD1* gene mutation. *Pediatric Neurology*. 2014;51:566–9.
46. Tokoro K, Nakajima F, Yamataki A et al. Infantile chronic subdural hematoma with local protrusion of the skull in a case of osteogenesis imperfecta. *Neurosurgery*. 1988;22:595–8.
47. Tucker J, Choudhary AK, Piatt J. Macrocephaly in infancy: Benign enlargement of the subarachnoid spaces and subdural collections. *Journal of Neurosurgery: Pediatrics*. 2016;18:16–20.
48. Wester K. Two infants boys misdiagnosed as 'shaken baby' and their twin sister: A cautionary tale. *Pediatric Neurology*. 2019;97:3–11.
49. Whitby EH, Griffiths PD, Rutter S et al. Frequency and natural history of subdural haemorrhages in babies and relation to obstetric factors. *Lancet*. 2004;363:846–51.
50. Whitehead MT, Lee B, McCarron A, et al. Reduced subarachnoid fluid diffusion in enlarged subarachnoid spaces of infancy. *Neuroradiology*. 2017;30:418–24.
51. Wittscheiber D, Karger B, Pfeiffer H, et al. Understanding subdural collections in paediatric abusive head trauma. *American Journal of Neuroradiology*. 2019;40:388–95.
52. Zahl SM, Wester K, Gabaeff S. Examining perinatal subdural haematoma as an aetiology of extra-axial hygroma and chronic subdural haematoma. *Acta Paediatrica*. 2019. https://doi.org/10.1111/APA.15072.
53. McLean LA, Frasier LD, Hedlund GL. Does intracranial venous thrombosis cause subdural hemorrhage in the pediatric population? *American Journal of Neuroradiology*. 2012;33(7):1281–4.

Chapter 9

How I Became a Shaken Baby Syndrome Sceptic Paediatrician

A Review of the Observations That Challenge the Existence of Shaken Baby Syndrome

Marvin Miller

Introduction

Paediatricians have been taught, and most have accepted, that there is a sound scientific foundation for the existence of shaken baby syndrome (SBS). Moreover, the extensive publicity and affirmation of SBS by reputable professional organisations have convinced much of society SBS is a real entity. However, my experience as a practising paediatrician for more than four decades suggests otherwise, namely SBS is not a valid diagnosis and, for the past five decades, many thousands of cases of legitimate medical conditions have been misdiagnosed as SBS.

An SBS diagnosis is based on the classical triad of (1) subdural haematoma (SDH), (2) retinal haemorrhages (RHs), and (3) neurologic abnormality (seizures, unresponsive state, acute life-threatening event (ALTE), prolonged apnoea) [1].

Shaking as a cause of the triad was originally suggested by Guthkelch and Caffey in the early 1970s [2, 3]. The proponents of SBS today posit that adults who become frustrated with caring for a demanding infant, especially one who cries excessively, will lose their temper and violently shake the infant, causing the triad.

I am a paediatrician and subspecialist in clinical genetics and have been in academic paediatrics for 40 years. For the first 15 years of my career, I believed in the validity of this diagnosis. In my responsibilities as an attending paediatrician caring for infants admitted to the hospital with the triad, I referred such infants to the child abuse paediatrician in my hospital. I presumed the scientific underpinning of their discipline was sound.

However, in 1997 I was asked to consult on a young infant who presented with the triad in whom SBS was diagnosed, but the accused parent adamantly denied wrongdoing. The infant had marked macrocephaly and had slipped on the living room floor and hit his head prior to presentation. I questioned if the large head and fall might have contributed to the causation of the triad. I concluded it could have and testified to this effect in court on behalf of the accused – the child was returned to his parents and did well over the next 17 years (case 1 in [28] describes this infant).

This experience led me on a journey in the course of which I found increasing evidence that SBS is not a valid diagnosis and that over the past four decades many diagnoses of child abuse based on the finding of the triad were wrong, leading to devastating consequences for both the family involved and for society in wasting millions of dollars in adjudicating these cases.

9.1 The Pathogenesis of Shaken Baby Syndrome As Posited by Its Proponents

Proponents of SBS believe violent shaking of an infant can cause the triad, which consists of the following [4]:

1. Rupture of a bridging vein in the brain leading to the SDH.
2. Rupture of small vessels in the retina leading to RHs.
3. The development of increased intracranial pressure (ICP) from the SDH leading to neurologic abnormalities.

As I read the scientific literature on SBS, communicated with likeminded SBS sceptics, and did my own clinical research on this issue, I made numerous observations that caused me to doubt the validity of SBS.

9.2 Observations That Challenge and Undermine the Existence of Shaken Baby Syndrome

In this section I raise 13 issues that challenge or undermine the existence of SBS.

9.2.1 The Neuropathology of Shaken Baby Syndrome

The gross and microscopic neuropathology findings appear counter to what violent shaking would produce (see Chapter 3). First, the gross neuropathology in the overwhelming majority of autopsy cases of SBS confirms the head imaging studies that show a thin SDH. Proponents of SBS suggest violent shaking causes a bridging vein to rupture, but this would lead to a large focal SDH, not the more commonly observed thin SDH [4, 5].

Second, in infants who die of alleged SBS, the brain neuropathology is usually not one of trauma, but rather of hypoxia [5–7]. Geddes et al. studied the neuropathology of infants alleged to have died from SBS. Of 53 infants studied with alleged non-accidental head injury, microscopy of the brain showed hypoxic changes in 81% (43/53) of the cases and showed diffuse axonal traumatic changes in only 3 of the 53 infants.

Cohen and Scheimberg found intradural haemorrhage was common in hypoxic foetuses and infants [8]. Hypoxia leads to intradural/thin subdural haemorrhage, which leads to inflammatory changes in the brain with increased ICP. Thus, hypoxia-related intradural haemorrhage is consistent with Geddes's hypothesis that most cases diagnosed SBS/AHT are consequences of hypoxia, not trauma. This would explain the high frequency of thin SDH that is most often found in autopsy cases of alleged SBS. The neuropathology of most autopsy cases of alleged SBS is not consistent with trauma, but rather hypoxia. This stunning observation is one of the two most compelling arguments for the statement that SBS is not a valid medical diagnosis.

9.2.2 The Biomechanics of Shaken Baby Syndrome

Biomechanical analyses have shown that shaking cannot produce sufficient forces to cause brain damage (see Chapter 14). Ommaya et al. determined the magnitude of rotational acceleration needed to produce SDH in the monkey and extrapolated their findings to the human. They estimated the minimal rotational acceleration to cause traumatic shaking injury with SDH in the human would be about 6,000 radian/sec^2 [9]. Using human cadavers and high-speed film, Löwenhielm estimated it would require an angular acceleration of at least 4,500 rad/sec^2 to produce SDH from a ruptured bridging vein while Depreitere et al. estimated the value is 10,000 rad/sec^2 in adult brains [10, 11]. Taken together, the best human data suggest it would require a rotational acceleration of 4,000–10,000 radian/sec^2 to cause a SDH from a ruptured bridging vein.

Using biofidelic dolls, three studies have shown the magnitude of rotational acceleration that results from shaking alone is far below this threshold of 4,000 radian/sec^2. The rotational accelerations (radian/sec^2) caused by shaking alone in the three studies were the following: Duhaime = 1,139, Prange = 2,600 (maximal in which head hit back and chest), and Lloyd = 1,068 [12–14].

Thus, the available biomechanical evidence strongly indicates shaking alone does not cause the triad, as the rotational acceleration from shaking falls far below what is required to cause an SDH. Lloyd found rotational acceleration from shaking was similar to that of an infant jumping in a Jumparoo [14]. Violent shaking in an infant would likely cause catastrophic neck injury such as cervical spine dislocation/fracture and ligamentous injury. Yet these neck injuries are conspicuously absent in most cases of alleged SBS.

For decades SBS proponents argued that short falls could not produce the triad (see Chapter 15). In 2001 the American Academy of Pediatrics (AAP) Committee on Child Abuse and Neglect published a technical report on SBS with the following statement: 'SBS injuries are the result of violent trauma. The constellation of these injuries does not occur with short falls' [4].

Yet biomechanical analysis clearly shows short falls cause forces on the brain that are far greater than shaking, and John Plunkett provided undisputable evidence that accidental short falls could cause the triad [15]. What is most telling is that in 2018 a group of child abuse specialists published a series of short fall cases with the triad and conceded these cases are not SBS and the short fall caused the triad [16]. Clearly, some individuals in the child abuse community have changed their thinking about short falls, but many families were dissolved and many adults were imprisoned prior to this 2018 article.

Note that in 2008 the AAP offered a position statement indicating it would now use the term *abusive head trauma* (AHT) instead of SBS as it became evident to some in the AAP that shaking alone could not cause the triad [17]. This name change is in itself incriminating as it underscores the scepticism within the community of child abuse paediatricians that SBS can be caused by shaking alone. Yet, for many years, this is what SBS proponents preached and many around the world continue to do so.

Thiblin reported a series of 36 infants who were the victims of witnessed or filmed evidence of shaking events [18]. However, in 30 of the infants there was no evidence of the triad and in the other 6 there was information indicating blunt force trauma immediately after the shaking event or extenuating medical circumstances causing intracranial pathology. This series provides compelling evidence that shaking does not cause the triad. The biomechanical analysis of infant shaking showing that shaking alone cannot produce the triad (see Chapter 14) is the second of the two most compelling observations that SBS is not a valid diagnosis.

9.2.3 The Pathogenesis of Retinal Haemorrhages

The finding of RHs is perhaps the single finding that reflexively leads many doctors to the diagnosis of SBS. A major contention – but a misconception – of SBS proponents is that shaking causes RHs and that RHs are pathognomonic of child abuse – that is, no other clinical situations can cause RHs. However, experimental animal studies have never confirmed such a causation [19]. Moreover, it is difficult to understand how shaking could cause bleeding in vessels that are so firmly encased in the surrounding retinal tissues. One might expect bleeding in the skin of the face if indeed capillaries could be compromised by shaking – such is not found, however.

A far more likely explanation that does have scientific grounding is that the RHs are caused by increased ICP [20]. In an infant with increased ICP (from whatever cause), the retinal veins are compressed, leading to back pressure in the small vessels of the retina, some of which then leak blood, causing the RHs. Likewise, the optic nerve sheath haemorrhages (ONSH) often found in alleged SBS autopsy cases are also a result of the increased ICP via the cerebrospinal fluid (CSF) within the optic nerve sheath [21]. Figure 9.1 illustrates the pathogenesis of RHs and ONSHs from increased ICP.

Forensic pathologist Dr Pat Lantz has devised a simple and ingenious method of indirect ophthalmoscopy for detecting RHs at the time of autopsy [22]. Unless child abuse is being considered in an infant, a formal eye exam by a paediatric ophthalmologist is usually not done while the infant is still alive. Thus it has not been possible to know if clinical situations other than child abuse can cause RHs in infants. Lantz's use of post-mortem ophthalmoscopy has changed this, as he has demonstrated that RHs can be seen at autopsy using this unique post-mortem ophthalmoscopy in non-child abuse cases where there is an acute increase in ICP, including the following [23, 24]:

1. 4-year-old who drowned in a swimming pool.
2. 2-month-old who died of hypoxia from pertussis.
3. 14-month-old who died after being mauled by a dog and had fatal blood loss.
4. 5-month-old who died in a fire from smoke inhalation.
5. 15-month-old who aspirated popcorn and died from hypoxia.
6. 4-year-old who died from a ruptured cerebral vascular malformation.

Thiblin et al. have reported a series of 148 infants with intracranial pathology from the Swedish National Patient Register in which there were 29 with RHs and 119 without RHs [25]. Their analysis showed non-birth-related RHs in infants can be secondary to a traumatic or a non-traumatic aetiology, RHs are associated with raised ICP and chronic or mixed-density subdural haemorrhage, and isolated shaking is unlikely to cause RHs independently of intracranial pathology [25, 26]. This epidemiologic evaluation of how RHs occur draws the same conclusions as Lantz did from his series of infants with RHs.

Because the medical community has accepted the SBS dogma that RHs are specific for SBS and have dismissed the critical observation that any situation that causes an acute increase in ICP in a young infant can cause RHs, non-child abuse diagnoses associated with RHs have been missed. This is the major reason the SBS myth has been perpetuated; the idea that RHs are pathognomonic of SBS has now been incorporated into mainstream paediatric and forensic medical thinking. However, this idea is not based on sound, existing science as

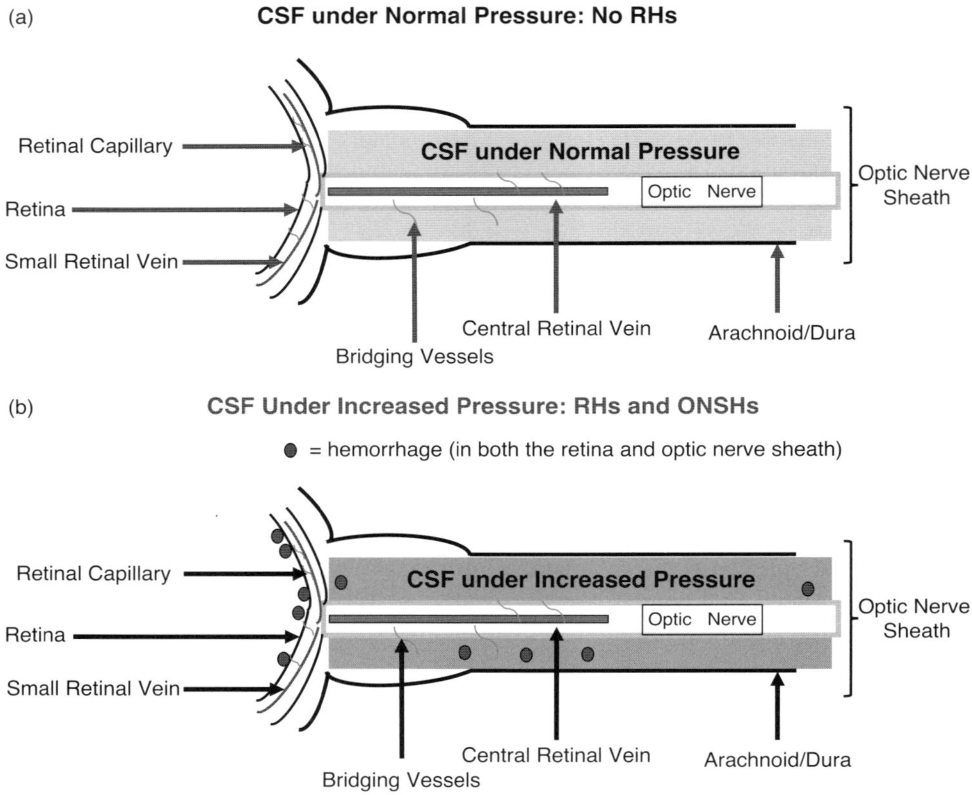

Figure 9.1 The aetiology of RHs in the triad: Increased ICP, not shaking
Figure 9.1a illustrates the normal anatomy and physiology of the eye relative to the ICP.
Both the optic nerve and the central retinal vein reside within the optic nerve sheath (anatomically the arachnoid/dura of the brain). Noteworthy, CSF is within the optic nerve sheath so the central retinal vein reflects the ICP. Under normal ICP there are no RHs.
Figure 9.1b illustrates the consequences of increased ICP. The increased ICP now causes a relative occlusion of the central retinal vein, leading to a high back pressure on the fragile retinal capillaries and causing RHs as shown in the figure. Thus, RHs are non-specific and any situation that leads to an acute increase in ICP can cause RHs in an infant. Moreover, RHs are *not* diagnostic of shaking an infant and vitreous traction from shaking is a highly unlikely cause of RHs. The increased ICP also causes small vessels/capillaries within the optic nerve sheath to leak leading to ONSH as shown in the figure.

the Lantz and Thiblin studies demonstrate. Even if the idea that RHs are pathognomonic for SBS remains part of the groupthink and public relations of SBS proponents, this idea is unfounded and should be rejected outright.

9.2.4 Alternative Causes of Shaken Baby Syndrome Discounted or Dismissed by Child Abuse Physicians

Proponents of SBS have dismissed several of the more common medical explanations that can cause the triad and thus have sometimes incorrectly diagnosed SBS. Four common alternative medical causes of SBS are not recognised by most SBS proponents:

1. An infant with an asymptomatic SDH from the trauma of birth that slowly increases in size until it becomes clinically significant and presents with the triad [27]. The overrepresentation of males with SBS is consistent with this as males have larger head circumferences than females at birth and thus have a greater chance of intracranial birth trauma.
2. An infant with benign external hydrocephalus (BEH) (also known as benign enlargement of the subarachnoid space and increased extra-axial fluid spaces; see Chapters 5 and 6) [28]. Multiple studies have clearly shown that infants with BEH are at increased risk to incur an SDH with minimal trauma or a spontaneous SDH that can enlarge.
3. Thrombosis of a cortical vein or intracranial sinus such as the sagittal sinus is another often missed alternative cause [29]. Appropriate brain imaging for vascular abnormalities and analysis by a paediatric radiologist trained in recognising such is essential in detecting cortical venous or sinus thrombosis.
4. Short falls are the fourth important alternative cause of SBS (see Chapters 14 and 15). For many years SBS proponents have dismissed short falls as a cause of the triad, but recently a study by Atkinson and other child advocacy paediatricians has shown that short falls can cause the triad [15, 16].

Finally, SBS proponents invariably state that their work-up addresses all of the rare, medical causes of SBS; however, there are many tragic cases that clearly indicate otherwise. I was indirectly involved in a case where Menkes disease was misdiagnosed as SBS with catastrophic consequences for the family [30]. Other rare medical causes of SBS include inherited bleeding disorders and ruptured aneurysms. Several articles provide rather detailed lists of rare but reported disorders that can cause SDH or the triad and thus be mistaken for SBS [31, 14].

9.2.5 Coerced Confessions in Shaken Baby Syndrome

Confessions of shaking have been the basis of several SBS convictions and an inclusion criterion for several published articles on SBS (see Chapter 12). However, it is now clear many of these confessions are exacted during plea bargaining or coerced (see Chapter 11) [32]. Not infrequently, a caregiver will admit to gently shaking an infant who was found unresponsive in an attempt to revive the infant, and such a statement is then turned into an admission of violent shaking causing SBS.

9.2.6 History Provided by Alleged Perpetrator

One of the basic tenets in sound medical practice is taking a comprehensive history and using the history as a starting point for laboratory and imaging testing in an effort to reach a diagnosis [33]. In cases of the triad, however, the history provided by the last person to be with the infant is typically dismissed and not believed by SBS proponents – a stunning violation of this basic tenet. The reason for this rejection of the history is that child abuse paediatricians and paediatric ophthalmologists believe SDH and RHs are diagnostic of SBS. Three common histories can be seen in the infant who presents with the triad:

- The infant was found by the caregiver to have apnoea or seizures or was having an ALTE while seeming normal immediately before. The last caregiver with the infant cannot provide an explanation for this unexpected neurologic event.

- The infant had a choking event and then became unresponsive.
- The infant had an ALTE immediately after a short fall or some time after a short fall with a lucid interval between the short fall and the ALTE presentation.

When the triad is eventually found with RHs and SDH, SBS protagonists typically dismiss the history provided by the caregiver who was last with the infant; that individual now becomes the alleged perpetrator. This judgement comes about because most SBS protagonists believe the following:

- Infants cannot present with the triad unless some serious historical event happened that the last caregiver with the infant should have known.
- A hypoxic event such as a severe choking episode cannot cause the triad (even though the Geddes et al. [5–7] studies suggest otherwise).
- Short falls cannot cause the triad (the 2018 Atkinson et al. article may change this misperception [16]).

Unfortunately, these three presentations can be associated with either medical diagnoses or accidental injury and SBS proponents wrongfully have diagnosed child abuse in many cases due to not considering a comprehensive differential diagnosis.

9.2.7 Lack of Witnessed or Videotaped Events of Shaken Baby Syndrome

It is estimated that there are some 1,300 cases of alleged SBS per year in the USA with a per capita incidence of approximately 30–35 cases per 100,000 infants $\leq$ 12 months of age [34]. Cases of SBS have been reported in most Western countries with a similar incidence to the USA. I estimate there are almost twice the number of infants in these Western countries, which would give a total yearly frequency of as many as at least 4,000 cases of SBS throughout the Western world.

In this modern time of cell phones with photographic capabilities and web cameras with video capabilities, one might think multiple, definitive episodes of shaking causing the triad would be recorded. Although many videos of shaking do exist (generally thanks to the presence of nanny cams), I am not aware of a single one in which the triad was produced by a filmed shaking incident. This is yet another compelling observation that indicates shaking may not be a valid cause of the triad.

9.2.8 The Multidisciplinary Team in Child Abuse Investigations

Almost all child abuse investigations are evaluated by a multidisciplinary team (MDT). Proponents of SBS often claim the MDT utilised in child abuse investigations ensures fair and impartial evaluations of cases of infants who present with the unexplained triad. Also called the Suspected Child Abuse and Neglect (SCAN) team, MDTs are usually called upon when there are allegations of child abuse. In SBS cases the team would typically consist of a child abuse paediatrician, paediatric radiologist, paediatric ophthalmologist, social worker, child protection worker, detective, and others.

My own experience in dealing with the various members of the MDT evaluating a case of the unexplained triad is that they all have similar thinking. Unless there is some history of confirmed trauma, the finding of the triad will generally lead to a diagnosis of SBS. While law enforcement officers are typically not official members of the MDT, they often participate in their evaluations and are likeminded. The MDT is a classic example of groupthink (see Chapter 13). Dr John Plunkett appropriately described the likely perilous consequences of such groupthink: 'The danger is for such a group to become a de facto star chamber unencumbered by accountability or self-doubt' [35].

9.2.9 Risk Profile for Committing Child Abuse

The child abuse literature contains studies that evaluate risk factors in an adult that can be used to generate a profile of the likelihood an individual might commit child abuse [36]. Risk factors include the following:

- Young age
- Unemployed
- Drug/alcohol use or addiction
- Themselves abused as a child
- Family stress

I have never seen an SBS advocate refer to this literature in the cases I have reviewed. I would think, if the last adult person caring for an infant who presents with the triad has a low risk profile for committing child abuse, then alternative medical explanations would be aggressively sought. Unfortunately, I have not found this to be the case.

I am aware of alleged SBS cases where the paediatrician knows the family well and believes child abuse is highly unlikely. Yet, because of fear of retribution from the child abuse community in their region, some families have told me that the paediatrician often remains silent and does not support the family in legal proceedings.

9.2.10 Quality of Evidence of the Shaken Baby Syndrome Literature

Independent analyses by Donohoe and, more recently, by the Swedish Agency (SBU) both concluded the scientific evidence that shaking alone could cause the triad was weak, indeed virtually non-existent, and plagued by circular reasoning (see Chapter 10) [37, 38]. The hundreds of published articles on SBS, many in peer-reviewed journals, may give the public the impression that SBS is a valid diagnosis. However, this impression and confidence is without scientific foundation.

One of the original physicians to publish about the possibility that shaking might cause the triad, Dr Norman Guthkelch, has adamantly insisted his observations have been misinterpreted and he too was sceptical about the existence of SBS [39]. The SBS literature is necessarily of poor quality since the scientific foundation upon which the diagnosis of SBS relies has never been properly established. To the contrary, as this chapter illustrates, when SBS is critically analysed from multiple angles, it can firmly be concluded 'SBS is not a valid diagnosis.'

9.2.11 Grants for Shaken Baby Syndrome Research and National Shaken Baby Syndrome Organisations

Over the years many large federal grants for SBS research have been awarded related to research on SBS. Moreover, there is a national organisation that promotes the existence and prevention of SBS. If there is no scientific foundation for the existence of SBS, then these many articles are meaningless and the National Center on Shaken Baby Syndrome is promoting and preventing an entity that is not scientifically justified. This represents a tremendous waste of resources.

9.2.12 Professional Society Consensus Statements

Proponents of SBS frequently point out the overwhelming consensus of professional organisations about the certainty of the diagnosis of SBS [40]. However, such organisations consist of groups of likeminded SBS proponents, so there is nothing surprising or convincing about this consensus, which is akin to the fox guarding the henhouse. These organisations are self-proclaimed star chambers.

9.2.13 Perpetuation of the Myth

The totality of evidence is compelling that SBS is not a valid diagnosis. I have long wondered why SBS proponents dismiss and discount all this evidence which would cause any impartial observer to question the existence of SBS. Proponents of SBS have spread this diagnosis for more than five decades, with far-reaching consequences for the accused, the affected child, and society: wrongful imprisonment of innocent parents and caregivers, unnecessary dissolution of intact families, ruined reputations, and extraordinary cost to society and families.

I can only conclude SBS proponents continue to believe in the existence of SBS so as to protect themselves and their reputations. If SBS proponents admitted the theory that shaking is the main – or even the only possible – cause of the triad is simply wrong, then the realisation their reports and legal testimony had wrongfully dissolved families and imprisoned innocent caregivers would be devastating to their careers and life's work. Thus, as a defence mechanism, they must protect themselves by being fanatical adherents to the theory of SBS, regardless of the massive evidence to the contrary. To paraphrase Upton Sinclair: 'It is hard to get someone to understand something when their reputation [my word] depends on them not understanding it.'

For this reason, I believe SBS proponents have doubled down by writing articles that, instead of countering the legitimate scientific objections to the SBS theory such as those raised here, attack the messengers seeking to refute SBS [41, 42]. The incredibly frequent position of 'attacking the messenger rather than the message' underscores the desperation of SBS proponents in keeping their theory alive.

The psychology literature also provides insight as to why SBS proponents hold so zealously to their theory; it is a classic example of the 'backfire effect'. 'When people encounter evidence that should cause them to doubt their beliefs, they often reject this evidence, and strengthen their support for their original stance. This occurs due to a cognitive bias known as the backfire effect' [43]. I presume, because SBS proponents have been responsible for dissolving families and incarcerating alleged perpetrators of SBS based on their reports and court testimony, they would find it excruciatingly painful if SBS were found to be erroneous and that they were responsible for these miscarriages of justice.

It is critical that the public understand the institutional power and influence members of the child abuse protection community (CAPC) exert. They are intricately linked to and supported by the AAP and in many communities the law enforcement community is a de facto part of the MDT. Originally, they promoted the idea that SBS was a valid and scientifically justified diagnosis and that there was no controversy on this matter. However, as mounting evidence from multiple fronts now unequivocally shows the falsehood of that stance, the CAPC's members now find themselves pushed to defend it. There is now little for them to stand on. Unfortunately, this self-serving attitude has been part of one of the saddest chapters in modern paediatrics: paediatricians and other healthcare providers conspiring with law officials to wrongfully remove children from their parents and to unjustly send adults to prison.

9.3 My Understanding of the Pathogenesis of the Triad

If shaking alone cannot cause the triad, what is the pathogenesis of the triad in those infants who have been diagnosed as victims of SBS/AHT? If there is no evidence of external head trauma and we accept that shaking alone *cannot* cause the triad, then one of the previously noted alternative causes is likely the primary cause. In some cases of the triad there may be two or more causative factors. As there are multiple causes of the triad, there is likely a single, unifying pathway of pathogenesis that leads to the triad through a cascade of events.

Certainly one aetiology is child abuse in which there is intentional, violent impact of the infant's head against some hard object or intentional dropping of the infant on the floor. A second aetiology is an accidental short fall. While the vast number of short falls do not cause the triad, it is now known that it can happen in rare cases. However, in both these aetiologies, evidence of external head trauma would be expected. In order to distinguish an accidental cause of the triad from an inflicted abuse, one must take into account the history provided by the caregiver who witnessed or caused the accidental event and the surrounding circumstances. For example, older siblings can sometimes inadvertently injure their younger sibling with or without parents witnessing the event [44].

9.4 The Influence of Child Abuse Dogmas on Law Enforcement and the Judicial System

In many communities the physicians directly involved in child abuse allegations of infants who present with the unexplained triad or unexplained fractures have unduly influenced both law enforcement and the judicial system. Too often, police interrogate an alleged parent, not with the goal of obtaining an accurate historical account of what happened, but rather with the idea of obtaining an admission of guilt. The CAPC has convinced authorities without question that child abuse has occurred and law enforcement must find the perpetrator, typically the last person with the child. Moreover, the tactic of playing one parent against the other and/or threatening parents separately that, if they do not tell law enforcement who is responsible, they will risk forever losing their children often results in a coerced confession.

Too often, judges side with prosecutors in these cases because of political influence and their acceptance of the CAPC as being correct. Unless they have read the latest medical literature regarding the shortcomings of the SBS/AHT diagnosis, both law enforcement and the judicial system are in a mode of truth default as described by Malcolm Gladwell [45]. The entire medical legal system is stacked against innocent parents accused of SBS/AHT even though the most recent and evolving science is often firmly on their side.

Conclusion

I have the same two goals as any child abuse physician involved in the disposition of cases of the unexplained triad:

1. If there is compelling evidence of child abuse, the child should be removed from the care of the perpetrator and the perpetrator should be appropriately prosecuted.

2. If there is no supporting evidence of child abuse and there is a medical or accidental explanation of the findings, then child abuse should not be diagnosed. Shaking alone is not sufficient to cause the triad. If child abuse is being considered, there should be evidence of external trauma since impact is needed to cause the triad.

Unfortunately, society has been fooled into believing a rigid version of SBS theory for the past five decades. Yet as noted earlier in this chapter, several unrefuted scientific studies have proved the triad cannot be produced by shaking alone. The medical profession has allowed this miscarriage of justice to exist for far too long and it must now disavow this theory. The cost of the injustices it has caused has been enormous with many children wrongfully removed from their parents and many adults wrongfully imprisoned. It is high time for the errors in SBS theory to be exposed and for true diagnoses to be actively sought when an infant presents with the triad.

References

1. Richards PG, Bertocci GE, Bonshek RE et al. Shaken baby syndrome. *Archives of Disease in Childhood*. 2006;91(3):205–6.
2. Guthkelch AN. Infantile subdural haematoma and its relationship to whiplash injuries. *British Medical Journal*. 1971;2(5759):430–1.
3. Caffey J. On the theory and practice of shaking infants: Its potential residual effects of permanent brain damage and mental retardation. *American Journal of Diseases of Children*. 1972;124 (2):161–9.
4. American Academy of Pediatrics. Shaken baby syndrome: Rotational cranial injuries. Technical report. *Pediatrics*. 2001;108 (1):206–10.
5. Geddes JF, Hackshaw AK, Vowles GH, Nickols CD, Whitwell HL. Neuropathology of inflicted head injury in children. I. Patterns of brain damage. *Brain*. 2001;124:1290–8.
6. Geddes JF, Vowles GH, Hackshaw AK et al. Neuropathology of inflicted head injury in children. II. Microscopic brain injury in infants. *Brain*. 2001;124:1299–1306.
7. Geddes JF, Tasker RC, Hackshaw AK et al. Dural haemorrhage in non-traumatic infant deaths: Does it explain the bleeding in 'shaken baby syndrome?' *Neuropathology and Applied Neurobiology*. 2003;29:14–22.
8. Scheimberg I, Cohen MC, Zapata Vazquez RE et al. Non-traumatic intradural and subdural haemorrhage and hypoxic ischaemic encephalopathy in fetuses, infants and children up to 3 years of age. Analysis of two audits of 636 cases from two referral centers in the United Kingdom. *Pediatric Development Pathology*. 2013;16:149–59.
9. Ommaya A, Fass F, Yarnell P. Whiplash injury and brain damage. *JAMA*. 1968;204:75–9.
10. Löwenhielm P. Strain tolerance of the Vv. Cerebri Sup. (bridging veins) calculated from head-on collision tests with cadavers. *Zeitschrift für Rechtsmedizin*. 1974;75 (2):131–44.
11. Depreitere B, Van Lierde C, Vander Sloten J et al. Mechanics of acute subdural hematomas resulting from bridging vein rupture. *Journal of Neurosurgery*. 2006;104 (6):950–6.
12. Duhaime AC, Gennarelli TA, Thibault LE et al. The shaken baby syndrome: A clinical, pathological, and biomechanical study. *Journal of Neurosurgery*. 1987;66 (3):409–15.
13. Prange MT, Coats B, Duhaime AC, Margulies SS. Anthropomorphic simulations of falls, shakes, and inflicted impacts in infants. *Journal of Neurosurgery*. 2003;99(1):143–50.
14. Lloyd J, Willey EN, Galaznik JG, Lee III WE, Luttner SE. Biomechanical evaluation of head kinematics during infant shaking versus pediatric activities of

daily living. *Journal of Forensic Biomechanics*. 2011;2(2):1–9.

15. Plunkett J. Fatal pediatric head injuries caused by short-distance falls. *American Journal of Forensic Medicine and Pathology*. 2001;22(1):1–2.
16. Atkinson N, Van Rijn RR, Starling SP. Childhood falls with occipital impacts. *Pediatric Emergency Care*. 2018;34 (12):837–41.
17. Christian CW, Block R. Abusive head trauma in infants and children. *Pediatrics*. 2009;123(5):1409–11.
18. Thiblin I, Andersson J, Wester K et al. Medical findings and symptoms in infants exposed to witnessed or admitted abusive shaking: A nationwide registry study. *PLoS One*. 2020;15(10):e0240182.
19. Finnie JW, Blumbergs PC, Manavis J et al. Neuropathological changes in a lamb model of non-accidental head injury (the shaken baby syndrome). *Journal of Clinical Neuroscience*. 2012;19(8):1159–64.
20. Muller PJ, Deck JH. Intraocular and optic nerve sheath hemorrhage in cases of sudden intracranial hypertension. *Journal of Neurosurgery*. 1974;41(2):160–6.
21. De Leeuw M, Beuls E, Jorens PG, Parizel P, Jacobs W. The optic nerve sheath hemorrhage is a non-specific finding in cases of suspected child abuse. *Journal of Forensic and Legal Medicine*. 2015;36:43–8.
22. Lantz PE, Adams GG. Postmortem monocular indirect ophthalmoscopy. *Journal of Forensic Science*. 2005;50(6): JFS2005137-3.
23. Lantz PE, Stanton CA. Postmortem detection and evaluation of retinal hemorrhages. In 58th Annual Scientific Meeting of the American Academy of Forensic Sciences, 2006.
24. Personal communications with Dr Pat Lantz.
25. Thiblin I, Andersson J, Wester K, Högberg G, Högberg U. Retinal haemorrhage in infants investigated for suspected maltreatment is strongly correlated with intracranial pathology. *Acta Paediatrica*. 2022;111(4):800–8.
26. Squier W. Infant retinal haemorrhages correlate with chronic subdural haemorrhage, not shaking. *Acta Paediatrica*. 2022; 111(4):714–15.
27. Miller R, Miller ME. Overrepresentation of males in traumatic brain injury of infancy and in infants with macrocephaly: Further evidence that questions the existence of shaken baby syndrome. *American Journal of Forensic Medicine and Pathology*. 2010;31:165–73.
28. Miller D, Barnes P, Miller M. The significance of macrocephaly or enlarging head circumference in infants with the triad: Further evidence of mimics of shaken baby syndrome. *American Journal of Forensic Medicine and Pathology*. 2015;36(2):111.
29. Krasnokutsky MV. Cerebral venous thrombosis: A potential mimic of primary traumatic brain injury in infants. *American Journal of Roentgenology*. 2011;197(3): W503–W507.
30. https://onsbs.com/prologue.
31. David TJ. Non-accidental head injury: The evidence. *Pediatric Radiology*. 2008;38:370–7.
32. Leestma JE. 'Shaken baby syndrome': Do confessions by alleged perpetrators validate the concept? *Journal of American Physicians and Surgeons*. 2006;11:14–26.
33. Hampton JR, Harrison MJ, Mitchell JR, Prichard JS, Seymour C. Relative contributions of history-taking, physical examination, and laboratory investigation to diagnosis and management of medical outpatients. *British Medical Journal*. 1975;2 (5969):486–9.
34. National Center on Shaken Baby Syndrome. www.dontshake.org/learn-more.
35. Plunkett J. Recognizing abusive head trauma in children. *Journal of the American Medical Association*. 1999;282(15):1421–2.
36. Flaherty EG, Stirling J, Committee on Child Abuse and Neglect. The pedian's role in child maltreatment prevention. *Pediatrics*. 2010;126(4):833–41.
37. Donohoe M. Evidence-based medicine and shaken baby syndrome. Part 1: Literature

review. 1966–1998. *American Journal of Forensic Medicine and Pathology.* 2003;24:239–42.

38. Lynøe N, Elinder G, Hallberg B et al. Insufficient evidence for 'shaken baby syndrome': A systematic review. *Acta Paediatrica.* 2017;106(7):1021–7.

39. Guthkelch AN. Problems of infant retino-dural hemorrhage with minimal external injury. *Houston Journal of Health Law and Policy.* 2012;12:201–8.

40. Choudhary AK, Servaes S, Slovis TL et al. Consensus statement on abusive head trauma in infants and young children. *Pediatric Radiology.* 2018;48(8):1048–65.

41. Strouse PJ. Child abuse: We have problems. *Pediatric Radiology.* 2016;46:587–90. https://doi.org/10.1007/s00247-016-3551-9.

42. Hymel KP. Denying the abusive head trauma denialists their day in court, one step at a time. *Pediatric Radiology.* 2019;49 (13):1710–11.

43. The backfire effect: Why facts don't always change minds. https://effectiviology.com/backfire-effect-facts-dont-change-minds.

44. Adelson L. The battering child. *JAMA.* 1972;222(2):159–61.

45. Gladwell M. *Talking to strangers: What we should know about the people we don't know.* Penguin UK, 2019.

Chapter 10

The Swedish Systematic Literature Review on Suspected Traumatic Shaking (Shaken Baby Syndrome) and Its Aftermath

Niels Lynøe and Anders Eriksson

10.1 Introduction

The Swedish Agency for Health Technology Assessment and Assessment of Social Services, known by its Swedish acronym, SBU, invites scientists and clinicians to identify knowledge gaps within the fields of medical and social sciences research. In 2012, the SBU received a proposal to examine the evidence supporting a mechanism later referred to as traumatic shaking of an infant. In the spring of 2014, an expert panel of six members was selected to undertake an appraisal of the relevant literature. Work began in autumn 2014.

The systematic review of literature undertaken for quality assessment of the observational studies on shaken baby syndrome (SBS) was mainly epidemiological. The experts who conducted the systematic literature review were not from the start altogether familiar with the theories about mechanisms and causes, other than that three findings – encephalopathy, subdural haemorrhage (SDH), and retinal haemorrhage (RH), referred to as the *triad* – were considered to be closely associated with traumatic shaking and included in the concept of SBS. We were aware the issue was controversial, but not of the exact nature of the controversy.

Reports on health technology assessments presented by the SBU are usually highly respected and readily accepted in clinical practice [1]. However, this time there was a massive and surprisingly critical international reaction, which led the authors to follow up their literature review with an investigation and analysis of the SBS controversy itself, presented in this chapter.

This controversy not only concerns a straightforward disagreement as to whether various scientific theories explaining the symptoms are correct, but is further complicated by the fact that proponents of the mainstream SBS theory deny the existence of any controversy. They also deny that there are problems with the epidemiological studies on which the theories rely for corroboration, unearthed by our literature review. We found that most of the published literature is not of sufficient quality to yield definitive conclusions about the mechanisms at work in SBS due to severe problems of study quality and circular reasoning, explained in detail in what follows.

10.2 The SBU Report on Traumatic Shaking

10.2.1 Background

The hypothesis that shaking a baby in a whiplash-like manner might cause SDH was suggested by the neurosurgeon Norman Guthkelch in 1971 [2]. A year later, the American paediatric radiologist John Caffey elaborated and reversed this hypothesis and suggested that if SDH and

RH were identified, one should suspect the infant had been shaken [3]. According to both Guthkelch and Caffey, these signs were often observed *without* signs of trauma to the infant head. In 1979, RH was suggested as pathognomonic for SBS [4]. Eventually encephalopathy [5] was added and the three symptoms and signs – SDH, RH, and encephalopathy – were subsequently referred to as the triad.

Biomechanical studies have indicated that very high energy forces are needed to cause the triad [6] (see Chapter 14). Despite some contradictory findings [7, 8], there seems to be consensus that the forces needed are much easier to attain if the infant's head is also exposed to impact – for example, slamming the infant's head against a hard surface. Eventually, however, it was stated that if the triad was identified with no signs of impact or trauma, then once a short and specific set of 'acceptable' medical explanations (such as leukaemia, brain tumour, or severe accidental trauma) was ruled out, the only explanation was that the infant must have been violently shaken [9, 10], a conclusion which represents the gist of mainstream SBS theory.

During the past 40 years there have been many studies on the family of related topics 'shaken baby syndrome', 'abusive head trauma' (AHT), 'inflicted head trauma', 'non-accidental head injury', and similar expressions. These studies are used to support the claim that SBS/AHT theory is based on a scientifically robust body of knowledge [11–13]. Yet since 2001, the validity of the link between the triad and shaking of an infant has also been increasingly questioned [14–22]. Among others, Norman Guthkelch himself has questioned the manner in which his original hypothesis was inverted and developed into a dogma [18].

Because the diagnostic accuracy in this context has serious medical, societal, and legal implications for the parties concerned, it is extremely important that the diagnostic accuracy should be as high as possible. This consideration was the starting point for the Swedish systematic review. The main objective of the review was to determine the diagnostic accuracy of the triad in establishing that an infant has been violently shaken [23–26].

10.2.2 Methods

The criteria for study eligibility were:

- Population (or subpopulation): Infants $\leq$ 12 months of age
- Index test: The triad in suspected traumatic shaking
- Reference test ('gold standard'): Confessed or witnessed shaking or other trauma
- Outcome measure: Diagnostic accuracy

The particular focus was on triad cases with no relevant signs of trauma, henceforth referred to as *isolated triad cases*. Studies including children older than 12 months or *with* external signs of trauma were included only if a subgroup of children under 12 months of age or a subset of cases of isolated shaking could be identified within the study cohort.

In accordance with Health Technology Assessment (HTA) standards, an adapted peer-reviewed protocol was applied [27–31]. The systematic review was conducted by the SBU. The members selected for the expert panel included two paediatricians, an epidemiologist, a forensic pathologist, a general practitioner and ethicist, and a neuroradiologist.

The first step of the review process was an electronic literature search, which included the databases PubMed, Embase, and the Cochrane Library through 15 October 2015. Search terms included but were not limited to *infant*, *subdural haematoma*, *retinal haemorrhage*, *cerebral oedema, encephalopathy, accidental/non-accidental injury, shaken baby/shaken baby syndrome.*

The six experts engaged in the process worked in pairs, independently screening the titles and abstracts identified through the search strategy. All studies of potential relevance according to the inclusion criteria were retrieved in full text, and each pair of reviewers independently assessed one third of the full text studies to determine their eligibility for relevance.

The second step of the process involved determining the risk of bias of each individual study (low, moderate, or high). For each study, this risk was assessed independently by two reviewers using an adapted version of the QUADAS 1 tool [28]. Risk assessment focused on the risk of systematic errors (bias) due to methodological flaws. Systematic literature reviews were assessed using AMSTAR [29].

In principle, studies were to be assessed as having a *low risk of bias* when the study cases were unequivocally confirmed as having been violently shaken and when the shaking preceded the symptoms associated with the triad, as proven either by video recording or by evidence from independent witnesses. A further requirement was that the control cases had to be age-matched and unequivocally subjected to other defined types of trauma.

Studies were assessed as having *moderate risk of bias* when the study cases were identified only by a detailed confession by the suspected perpetrator and/or when there were shortcomings regarding controls – for example, no age match – or even lack of controls. Each individual study was assessed overall with respect to the significance of such shortcomings.

Studies were assessed as having *high risk of bias* when further shortcomings were identified – for example, insufficient justification that the cases under study were truly cases of shaking – and the consequent problem of circular reasoning, and it was considered that, in the presence of these and/or other defects, the results could not provide reliable information in answering the questions addressed in the systematic review.

In a large number of the studies included in the review, the authors classified cases as SBS or control by referring to the opinion of a child protection team. However, the child protection teams often now take for granted that, in the presence of the triad and the absence of the other 'acceptable' explanations such as those mentioned earlier in this chapter, the infant was violently shaken [9, 10, 25]. Other authors developed their own criteria for an 'acceptable' explanation and classified cases as SBS by default whenever those criteria were not fulfilled [9, 10]. Since the systematic review addressed the research question of *the certainty with which it can be concluded that, when the triad is present, the infant has been violently shaken*, a study in which it is assumed from the start that the presence of the triad means an infant has been shaken cannot be used due to circular reasoning.

10.2.3 Results

The literature search generated 3,773 records, of which 1,065 were original papers of potential relevance and were read in full text. Of these, 1,035 did not fulfil the inclusion criteria and were subsequently excluded, leaving 30 papers. Of these, 28 were assessed as having high risk of bias, 2 as having moderate risk, and none (0) as having low risk [25].

The strength of the two studies (one retrospective and one prospective) with moderate risk of bias [32, 33] was the fact that their study groups were based on confessions. One study provided detailed information about the shaking event in 14 out of 29 cases [32], while in the other study the control group entailed witnessed accidents in public areas [33]. One methodological weakness of both studies was that the risk of false confessions was not considered (see Chapters 11 and 12); there were also other methodological flaws [2, 25].

In the retrospective case-control study [32], the group of confessed shaking cases was compared to a group of people who were suspected suspected of, but denied, having shaken the infant. In the group of confessed shaking, 13 of 29 cases were allegedly injured through *isolated* shaking, and detailed information about the shaking event was provided in 14 cases. In all these cases, the caregiver explained that shaking was due to the infant's crying [32]. A corresponding specification was not provided in the denial group, which included 83 cases of which 19 admitted that they did shake the baby but as a resuscitation attempt *after* the infant's sudden loss of consciousness – that is, due to an apparent life-threatening event (ALTE). Twenty-eight were caused by minor trauma, and in the remaining 36 cases no explanation was provided [32]. The authors found no statistically significant differences between the two groups regarding age, sex, mortality, symptoms, and so forth. The authors concluded that '[a]s these 2 groups were similar, the causal mechanism may well have been the same despite the incomplete or absent confessions' [32].

In the prospective study [33], Vinchon et al. compared a group of 45 infants in which someone had confessed to or had been convicted of shaking the baby with a group of 39 infants who had been exposed to witnessed accidental trauma in a public area. 'Information on the confessions was obtained by a forensic paediatrician from judicial sources during expertise or after the judicial hearings were made public' [33]. No detailed information was provided in the study as to what had been confessed or under what circumstances the confessions had been obtained. The authors used a new 'triad' that included SDH, *diffuse* RH, and an *absence of scalp swelling*. For the applied triad the authors reported a sensitivity of 0.244, a specificity as well as positive predictive value of 1 (or 100%), and a negative predictive value of 0.534 [33].

Vinchon et al. excluded from their study cases with conditions or events that might cause the triad or its components, such as accidental trauma (fall, motor vehicle crash, etc.), sequelae of normal delivery, prematurity, macrocephaly and external hydrocephalus, coagulopathies, infections, metabolic diseases, leukaemia, immunological conditions, vascular malformations in the brain, asphyxia, and so forth [33].

10.2.4 Limitations of the 30 Studies Retained for the Review

The studies were mostly observational, using comparison groups derived primarily from retrospective case-control studies extracted from medical records or registers. Other studies were designed as prospective cohort studies. Apart from the usual methodological bias issues associated with retrospective case-control studies, other issues were also observed. For example, in most of the studies, the average age of the control group (often accidental falls) was significantly higher than that of the SBS/AHT group. Furthermore, the radiological and ophthalmological interpretations were not blinded.

The criteria for classifying cases as SBS or control varied. Sometimes the composition of the comparison group was presented explicitly, but very often the criterion was simply the assessment of a child protection team (or a 'multidisciplinary team'), leading to the aforementioned circular reasoning bias. Sometimes the criteria for SBS/AHT cases were related to the height of a fall, with falls of less than 1 or 1.5 meters classified automatically as

SBS cases despite the fact that there are known cases of witnessed short falls causing the triad [34, 35]. These insufficient classification criteria result in uncertainty as to whether the study group also included accidental injury cases and/or whether the control group also contained SBS/AHT cases.

10.2.5 Main Findings and Conclusions

From the fact that, of the 30 studies included in the systematic review, 28 were assessed as at high risk of bias, 2 at moderate risk, and none at low risk, the following two major conclusions were drawn:

(i) There is **insufficient** ('very low' according to GRADE) **scientific support** to assess the diagnostic validity of the triad in identifying shaken baby cases [27, 30].
(ii) There is **limited** ('low' according to GRADE) **scientific support** to conclude that shaking is associated with the triad [27, 30].

In order to assess the strength of evidence provided by each study, we used a two-step process. First, the strength of evidence was given a preliminary score depending on the study design, following the internationally accepted guidelines from the GRADE Working Group [30]:

Evidence grade	Study design
Strong	Randomised controlled studies
Moderate	-
Low	Observational studies, e.g., cohort and case-control studies
Very Low	Case studies

Next, the score could be decreased in the presence of deficiencies in study quality, lack of concordance between studies, and/or high risk of publication bias, or increased in the presence of significant outcome effects, low risk of confounders, distinct dose-response correlation, and so forth.

Since only two studies were assessed as having a moderate risk of bias, and only the prospective study [33] is truly relevant for calculating the diagnostic accuracy we were investigating, our final conclusion was that the presence of the isolated triad was insufficient evidence for the determination of traumatic shaking [25, 27] and that, due to the low quality of the reviewed studies, *the incidence and prevalence of SBS remain unknown.*

The purpose of evidence-based medicine is not only to identify studies with high, low, or moderate risk of bias; a major aim of any systematic literature review is to disclose 'rubbish research' and demonstrate 'the enormous amount of research waste caused by poor quality studies' [36]. In the SBS/AHT context, this is worse than just wasting resources in research, in the judicial system, and in society; overdiagnosis of abuse in poor-quality studies and in real life has contributed to too many human tragedies for children, families, and caregivers [37].

10.3 The Nature of Scientific Controversy

A scientific controversy is more than a simple disagreement about which of two theories is correct. Freudenthal [38] gave the following definition which specifies when a disagreement crosses the line and becomes an actual scientific controversy: 'a persistent antagonistic discussion about a disagreement concerning a substantial scientific issue that is not resolvable by standard means of the discipline involved'.

In the present context, the disagreement concerns not only the actual mechanisms that can produce the isolated triad, but also the question of whether there is a controversy over SBS/AHT at all. In 2018, a group of paediatric researchers and other concerned people presented a 'consensus' statement in which they claimed that there is no scientific controversy within the field of AHT research [11]. According to this 'consensus' statement, the determination of whether an infant has been violently shaken, with or without impact, is based on pure scientific reasoning – that is, it is a purely evidence-based medical conclusion [11].

Denying the existence of the controversy can be considered a symptom of a crisis within the prevailing AHT research field. Although critical researchers have recognised its existence, the majority of SBS proponents still deny it completely and remain ignorant of the competing theories [11]. There are, in fact, several theories presenting alternative aetiologies and pathogeneses of subdural and retinal bleeding, as well as of encephalopathy [5, 14–17]. While the traditional SBS theory relies on shaking as the only explanation once a list of 'accepted' causes is ruled out, more recent theories suggest that the triad can actually occur spontaneously – for example, [14–17], in particular the theory of Geddes et al. [14–16], which has been essentially ignored by SBS proponents.

For clarification, we briefly present some relevant distinctions about scientific knowledge. Scientific knowledge can be divided into *knowing that* and *knowing how* [39]. In medicine, *knowing that* can be further subdivided: (i) knowledge and research about mechanisms – for example, theories about aetiology and pathogenesis – and (ii) epidemiological research about statistical associations/correlations. Usually there is an interaction between mechanism knowledge and correlation knowledge. Sometimes epidemiological studies precede mechanism studies – for example, in the discovery of the aetiology of AIDS – and sometimes mechanism theories are the point of departure for conducting randomised controlled trials of the effect of a theoretically interesting new treatment [39].

Knowing how is usually considered the practical application of *knowing that*, although it can also imply a tacit dimension acquired by long personal experience as a clinician, which means that it is often not possible to explain exactly why certain conclusions are reached or decisions are made. Usually *knowing that* is the basis for developing *knowing how*, but sometimes *knowing how* becomes the point of departure for *knowing that* (Figure 10.1).

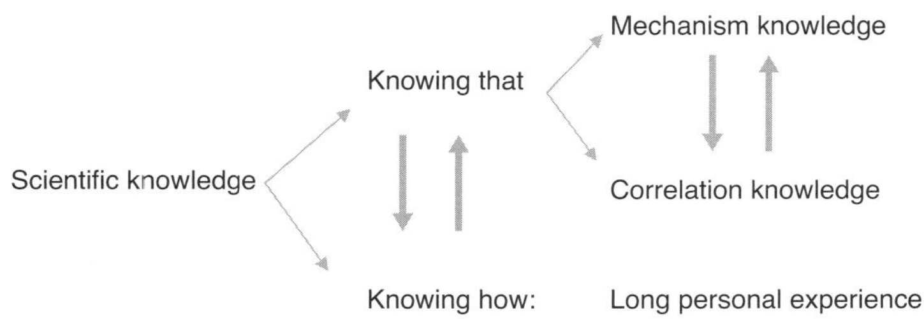

Figure 10.1 The interaction between 'knowing that' and 'knowing how' on the one hand and mechanism knowledge and correlation knowledge on the other. The main problem with respect to the issue of traumatic shaking is that 'knowing how' (in terms of non-evidence-based medicine) seems to influence 'knowing that' [39].

Within the field of SBS research, mechanism research typically concerns neuropathology and biomechanics. The purpose of this research is to generate theories about causes, pathogenesis, and development of various conditions. Researchers within such a field do not necessarily depend on epidemiological studies or what is here referred to as correlation knowledge. This does of course not imply that, for example, neuropathologists do not make observations. A pathologist can study the macro-micro anatomical structures in the brain or the intracranial vessels when conducting an autopsy. In a series of such autopsies – for example, from infants with SDH and RH as well as signs of encephalopathy (the triad) – the pathologist might systematically compare a series of cases of the triad without signs of trauma to a series of cases with signs of trauma (bruises, fractures, etc.). In just such a study, the English pathologist Jennian Geddes and her co-workers found that only 2 out of 37 fatal cases had direct mechanical brain damage (disrupted nerve fibres) and signs of impact with skull fractures; all the remaining cases had only findings associated with brain hypoxia [15, 16]. On the basis of these observations, Geddes et al. developed the hypoxia/brain swelling/increased intracranial pressure cascade theory to explain the isolated triad findings (see Chapter 3).

Correlation knowledge can be obtained by means of studies, optimally randomised controlled trials. Since such studies start with an experimental design, they will, if properly conducted, result in high-quality evidence and low risk of bias. However, it is obviously not possible to conduct experimental studies in which infants are shaken, so the only available alternative is to perform observational studies on past cases: observational studies can be case studies or series of these: cohort studies, case-control studies, or cross-sectional studies. The latter is preferable for calculating the diagnostic accuracy with respect to predictive values, because the prevalence of cases in the actual population is known. The lower the prevalence, the higher the number of false positives, resulting in a lower positive predictive value. Researchers who conduct observational studies are typically clinical epidemiologists. Such studies are not comparable with randomised controlled trials; because they can never be assessed as higher than a moderate risk of bias.

The SBU report on traumatic shaking was based on assessment of a systematic compilation of observational studies – that is, only correlation knowledge. Theories about mechanisms of aetiology and pathogenesis were referred to only in the context of considering the criteria applied by child protection teams and the associate risks of circular reasoning when researchers used the teams' determinations as reference standard.

In the context of SBS, a child protection professional has explained their procedure as follows: '[we] put all the information together and spit out the probability [of AHT] based on our experience' [40]. This clearly shows that decision-making in this context is based on the personal experience that usually comprises knowing how, rather than being evidence-based. When this attitude is adopted by whole teams, the issue of groupthink may arise [9, 41]. Members of a child protection team (or a similar team) may consider that they are the only ones who are competent, the only ones with the right experience, the only ones who really care about protecting children. In this situation, there is a significant risk that members of a team will come to rely on each other's opinion, eventually developing complete immunity to criticism from outside, and even becoming extremely antagonistic to anyone who questions the team's consensus-based decisions. If the team rules out the 'accepted' causes in a given case, they are certain that their conclusion of violent shaking is correct and anybody who questions it or suggests further potential causes for the symptoms is wrong, and often even called a 'child abuse denialist' [12]. This appellation in itself reveals the psychological presence of groupthink, since it does not in general correspond to any reality, given that medical researchers suggesting alternative causes for the isolated triad have never even thought of denying the existence of child abuse (see Chapter 1).

The combination of long personal experience and groupthink, each reinforcing the other to the exclusion of any openness to new theories, clearly jeopardises impartial decision-making. In an isolated triad case, a child protection team decreeing shaking may cause far more harm than good to the infant and its family, resulting in infants being unnecessarily removed from safe environments, innocent parents imprisoned, and families split up [9, 37].

10.4 National and International Reaction to the SBU Report

Before the report was even published, no fewer than seven organisations of paediatricians and paediatric radiologists approached the SBU and eagerly offered to scrutinise the report and 'correct' what they considered erroneous [42]. In several cases, the language was abrasive. These approaches, by emails, letters, and meetings with the director general of the SBU, occurred *before* any results were released.

How could so many people even be aware of the report? The preliminary Swedish draft was sent to external reviewers in Sweden and Norway; in spite of the fact that they were told that as a preliminary draft it was supposed to be confidential (as always in the peer review process), its content and preliminary conclusions were clearly unofficially translated into English and it was forwarded to several organisations inside and outside Sweden.

Since the SBU has its own review process, it declined all offers to review the report before publication. The final report was published in Swedish in October 2016 [23], and a shorter version was published in English in *Acta Paediatrica* in February 2017 [24]. The full report was published in English by the SBU in March 2017 (www.sbu.se) and as a supplement in *Acta Paediatrica* in 2018 [25]. After publication of the shorter version, critical comments appeared in a number of scientific journals. Leaving aside reactions of pure hostility, the various issues critics raised are presented in Table 10.1.

One of the critical groups correctly pointed out one instance of misquotation ('mean age' instead of 'peak age') and criticised the fact that the SBU had used only certain types of observational studies when calculating the diagnostic accuracy [43]. While these observations were justified, neither of them had any influence on the search strategy, the assessment, or the conclusions of the report. Apart from these minor issues, no specific errors were identified. In particular, the comparison with the 1998 study by Wakefield, which concluded that children vaccinated against measles, mumps, and rubella (MMR) had contracted autism, is entirely unjustified by any substantive argument: it would seem that the only similarity between the two reports is that mainstream medical professionals disagreed with their conclusions [44].

10.4.1 Four Most Frequent Critical Comments

i 'Analysis of isolated triad cases is not relevant and of no practical use.'

Several critics have claimed that focusing on triad cases with no signs of trauma (*isolated* triad cases) has no relevance for clinical practice [43, 45–47], asserting that infants classified as SBS/AHT cases (almost) always also exhibit signs of trauma (bruises or fractures). These

Table 10.1 Critical comments presented by paediatricians, paediatric ophthalmologists, and paediatric radiologists

Issues of criticism	Paediatricians	Paediatric ophthalmologists	Paediatric radiologists
Wrongful research question	+		
Wrongful terminology	+		
Wrongful literature search	+		
Wrongful choice of population	+	+	+
Wrongful choice of index test	+	+	
Overlapping population and index test	+		
Wrongful choice of reference test	+	+	
Wrongful choice of outcome measure	+	+	
Double standards applied	+	+	
Isolated triad cases rare and not relevant	+	+	+
Subdural bleedings are most important	+		
Retinal bleedings are pathognomonic	+	+	
Catastrophic consequences will follow	+		+
Circular reasoning is no or a minor problem	+	+	
Report ordered by defence lawyers	+		+
Expert panel is unqualified	+	+	
Classifying cases is a purely scientific task	+		+
Neonatal bleedings are not relevant			+
Analogy with Wakefield's MMR study	+		+

A '+' indicates that criticism arose in that group on that issue.

critics claimed that the expert panel had been working in an 'ivory tower with no contact with clinical practice' [46].

This claim is completely unfounded. One of the pioneers within the field, John Caffey, stated that it was remarkably common for SDH and RH to be observed without signs of trauma to infants' heads [3]. Since then, numerous studies of collected cases of AHT have reported about two thirds showing signs of impact (see [14–16], in which all cases with impact had a fatal outcome. In this study [15], 13 out of 37 infants were isolated triad cases with no signs of trauma and no injuries in the neck region, while a more recent study [58] contained 28 isolated triad cases out of a total of 67. The panel identified four further studies and found that a range of 20–46% (average 33%) of all alleged SBS/AHT cases were isolated triad cases [48]. Indeed, even if some two thirds of published cases do show signs of impact, it is of course possible that some of these are cases of accidents misclassified as abuse. Many SBS/AHT proponents reject short falls (less than 1 or 1.5 meters) as possible causes of the triad and automatically classify these cases as abuse on the basis of biomechanical models which are in fact contradictory [6, 7, 25], and in denial of the existence of actual published cases where a witnessed short fall did result in the triad [34, 35] (see Chapters 14 and 15).

The claim by SBS/AHT proponents that the isolated triad is extremely rare is inexplicable. In one qualitative study in which paediatricians were asked about medical factors in AHT identification, a participant stated that 'I had it drummed into me that if there's subdural haemorrhaging, retinal haemorrhage, it's abuse' [40]. Doctors have been provided with clinical guidelines which stress that the presence of the triad is an extremely strong indication of violent shaking, particularly RH, supposed to be pathognomonic. This statement was found in Swedish guidelines from 2008 and 2011 – now withdrawn – and a similar statement still exists in the French guidelines [49] (see Chapter 22). Furthermore, although called guidelines, these documents actually constitute injunctions; a clinician who ignores them may find their professional practice under threat.

One remarkably indicative hint that the link between shaking and the triad is not as strong as claimed is given by the results of preventive 'do not shake' programmes for parents, teaching them to put an inconsolably crying baby in its cot and leave the room if they feel themselves becoming impatient [50]. A collection of seven studies assessing these programmes showed contradictory results with an overall tendency of no effect [50]. One study [51] included three other preventive programmes addressing other problems (positioning infants in car seats, positioning infants on their back lying down, and verifying correct bath water temperatures); these were expected to have no influence on the incidence of AHT [51]. Contrary to expectations, all three of these other preventive programs resulted in a significant ($p < 0.001$) decrease in AHT incidence – but the 'do not shake preventive program' did not. It is difficult to hypothesise any interpretation of these findings other than that AHT is being misdiagnosed and overdiagnosed; indeed, if a reduction in the frequency of shaking is not diminishing the incidence of alleged SBS, then it would seem that shaking is not the true cause. It seems likely that including the isolated triad cases in the overall AHT group is skewing the results, hiding the potentially preventive effect of the programme. We suggest that *if* there is a causal relation between shaking and alleged AHT, and *if* in studying the effect of the preventive programme the researchers were to separate isolated triads from those with signs of trauma, then a preventive effect might be detectable in the latter group [50, 51].

Benign external hydrocephalus (BEH) is an important but often unrecognised element in causing the triad (see Chapters 5 and 6). Vinchon et al. excluded BEH cases when they conducted their study [33], but in many countries, such as Norway and Sweden, BEH is not considered by child abuse paediatricians to be one of the 'acceptable' causes for the triad [52, 53]. In one Norwegian case, two pairs of 3-month-old premature dizygotic twins were separated from their biological parents for 3 years under the assumption that they had been vigorously shaken, an assumption based solely on the finding of the triad in the two boys whereas their twin sisters had only chronic subdural hematomas/hygromas [53]. It was considered that all four twins suffered from the same condition that had manifested more severely in the males. An almost similar case of monozygotic twin boys was reported from Sweden; the first born displayed the triad and the second born a dyad of SDH and RH [52]. Cases such as these end up in court, so the claim that concentrating on the isolated triad (or dyad) has no practical relevance is simply false.

ii 'Retinal haemorrhage is pathognomonic of violent shaking.'

Paediatric ophthalmologists in particular have criticised the report because it did not consider the ophthalmological issue more thoroughly and drew attention to what was – and by some still is – considered a fact – that is, that retinal bleeding is pathognomonic for SBS/AHT [55, 56]. This opinion seems to be reflected also among child protection professionals in the United States. Child protection professionals consider that RH is significantly more likely to indicate SBS (approximately 60% of respondents to a questionnaire stated so) than SDH and coma/death (approximately 30% for each) [57].

While the SBU expert panel initially accepted this claim regarding RH as pathognomonic, it later found the claim untenable. In one randomised, blinded study [58] based on RetCam images of RH in children caused by a variety of (supposed) mechanisms such as disease processes, accidental trauma, and violent shaking, ophthalmologists were asked to classify the cause in each case using only the images but blinded to the (supposed) aetiology. The level of inter-observer agreement was between 'poor' and 'bad', with a Kappa value[1] of 0.219 [58]. If ophthalmologists have such difficulty in differentiating the causes of RH when blinded to the supposed mechanism, it is obvious that either proponents exaggerate their own capacity or that the retinal bleeding associated with alleged traumatic shaking is far from pathognomonic.

An ophthalmological study published after the SBU report indicated that the retinal bleeding supposed to be associated with traumatic shaking merely represents the result of increased intracranial pressure caused by brain swelling and hypoxia, in which case retinal bleeding is not pathognomonic for SBS/AHT, but rather represents a non-specific effect of increased intracranial pressure [59, 60]. Indeed, it has long been known that increased intracranial pressure due to brain swelling can cause retinal bleeding, both from medical conditions such as subarachnoid bleeding (Terson's syndrome) [61], and from effects such as hypoxia in healthy mountaineers who develop brain swelling, increased intracranial pressure, and subsequent retinal bleeding [62].

In a recent Swedish study of 36 infants [63], three caregivers had on arrival at the hospital spontaneously admitted shaking the infant violently, while in the other 33 cases, the shaking was witnessed and/or video recorded. Although the shaking was described as violent and repeated in several cases, only 2 of the 32 infants with brain imaging had intracranial subdural fluid collections, which were described as chronic hematoma in one case and as acute and (possibly) chronic hematoma in the other [63]. The former case had a history of shaking only, the latter of both shaking and impact. Extensive RH was not observed in any of the 30 infants with shaking only. This study does not support the claim that RH is pathognomonic for violent shaking – on the contrary [64].

---

1 Kappa values > 0.81 are considered very good, 0.61–0.80 good, < 0.41–0.60 moderate, 0.21–0.40 poor, and < 0.20 bad. The actual Kappa value of 0.219 is barely better than pure random choice.

iii 'Circular reasoning is not a major problem.'

Several critics have claimed that circular reasoning is not a problem when calculating diagnostic accuracy, or at least not an important issue. Hence, according to this critique, the SBU report wrongly and unnecessarily disqualified a number of studies [11, 43, 45–47, 54], essentially those in which the judgement of a child protection team was used as the gold standard/reference test when researchers classified *all* triad cases as true positive SBS/AHT cases [65]. Obviously, if this classification is used as a reference to determine true cases of AHT/SBS, then 100% of isolated triad cases will automatically be classified as AHT/SBS – especially since any case where one of the 'acceptable' alternative causes was found is generally excluded from these studies, thus eliminating all false positives by definition. Clearly the diagnostic criteria used in the studies need to be separate (ideally mutually independent) from the criteria whose diagnostic accuracy is being evaluated by considering the studies.

When the predictive accuracy of diagnostic criteria is too perfect to be true (e.g., 100%), one would be wise to suspect and seek for instances of circular reasoning. If this is not done, the continued use of circular reasoning is nothing other than a series of self-fulfilling prophecies [66] (see Chapter 17). This is precisely what the SBU expert panel discovered in the course of its systematic literature review. Voluntarily ignoring this major issue is a form of scientific misconduct [66].

Nor is it true, as some critics have claimed [11, 46, 47], that the problem of circular reasoning has never been raised in the context of AHT/SBS except in the SBU report. To the contrary, several researchers have previously commented on the issue and taken specific measures to avoid it (see, e.g., [67, 68]). Moreover, in 5 out of 7 meta-analyses included in the SBU report, the authors were aware of the circularity issue [25]. Nevertheless, of all the critical comments levelled at the SBU report, only a single one admitted the existence of the problem of circular reasoning [69].

iv 'Classifying triad cases as abuse is a purely scientific matter.'

The authors of an influential so-called consensus statement, published in 2018, state that diagnosing SBS/AHT is a purely medical matter based on evidence and scientific reasoning, despite the fact that the main priority of child protection teams is to protect children from abuse and that the balance of doubt will always tilt that way in their assessments [11]. Anyone who questions whether the end justifies the means in this context is accused of child abuse denialism or worse [12, 43]. These priorities may not be openly declared in scientific settings, but they are present, and, subconsciously, paediatricians and child protection teams have succeeded in inserting them into the scientific reasoning by accepting their own decisions as the scientific gold standard of diagnostic accuracy, leading to the circular reasoning described earlier in this chapter. What is happening here is that, for the sake of protecting children, *values* are being declared as *pure scientific reasoning* – yet, given the separation of babies from their families and the conviction of innocent parents, this process is not even protecting children [11, 7].

If medical practitioners really treated the classification of triad cases as a purely scientific matter, they would be obliged as a matter of science to take account of the alternative theories explaining how the isolated triad can arise through spontaneous and natural causes (e.g., [14–16]) – the 'non-shaken baby theory'. Indeed, one article used standard Bradford Hill criteria to compare the two theories as causes for the isolated triad and actually found that the 'non-shaken baby theory' has *higher plausibility* than the 'shaken baby theory', implying that it could be the correct explanation in many cases [22]. In fact, part of what casts doubt on the standard SBS theory is the need to adjoin a number of more or less desperate ad hoc hypotheses [71]. Certainly, adding these is a common and normal part of scientific procedure [39], but the SBS theory has too many and too far-fetched auxiliary and ad hoc hypotheses [71].

One would think that, when paediatricians act as scientific researchers, they should relinquish their other hat as members of child protection teams and cease to use the teams' assessments as the gold standard. Almost all paediatric researchers have failed to do this, however. The two articles assessed as 'at moderate risk' by the expert panel [32, 33] were the only two articles found that appeared to circumvent this issue and be aware of this problem, and two previously conducted systematic literature review also took the risk of circular reasoning into consideration [20, 68].

The same risk of circular reasoning arises when a member of a child protection team cannot separate this role from the role of the expert witness in the judicial process and presents the team's assessment as a scientifically validated result. This problem reverberates through the system, since if a judge accepts the protection team's assessment as scientifically valid, the accused will be convicted; if a police interrogator accepts the team's assessment that the infant has necessarily been shaken, it may lead to strong pressure and police-induced confessions. According to Dr P. Strouse, the editor of *Pediatric Radiology*, it is 'child abusers who tear families apart, not hospital child protection teams' or other concerned authorities – a statement which supports the unjustified assumption of zero-error procedures on the part of the protection teams [12]. It is of course understandable that it is difficult for researchers as well as many engaged clinicians to accept that almost all studies conducted during the past 40 years have been a waste of time and resources, and to accept that what previously was 'true' actually represents a misconception. Even harder to accept is the obvious and tragic consequence that paediatricians and child protection teams have overdiagnosed SBS/AHT, torn families apart, and sent innocent caregivers to prison [37]. This difficulty is undoubtedly one of the main reasons behind the hostile reactions to the SBU report.

If classifying AHT cases were truly a scientific matter, then a scientific fact that is easy to establish from a literature review, namely the fact that about one third or more of triad cases are isolated, would not be systematically denied by proponents of the SBS/AHT concept, who continue to maintain that triad cases are (almost) always accompanied by external signs of trauma. In fact, it seems as if the claim that isolated triad cases are so rare that 'the SBU report is of no practical value' [46, 47] emerged only *after* the publication of the report. Possibly it represents nothing more than a reaction intended only to undermine the importance of the SBU report. But this attitude does certainly not support the claim that classification is a purely scientific matter.

10.5 Concluding Remarks and Suggestions for Future Directions

The results of the SBU report and of the analysis in this chapter of its hostile reception have suggested several directions for future research which seem very important in order to move beyond the controversy and nearer to the truth of the scientific explanation for the triad.

The first suggestion is that denialism must stop: denial of the existence of a controversy, denial of other possible aetiologies for the triad, denial that it is important to consider the isolated triad separately from the triad with relevant trauma and that this separation could explain many observations such as the lack of efficacy of the shaking prevention programmes. In particular we suggest that studies henceforth separate cases of isolated triad from triad with relevant trauma, and also the youngest infants (< 6 months) from older infants.

The second suggestion is that circular reasoning must be avoided in that the assessments by child protection teams, based on the SBS theory 'triad means violent shaking' (in the absence of a small number of other 'acceptable' explanations), must not be used in studies intended to assess the correlation of the triad with actual shaking. Rather, we suggest that such studies use as true positives only witnessed (preferably video-taped) cases or cases where confession is made spontaneously, with circumstantial detail, before the professional assessment of shaking is revealed to the caregiver. Moreover, caregivers might be telling the truth when they claim that they did shake the baby, but *after* the appearance of encephalopathy symptoms and as a resuscitation attempt. The reason why such a baby collapses might be due to a prolonged ALTE [72].

The third suggestion is to put the claim of scientific evidence-based medicine into practice by studying the existing research and pursuing further research on alternative aetiologies for the triad and being ready to accept the validated results of such research. The fourth suggestion is that the people who conduct research on the aetiology of the triad, those who assess children for signs of abuse, those who dictate government health policy and medical guidelines, and those who testify as expert witnesses at trials, should not be one and the same restricted group of people, who end up yielding to a system of groupthink that excludes any outside information.

The main conclusion of the SBU report was that, due to the problems described throughout this chapter, there is *insufficient* and very low level evidence for the claim that the isolated triad accurately indicates traumatic shaking.

References

1. Swedish Agency for Health Technology Assessment and Assessment of Social Services (SBU).*SBU reports' influence of the healthcare system*. Stockholm, 2012 (in Swedish). https://bit.ly/3NBrBow.
2. Guthkelch AN. Infantile subdural haematoma and its relationship to whiplash injuries *British Medical Journal.* 1971;2:430–1.
3. Caffey J. On the theory and practice of shaking infants: Its potential residual effects of permanent brain damage and mental retardation. *American Journal of Diseases of Children.* 1972;124:161–9.
4. Eisenbrey AB. Retinal hemorrhage in the battered child. *Pediatric Neurosurgery.* 1979; 5:40–4.
5. Squier W, Mack J, Green A, Azis T. The pathophysiology of brain swelling associated with subdural hemorrhage: The role of the trigeminovascular system. *Child's Nervous System.* 2012;28:2005–15.
6. Duhaime AC, Christian CW, Rorke LC, Zimmerman RA. Nonaccidental head injury in infants: The 'shaken-baby syndrome'. *New England Journal of Medicine.* 1998;338:1822–9.
7. Prange MT, Coats B, Duhaime AC, Margulies SS. Anthropomorphic simulations of falls, shakes, and inflicted impacts in infants. *Journal of Neurosurgery.* 2003;99:143–50.
8. Duhaime AC, Alario A, Lewander WJ et al. Head injuries in very young children: Mechanism, injury type and ophthalmological findings in 100 hospitalized patients younger than 2 years of age. *Pediatrics.* 1992;90:179–85.
9. Lynøe N, Juth N, Eriksson A. From child protection to paradigm protection: The

genesis, development and defence of a scientific paradigm. *Journal of Medicine and Philosophy*. 2019;44:378–90.

10. Lynøe N, Eriksson A. The unspoken shaken baby lie detector algorithm: An analysis of diagnostic procedures in cases of allegedly abusive head trauma without external signs of trauma. *Journal of Research in Philosophy and History*. 2020;3 (2). www.scholink.org/ojs/index.php/jrph/article/view/3224.
11. Choudhary AK, Servaes S, Slovis TL et al. Consensus statement on abusive head trauma in infants and young children. *Pediatric Radiology*. 2018;48(8):1048–65.
12. Strouse PJ. Child abuse: We have problems. *Pediatric Radiology*. 2016;46:587–90.
13. Ludvigsson J, Steinwall Larsen S, Van Agthoven G et al. The presence of shaken baby syndrome is scientifically robust. *Swedish Medical Journal*. 2015;112:DE6U.
14. Geddes JF, Hackshaw AK, Vowles GH, Nickols CD, Whitwell HL. Neuropathology of inflicted head injury in children. I. Patterns of brain damage. *Brain*. 2001;124:1290–8.
15. Geddes JF, Vowles GH, Hackshaw A et al. Neuropathology of inflicted head injury in children. II. Microscopic brain injury in infants. *Brain*. 2001;124:1299–1306.
16. Geddes JF, Whitwell HL. Inflicted head injury in infants. *Forensic Science International*. 2004;146:83–8.
17. Zahl SM, Wester K, Gabaeff S. Examining perinatal subdural haematoma as an aetiology of extra-axial hygroma and chronic subdural haematoma. *Acta Paediatrica*. 2020;109(4):659–66.
18. Guthkelch AN. Problems of infant retino-dural hemorrhage with minimal external injury. *Houston Journal of Health Law and Policy*. 2012;12:201–8.
19. Findley KA, Barnes PD, Moran DA et al. Shaken baby syndrome, abusive head trauma, and actual innocence: Getting it right. *Houston Journal of Health Law and Policy*. 2012;12:209–312.
20. Donohoe M. Evidence-based medicine and shaken baby syndrome: Part I. Literature review, 1966–1998. *American Journal of Forensic Medicine and Pathology*. 2003;24 (3):239–42.
21. Riggs JE, Hobbs GR. Infant homicide and accidental death in the United States, 1940–2005: Ethics and epidemiological classification. *Journal of Medical Ethics*. 2011;37:445–8.
22. Acres M, Morris JA. The pathogenesis of retinal and subdural haemorrhage in non-accidental head injury in infancy: Assessment using Bradford Hill criteria. *Medical Hypotheses*. 2014;82:1–5.8.
23. Swedish Agency for Health Technology Assessment and Assessment of Social Services (SBU). Traumatic shaking: The role of the triad in medical investigations of suspected traumatic shaking. A systematic review. SBU assessment. Report 255E/2016 (in Swedish and English). https://bit.ly/3DGrvaC.
24. Lynøe N, Elinder G, Hallberg B et al. Insufficient evidence for 'shaken baby syndrome': A systematic review. *Acta Paediatrica*. 2017;106(7):1021–7.
25. Elinder G, Eriksson A, Hallberg B et al. Traumatic shaking: The role of the triad in medical investigations of suspected traumatic shaking. *Acta Paediatrica*. 2018;107(S472):3–23.
26. Elinder G, Eriksson A, Hallberg B et al. Gaisho sei no yusaburi: Gaishosei no yusaburi ga utagawareru jian no igakuteki chosa ni okeru san. Choko no yakuwari [Traumatic shaking: The role of the triad in medical investigations of suspected traumatic shaking. A systematic review]. (Translation by Kana Sasakura). *Ryukoku Hogaku*. 2018;50(3):670–95.
27. SBU Handbook (including appendix 10 regarding statistical concepts and chapter 10, page 130, regarding the assessment of grading studies). www.sbu.se/upload/ebm/metodbok/SBUsHandbok.pdf.
28. Whiting P, Rutjes AW, Reitsma JB, et al. The development of QUADAS: A tool for the quality assessment of studies of diagnostic accuracy included in systematic

reviews. *BMC Medical Research Methodology*. 2003;3:25.

29. Shea BJ, Grimshaw JM, Wells GA et al. Development of AMSTAR: A measurement tool to assess the methodological quality of systematic reviews. *BMC Medical Research Methodology*. 2007;7:10. https://doi.org/10.1186/1471-2288-7-10.
30. Gordon Guyatt G, Oxman AD, Elie A et al. GRADE guidelines: 1. Introduction. GRADE evidence profiles and summary of findings tables. *Journal of Clinical Epidemiology*. 2011;64:383–94.
31. Rutjes AWS, Reitsma JB, Coomarasamy A, et al. Evaluation of diagnostic tests when there is no gold standard. A review of methods. *Health Technology Assessment*. 2007;11(50).
32. Adamsbaum C, Grabar S, Mejean N, Rey-Salmon C. Abusive head trauma: Judicial admissions highlight violent and repetitive shaking. *Pediatrics*. 2010;126:546–55.
33. Vinchon M, de Foort-Dhellemmens S, Desurmont M, Delestret I. Confessed abuse versus witnessed accidents in infants: Comparison of clinical, radiological, and ophthalmological data in corroborated cases. *Child's Nervous System*. 2010;26:637–45.
34. Gardner HB. A witnessed short fall mimicking presumed shaken baby syndrome. *Pediatric Neurosurgery*. 2007;43:433–5.
35. Denton S, Mileusnic D. Delayed sudden death in an infant following an accidental fall: A case report with review of the literature. *American Journal of Forensic Medicine and Pathology*. 2003;24(4):371–6.
36. Clarke M, Chalmers I. Reflections on the history of systematic reviews. *BMJ Evidence-Based Medicine*. 2018;23(4):121–2.
37. Högberg U, Eriksson G, Högberg G, Wahlberg Å. Parents' experiences of seeking health care and encountering allegations of shaken baby syndrome: A qualitative study. *PLoS One*. 2020;15(2): e0228911.
38. Freudenthal G. A rational controversy over compounding forces. In *Scientific controversies: Philosophical and historical perspectives*. P Machamer, M Pera, A Baltas, eds. Oxford University Press, 2000.
39. Johansson I, Lynøe N. *Medicine & philosophy: A twenty-first century introduction*. Ontos, 2008.
40. Cowley LE, Maguire S, Farewell DM et al. Acceptability of the predicting abuse head trauma (PredAHT) clinical prediction tool: A qualitative study with child protection professionals. *Child Abuse and Neglect*. 2018;81:192–205.
41. Breger ML. Making waves or keeping the calm: Analyzing the institutional culture of family courts through the lens of social psychology groupthink theory. *Law and Psychology Review*. 2010;34:55–90.
42. Offiah AC, Servaes S, Adamsbaum CS et al. Initial response of the European Society of Paediatric Radiology and Society for Pediatric Radiology to the Swedish Agency for Health Technology Assessment and Assessment of Social Services' document on the triad of shaken baby syndrome. *Pediatric Radiology*. 2017;47:369–71.
43. Debelle GD, Maguire S, Watts P, et al. Abusive head trauma and the triad. A critique on behalf of RCPCH of 'Traumatic shaking: The role of the triad in medical investigations of suspected traumatic shaking'. *Archives of Disease in Childhood*. 2018;103(6):606–10.
44. Lynøe N, Eriksson A. No similarities between the Wakefield report on measles, mumps and rubella vaccine and the Swedish report on traumatic shaking. *Acta Paediatrica*. 2020;109(7):1326–9.
45. Saunders D, Raissaki M, Servaes S et al. Throwing the baby out with the bath water: Response to the Swedish Agency for Health Technology Assessment and Assessment of Social Services (SBU) report on traumatic shaking. *Pediatric Radiology*. 2017;47(11):1386–9.
46. Bilo RAC. The Swedish Agency for Health Technology. Report about traumatic shaking: Much ado about nothing? *Forensic*

Science, Medicine and Pathology. 2018;14 (4):541–4.

47. Laurent-Vannier A, Adamsbaum C, Raul JS, et al. Flawed Swedish study on traumatic shaking is already being used by defence lawyers and its findings must be ignored. *Acta Paediatrica*. 2018;107 (12):2048–50.
48. Lynøe N, Eriksson A. Is focusing on the triad really irrelevant and of no practical use? *Acta Paediatrica*. 2018;107 (10):1675–6.
49. Laurent-Vannier A, Nathanson M, Quiriau F et al. A public hearing on 'Shaken baby syndrome: Guidelines on establishing a robust diagnosis and the procedures to be adopted by healthcare and social services staff'. Guidelines issued by the Hearing Commission. *Annals of Physical and Rehabilitation Medicine*. 2011;54:600–25.
50. Lynøe N, Eriksson A. Why programs for managing colicky crying fail to prevent abusive head trauma and suggestions for improvement. *JAMA Pediatrics*. 2021, 26 April. https://doi.org/10.1001/jamapediatrics.2021.0455.
51. Keenan HT, Leventhal JM. A case-control study to evaluate Utah's shaken baby prevention program. *Academic Pediatrics*. 2010;10:389–94.
52. Wester K, Wikström J, Lynøe N, Eriksson A. Unsubstantiated belief in the diagnostic accuracy of the triad of abusive head trauma may lead to incorrect diagnoses of alleged abuse cases. *Acta Paediatrica*. 2021. https://doi.org/10.1111/apa.15892.
53. Wester K. Two infant boys misdiagnosed as 'shaken baby' and their twin sisters: A cautionary tale. *Pediatric Neurology*. 2019;97:3–11. https://doi.org/10.1016/j.pediatrneurol.2019.02.024.
54. Levin AV. The SBU report: A different view. *Acta Paediatrica*. 2017;106 (7):1037–9.
55. Hellgren K, Hellström A, Hård AL et al. The new Swedish report on shaken baby syndrome is misleading. *Acta Paediatrica*. 2017;106(7):1040.
56. Hylton C, Goldberg MF. Circumpapillary retinal ridge in the shaken-baby syndrome. *New England Journal of Medicine*. 2004;351:170.
57. Narang SK, Estrada C, Greenberg S, Lindberg D. Acceptance of shaken baby syndrome and abusive head trauma as medical diagnoses. *Journal of Pediatrics*. 2016;177:273–8.
58. Mulvihill AO, Jones P, Tandon A, Fleck BW, Minns RA. An inter-observer and intra-observer study of a classification of RetCam images of retinal haemorrhages in children. *British Journal of Ophthalmology*. 2011;95:99–104.
59. Minns RA, Jones PA, Tandon A et al. Raised intracranial pressure and retinal haemorrhages in childhood encephalopathies. *Developmental Medicine and Child Neurology*. 2017;59:597–604.
60. Squier W. Retinal haemorrhage: A red flag for raised intracranial pressure. *Developmental Medicine and Child Neurology*. 2017;59:565.
61. Medele RJ, Stummer W, Mueller AJ, et al. Terson's syndrome in subarachnoid hemorrhage and severe brain injury accompanied by acutely raised intracranial pressure. *Journal of Neurosurgery*. 1998;88 (5):851–4.
62. Frayser R, Houston C, Bryan AC, et al. Retinal hemorrhage at high altitude. *New England Journal of Medicine*. 1970;282 (21):1183–4.
63. Thiblin I, Andersson J, Wester K et al. Medical findings and symptoms in infants exposed to witnessed or admitted abusive shaking: A nationwide registry study. *PLoS One*. 2020 15(10):e0240182.
64. Thiblin I, Andersson J, Wester K, et al. Retinal haemorrhage in infants investigated for suspected maltreatment is strongly correlated with intracranial pathology. *Acta Paediatrica*. 2022;111 (4):800–8. https://doi.org/10.1111/apa.16139.
65. Lynøe N, Eriksson A. A diagnostic test can prove anything if you use incorrect assumptions and circular reasoning. *Acta Paediatrica*. 2018;107(12):2051–3.

66. Lynøe N, Elinder G, Hallberg B et al. Is accepting circular reasoning in shaken baby studies bad science or misconduct? *Acta Paediatrica*. 2017;106(9):1445–6.

67. Squier W, Mack J, Lantz PE et al. Circular reasoning. *Minnesota Medicine*. 2010;93(3):8.

68. Leestma J. Case analysis of brain-injured admittedly shaken infants. 54 cases, 1969–2001. *American Journal of Forensic and Medical Pathology*. 2005;26:199–212.

69. Ludvigsson J. Extensive shaken baby syndrome review provides a clear signal that more research is needed. *Acta Paediatrica*. 2017;106(7):1028–30.

70. Lynøe N, Eriksson A. Hidden clinical values and overestimation of shaken baby cases. *Clinical Ethics*. 2019;14 (3):151–4.

71. Lynøe N, Brooks CB, Juth N, Eriksson A. Do child abuse pediatricians search for a 'Pediatric Vulcan planet'? Comparison of controversies about the Vulcan-must-exist-theory and the infant-must-have-been-shaken-theory. *Journal of Research in Philosophy and History*. 2020;3 (2):162–93.

72. Lynøe N, Eriksson A. Can a prolonged unexplained event change a reliable resuscitator into an unreliable perpetrator? Submitted.

Chapter 11

Interrogation and the Infanticide Suspect

Mechanisms of Vulnerability to False Confession

Deborah Davis and Richard Leo

Doctors and prosecutors who defend the diagnosis of shaken baby syndrome (SBS) point, among other things, to the many confessions obtained from parents and other caregivers as evidence of the reality of the diagnosis [1–5]. But are such confessions really good evidence either of the actual guilt of the suspects or of the validity of a shaken baby diagnosis (see Chapter 12)? The link between the behaviour of shaking a baby and the medical injuries in question is, of course, subject to widespread criticism (see Chapters 3–10, 14, 16, 17) [2, 4]. In addition, however, the large and growing body of proven police-induced false confessions and the substantial research base further documenting the reality of false confessions and examining their causes clearly show that confessions are not reliable indicators of guilt [6–12].

If, as many argue, the shaken baby diagnosis is not valid, it follows that, among the many confessions of parents and caregivers, many, if not most, are false [2, 13, 14]. Indeed, we suggest that (even if the shaken baby diagnosis is valid in general) suspects in alleged shaken baby cases are arguably more vulnerable to false confession than those suspected of other crimes.

The purpose of this chapter is to examine the questions of (1) how, if at all, interrogations of those suspected of injuring or killing a child are conducted differently than other interrogations, and (2) what, if anything, would render such suspects more or less vulnerable to confession (true or false) than other suspects. That is, what might be unique about the experience of such suspects in police interrogation? To engage this analysis it is necessary to first consider how interrogations are typically conducted, and the primary reasons suspects confess, keeping in mind that their confessions can be either true or false.

11.1 The Basics of Interrogation Strategy

Although research has steadily accumulated in support of the reform of interrogation procedures, and although some reforms have slowly been adopted by select police departments, most interrogations in America are still conducted using methods taught by John Reid and Associates, or methods very similar to (and typically inspired by) the Reid method [10–12, 15]. This has certainly remained true among the cases we have reviewed as experts on interrogation and confession. We will therefore discuss our two questions using the context of Reid-like interrogation methods.

Space does not permit an extensive summary of these methods [12, 16]. For our purposes here, it is sufficient to note that interrogations consist of three broad strategies among the Reid 9-Steps: establishing hopelessness, selling confession, and taking the confession [10–12]. These strategies are specifically designed to convince suspects that confession is in their best interests and that it will produce the best legal outcomes, and potentially better social outcomes of other types (such as preserving relationships with others). Thus, in the following sections, we discuss the first two of these broad strategies, noting both ways in which they are differently employed in interrogations of those suspected of killing of injuring children, and mechanisms of vulnerability to the strategies that are unique to such suspects. That is, why might these suspects be easier to convince that confession is in their best interests? In a final section, we consider other reasons suspects confess and discuss whether child abuse suspects might be more vulnerable to confessions for such reasons as well. Keeping in mind that the considerations we discuss will apply to those suspected of any mechanism of child killing, for simplicity we use 'shaken baby' to reference all such suspects.

11.2 Establishing Hopelessness

Presumably, if suspects' attention can be diverted from trying to establish innocence, the interrogator can better sell confession as the best way to achieve optimal outcomes. Therefore, the intent of the interrogator is to first convince suspects that their situation is hopeless, that there is no way to prove or to convince others that they are innocent (and, moreover, that there is strong, even overwhelming, evidence of guilt).

However, it is necessary to look at this concept more broadly as undermining suspects' 'self-efficacy for defence', meaning suspects' sense of their overall ability to defend themselves against the allegations [17]. This includes not only perceptions of the strength of evidence against them, but also additional factors such as the sense that one is a person others are likely to find credible or to judge fairly, and other resources to support the defence (such as financial resources, skilful attorneys, investigators, expert witnesses, supportive witnesses, and so on). That is, considering all such factors, what is the person's assessment of his or her ability to successfully defend against the allegations? Though suspects' attention during interrogation is likely to focus disproportionately on their ability to convince the interrogator through their own assertions of and arguments for innocence, suspects are likely to consider the other elements of self-efficacy as well. With this in mind, one can ask in what ways might the self-efficacy for defence be affected by the nature or circumstances of the allegation?

11.3 Perceived Strength of Evidence

First is the issue of the evidentiary situation of such suspects. That is, what is the nature and strength of evidence apparently implicating them? What evidence might be available that might exonerate the suspect, or at least provide some evidence of innocence? Davis and Leo have argued that some classes of suspects suffer a disadvantage in self-efficacy for defence simply because of the nature of the accusation itself, along with a compromised evidentiary situation: the latter referring to the way the nature and circumstances of the crime seem to implicate suspects while simultaneously making it very difficult for suspects to marshal evidence in their defence [18]. Here, we argue that suspects in shaken baby cases and some other instances of severe child injury or death are among the class of suspects suffering impaired self-efficacy for defence: a deficit that begins with the nature of their evidentiary situations.

The evidentiary situation begins with the undeniable fact of the death or severe injury of the child. It is the cause of the injury and the involvement of the suspect that is in question.

However, at one level, the involvement of the suspect is also not in question. That is, the suspect has had the opportunity to injure the child. The suspect might have been present when the injury occurred or might have had the opportunity over a period of time to injure the child in a way that led to the ultimate crisis prior to death. In many instances, an acute injury occurs when the accused is the only person present, or at least the only plausible culprit (e.g., when only other young children are in the house). If the child has other non-fatal bruises or injuries, or has a medical history of (especially repeated) injuries, this creates an appearance of a pattern of abuse – even if the injuries are accidental or caused by underlying medical issues – and therefore also becomes a basis for interrogators to argue for the likely guilt of the suspect.

With this background of apparently strong existing circumstantial evidence supporting suspects' guilt, interrogators can add to suspects' sense of hopelessness. This occurs at first, of course, by the confident and unwavering accusation of guilt that occurs when the accusatory phase of the interrogation commences, and that is maintained throughout. This is supplemented by interrogators' references to actual or fabricated evidence to support the accusation [19]. In cases involving an injured or deceased child, interrogators commonly (in our experience) claim to have reports from doctors who have examined the child and who claim that their findings support the accusation of caregiver-inflicted rather than of accidental injuries or natural causes (see also Chapter 22).

The doctors may make claims supporting a shaken baby determination or non-accidental head trauma that lack empirical support but that are then repeated to suspects by interrogators. Most suspects will feel at a disadvantage in trying to dispute the findings of a doctor who has greater medical expertise. These include such claims as 'minor falls cannot cause the head injury in question (and therefore the suspect is lying about how the injury came about)', 'the current minor fall must have caused an exacerbation of injuries caused by previous shaking or abuse', 'they have ruled out every other cause of the symptoms in question, leaving only shaken baby as the explanation', and others. In other words, the interrogators explain, in effect, that doctors have already proven suspects' guilt.

In the case of a shaken baby allegation, the cause of the injuries is purportedly established by their nature. That is, a *constellation* of symptoms said to result from shaking is present, most commonly the triad of subdural haematoma, retinal haemorrhages, and encephalopathy. The notion that this combination of injuries can only occur through shaking creates the presumption that, when the baby has such symptoms, the last caregiver in contact with the baby must be guilty. The logic of symptoms equals shaken baby equals guilty caregiver is used throughout the interrogation of SBS suspects. Suspects are often told by doctors, interrogators, prosecutors, and even their own attorneys that the medical evidence is conclusive and the odds of acquittal are next to zero, promoting not only (potentially false) confessions, but also (potentially false) guilty pleas (see also Chapter 12) [2]. In many cases, this seemingly damning set of circumstances and lack of ability to marshal exculpatory evidence is supplemented by two potentially self-incriminating circumstances, one occurring prior to the interrogation and one as part of it.

11.4 The Role of 'Pretext Calls'

The first consists of any incriminating statements the suspect may have made during a 'pretext call' [20, 21]. Such calls (or other arranged and recorded interactions) are made at the behest of police and the caller is advised by police concerning how to conduct the call, what admissions are needed, and how to best try to elicit incriminating admissions from the suspect. The call is typically made by the victim or someone close to the victim and/or suspect – someone who, it is hoped, will not be suspected of collaborating with police and whom the suspect might trust as sincere. In cases of shaken baby or child abuse allegations, the call is most often made by a parent of the child. The task of the caller is to cause the suspect to admit culpability and to fully explain what happened, and, if not, to cause him or her to make other incriminating statements consistent with guilt that will be perceived as inculpatory and support prosecution.

Such calls are often used in cases where the victim and/or an advocate of the victim knows the suspect, including prominently child abuse, child sex abuse, and adult sexual assault or sexual harassment cases. Though confessions are important in solving and prosecuting any case, they are particularly important in cases where guilt might be otherwise difficult to prove – for example, when the cause of death might be apparent, but the mechanism producing the injury causing death is hard to prove (e.g., accidental fall versus pushing or throwing the child, causing head trauma).

Davis et al. have identified many of the advantages and disadvantages of pretext callers in eliciting admissions from suspects, the similarities and differences between the tactics used by pretext callers versus interrogators, and many of the most common tactics pretext callers use to attempt to elicit admissions [20–22]. Among the most common tactics for pretext callers when a child has died or been seriously injured are displays of extreme distress, expressions of great need (or the right) to know and understand what happened to one's child, claims that doctors need to know what happened to treat adequately, and threats and promises regarding continuation of the relationship with the suspect contingent on the suspect 'explaining' or admitting what happened.

Arguably, suspects can be less reluctant to make admissions to pretext callers, as mostly they are persons with whom the suspect has an ongoing relationship, often as a lover or spouse. Thus, additional motives come into play that can lead the suspect to want to comply with the caller's demands (sometimes even if innocent), such as soothing the caller's feelings, attempts to repair or maintain the relationship with the caller, and sometimes to keep the caller from involving law enforcement. Suspects often do make admissions during such pretext calls, even though some are false, so as to appease the caller. If they do make admissions during the call, these admissions become central to interrogator tactics in the police interrogation that typically follows [20]. The interrogator will continually remind the suspect of them to support claims of the suspect's guilt, thereby adding to the many factors contributing to the suspect's hopelessness during the police interrogation.

11.5 The Role of Failed Polygraph Examinations

The second potentially self-incriminating factor comes into play if the suspect agrees to take a polygraph examination. Interrogators often offer such an option to suspects, purportedly as a means to clear themselves from suspicion, and suspects often comply. The suspect may then actually fail the polygraph or may be told falsely that he or she failed [10, 12]. The alleged failure of the polygraph is then used by the interrogator as seeming proof of guilt, further cementing the suspect's sense of hopelessness.

Notably, many scholars have suggested that defendants belonging to social groups stereotyped as more likely to commit certain crimes are likely to appear more deceptive when assessed through procedures based on behavioural cues of anxiety and arousal [18, 23–28]. Presumably, such group members' awareness of the criminal stereotypes associated with their social category creates more anxiety that they will personally be presumed guilty. The National Research Council report on the polygraph first raised the issue of how this 'stereotype threat' would affect performance on the polygraph [28–30]. The authors of the report noted that, because the polygraph relies on indices of arousal and anxiety, innocent persons belonging to criminally stereotyped social categories will suffer greater risk of false positives for deception. While many caregivers of children may not be subject to this risk, it is well known that non-biological parents (in particular, males) in fact are more likely to kill or injure stepchildren [31]. Awareness of this fact, or of this belief among the public, will arguably render such defendants more likely to fail the polygraph exam and thereby to give interrogators more seeming 'evidence' of their guilt. It is important to note as well, however, that enhanced anxiety need not be the result of stereotype threat. Anything leading the suspect to feel that others will presume him or her guilty will arguably also produce greater anxiety during the polygraph and therefore greater vulnerability to false positives for deception.

11.6 Other Threats to Self-Efficacy for Defence

As noted earlier, self-efficacy for defence can be described as the suspect's overall sense that he or she can successfully defend against the accusations of guilt. In addition to the previously discussed contributors to hopelessness, the sense of self-efficacy includes the suspect's ability to recruit resources for defence, as well as expected reactions from prosecutors, judges, and juries. Suspects may consider their financial resources, where (or from whom) they might get financial help, how others are likely to react to them, and so on. Given the horrific nature of injury to or death of a child, many suspects might assume that their social resources might be withdrawn and that prosecutors, judges, and juries are likely to judge them unfavourably and perhaps unfairly.

In summary, the shaken baby suspect can be caught in a web of apparently overwhelming evidence of guilt that seems inescapable and that, in combination with other determinants of self-efficacy, can lead him or her to feel there will be no avenue for convincing others of innocence or of providing proof (or even supportive evidence) of innocence. If the interrogator has been able to convince the suspect that the injuries *had* to have been caused by his or her own (inappropriate) actions (or will be perceived in this way), it becomes easier to convince the suspect that confession is the best choice and to induce him or her to confess to actions that could plausibly cause the injuries: shaking too hard, deliberately inflicting or causing blunt force trauma through negligence, or others.

11.7 Selling Confession

'Psychologically speaking, a successful interrogation is analogous to selling a resident of the Yukon air conditioning in January; for a suspect to acknowledge a criminal act involving negative consequences requires that the suspect believe a confession is in his best interest' [32].

Interrogators explicitly acknowledge that they must convince suspects of a big lie: that confession will be good for them and result in better legal outcomes [32]. This is done through strategies designed to lower the perceived net costs of confession and to raise the perceived costs of denial [12, 33]. Though we do not review such strategies in full here, we point out several commonly used in shaken baby cases.

The Reid 9-Steps suggest the use of exculpatory 'themes' to help lower the perceived costs of confession [15]. The intent is to suggest to the suspect exculpatory scenarios for how and why the alleged actions occurred that make them seem less morally (and seemingly legally) reprehensible and more justifiable, make the suspect seem less culpable, and so on. If the suspect believes the alleged actions are not that serious, confessions will seem to result in less serious legal outcomes.

In SBS and other child abuse cases, the interrogator, having established that the medical evidence conclusively indicates that the causes of injuries was SBS or otherwise not natural, will make suggestions concerning how and why it happened: the injury was caused by the suspect but was accidental, the child is at fault due to excessive crying or misbehaviour, the stresses of having the child are severe and it is understandable to become frustrated and angry and to shake (push, slap, etc.) the child, the child was shaken for a good reason (such as trying to awaken, revive) but was unintentionally shaken too hard, the head was moved too violently during play or rocking, and so on. The suspect is arguably trying to understand what he or she might have done that could have been severe enough to create the injuries in the manner the medical expert has determined to have occurred. As such, the suspect may begin to speculate and to offer up things that might approximate in some way what the doctor and interrogator claim happened.

If the suspect agrees that (s)he might have burped, bounced, played too vigorously, swung the child in a swing forcefully, tripped or fell with the child, held the child too tightly, or shaken the child in any degree, these admissions might be taken as a confession of criminal liability [34]. They may also form the basis of the 'stepping stone' approach to eliciting a more inculpatory admission [35]. The interrogator may, for example, tell the suspect who has admitted that he gently shook the child to try to revive or arouse him that the evidence clearly shows that this was not a gentle shaking, and attempt to induce the suspect to admit to more vigorous shaking instead.

The strategy that is perhaps most unique to SBS suspects occurs when the suspect might plausibly believe that the child has not yet died. That is, we have often seen interrogators tell suspects that the doctor absolutely must know exactly what happened to the child in order to be able to treat the injuries successfully (otherwise the child might die). If the suspect has actually committed a form of violence that could cause the injuries, (s)he may then confess accurately. However, a suspect who did not act inappropriately may still try to help save the child by offering up scenarios as discussed earlier in this chapter that are the best guess as to something that could possibly cause the injury, only to have the interrogator follow up by trying to convince the suspect that the actions had to have been more forceful than claimed to result in the injury at hand.

Together, the perceived evidentiary situation of the suspect and the aforementioned strategies can cause the suspect to come to believe falsely that he or she actually did cause the injuries through shaking or other inappropriate/illegal actions, and to confess accordingly. Combined with other tactics emphasising potential costs of denial (such as being thought a remorseless, cold-hearted liar who won't take responsibility, causing judges and juries to look more harshly upon the suspect, having to believe the worst motives and actions because the suspect won't 'tell his side of the story', and others), the suspect may also become convinced that it is better to confess (even falsely) than to be perceived as not only guilty, but as a hopelessly reprehensible person who deserves no mercy.

11.8 Vulnerability to False Confession: What Is Unique about the Shaken Baby Suspect?

Interrogation scholars have identified a number of dispositional and situational variables that can render suspects more likely to confess during interrogation [18, 23, 24, 35]. Because we are not aware of reasons to believe that shaken baby suspects are more or less likely to possess vulnerable personalities, we focus here on situational influences that might be different for such suspects.

First, it is important to consider the reasons most suspects confess and what personal resources are necessary to resist confession for these reasons. Interrogation scholars widely point to three reasons that account for most confessions. The person might confess to escape the aversive interrogation, because he or she has become convinced that confession will result in better legal (and sometimes personal) outcomes, or because he or she has become convinced by the arguments and 'evidence' of the interrogator that (s)he 'must have' committed the crime as suggested [7, 11, 36]. Villalobos and Davis point to a reason that is much less common, but that must be considered for bereaved suspects: lack of motivation [17]. Because it is likely to be most unique to shaken baby suspects, we consider the latter first.

> I found my daughter. She didn't even have eyes in her head. I was already broken. They didn't have to break me. [37]

To resist the many pressures to confess inherent to police interrogation, one must care. Suspects must care about what happens to them, care whether they live or die (and where), care about the truth and what will be believed, care about achieving justice, and more. Without that motivation it will be easier in the moment to simply comply and say what interrogators want and expect to hear. But what can we expect of the motivations of a shaken baby suspect, particularly one who is the child's parent? Many are likely to feel as did Jerry Hobbs: essentially that nothing matters once one's child has died. There is no motivation left for self-protection and no strength to try. Prison might seem attractive as a means of escape or self-punishment. Guilt is likely to be an overwhelming emotion for many parents, even those who had no role in inflicting injury (who feel that they have failed in their duty to protect the child). Such parents might feel that they are in some way actually guilty and deserving of punishment (feelings that we have seen overtly expressed many times in interrogations of shaken baby suspects).

These kinds of thoughts and lack of motivation are exacerbated by the enormous distress and compromised physical condition of many shaken baby suspects. Whereas most suspects are distressed by allegations against them and the potential for incarceration, shaken baby suspects, particularly parents, are likely to suffer intense distress over the condition or death of the child. Many suffer striking levels of emotional breakdown and despair and poor physical condition. Many come into the interrogation physically depleted as well, having not slept for hours or days, often not having eaten properly, and sometimes drug or alcohol impaired in their efforts to drown their grief. Many suffer severe anxiety because the fate of the severely injured child is not yet known.

While such physical and mental distress can undermine motivation to resist confession, it can also undermine the ability to resist [18, 23, 24]. When already distressed, a person is less able to tolerate further distress. Thus, the likelihood that a suspect will confess just to escape the distressing interrogation (regardless of long-term consequences) will increase. Moreover, distress undermines the ability to think clearly, to recognise flaws in what one is told by the interrogator, to remember information that would suggest confession is unwise, to be able to handle the conversation adequately, to remember potential sources of evidence of innocence, and much more. As a result, it becomes easier to convince suspects that confession will result in better outcomes for them – or even that they might have actually done what the interrogator suggests.

All in all, the impact of the extreme anxiety, distress, and despair of those whose children have died or been severely injured cannot be underestimated. It renders them more vulnerable to (potentially false) confession through all major pathways to false confession: the need to escape, becoming convinced that confession is advantageous, becoming convinced one must have acted as accused, and the less common pathway of lack of caring/motivation.

11.9 The Significance of the Confession

We have presented a number of reasons to expect that those accused of causing severe injury or death to a child might be more susceptible than many other suspects to confessing during interrogation, including to confessing falsely. Given the strong reasons to expect a greater rate of false confession among these suspects, the potential for any confession to be false must be carefully considered (see Chapter 12). It is crucial to carefully inspect the content of the interrogation, to consider and give weight to the felt hopelessness and the physical and emotional condition of the suspect during interrogation (as discussed earlier), and to consider the content of the confession to better assess the potential that the confession is false.

In particular, it is important to track the evolution of the suspect's confession. In many SBS interrogations, the suspect is essentially fed the confession. Few suspects are aware of SBS before their interrogations and are unlikely to formulate a confession around shaking without repeated and insistent references to and explanations of the SBS phenomenon and alleged 'diagnosis' for the suspect's alleged victim. Thus, a long process occurs during which the interrogator (1) provides seemingly overwhelming evidence that the suspect is responsible for the injuries and that they occurred in a specific manner (e.g., shaking), and (2) tries to elicit an account of how the violent shaking sufficient to cause the injuries occurred. The interrogators suggest many possibilities, elicit possibilities from the suspect, and argue that any minimally violent actions the suspect suggests *had* to have been more violent. In the end, even if suspects do confess, it is important to ask whether they are admitting to actions they do remember performing as claimed or simply agreeing that (given all the medical 'evidence' and conclusive diagnoses of the medical professionals) they *must have* performed them.

References

1. Adamsbaum C, Grabar S, Mejean, N, Rey-Salmon C. Abusive head trauma: Judicial admissions highlight violent and repetitive shaking. *Pediatrics*. 2010;126:546–55.
2. Brook C. Wrongful Convictions Report. Is there evidentiary basis for shaken baby syndrome? The conviction of Joby Rowe. 2019. https://wrongfulconvictionsreport.org/2019/09/10/is-there-evidentiary-basis-for-shaken-baby-syndrome-the-conviction-of-joby-rowe.
3. Cenziper D. Shaken science: Prosecutors build murder cases on disputed shaken baby syndrome diagnosis. *Washington Post*. 2015. www.washingtonpost.com/graphics/investigations/shaken-baby-syndrome.
4. Findley KA, Barnes PD, Moran DA, Squier W. Shaken baby syndrome, abusive head trauma, and actual innocence: Getting it right. *Houston Journal of Health Law and Policy*. 2012;12(2):209–312.
5. Vinchon M, De Foort-Dhellemmens S, Desurmont M, Delestret I. Confessed abuse versus witnessed accidents in infants: Comparison of clinical, radiological, and ophthalmological data in corroborated cases. *Child's Nervous System*. 2010;26:637–45.
6. Drizin, SA, Leo RA. The problem of false confessions in the post-DNA world. *North Carolina Law Review*. 2004;82:891–1007.
7. Leo RA, Ofshe RJ. The consequences of false confessions: Deprivations of liberty

and miscarriages of justice in the age of psychological interrogation. *Journal of Criminal Law and Criminology.* 1998;88:429–96.

8. Garrett BL. *Convicting the innocent: Where criminal prosecutions go wrong.* Harvard University Press, 2011.
9. Innocence Project. https://innocenceproject.org.
10. Woody WD, Forrest KD. *Understanding police interrogation: Confessions and consequences.* New York University Press, 2020.
11. Kassin SM, Drizin SA, Grisso T et al. Police-induced confessions: Risk factors and recommendations. *Law and Human Behavior.* 2010;34:3–38.
12. Leo RA. *Police interrogation and American justice.* Harvard University Press, 2009 (for reviews).
13. Papetti R. *The forensic unreliability of the shaken baby syndrome.* Academic Forensic Pathology International, 2018.
14. Tuerkheimer D. *Flawed convictions: Shaken baby syndrome and the inertia of injustice.* Oxford University Press, 2015.
15. John E. Reid and Associates, Inc. http://reid.com.
16. Kozinski W. The Reid interrogation technique and false confessions: A time for change. *Seattle Journal for Social Justice.* 2018;16:301–45 (for reviews).
17. Villalobos JG, Davis D. Interrogation and the minority suspect: Pathways to true and false confession. In *Advances in psychology and law* (Vol. 1). M Miller, B Bornstein, eds. Springer, 2016.
18. Davis D, Leo RA. Interrogation-related regulatory decline: Ego depletion, failures of self-regulation, and the decision to confess. *Psychology, Public Policy, and Law.* 2012;18(4):673–704.
19. Inbau FE, Reid JE, Buckley JP, Jayne, BC. *Criminal interrogation and confessions* (5th ed.). Jones & Bartlett, 2013.
20. Davis D, Leo RA, Livingston TN, Rerick PO. Interrogation and the sexual assault suspect: On the synergy between pretext caller and police interrogator. In *Criminal investigations of sexual offenses: Investigative techniques and operational challenges.* N Deslauriers-Varin, C Bennell, eds. Springer, 2021, pp. 1–41.
21. Livingston T, Rerick PO, Villalobos JG, Davis D. Deception induced confession: Strategies of police interrogators and their lay collaborators. In *Palgrave handbook of deceptive communication.* T Docan-Morgan, ed. Springer, 2019, pp. 747–67.
22. Davis D, Villalobos JG. Language and the law: Illustrations from cases of disputed sexual consent. In *Oxford handbook of language and social psychology.* T Holtgraves, ed. Oxford University Press, 2014, pp. 438–58.
23. Davis D, Leo RA. To walk in their shoes: The problem of missing, misrepresented and misunderstood context in judging criminal confessions. *New England Law Review.* 2012;46(4):737–67.
24. Davis D, Leo RA. Acute suggestibility in police interrogation: Self-regulation failure as a primary mechanism of vulnerability. In *Suggestibility in legal contexts: Psychological research and forensic implications.* A Ridley, F Gabbert, DJ La Rooy, eds. Wiley, 2012, pp. 171–97.
25. Davis D, Leo RA. Interrogation through pragmatic implication. In *The Oxford handbook on language and law.* L Solan, P Tiersma, eds. Oxford University Press, 2012, pp. 354–66.
26. Davis D, Leo RA. Stereotype threat and the special vulnerabilities of sexual abuse/assault suspects to false confession. In *Vilified: Wrongful allegations of person abuse.* R Burnett, ed. Oxford University Press, 2016, pp. 175–90.
27. Najdowski CJ. Stereotype threat in criminal interrogations: Why innocent black suspects are at risk for confessing falsely. *Psychology, Public Policy and Law.* 2011;17(4):562–91.
28. National Research Council of the National Academies. *The polygraph and lie detection.* National Academies Press, 2003.

29. Steele CM. *Whistling Vivaldi: How stereotypes affect us and what we can do.* W. W. Norton, 2011.

30. Steele CM, Aronson J. Stereotype threat and the intellectual test performance of African Americans. *Journal of Personality and Social Psychology.* 1995;69(5):797–811.

31. Harris GT, Hilton NZ, Rice ME, Eke AW. Children killed by genetic parents versus stepparents. *Evolution and Human Behavior.* 2007;28(2):85–95.

32. Jayne BC, Buckley JP. *Investigator anthology: A compilation of articles and essays about the Reid technique of interviewing and interrogation.* John E. Reid & Associates, Inc., 1999.

33. Davis D, Leo RA, Follette WC. Selling confession: Setting the stage with the 'sympathetic detective with a time-limited offer. *Journal of Contemporary Criminal Justice.* 2010;26(4):441–57.

34. Cronkright M. What if a parent confesses to shaking a baby? Part two. 2020. www.Michiganparentdefense.com/blog/2020/January/what-if-a-parent-confesses-to-shaking-a-baby-par2.

35. Gudjonsson GH. Mental vulnerabilities and false confession. In *Investigative interviewing: The essentials.* M St.-Ives, ed. Carswell, 2014, pp. 191–222.

36. Gudjonsson GH. *The psychology of interrogations and confessions: A handbook.* Wiley, 2003.

37. Martin A. Jerry Hobbs' confession. *New York Times Magazine.* 25 November 2011.

Chapter 12

Can Confession Substitute for Science in Shaken Baby Syndrome/Abusive Head Trauma?

Keith Findley

For any medical diagnosis, high-quality research is critical. Shaken baby syndrome/abusive head trauma (SBS/AHT), as a medico-legal determination that goes beyond diagnosis, is no different. Indeed, a solid scientific foundation is especially critical in SBS/AHT because erroneous determinations can have catastrophic consequences from both false negatives – severe injury or death to a child – and false positives – erroneous destruction of a family and/or imprisonment or even a death sentence for an innocent caregiver. Moreover, in the legal world, medical determinations of SBS/AHT can have outsized effects – unlike virtually any other type of expert opinion evidence, a medical expert's opinion is often used to prove all of the elements of the offence – what happened, who did it (based on timing the injuries), and even what mental state the suspect had ('knowing', 'intentional', 'reckless', or the like) [1]. While proponents of the SBS/AHT hypothesis insist that SBS/AHT is purely a medical determination, not a legal one [2], the reality is that these physicians explicitly address their arguments to the courts and their opinions are in many cases used to satisfy the entire legal case [3].

12.1 The Research Challenge: Circularity

Unfortunately, research on abuse is inherently difficult. Because randomised controlled studies are impossible, the dominant research methodology has been retrospective studies of children with intracranial injuries who are sorted into two categories – abused (children thought to have been subjected to shaking or shaking with impact) and non-abused (children injured or killed by accidents or natural conditions). Once sorted, the cases are then analysed to confirm that shaking can cause such injuries, to identify typical characteristics of abusers, and to identify diagnostic features to distinguish abuse from non-abuse. But because there are no gold-standard diagnostic criteria or laboratory tests for SBS/AHT [4], researchers typically rely on the presumed features of abuse – for example, the presence of subdural haematoma, retinal haemorrhages, and encephalopathy, or some combination of this triad and other features. Therein lies the circularity confound that is present in virtually all the foundational research on SBS/AHT – the very signs being studied are used as the inclusion criteria for the abuse cohort in the research.

Circularity in SBS/AHT research is universally recognised. Narang, a leading proponent of the hypothesis, acknowledges that 'some circularity is inevitable' [5]. Vinchon, another leading proponent, has conceded that '[s]ince in most series the diagnosis of [AHT] is based on the presence of [SDH, encephalopathy, and RH], evaluation of the diagnostic value of these criteria is flawed by a bias of circularity' [6]. Meta-analyses attempting to identify diagnostic criteria for SBS/AHT have similarly acknowledged the circularity. Despite efforts to select only what they deemed to be the very best research in the field, Maguire et al. noted that they could not avoid circularity:

> Diagnostic studies in this field are open to criticism of circularity because of their dependence on a constellation of clinical features, as opposed to a single gold-standard diagnostic test, which does not exist . . . [E]xcept in cases of independently witnessed injury, a diagnosis must rest on a probabilistic assessment of how likely it is that AHT took place. It is not possible to restrict research in this field to independently witnessed abuse, which represents a tiny proportion of cases. [7]

A similar meta-analysis by Piteau et al. used the same standards for selecting 'confirmed' cases. Like Maguire et al., Piteau et al. acknowledged that circularity is unavoidable:

> As there are no standardized criteria for the definition of abuse, most authors developed their own criteria, and many of these are fraught with circular reasoning. The diagnosis of AHT relies on historical features, clinical findings, and radiologic interpretations, and it is these same criteria that are used to categorize head trauma as abusive or nonabusive. [8]

Indeed, the only independent governmental examination of the SBS/AHT research base, undertaken in 2016 by the Swedish Agency for Health Technology Assessment and Assessment of Social Services (SBU) (see Chapter 10), determined, precisely because of this circularity confound, that *none* of the research in this field is of high quality, and that in sum the evidentiary foundation for the 'diagnosis' of SBS is of 'very low quality' [9].

12.2 Reliance on Confessions

To overcome the circularity problem, researchers have looked for sorting criteria that do not depend on the variables that are themselves being studied [10]. For example, expressly 'to minimize circularity by dependence purely on the clinical features alone to determine if abuse had taken place', Maguire et al. included only cases in which abuse was 'confirmed'. They considered cases 'confirmed' (1) if deemed so 'at case conference or civil, family, or criminal court proceedings or admitted by perpetrator or independently witnessed'; or (2) if deemed confirmed 'by stated criteria, including multidisciplinary assessment' [7]. Such conclusions, however – apart from 'independently witnessed' incidents (of which there are none in the literature involving shaking leading to brain injury) – are themselves necessarily dependent on the diagnostic criteria being evaluated and hence still subject to circularity.

Ultimately, researchers settled on confessions as the gold standard for identifying cases in which a child was abused [6, 11, 12]. The SBS hypothesis has become so dependent on confessions that Dias's chapter in a prominent textbook that strives to make 'the case for shaking' proclaims that 'confessed shaking . . . *is* the evidentiary basis for shaking' (emphasis in original) [14]. Similarly, in an article intended in part to establish that pure shaking can injure the infant brain, Minns has argued that '[e]ven a single, carefully documented case of shaking alone is sufficient to establish the possibility that shaking alone can result in head injury' [15]. He then cited exactly one such case, involving a 4-month-old child, which he deemed 'carefully documented' because the caregiver acknowledged 'that the child was shaken angrily "in the air" (without impacting on any hard or soft surface) for between five and ten seconds'. Without any further analysis of the purported confession, Minns concluded: 'From this single case it is clear that adults can and do shake infants and this does cause brain damage in the form of an encephalopathy with subdural and retinal haemorrhages, and that impaction on any type of surface is not necessarily required.'

Vinchon et al. have contended that confessions can be employed to overcome the circularity bias: their solution was to 'classify infantile head traumas along a spectrum, from certain abuse (confessed) to certain accident (witnessed)' [6]. Subsequently, Vinchon et al. listed and then sought to discredit what they called '12 fake news [*sic*]' about SBS/AHT – 12 criticisms of the SBS/AHT hypothesis. A primary reason they cited for rejecting these criticisms was that 'Violent and repeated shaking is the main mechanism reported by perpetrators' [16]. Addressing the concern that these confessions might be unreliable, Vinchon et al. asserted simply that 'the confessions are stereotyped' (i.e., consistent) – apparently believing that this makes them accurate and reliable.[1] Moreover, Vinchon et al. appeared to believe that confessions are likely to be coerced and false only if produced through formal plea bargaining. 'Plea-bargaining is not a legal practice in all countries. It does not exist in France, where confessions are obtained during close cross-interrogation, under no physical pressure' (see Chapter 22). Both of these points reveal serious misconceptions about interrogations and confessions, as addressed in what follows.

Others have also looked to confessions as the gold standard. Starling, Holden, and Jenny created a hierarchy of certainty intended to overcome circularity, in which confession sits at the top as the gold standard, followed by convictions, then cases in which the caregiver was charged but not convicted, and finally cases in which caregivers provided what the researchers deemed an inadequate or 'discrepant' explanation [13].

In 2020, Edwards et al. published a systematic review of all confession-based SBS/AHT research from 1963 to 2018 [17]. They found 55 studies with a total of 434 confessions over 55 years. They acknowledged that the vast majority of the confessions contained only bare information merely identifying the mechanism of injury and nothing more (82.7% described only the mechanism, while only 17% provided at least one additional detail and only 2.3% provided three details or more beyond the mechanism). They also acknowledged that 'it is possible that some of the reported confessions were false'. But without any other analysis of the nature of the interrogations and confessions, they concluded that 'confessions can provide important details about what happened, including the mechanism of the injury and the characteristics of the perpetrator'.

Even critics of the SBS/AHT hypothesis have given confessions heightened credence. As noted, in 2016 in Sweden, the SBU panel of leading paediatricians and experts in forensic medicine, radiology, medical epidemiology, and medical and research ethics undertook a systematic review of the medical literature on SBS/AHT (see Chapter 10). After retrieving 3,773 SBS-related medical papers, the SBU found that only 30 were relevant to assessing the diagnostic value of the triad. Of those, none were of high quality, only 2 were of moderate quality, and all the rest were low quality. What distinguished the 2 the SBU deemed of moderate quality? Those studies at least tried to avoid circularity *by relying upon confessions* (the SBU found no studies with witnessed or videotaped cases) [9].

[1] In science, this would be called *reliability* – the ability to get the same result from the same process every time. But it would not constitute *validity* – a showing that a procedure or technique accurately measures what it purports to measure. Vinchon et al. overlook that both reliability and validity are required to establish scientific bona fides of a method or technique. Without a showing of validity, merely showing similarity between confessions across cases does not ensure that the interrogation process is *accurately* capturing what produced a child's injuries.

Yet none of the research – not even the SBU report – has examined the confessions themselves to determine if they are reliable and whether they truly are independent of the triad, so that they avoid circularity (although, to its credit, the SBU recognised that the confession-based research still did not achieve high-quality status and should be approached with caution).[2] Starling et al., for example, acknowledged that 'an argument could be made that the perpetrators were coerced in some manner or that mechanisms were suggested to them' [11]. But she explored the issue no further, stating: 'An analysis of the investigative techniques involved in eliciting the admissions is beyond the scope of this article.'

Similarly, Biron and Shelton acknowledged the possibility of unreliable confessions but dismissed the concern without further inquiry. 'There is clearly an inherent unreliability in the content of perpetrator statements, yet they remain the only available window through which the abusive act can be directly observed' [12]. Biron and Shelton then identified five cases in which the accused allegedly confessed. From those 'confessions', without any analysis of the interrogations, they concluded that '[t]he abusive shaking of an infant by an adult caregiver can result in death or serious neurological impairment even when no associated impact takes place'.

Minns also acknowledged that '[t]he reliability of confessions or acknowledgement by perpetrators of any sort of injury can be questioned', but without any analysis he also dismissed any concerns about reliability. He asserted simply, 'there is no reason to believe that any of the ... cases [he examined from a Scottish database] were anything but uncoerced confessions' [15].

Adamsbaum et al. acknowledged that 'perpetrator admissions are not scientific evidence' [18]. They also conceded that some of the confessions in their study had to be in some respects false because some claimed shaking with no impact yet the medical findings included skull fractures. They also noted that '[n]o correlation was found between repetitive shaking and SDH densities', suggesting that confessions related to repetition of shaking was not consistent with the medical data. Nonetheless, without further analysis, they concluded that confessions 'confirm[] the pathogenic nature of shaking in and of itself'. Similarly, Vinchon et al. acknowledged that '[d]etails of abuse as reported by abusers may be unreliable'; nonetheless, without more they concluded simply, 'we think the information on confessions obtained from the judiciary can be trusted' [6].

Dias likewise, without any empirical data, has dismissed the possibility that confessions provide an unreliable foundation for the hypothesis:

> This common and consistent admission by the perpetrator to shaking the infant (whether or not cranial impact injury is described or discovered by physical examination, radiographic studies, or autopsy) overwhelmingly suggests that shaking is an important component of infant abusive TBI [traumatic brain injury] and is, in fact, sufficient to cause the intracranial injuries found in AHT. To suggest otherwise (as required by the biomechanical evidence) would require that every confessed perpetrator has to have been consistently and universally lying about the same phenomenon, something that defies logic and common sense. [14]

---

[2] While 'reliability' and 'validity' have distinct meanings in science, this chapter uses the term 'reliability' broadly in the lay sense that encompasses notions of both reliability and validity because that is the sense in which both medical researchers and the legal system have used the term.

Dias might be correct about that, but without investigating the interrogations and confessions, his claim is pure speculation. It also likely is *not* correct. Contrary to Dias's intuition, it is entirely possible that most confessions in shaking cases are false to some degree or entirely. If all suspects are questioned in a similar manner, using interrogation tactics known to induce false confessions, and if all are fed the same medical information about what must have happened to cause such injuries – as is common – then it would not be surprising that a certain percentage of innocent suspects succumb and confess and then repeat similar stories about what happened. This possibility is enhanced by the reality that there are very few documented SBS confessions in the literature [19–21]; even SBS proponents concede that '[c]onfessions are uncommon' [19, 21]. As Minns observed, 'this is almost always an unwitnessed injury and is mostly denied by the perpetrator' [15]. The risk of relying on confessions to break free of circularity is compounded by the recognition in the literature that almost all – if not all – confessions come not spontaneously and promptly, but only after the caregiver has been subjected to the interrogation process, with attending risks and likelihood of contamination and psychological coercion [10, 11]. In the end, because it is impossible for interrogators to ignore the existence of a medical determination of SBS/AHT, confession-based evidence will never reach the level of double-blind placebo control studies that is considered the gold standard in evidence-based medicine.

12.3 The Study of Interrogations and Confessions

The sanguinity about confessions in SBS research ignores the extensive body of interrogations and confessions scholarship of the past three-plus decades (see Chapter 11). Although counter-intuitive, we now know that police interrogations can induce wholly innocent individuals to confess to serious crimes. Among the cases in which a convicted individual was exonerated by post-conviction DNA testing, more than 25% of the innocent suspects had confessed falsely [22, 23]. Notably, 99% of these DNA cases involved the most serious crimes – murders, rapes, and rape/murders. Expanding the pool of wrongful convictions beyond those established by DNA testing, the National Registry of Exonerations lists approximately 12% of the exonerations in its database of 2,879 cases (as of October 2021) as involving false confessions [24].

Extensive research reveals that false confessions are produced in part by psychological pressures in the interrogation process [25–32]. Most police in America are trained in the 'Reid Technique' of interrogation or a variant [33]. The technique involves a nine-step process designed to break down suspects and elicit an admission. Several steps involve 'maximisation' techniques – strategies designed to make suspects believe their situation is hopeless, that they will be convicted, and that they are facing dire consequences. Part of this process can include presentation of real or fabricated proof of guilt [26, 28, 32]. Police then counter the maximisation strategies with minimisation techniques. Through minimisation, interrogators offer suspects a way out – a way to minimise the moral culpability or legal consequences of the alleged conduct. Interrogators do this through a process of 'theme building' in which they suggest, for example, that the suspect is a good person who understandably and unintentionally lost control, that the victim had it coming, or that the offence was an accident. Suspects who are convinced that they will be convicted and believe that confessing will minimise the consequences (or at least put an end to the questioning) may well make a rational choice to confess, even falsely – a type of confession recognised in the literature as coerced-compliant false confessions. Alternatively, the interrogation may be so intense that suspects come to doubt their own memory and begin to believe they must have committed the crime – a type of confession known as persuaded false confessions [31, 32].

In 2010, the American Psychology-Law Society of the American Psychological Association published a 'white paper' on police-induced confessions [32]. Drawing on decades of social-psychological research, the expert-authors concluded that certain interrogation tactics are correlated to false confessions, including presentation of false evidence and minimisation.

Of particular significance in the SBS context is that researchers have identified two fundamental errors that can produce false confessions: misclassification and contamination [34]. Misclassification arises from the distinction police make between an interview and an interrogation. An interview is a fact-developing process in which the objective is to learn what the subject knows. An interrogation, by contrast, is a guilt-presuming process in which the objective is solely to obtain a confession or incriminating statement. Investigators move from an interview to an interrogation when they are satisfied that the subject is guilty; at that point, the objective is to get statements that confirm guilt. Indeed, interrogators are trained to cut off all denials and assertions of innocence.

Misclassification arises when investigators misjudge the culpability of the subject and shift from interviewing to interrogating when the subject is in fact not guilty. At that point, the risk arises that the psychologically powerful interrogation techniques might induce the sought-after result – a confession – even though the subject in fact is innocent.

Contamination occurs when, during the ensuing guilt-presuming interrogation, interrogators reveal facts about the case that provide even an innocent suspect with the information needed to develop a factually rich confession statement. Interrogators push suspects to provide details, including 'inside information' that only the true culprit could have known. As Garrett explains it, 'the power of a confession derives from the lengthy narrative describing what happened, and not from the bare statement that "I did it"' [22]. But many of the interrogation techniques – such as confronting the suspect with real or fabricated evidence of guilt – run the risk of 'leaking' insider information to the suspect, providing the appearance that the suspect has detailed knowledge of the crime, when the suspect may have none. Garrett's study of the first 250 individuals convicted of serious crimes whose actual innocence was later established by DNA testing identified 40 cases in which the innocent suspect had falsely confessed. In 38 of those 40 cases, 'detectives testified that these defendants did far more than say "I did it." According to the detectives, the suspects had "guilty" or "inside knowledge"' – knowledge the detectives swore they had not revealed to the innocent suspects. Because DNA proved that these suspects were all innocent, however, all of that insider information had to have come from the detectives, not the guileless suspects.

12.4 Interrogations and Confessions in Shaken Baby Syndrome/Abusive Head Trauma Cases

Given all of this, the unquestioning reliance on purported confessions to substitute for scientific evidence is dubious at best. To begin, confessions are not scientific evidence. They are not generally amenable to testing for validity or reliability, and the circumstances that induce them are not subject to control by the researcher. They also may be misleading, for three reasons. First, they could be false in whole or in part. Second, they may be the product of interrogations that rely upon the medical findings to convince the caregiver to confess and that provide the substance of those confessions – the consistent narrative across cases that Dias finds so unlikely if the confessions are false. In such cases, the purported confessions are the product of the medical findings, not an independent source of verification that allows researchers to break free from circular reasoning. Third, even if they bear some truth, many of the confessions that researchers rely upon are not truly confessions because they involve statements about minor shaking or shaking *after* a child has collapsed in an effort to revive the child, neither of which could be the cause of the child's catastrophic distress.

12.4.1 Reliability and Dependence on the Medical Findings

One cannot assume reliability of SBS/AHT confessions in part because both misclassification and contamination are serious risks in such cases – indeed, as Davis and Leo demonstrate in this book (Chapter 11), they are especially fraught risks in such cases. Misclassification will occur if the interrogators conclude erroneously – based on the triad-driven hypothesis – that the medical findings show that the child was shaken or shaken and slammed. It will not suffice to say that, if physicians determine that the child was abused, then there is no misclassification, because the very basis for relying on the confessions is to verify that the hypothesis-driven determination is correct. Its validity cannot be assumed. If, in fact, the hypothesis is wrong, then the medical determinations of abuse will indeed lead to misclassification of innocent suspects and improper initiation of guilt-presuming interrogations.

Moreover, because any misclassification will be based on medical findings that correlate to a specific mode of abuse, confronting the suspect with that medical evidence produces contamination – providing the suspect with details of what the interrogators believe must have happened, thereby providing the information needed for a factually rich confession. Typically, for example, interrogators will reject claims of an accident or other innocent mechanism of injury, informing the suspect that the doctors have found, for example, subdural haematoma and retinal haemorrhages, and that, absent a major motor vehicle crash, the only way to produce those findings (or other combinations of findings) is through the rapid acceleration/deceleration forces from shaking or shaking and slamming. And they will often inform the suspect that, according to doctors, the forces applied had to have been massive – the equivalent of throwing a child from a multi-story building or hitting the child with an automobile at 35 miles per hour. When confronted with such indisputable 'medical' evidence, it is not surprising that caregivers, if they are induced to confess, come up with very similar statements describing violent shaking or slamming.

For example, in a New York case examined in a compelling documentary, *Scenes of a Crime*, with a video-recorded interrogation, detectives repeatedly told the suspect to demonstrate throwing the child down and to do it with greater force until they were satisfied with his demonstration. New York's highest court vacated the conviction and ordered suppression of the confession, finding it both coerced and unreliable. The court noted: 'Every scenario of trauma induced head injury equal to explaining the infant's symptoms was suggested to defendant by his interrogators. Indeed, there is not a single inculpatory fact in defendant's confession that was not suggested to him' [35].

For these reasons, all of the justifications posited by Vinchon, Dias, and others for accepting confessions are inadequate. First, that the alleged confessors describe the same mechanism of injury means little if that mechanism is fed to them, as appears to be the case in virtually every interrogation. Second, that some countries do not rely on plea bargaining, so that, as Vinchon et al. put it, in those countries, confessions are obtained not during plea bargaining but 'during close cross-interrogation, under no physical pressure', ignores that *most* false confessions even in plea-bargain jurisdictions occur prior to plea bargaining, 'during close cross-interrogation, under no physical pressure' [16]. It is that 'close cross-interrogation' that generates *psychological* pressure that induces most false confessions today.

Recent data confirm that the coercive interrogation process is very much alive not only in the United States, but also in countries like France, which claim to have no plea bargaining (see Chapter 22). *Le Monde* has described a study that shows that French interrogators employ maximisation and minimisation and exhibit both misclassification and contamination, just as elsewhere [36]. One French caregiver reported, for example, that 'by the third interrogation, I was shown an expert report of the hospital concluding that [the child] had been shaken. I was told that there was proof it was either me or my husband'. The study found that 95 out of 115 French caregivers were interrogated in police custody and 'the diagnosis of child abuse was presented to them as absolutely certain in 80% of cases (76 out of 95)'. Similarly, a qualitative content analysis of interviews with 12 parents in Sweden who were wrongly accused of SBS/AHT reported that parents said their 'interrogations were performed without the presence of legal representatives, and were harsh and brutal. They were told "We know that you are 100% guilty" and were subjected to intense pressure and questioning' [37].

In another paper, Vinchon et al. cited a study examining the features of AHT cases (again, the determination of AHT was marred by the typical – but unacknowledged – circularity confound) in which the 'perpetrators' confessed compared to those in which they did not [38]. The only statistically significant difference between the two groups was that 'the severity of RH and the prevalence of brain lesions was significantly higher in the confession group'. Without explanation, Vinchon et al. concluded, 'Our interpretation of these results is that the diagnosis of AHI [abusive head injury] was correct in both groups, but denial was more prevalent in the less severe cases. We also think that these results validate the diagnostic protocol currently in use.' Given that the study included no measure of the validity of either the diagnostic process or the confessions themselves, this conclusion is startling and inexplicable.

Similarly mystifying is Vinchon et al.'s surmise that caregivers likely confessed more frequently in cases with serious injuries because in the less serious cases the 'perpetrator' was able 'to convince himself that "nothing happened; hence I did nothing"'. According to Vinchon et al., in cases with more severe lesions, the injuries 'made it all the more difficult to deny the evidence'. Without any supporting evidence, Vinchon et al. wrote that 'our opinion is that the perpetrator confesses with the sole purpose of relieving his conscience'.

Vinchon et al. reached these conclusions without any apparent awareness of the research on the psychology of interrogations and confessions or any inquiry into or analysis of what the suspects were told in the interrogations, what the perpetrators actually said, whether the perpetrators recanted once freed from the pressures of the interrogation, or the myriad other questions that would be required to draw meaningful conclusions from the data.

The research on interrogations and confessions teaches that it is equally if not more likely that, with more severe retinal haemorrhages and brain lesions, interrogators are motivated to push hard against denials and to insist that the child had to have been shaken/slammed. That in turn increases the psychological pressures on the caregivers; as noted later in this chapter, research shows that interrogators are more aggressive in their interrogations when convinced of guilt. And it increases the likelihood that suspects were told the 'facts' that provided the content of the resulting confessions. Vinchon et al.'s rush to conclude the contrary reflects not science or evidence but an apparent advocacy bias or confirmation bias (see Chapter 13).

Even if child abuse physicians, rather than members of law enforcement, question the caregiver and obtain a confession, the psychological pressures that can induce false confessions and cue suspects about what to say are prevalent. Edwards et al. thought it significant that they found no statistically significant difference between confessions elicited by police and those elicited by medical personnel [17]. Of the 434 confessions they found in the literature, 50.9% were obtained during investigation by law enforcement, while 13.6% were obtained during medical questioning (35.5% were unknown).

They concluded that the similarity in the confessions across categories validated the confessions because they assumed that '[n]either psychological techniques of interrogation nor plea bargains are part of a medical evaluation'. Not only did they cite no data for their claim about what happens during medical questioning, but their assumption misapprehends the nature of the psychological pressure at issue. Although physicians are not trained as interrogators, they naturally adopt many of the Reid strategies simply because, based on the medical orthodoxy to which they likely adhere, they *believe* that nothing is likely to explain the symptoms except SBS/AHT, and hence they will likely engage in the same guilt-presumptive processes as will police, complete with rejecting claims of innocence and suggesting to the caregiver the mechanism they believe would have caused the medical conditions.

Indeed, caregivers routinely complain that medical personnel questioned them in guilt-presuming and accusatory ways. According to a survey by a French association of parents in 2021, 72% of 150 respondents said they felt medical personnel had an accusatory attitude against them [39]. Similarly, Högberg et al.'s qualitative analysis of the experiences of 12 wrongly accused parents found that '[o]ur participants, when seeking care for their infants, instead experienced harm inflicted by healthcare service', partly because healthcare providers treated them with 'disrespect, manipulation and deception' [37]. Beyond that, no representative sampling data exist to tell us what happens in most SBS/AHT interrogations. No one has studied the process in a systematic way. Without that inquiry, reliance on confessions to prove SBS/AHT is unjustified and dangerous.

The unblinking reliance on confessions is even more inappropriate given what we *do* know about the process. Because the presumption of abuse that the traditional hypothesis attaches to any case in which a baby presents with the 'triad' or its variants, police (and child abuse physicians) approach their questioning with a presumption of guilt. Empirically, we know that such guilt-presuming interrogations evoke aggressive questioning tactics and that even innocent suspects respond to such tactics in ways that make them appear guilty to neutral observers (ironically, that is even more true for the innocent than guilty) [40]. Moreover, as Davis and Leo explain in Chapter 11, caregivers are especially vulnerable during these interrogations because they have just lost a child in their care and have fewer emotional reserves to draw upon to resist psychological pressures to confess. Stress is an empirically established contributor to false confessions.

Additionally, while there are no generalisable data, there is considerable anecdotal data in SBS/AHT cases that support the likelihood that the risk of false confession in these cases is significant, or at least that we cannot assume that confessions are independent of the medical findings. Without that independence, we cannot assume that the confessions permit researchers to break free from the circularity that infects the research.

Tuerkheimer, for example, has analysed confessions in several cases and provides rich examples of the methods used to induce confessions. She shows that the interrogations in each case she examined relied heavily on the medical findings and opinions of child abuse physicians, and on the guilt-presuming psychological interrogation tactics known to cause false confessions [41].

I have collected a random sample of recorded interrogations in SBS/AHT cases from across the United States, and, in every case, the interrogations conform to this pattern. In not a single SBS/AHT case have my colleagues or I yet seen a caregiver spontaneously and without prompting by medical evidence confess and describe shaking or shaking with impact as the mechanism of injury. Without exception these interrogations involve maximisation, including presentation of purported inculpatory evidence, such as triad-based medical opinions. While the medical sources of those opinions, and the police interrogators who rely upon them, typically believe those statements, if incorrect, then those statements would have the same effect as presenting false evidence. Moreover, in some cases, police have indeed fabricated medical evidence of SBS [42].

Illustrating this use of maximisation and medical evidence, when a parent in one fairly typical interrogation insisted that abuse 'didn't happen. It didn't happen', the investigating detective deployed the medical evidence. According to the detective, 'At this time, I told him, "It did happen. All you have to do is go to the hospital and see him lying there. The doctors aren't lying. They aren't making this up. Your son has been shaken"' [42]. In another typical interrogation, after the parent denied harming the child, the detective told him that, according to the doctors, the child has 'got what's called subdural hemorrhaging in her brain. That's usually indicative of some kind of inertial force. Not blunt trauma to the head, but either some kind of violent shaking, some type of large fall, some type of violent action that occurred against her' [43].

Judge Richard Posner of the US Court of Appeals for the Seventh Circuit has identified the problematic nature of such interrogation tactics. In *Aleman v Village of Hanover Park* (2011), he wrote:

> Not being a medical expert, Aleman could not contradict what was represented to him as settled medical opinion. He had shaken Joshua, albeit gently; but if medical opinion excluded any other possible cause of the child's death, then, gentle as the shaking was, and innocently intended, it *must* have been the cause of death. Aleman had no rational basis, given his ignorance of medical science, to deny that he had to have been the cause. [42]

Judge Posner accordingly concluded, 'A confession so induced is worthless as evidence'.

Yet such exchanges are the norm and demonstrate both the ways in which maximisation puts pressure on caregivers to come up with some explanation that includes abuse and the contamination error – the interrogators lead the suspects to describe the hypothesised shaking/slamming. The near ubiquity of such exchanges suggests powerfully that, contrary to Dias's intuition, it would not be at all surprising if all or most such confessions were false and included similar (stereotypical) descriptions of what supposedly happened.

The SBS interrogations also mix in minimisation, typically an assertion by the interrogators that they know the suspect is not a monster, that the suspect loves the child, that it was not intentional, that the suspect just snapped and shook the child when the child would not stop crying, that it was just a shake not a beating, that it was an accident, that police could help the suspect or doctors could treat the child if the suspect would explain how he or she abused the child, and that if the suspect did not confess authorities would have no choice but to conclude the act was intentional and the suspect was heartless.

In the last of these interrogations quoted above, for example, after telling the father that the medical evidence proved violent 'inertial' forces like shaking, the detective offered the father a culpability-minimising way to start admitting responsibility:

> [DETECTIVE]: Okay. Is it just that maybe you guys got frustrated with her and somebody, you know, dropped her harder than they should've? You know, picked her up hard, you know, something more than you guys would normally do? I know at 4:30 in the morning –
>
> [CHILD'S FATHER]: Oh –
>
> [DETECTIVE]: – it can be frustrating to have a child crying, you've got to get up, everybody's tired.
>
> [FATHER]: Not that I can think of.
>
> [DETECTIVE]: Is this an accident that could have happened somehow?
>
> [FATHER]: Maybe. It had to have been an accident that have happened at some point in time, but I don't –
>
> [DETECTIVE]: Maybe like how? When you say –
>
> [FATHER]: – understand like –
>
> [DETECTIVE]: When you say 'maybe', how – how could this have happened maybe?
>
> [FATHER]: Well, obviously something happened, and I don't know what happened. Like I know she hasn't been dropped. . . .. . .
>
> [DETECTIVE]: If it's not you, David, then it has to be [your wife,] Jacqueline. There's nobody else that's caring for you guys' child but you guys [44].

12.4.2 Confessions That Are Not Confessions

Some 'confessions' relied upon by researchers are also problematic even if in some sense true because the acts the suspects 'confess' to might not in fact support the SBS/AHT hypothesis. A natural (indeed, recommended) response to finding a child who is unresponsive is to give her a shake to rouse her [45]. At times, admissions to such acts are deemed 'confessions' to abuse. Caffey's seminal 1972 article – one of the foundational articles underlying the SBS hypothesis – includes 'burpings', a 'confession' that a mother merely said 'she and her husband "might have shaken [the infant] when he cried at night"', and a case in which a mother said she 'yanked a child to prevent him from falling off a bassinet onto the floor' [46]. Imwinkelried observes that '[i]t is debatable whether such conduct should be characterized as the kind of major, violent shaking events that supposedly cause shaken baby syndrome' [47].

Biron and Shelton described the 'confessions' in their study of five shaking cases:

- Case 1: '[H]e gave her a bit of a shake.'
- Case 2: 'He stated that he had shaken the infant "out of anger" for 2–3 minutes, supporting his head with his hands, although it still "rocked back and forth" (he later indicated that the shaking may not have taken that long).'

- Case 3: '[G]ave him a little shake.'
- Case 4: Gave her 'a bit of a shake to stop her crying'. It was a 'fairly vigorous shake'.
- Case 5: Father said he 'often vigorously bounced the infant on his knee after feeding, causing her head to move "up and down and back and forth"' [12].

Despite the minimal force admitted in these statements, Biron and Shelton concluded: 'Together, the medical and perpetrator evidence pertaining to all five incidents provides strong evidence of shaking in the absence of any type of impact trauma'.

One additional paper is worth noting because it reports a single confession that appears to bear more indicia of reliability than most. In the single case described in that paper, after the accused parent abruptly pled guilty, the accused agreed to be interviewed for purposes of research with assurances that his statements would be held in confidence and could not affect his sentencing [21]. In response to what the paper describes as 'non-directive' questioning, the accused tearfully described shaking a 3-year-old child 5–15 times, repeated in three bursts. He said he then set her down in the tub and turned away, and he heard her fall and apparently hit her head on the tub. Medical examination confirmed that the child not only had a subdural haematoma, retinal haemorrhages, and cerebral oedema, but also a haematoma on the left side of her head from the impact.

While this confession seemingly avoided the suggestion and contamination of most SBS/AHT interrogations, it too cannot prove the SBS/AHT hypothesis. First, it is a single case report – the lowest form of research for validating a hypothesis under accepted quality-of-evidence standards, which, standing alone, has almost no statistical power. Second, while the interrogation apparently avoided suggestion, it came late in the criminal process, after the accused unavoidably would have been exposed to the prosecution's theory of the case and the medical opinions underlying it. Third, while the accused may have been assured that his confession could not be used against him in the criminal case, that cannot eliminate the possibility that his own sense of moral self-worth might have induced him to minimise the degree to which he might have engaged in even more violent behaviour than shaking. Fourth, this case involved not an infant, but a 3-year-old, which makes it far less plausible that shaking alone could have generated sufficient forces, given that biomechanical research has established that shaking a toddler generates 10 times *less* acceleration than shaking an infant [47]. Finally, and perhaps most importantly, this case was not a pure shaking case; by all accounts it involved both shaking and impact. Given the impact, it is impossible to know which insult – shaking or impact – caused the child's brain and eye findings. In sum, while there may be some truth in this confession, it provides no assurances of validity in the SBS/AHT hypothesis.

12.4.3 False Confessions by the Guilty

Ironically, some confessions are unreliable not because the suspect is innocent, but because the suspect is guilty – but guilty of something more culpable than shaking. The research that depends on confessions for validation overlooks that individuals who are guilty of more violent conduct, including beating, throwing, or slamming a child, will have every incentive to minimise their culpability by confessing to something seemingly less heinous – shaking – especially when interrogators offer shaking as a minimisation theme.

While these confessions might be true to the extent that guilty caregivers admit abuse, those admissions cannot validate shaking as the mechanism of injury. And if in fact the perpetrators impacted the head, then the confessions become useless not only for validating shaking as a mechanism, but for validating any particular findings or symptoms as independently diagnostic of abuse – because once the mechanism is impact, there is no way medically to differentiate between inflicted and accidental impacts.

Not only does this risk – that the guilty will mask more culpable conduct by claiming all they did was shake the child – seem likely as a matter of logic, especially since interrogator minimisation strategies encourage such responses, but the confession cases that researchers rely upon confirm that some suspects hide behind shaking to mask more egregious conduct. After noting that confessions in AHT cases are rare, Adamsbaum et al. acknowledged that among their 29 confession cases – all obtained after the suspects were subjected to police and judicial-process questioning – two of the children had skull fractures, yet the suspect made 'no admission of head impact, which suggests incomplete confessions' [18].

Similarly, Starling et al. acknowledged that 4 of their 32 cases involving confession to shaking with no impact had medical evidence of impact, 'indicating incomplete admissions to the mechanism of injury' [11]. Leestma, whose search of the literature from 1969 to 2001 found a total of 54 cases with confessions to shaking, reported that 43 showed signs of cranial impact [19]. In a response to the SBU report, Vinchon acknowledged the risk that suspect admissions might understate the nature of the abuse, conceding that the 'scientific value [of confessions data] should not be pushed too far however, regarding in particular the dating of trauma, since child abusers are generally unreliable record keepers, and many cases are confessed as a single episode whereas evidence suggests repeated insults' [49].

12.4.4 Confessions That Challenge the Shaken Baby Syndrome Hypothesis

At least one type of confession bears some greater indicia of reliability and has the potential for breaking free of circularity. Those confessions, however, suggest that shaking is not the culprit in these cases.

To date, just one paper has sought confessions that are not tainted by the interrogation or judicial process – confessions made prior to any pressure, prompting, or suggestion from interrogators. To avoid circularity, Thiblin et al. collected 36 cases from the Swedish National Patient Register in which shaking was established not by medical findings, but either by a witnessed or video-recorded account (33 cases) or by admission (3 cases) [50]. Admitted shaking was defined as 'a spontaneously delivered history of shaking before or in direct connection with seeking care before diagnostic procedures . . . were performed. In the case of admitting shaking before seeking care, e.g., to social services, the history of shaking had to be maintained when seeking care at the hospital'. In 30 of the 36 shaking cases, 'no medical findings or symptoms were reported' and the 6 who had some medical findings all also had predisposing medical conditions (as well as, in some cases, signs of impact such as skull fractures). Importantly, 'no infant subjected to shaking with or without blunt force trauma and without any possibly predisposing factors had any of the findings regarded as highly specific for AHT'. These data contrast starkly with the research that relies upon interrogation-marred confessions, suggesting that shaking is not a likely cause of these injuries.

12.5 Conclusion

If confessions are the evidence base for SBS, as proponents contend, then they must be evaluated to determine if they form a solid base or if they are themselves the product of circularity – that is, to determine if confessions might themselves be generated by investigators' belief that the suspect committed abuse based upon diagnostic findings like the triad. That analysis, however, has not been undertaken. To the contrary, the available evidence suggests strongly that SBS confessions are not independent of the diagnostic findings, but are products of the circularity that so undermines most research in this field. If, therefore, confessions cannot sustain the hypothesis, then untold numbers of innocent parents and other caregivers might be suffering wrongful convictions, lengthy terms in prison, and even death sentences. And surviving children are being inappropriately removed from their homes and their parents. Simply put, on the current state of knowledge, purported confessions cannot be relied upon as providing the scientific foundation for the hypothesis that is to date missing.

References

1. Findley KA, Barnes PD, Moran DA, Squier W. Shaken baby syndrome, abusive head trauma, and actual innocence: Getting it right. *Houston Journal of Health Law and Policy*. 2012;12:209–312.
2. Choudhary AK, Servaes S, Slovis TL et al. Consensus statement on abusive head trauma in infants and young children. *Pediatric Radiology*. 2018;48(8):1048–65.
3. Findley KA, Risinger DM, Barnes PD et al. Feigned consensus: Usurping the law in shaken baby syndrome/abusive head trauma prosecutions. *Wisconsin Law Review*.2019:1211–67.
4. Hymel KP et al. for the Pediatric Brain Injury Research Network. Derivation of a clinical prediction rule for pediatric abusive head trauma. *Pediatric Critical Care Medicine*. 2013;14:210–20.
5. Narang, SA. A Daubert analysis of abusive head trauma/shaken baby syndrome. *Houston Journal of Health Law and Policy*. 2011;11:505–633.
6. Vinchon M, de Foort-Dhellemmes S, Desurmont M, Delestret I. Confessed abuse versus witnessed accidents in infants: Comparison of clinical, radiological, and ophthalmological data in corroborated cases. *Child's Nervous System*. 2010;26: 637–45.
7. Maguire SA, Kemp AM, Lumb RC, Farewell DM. Estimating the probability of abusive head trauma: A pooled analysis. *Pediatrics*.2011;128:e550–e564.
8. Piteau SJ, Ward MGK, Barrowman MJ, Plint AC. Clinical and radiographic characteristics associated with abusive and nonabusive head trauma: A systematic review. *Pediatrics*. 2012;130:1–9.
9. Swedish Agency for Health Technology Assessment and Assessment of Social Services. Traumatic shaking: The role of the triad in medical investigations of suspected traumatic shaking. A systematic review. 2016. https://bit.ly/3DGrvaC.
10. Matschke J, Voss J, Obi N et al. Nonaccidental head injury is the most common cause of subdural bleeding in infants < year of age. *Pediatrics*. 2009;124:1587–94.
11. Starling SP, Patel S, Burke BL et al. Analysis of perpetrator admissions to inflicted traumatic brain injury in children. *Archives of Pediatric and Adolescent Medicine*. 2004;158:454–8.
12. Biron D, Shelton D. Perpetrator accounts in infant abusive head trauma brought about by a shaking event. *Child Abuse and Neglect*. 2005;29:1347–58.
13. Starling SP, Holden JR, Jenny C. Abusive head trauma: The relationship of perpetrators to their victims. *Pediatrics*. 1995;95:259–62.
14. Dias MS. The case for shaking. In *Child abuse and neglect: Diagnosis, treatment, and evidence*. C Jenny, ed. Elsevier Saunders, 2010, pp. 362–70.
15. Minns RA. Shaken baby syndrome: Theoretical and evidential controversies. *Journal of the Royal College of Physicians of Edinburgh*. 2005;35:5–15.

16. Vinchon M, Noulé N, Karnoub MA. The legal challenges to the diagnosis of shaken baby syndrome or how to counter 12 common fake news. *Child's Nervous System*. 2022;38(1):133–45. https://doi.org/10.1007/s00381-021-05357-8.

17. Edwards GA, Maguire SA, Gaither JR, Leventhal JM. What do confessions reveal about abusive head trauma? A systematic review. *Child Abuse Review*. 2020;29:253–68.

18. Adamsbaum C, Grabar S, Mejean N, Rey-Salmon C. Abusive head trauma: Judicial admissions highlight violent and repetitive shaking. *Pediatrics*. 2010;126:546–55.

19. Leestma JE. Case analysis of brain-injured admittedly shaken infants: 54 cases, 1969–2001. *American Journal of Forensic Medicine and Pathology*. 2005;26:1–14.

20. Leestma JE 'Shaken baby syndrome': Do confessions by alleged perpetrators validate the concept? *Journal of American Physicians and Surgeons*. 2006;11:14–16.

21. Bell E, Shouldice M, Levin A. Abusive head trauma: A perpetrator confesses. *Child Abuse and Neglect*. 2011;35:74–7.

22. Garrett BL. The substance of false confessions. *Stanford Law Review*. 2010;62:1051–1119.

23. Innocence Project. The causes of wrongful conviction. https://innocenceproject.org/causes-wrongful-conviction.

24. National Registry of Exonerations. www.law.umich.edu/special/exoneration/Pages/detaillist.aspx.

25. Leo RA. Inside the interrogation room. *Journal of Criminal Law and Criminology*. 1996;86:266–303.

26. Kassin SM, Kiechel KL. The social psychology of false confessions: Compliance, internalization, and confabulation. *Psychological Science*. 1996;7(3):125–8.

27. Ofshe RJ, Leo RA. The social psychology of police interrogation: The theory and classification of true and false confessions. *Studies in Law, Politics, and Society*. 1997;16:189–251.

28. Ofshe RJ, Leo RA. The decision to confess falsely: Rational choice and irrational action. *Denver University Law Review*. 1997;74:979–1122.

29. Davis D, Leo RA. The problem of interrogation-induced false confession: Sources of failure in prevention and detection. In *Handbook of forensic sociology and psychology*. SJ Morewitz, ML Goldstein, eds. Springer Science + Business Media, 2014, pp. 47–75.

30. Drizin SA, Leo RA. The problem of false confessions in the post-DNA world. *North Carolina Law Review*. 2004;82:891–1004.

31. Kassin SM. The social psychology of false confessions. *Social Issues and Policy Review*. 2015;9:25–51.

32. Kassin SM, Drizin SA, Grisso T et al. Police-induced confessions: Risk factors and recommendations. *Law and Human Behavior*. 2010;34(1):3–38.

33. Inbau FE, Reid JE, Buckley JP, Jayne BC. *Criminal interrogation and confessions*. 5th ed. Jones & Bartlett Learning, 2013.

34. Leo RA, Drizin SA. The three errors: Pathways to false confession and wrongful conviction. In *Police interrogations and false confessions: Current research, practice, and policy recommendations*. GD Lassiter, CA Meissner, eds. American Psychological Association, 2010, pp. 9–30.

35. *People v Thomas*, 8 N.E.3d 308 (N.Y. 2014).

36. Cabut S. Shaken babies: Doubts about the reliability of self-incriminations. *Le Monde*. 15 November 2021. https://bit.ly/3UvJZ4m.

37. Högberg U, Eriksson G, Högberg G, Wahlberg A. Parents' experiences of seeking health care and encountering allegations of shaken baby syndrome: A qualitative study. *PLoS One*. 2020;15(2):e0228911. https://doi.org/10.1371/journal.pone.0228911.

38. Vinchon M, Karnoub MA, Noulé N et al. Confessed versus denied inflicted head injuries in infants: similarities and differences. *Child's Nervous System*. 2021;38(1):147–52. https://doi.org/10.1007/s00381-021-05381-8.

39. Rossant C. Personal communication. 2021.
40. Kassin S. On the psychology of confessions: Does innocence put innocents at risk? *American Psychologist*. 2005;60:215–28.
41. Tuerkheimer D. *Flawed convictions: Shaken baby syndrome and the inertia of injustice*. Oxford University Press, 2014.
42. *Aleman v Village of Hanover Park*, 662 F. 3d 897 (7th Cir. 2011).
43. National Registry of Exonerations, Clarence Jones III. https://bit.ly/3UjlWWu.
44. *State v Paul*, Superior Court for Alaska, First Jud. Dist. at Juneau, Case No. 1JU-11-00823CR. Interviews of David Paul, 2010.
45. Medline Plus. CPR-Infant. https://bit.ly/3UoD11P.
46. Caffey J. On the theory and practice of shaking infants: Its potential residual effects of permanent brain damage and mental retardation. *American Journal of Diseases of Children*. 1972;124:161–9.
47. Imwinkelried EJ. Shaken baby syndrome: A genuine battle of the scientific (and non-scientific) expert. *Criminal Law Bulletin*. 2010;46:1–44.
48. Ibrahim N, Margulies S. Biomechanics of toddler head during low-height falls: An anthropomorphic dummy analysis. *Journal of Neurosurgery and Pediatrics*. 2010;6:57–68.
49. Vinchon M. Response to Lynøe: Questions about isolated trauma shaking and confessions. *Child's Nervous System*. 2017;33(9):1423–4.
50. Thiblin J, Andersson K, Wester, J et al. Medical findings and symptoms in infants exposed to witnessed or admitted abusive shaking: A nationwide registry study. *PLoS One*. 2020;15(10):e0240182. https://doi.org/10.1371/journal.pone.0240182.

Chapter 13

Cognitive Bias in Medico-legal Judgments

Jeff Kukucka and Keith Findley

13.1 What Is(n't) Cognitive Bias?

Psychologists have long known that people do not evaluate information in an objective way. Rather, our judgments are often unknowingly coloured by our pre-existing beliefs and/or contextual factors [1]. Accordingly, people with differing mind-sets often interpret the same information in markedly different ways. For example, studies have found that people perceived greater resemblance between unrelated individuals who they thought were close family compared to close family who they thought were unrelated [2], formed different impressions of the same individual after reading the same list of traits either forward or backward [3], and interpreted the same drawing as either a seal or horse depending on which interpretation produced a favourable outcome [4] – all of which represent examples of *cognitive bias*.

Cognitive bias refers to 'a set of influences that may affect the reliability [i.e., consistency] and validity [i.e., accuracy] of one's observations and conclusions' [5]. Simply put, extraneous factors can produce errors in our perceptions and judgments. Moreover, cognitive bias is an innate and subconscious phenomenon, and as such, it does not reflect incompetence, malfeasance, or deliberate prejudice [6–7]. Rather, cognitive bias affects all people, especially when the information in question is ambiguous [8].

13.2 Sources of Cognitive Bias

Kassin et al. [9] reviewed literature showing that cognitive bias can affect the collection and/or interpretation of evidence during criminal investigations and trials – including judgments of physical evidence made by forensic science experts. Likewise, it is now well known that medical experts also make mistakes, often at alarming rates [10, 11], sometimes due to cognitive bias [10, 12]. As research on cognitive bias in forensic contexts has proliferated, scholars have identified various sources of bias that can affect expert decision-making [13].

Of primary importance, irrelevant contextual information (i.e., knowledge of extraneous facts or theories, including peer opinion) can influence expert opinions. In one study, for example, fingerprint experts changed 17% of their own prior judgments of the same fingerprints after learning that the suspect confessed or provided an alibi [14]. Additionally, base rate expectations can affect decision-making; Growns and Kukucka found that individuals who primarily viewed matching fingerprints developed a response bias that rendered them more likely to misjudge non-matching prints as matches [15]. Finally, organisational factors – such as job-related stress or adversarial allegiance – can affect forensic expert decision-making [16, 17]. While some laboratories have taken proactive steps to mitigate cognitive bias [18–20], others insist that they are immune to bias. Kukucka et al. [21] found that 71% of forensic experts believed that cognitive bias is a cause for concern in forensic science generally, but only 52% felt it is a cause for concern in their own discipline, and only 26% felt that they are personally susceptible to bias.

In this chapter, we will explain how these sources of cognitive bias can likewise affect the judgment of medico-legal experts and thus increase the risk of potentially devastating errors. In so doing, we will also recount how these findings have been met with both positivity and hostility from the medical community, and we will describe best practices for mitigating cognitive bias in medico-legal decision-making.

13.3 Are Medical Judgments Vulnerable to Bias?

As noted already in this chapter, cognitive bias is especially apt to affect judgments of information that permits multiple plausible interpretations, which is often true of medical data. To illustrate, Oliver and Fang showed medical experts images of 'classic' skin injuries (i.e., images used for training purposes) and asked them to determine the class, kind, and object of each injury [22]. They found that consensus ranged from 68% to 77%, which the authors described as 'surprising[ly]' low, given that the images were specifically chosen for their apparent clarity and prototypicality. From these data, the authors ultimately concluded that '"classic" patterned injuries may not be so classic' after all.

In the legal system, where physicians are often asked to determine whether a given injury was unintentional (e.g., natural or accidental) or criminal, these subjective judgments can produce costly errors. In one study, for example, paediatric emergency doctors misjudged 60% of accidental childhood fractures as abuse and 15% of non-accidental fractures as accidents – which could prompt false allegations or re-victimisation, respectively [23]. More recently, Wester et al. [24] asked independent medical experts to review medical records from 17 shaken baby syndrome/abusive head trauma (SBS/AHT) cases – 16 of which resulted in criminal convictions. In all but one case, the independent experts concluded that the child's injuries 'possibly, or even probably, had a non-traumatic cause'. Thus, medical experts frequently form differing opinions of the same medical data – one of which must be erroneous – which in turn produce dramatically different legal outcomes (see also Chapter 6).

Importantly, determinations like SBS/AHT are especially susceptible to cognitive bias because they are highly subjective. Child abuse physicians have acknowledged that there are no accepted diagnostic criteria for SBS/AHT, let alone objective laboratory tests [25] (see also Chapter 10). Instead, they argue that the determination hinges on clinical judgment – that is, their assessment of the totality of the circumstances and their experience-based opinion about whether a child was abused [26]. However, child abuse physicians' experience-based opinions are critically limited by the fact that they work in an 'open-loop system' where they rarely receive feedback on their judgment and therefore cannot learn from experience [27].

In contrast to other medical domains where a patient's response to a treatment provides feedback on the validity of the diagnosis, there is no mechanism to inform these physicians whether a child's injuries were intentional or accidental and thus whether their SBS/AHT determination was accurate [28]. Hypothetically, a physician could have consistently 'diagnosed' SBS/AHT for decades and been wrong in every single instance, but they would have no way of knowing it because there are no ready checks on erroneous clinical judgments about SBS/AHT to reveal errors and prompt corrective countermeasures.

Given this subjectivity, it is unsurprising that medical doctors' diagnostic and treatment decisions are subject to cognitive bias [29, 30]. To their credit, some medical experts have long acknowledged this reality and proposed measures to address it, even while others remain obstinate [31, 32]. In what follows, we review evidence that the aforementioned sources of cognitive bias – base rates, stress, allegiance, and extraneous information – can and do influence the judgment of medico-legal experts.

13.4 Effects of Base Rates, Stress, and Allegiance

13.4.1 Base Rates

The *prevalence effect* is a phenomenon where people fail to detect rare stimuli in visual search and comparison tasks. For example, airport security officers more often failed to notice weapons in travellers' luggage when only 5% of bags contained weapons (compared to 50% [33]) and people were less adept at detecting fake IDs when only 10% of individuals presented fake IDs (compared to 50% [34]).

Meta-analytic evidence suggests that expertise does not protect against prevalence effects [35]. Accordingly, prevalence effects can impact the judgments of medical professionals. In one study, cytologists more often failed to detect cervical cancer when its incidence was low rather than high [36]. In two others, radiologists spent less time searching for – and more often failed to detect – lesions that they believed were rare, even if those lesions were medically important [37, 38]. Taken together, these findings suggest that medical experts' experience in past cases can undermine their judgment in the present case.

In SBS/AHT, the prevalence effect can influence a physician's choice of diagnostic tests as well as their ultimate opinion. Because medical doctrine has long held that retinal haemorrhages (RH) are prevalent and diagnostically significant in SBS/AHT, physicians tend to order fundoscopic examinations to look for RH when child abuse is suspected, but not when other aetiologies are suspected. The inevitable consequence is that RH are discovered more often in suspected SBS/AHT cases, which then reinforces the prevalence expectation, creating a sort of self-fulfilling prophecy. Likewise, because some alternative explanations for medical findings attributed to SBS/AHT are quite rare (e.g., short-fall deaths, coagulopathies, inherited disorders), the prevalence effect will predispose physicians to posit abuse and render them less likely to consider these alternatives, even if one of them is the true cause.

13.4.2 Stress

Psychologists have long known that stress hinders performance [39], including among medical doctors specifically [40], and that implicit (i.e., unconscious) racial biases are pervasive, including in healthcare [41]. Burgess [42] hypothesised that these factors may interact, such that heightened stress may further exacerbate physicians' pre-existing implicit biases against non-White patients. Sure enough, Johnson et al. [43] found that physicians showed a moderate pro-White bias overall – and this bias was stronger among physicians who had just finished working a particularly busy shift. Thus, it appears that workplace-related stressors can indeed intensify physicians' unconscious racial biases.

13.4.3 Allegiance

Gitlin et al. [44] found evidence that medical experts' judgments tend to favour the party that retained them in a legal dispute. First, they obtained 492 chest radiographs from lawsuits in which the plaintiff claimed to have respiratory damage from asbestos exposure. In 95.9% of these cases, a medical expert hired by the plaintiff found abnormalities in their radiograph. However, the authors then gave these same radiographs to independent experts and found that only 4.5% found abnormalities, suggesting that the original experts were inclined to give an opinion that benefitted the plaintiff.

Such allegiance effects appear especially powerful among child abuse physicians, who, unlike physicians in other diagnostic contexts, tend to overtly eschew neutrality and endorse what can be described as an 'advocacy bias', as illustrated by common assertions in the SBS/AHT literature (see also Chapter 19):

- 'Bias should be in favor of the child's safety' [45].
- 'The medical expert, although theoretically a neutral in the courtroom, must be the advocate for the child' [46].
- 'In other children, sufficient suspicions are raised that protection of the child is prioritized, even if the determination cannot be made definitively' [47].
- '[W]hen we prioritize saving lives over, say, the risks of overdiagnosis, we are adhering to our strongly held values – not empirical truth' [48].

A diagnostic process that values protection of the child over truth (and that ignores the fact that removing children from non-abusive homes is itself damaging to them) inevitably – and indeed by design – biases determinations in favour of abuse findings.

13.5 Effects of Non-medical Information

The aforementioned sources of cognitive bias are presumably difficult to eliminate insofar as they are endemic to medical experts' work. In contrast, a priori knowledge of biasing non-medical information is arguably a more pernicious – but also more avoidable – source of bias. All too often, medical experts consider information that should have no bearing on their opinion, which then guides how they prioritise and evaluate other information and thereby undermines the independent value of their opinion [9, 49]. Moreover, in the forensic sciences, extraneous information has been shown to influence decision-making regardless of whether it does (e.g., inculpatory DNA [50]) or does not (e.g., gruesome photographs [51]) imply a particular outcome. In what follows, we review studies in which a priori knowledge of extraneous non-medical information likewise improperly influenced medical experts' opinions.

13.5.1 Non-experimental Studies

Early research in this area was mostly archival in nature, analysing historical records for trends that suggest bias in the evaluation and/or reporting of child abuse. For example, studies found that illnesses were more often misdiagnosed as abuse among Black children [52], that non-White and children of low socioeconomic status (SES) were more often referred to child protective services for suspicion of abuse [53–56], and that abuse more often went unrecognised among White children, many of whom went on to be re-victimised [57]. Taken together, these findings imply that child abuse may be over-suspected among Black or low-SES children – and/or under-suspected among White or affluent children – due to physicians' stereotypic beliefs about who commits abuse. However, given the non-experimental nature of these studies, we must be cautious in interpreting these data; these findings may not reflect cognitive bias but rather an actual difference in rates of abuse between demographic groups.

13.5.2 Experimental Studies

With that in mind, we now review experimental data showing that extraneous non-medical information can unduly influence medical judgments. In perhaps the earliest such experiment, Laskey et al. [58] found that physicians were more likely to believe that a paediatric femoral fracture was due to abuse if the child's family was thought to be of low (rather than high) SES, even though the injury itself was identical. Similarly, Anderst et al. [23] found that medical experts more often misjudged the same accidental femoral fracture as indicative of abuse if led to believe that the child came from a 'high-risk' home (i.e., unmarried parents and a history of intimate partner violence, depression, drug use, and financial strain) rather than a 'low-risk' home (i.e., married parents and financial stability). Finally, Loos et al. [59] found that medical professionals – all of whom viewed the same radiographs – were more likely to believe that a childhood fracture was the result of abuse if also told that the child's parents were immigrants, unmarried, or on welfare. In each case, the data provided clear evidence that medical experts' opinions of the same medical data were inappropriately influenced by non-medical information.

More recent studies have attempted to illuminate the psychological mechanism(s) that underlie this phenomenon. For instance, Najdowski et al. [60] found that emergency medical professionals who read a clinical vignette about an unresponsive infant remembered more abuse-relevant details – both true and false – if led to believe that the family was Black and had prior involvement with child protective services. This finding suggests that doctors may be more likely to notice, remember, and/or confabulate information that corroborates their pre-existing stereotypes about abusers.

However, Fawver et al. [61] found that cognitive bias did not affect what information experts noticed, but it did affect how they used that information. In their study, radiologists read case notes that were either accurate or misleading and then analysed a radiograph while their eye movements were recorded. Among those who read misleading case notes, diagnostic accuracy decreased by 40% – despite the fact that most radiologists did look at the area of the image that should have revealed the correct diagnosis. In other words, it appears that the radiologists who read misleading case notes did notice the relevant diagnostic information but failed to interpret it correctly.

13.5.3 Implications

Notably, Fawver et al. concluded that medical experts should only receive case information that is known to be accurate and complete. Alternatively, some have argued that unfettered access to case information benefits medical diagnosis. For instance, Oliver found that pathologists showed greater consensus in their judgments of skin injuries when they also received contextual information (e.g., toxicology results, eyewitness accounts) [62]. Oliver later cited this finding as evidence that 'access to history and context ... significantly decreased error' ([63], p. 161). However, this conclusion is unjustifiable, as Oliver himself explained that 'it was not possible to independently determine the ground truth' of the injuries in the study. In other words, experts who receive the same contextual information may well show greater consensus, but consensus is not synonymous with accuracy [62].

Oliver also asserted that 'forensic pathologists do not consider this particular kind of cognitive bias as serious a problem' as psychologists do [64]. Fortunately, not all medical professionals share this sentiment. In two large Medscape surveys, 40–50% of physicians – largely irrespective of gender, age, and race – reported that they held 'biases toward specific types or groups of patients' [65, 66]. However, there were sizeable disparities between specialties, with emergency room doctors being most likely (62%) and pathologists least likely (10%) to acknowledge their own biases. In the next section, we describe a recent publication that provided the first evidence of cognitive bias in expert manner-of-death opinions, which has prompted enthusiasm from some forensic pathologists and hostility from others.

13.6 Bias in Manner-of-Death Decisions: Data and Backlash

Dror et al. [67] theorised that cognitive bias would affect post-mortem judgments just as it affects medical judgments of living individuals. Depending on the case or jurisdiction, manner-of-death decisions are made by forensic pathologists, medical examiners, physicians, or coroners, who classify deaths in five categories: natural, suicide, accident, homicide, or undetermined. These judgments often carry significant legal implications insofar as they imply that a crime did or did not occur.

In their first study, Dror et al. obtained every death certificate for children who died before age 6 in the state of Nevada from 2009 to 2018, and they focused on Black and White children whose deaths were ruled unnatural (i.e., accidents or homicides). As predicted, unnatural childhood deaths were ruled as homicides more often if the child was Black (36%) rather than White (24%). Again, however, the archival nature of this study precludes causal inferences; it may be true that Black children truly are killed more often than White children.

To address this limitation, Dror et al. then conducted an experiment in which the participants were members of the National Association of Medical Examiners (NAME). Each participant read one of two versions of a vignette in which a child was found unresponsive in her home, was brought to the hospital with head injuries, and died. The two versions differed with respect to the child's race and caretaker. In one, the child was White and was found unresponsive by her maternal grandmother, and in the other, the child was Black and was found by her mother's boyfriend. Participants therefore received the same medical information about the child's injuries but different non-medical information, and they were asked to opine as to the child's manner of death. Although most participants (59%) ruled the death 'undetermined', clear evidence of bias emerged among the remaining participants. When told that the child was Black and found by her mother's boyfriend, participants were about five times more likely to rule the death a homicide (35%) than an accident (6%), but when told that the child was White and found by her grandmother, participants were only half as likely to rule the death a homicide (13%) than an accident (28%). While it is unclear whether the child's race and/or caretaker was responsible for the bias, it is abundantly clear that these experts' manner-of-death opinions were biased by irrelevant non-medical information.

13.6.1 Aftermath

Following its publication, NAME leadership launched fierce attacks against this paper, including demands for retraction and allegations of data fraud and ethics violations – all of which were thoroughly investigated and dismissed. Instead, the journal invited letters to the editor from interested parties – some of which praised the paper for drawing attention to an important and understudied issue while others were vitriolic and rooted in misconceptions about cognitive bias [68–70].

Gill et al. [71] argued that the data were invalid because it was unknown whether all participants were 'board-certified forensic pathologists' (see also [72]). While this is true, the studies were intended to represent all individuals with the authority to make real-world manner-of-death decisions, which includes not only pathologists but also medical examiners and coroners. More importantly, their argument implies that expertise grants immunity from bias, which is not only untrue [73, 74] but also exemplifies the phenomenon of the *bias blind spot* – that is, the tendency to recognise bias in others but not in oneself [75].

Peterson et al. [76] argued that the child's relationship to their caretaker is relevant given that children are historically more often killed by biologically unrelated men than by grandmothers. This claim is dangerous for three reasons. First, the application of population data to individual cases is an *ecological fallacy*. Even if true, the fact that unrelated men kill more children in general does not prove that this man killed this child. Second, extraneous information can lead experts to the correct decision, but for the wrong reasons [77]. For example, Stevenage and Bennett [50] found that non-experts were more accurate at identifying non-matching fingerprints if they knew in advance that DNA excluded the suspect – but that accuracy is incidental and does not reflect expertise.

Third, and relatedly, this practice is problematic from a Bayesian standpoint in that it leads fact-finders (e.g., jurors) to unwittingly double-count information. That is to say, jurors may consider the race of the child and/or their relationship of the caregiver in assessing the prior odds of guilt. Then the jury will hear the expert's opinion that the death was a homicide and use it to adjust their assessment of guilt – but they will treat these as independent pieces of evidence, not realising that the expert also considered race and relationship information in opining that the death was a homicide. Consequently, race and relationship information will be factored twice into jurors' assessments of the posterior odds of guilt – once of their own accord and then again as a part of the medical expert's opinion. For these reasons, manner-of-death opinions must be made independently of any other information that the jury will also independently consider. This is why, in general, expert opinions are most probative when they are based solely on information that the expert is uniquely qualified to evaluate. Indeed, that is in part why most legal rules of evidence limit the admissibility of expert opinions to those matters the experts are uniquely qualified to assess [88].

Lastly, several commentaries were surprisingly candid about the limitations of manner-of-death determinations, calling it 'not a scientific determination' [78] and noting that 'there is no "right" answer [or] criteria for correctness' [76] such that 'any individual determination is questionable' [78]. Instead, they claimed that manner-of-death decisions are 'misused . . . by the courts' – but the reality is that their decisions do carry considerable weight in criminal investigations and trials, and they do not typically communicate these limitations when testifying in court [76]. Consequently, erroneous manner-of-death opinions have contributed to miscarriages of justice, thus highlighting the need for practical reforms to minimise the risk of bias and error in death investigations, as we explain in what follows.

13.7 Best Practices for Mitigating Bias

Although experts may feel that they can avoid cognitive bias by simply making a conscious effort to set aside their beliefs [21], awareness and willpower are not enough to eradicate bias

[79]. Similarly, while implicit bias training may increase medical professionals' awareness of their own biases [80, 81], it is unclear whether such training produces lasting behavioural change [82, 83]. While awareness is an important first step, additional steps will be needed to combat bias and error in medico-legal decision-making [31]. In light of the aforementioned research, the ostensibly obvious solution would be to deny or limit experts' access to irrelevant and potentially biasing information. However, we must also balance the ideal with the practical; for instance, it is presumably impossible for a pathologist to conduct an autopsy on an individual and judge their manner of death without knowing their race.

Instead, we urge medical experts to thoughtfully consider what information is relevant to their decision-making and when they should consider non-medical information. For instance, Simon [84] described four types of information that death investigators typically consider:

(1) Medical history (e.g., medical records, statements from physicians or family).
(2) Findings from the death scene (e.g., the position of the body, the presence of weapons).
(3) Social history (e.g., risk-taking behaviour and economic status as reported by family and friends).
(4) Investigative facts (e.g., eyewitness statements, criminal history, investigators' theories).

The former two categories are typically relevant and beneficial to medical decision-making [85], but the aforementioned studies found that information from the latter two categories can prompt bias and error [58, 59, 67], such that one might wonder if medical experts should ever consider it – especially since such information is also typically presented as independent evidence in court and thus runs the risk of being double-counted.

Rather than flatly denying experts access to potentially helpful information, Dror and Kukucka [86] proposed a balanced approach to strengthening expert decision-making called *Linear Sequential Unmasking – Expanded* (LSU-E), which is grounded in psychological research showing that the order in which decision makers encounter information is critical, such that information encountered earlier tends to have more impact. Thus, rather than considering information in a random or incidental order, LSU-E asks experts to be strategic about how they sequence information. First, experts should form (and document) their initial opinion based solely on the raw data/evidence. Then, experts may consider other relevant information, and in so doing, they should prioritise information that is more relevant, more objective, and/or lower in biasing power.

For example, a medical examiner should first form an initial opinion as to a person's manner-of-death based solely on the anatomical data and nothing else; only then may they consider other information such as video recordings (*higher* objectivity) or eyewitness accounts (*lower* objectivity) of the death. Along the way, experts must also carefully document and justify any changes to their opinion, thereby creating transparency in how their opinion came about.

Some forensic science laboratories have proactively implemented variants of LSU-E and reported that it has been beneficial and not 'complex, overly time-consuming, or expensive' [18–20]. Quigley-McBride et al. [87] recently published a practical and research-based LSU-E toolkit in the hopes of encouraging more forensic examiners and labs to implement the procedure; the toolkit includes a worksheet that examiners can use to document and justify their decisions about what information to consider and in what order, as well as document any steps they took to combat its potential biasing effects, thereby increasing transparency about their decision-making processes. In the medico-legal arena, however, many experts continue to insist that unrestricted access to non-medical information is essential and that they are impervious to cognitive bias, despite undeniable evidence to the contrary.

13.8 Conclusion

Simply put, even the most qualified, experienced, and honest professionals are still human. As such, they are subject to the same cognitive biases as everyone, and those biases sometimes spawn errors. For medico-legal experts, a mistake can carry devastating consequences such as wrongfully imprisoning an innocent person or allowing a perpetrator to reoffend. For these reasons, we believe that maximising the validity of medico-legal decision-making is of paramount importance to society as a whole.

Empirical research leaves no doubt that knowledge of irrelevant non-medical information can undermine the independence and validity of medical experts' judgments. Accordingly, we urge medical professionals to take precautions to minimise the risk of bias and error, such as relying solely on medically relevant information in their decision-making and carefully optimising the sequence of that information. Moreover, we urge medical professionals to involve psychologists and other experts in these efforts. By pooling our complementary expertise, we can develop protocols that balance idealism and practicality and further our common goal of maximising the reliability and validity of medico-legal judgments.

References

1. Kahneman D, Sibony O, Sunstein CR. *Noise: A flaw in human judgment*. Little Brown Spark, 2021.
2. Bressan P, Dal Martello MF. 'Talis pater, talis filius': Perceived resemblance and the belief in genetic relatedness. *Psychological Science*. 2002;13:213–18.
3. Asch SE. Forming impressions of personality. *Journal of Abnormal and Social Psychology*. 1946;41:258–90.
4. Balcetis E, Dunning D. See what you want to see: Motivational influences on visual perception. *Journal of Personality and Social Psychology*. 2006;91:612–25.
5. Organization of Scientific Area Committees for Forensic Science (OSAC). (2020, 1 April). OSAC preferred terms. www.nist.gov/document/osac-preferred-terms-april-2020.
6. Klayman J, Ha Y-W. Confirmation, disconfirmation, and information in hypothesis testing. *Psychological Bulletin*. 1997;94:211–28.
7. Nisbett RE, Wilson TD. Telling more than we can know: Verbal reports on mental processes. *Psychological Review*. 1977;84 (3):231–59.
8. Kunda Z. The case for motivated reasoning. *Psychological Bulletin*. 1990;108:480–98.
9. Kassin SM, Dror IE, Kukucka J. The forensic confirmation bias: Problems, perspectives, and proposed solutions. *Journal of Applied Research in Memory and Cognition*. 2013;2:42–52.
10. Berner ES, Graber ML. Overconfidence as a cause of diagnostic error in medicine. *American Journal of Medicine*. 2008;121(5): S2–S23.
11. Graber ML, Wachter RM, Cassel CK. Bringing diagnosis into the quality and safety equations. *JAMA*. 2012;308 (12):1211–12.
12. Groopman J. *How doctors think*. Houghton Mifflin Harcourt, 2007.
13. Kukucka J, Dror IE (2023). Human factors in forensic science: Psychological causes of bias and error. In *The Oxford handbook of psychology and law*. D DeMatteo, KC Scherr, eds. Oxford University Press.

14. Dror IE, Charlton D. Why experts make errors. *Journal of Forensic Identification.* 2006;56:600–16.

15. Growns B, Kukucka J. The prevalence effect in fingerprint identification: Match and non-match base rates impact misses and false alarms. *Applied Cognitive Psychology.* 2021;35:751–60.

16. Almazrouei MA, Morgan RM, Dror IE. Stress and support in the workplace: The perspective of forensic examiners. *Forensic Science International: Mind and Law.* 2021;100059.

17. Murrie DC, Boccaccini MT, Guarnera LA, Rufino KA. Are forensic experts biased by the side that retained them? *Psychological Science.* 2013;24:1889–97.

18. Archer MS, Wallman JF. Context effects in forensic entomology and use of sequential unmasking in casework. *Journal of Forensic Sciences.* 2016;61:1270–7.

19. Found B, Ganas J. The management of domain irrelevant context information in forensic handwriting examination casework. *Science and Justice.* 2013;53:154–8.

20. Mattijssen EJAT, Kerkhoff W, Berger CEH, Dror IE, Stoel RD. Implementing context information management in forensic casework: Minimizing contextual bias in firearms examination. *Science and Justice.* 2016;56:113–22.

21. Kukucka J, Kassin SM, Zapf PA, Dror IE. Cognitive bias and blindness: A global survey of forensic science examiners. *Journal of Applied Research in Memory and Cognition.* 2017;6:452–9.

22. Oliver WR, Fang X. Forensic pathologist consensus in the interpretation of photographs of patterned injuries of the skin. *Journal of Forensic Sciences.* 2016;61:972–8.

23. Anderst J, Nielsen-Parker M, Moffatt M, Frazier T, Kennedy C. Using simulation to identify sources of medical diagnostic error in child physical abuse. *Child Abuse and Neglect.* 2016;52:62–9.

24. Wester K, Stridbeck U, Syse A, Wikström J. Re-evaluation of medical findings in alleged shaken baby syndrome and abusive head trauma in Norwegian courts fails to support abuse diagnoses. *Acta Paediatrica.* 2022;111(4):779–92. https://doi.org/10.1111/apa.15956.

25. Hymel KP, Willson DF, Boos SC et al. Derivation of a clinical prediction rule for pediatric abusive head trauma. *Pediatric Critical Care Medicine.* 2013;14(2):210–20.

26. Narang S. A Daubert analysis of abusive head trauma/shaken baby syndrome. *Houston Journal of Health, Law, and Policy.* 2011;11:505–633.

27. Schiff GD. Minimizing diagnostic error: The importance of follow-up and feedback. *American Journal of Medicine.* 2008;121(5):S38–S42.

28. Findley KA, Risinger DM, Barnes PD et al. Feigned consensus: Usurping the law in shaken baby syndrome/abusive head trauma prosecutions. *Wisconsin Law Review.* 2019;5:1211–68.

29. Bornstein BH, Emler AC. Rationality in medical decision-making: A review of the literature on doctors' decision-making biases. *Journal of Evaluation in Clinical Practice.* 2001;7(2):97–107.

30. Saposnik G, Redelmeier D, Ruff CC, Tobler PN. Cognitive biases associated with medical decisions: A systematic review. *BMC Medical Informatics and Decision-Making.* 2016;16(1):1–14.

31. Croskerry P. The importance of cognitive errors in diagnosis and strategies to minimize them. *Academic Medicine.* 2016;78(8):775–80.

32. Doherty TS, Carroll AE. Believing in overcoming cognitive biases. *American Medical Association Journal of Ethics.* 2020;22(9):773–8.

33. Wolfe JM, Brunelli DN, Rubinstein, J, Horowitz TS. Prevalence effects in newly trained airport checkpoint screeners: Trained observers miss rare targets, too. *Journal of Vision.* 2013;13:1–9.

34. Papesh MH, Goldinger SD. Infrequent identity mismatches are frequently undetected. *Attention, Perception, and Psychophysics.* 2014;76:1335–49.

35. Horowitz TS. Prevalence in visual search: From the clinic to the lab and back again. *Japanese Psychological Research*. 2017;59 (2):65–108.

36. Evans KK, Tambouret RH, Evered A, Wilbur DC, Wolfe JM. Prevalence of abnormalities influences cytologists' error rates in screening for cervical cancer. *Archives of Pathology and Laboratory Medicine*. 2011;135(12):1557–60.

37. Reed WM, Ryan JT, McEntee MF, Evanoff MG, Brennan PC. The effect of abnormality-prevalence expectation on expert observer performance and visual search. *Radiology*. 2011;258(3):938–43.

38. Nakashima R, Watanabe C, Maeda E et al. The effect of expert knowledge on medical search: Medical experts have specialized abilities for detecting serious lesions. *Psychological Research*. 2015;79(5):729–38.

39. Lazarus RS, Deese J, Osler SF. The effects of psychological stress upon performance. *Psychological Bulletin*. 1952;49 (4):293–317.

40. Motowidlo SJ, Packard JS, Manning MR. Occupational stress: Its causes and consequences for job performance. *Journal of Applied Psychology*. 1986;71(4):618–29.

41. Dovidio JF, Penner LA, Albrecht TL et al. Disparities and distrust: The implications of psychological processes for understanding racial disparities in health and health care. *Social Science and Medicine*. 2008;67(3):478–86.

42. Burgess DJ. Are providers more likely to contribute to healthcare disparities under high levels of cognitive load? How features of the healthcare setting may lead to biases in medical decision-making. *Medical Decision-Making*. 2010;30(2):246–57.

43. Johnson TJ, Hickey RW, Switzer GE et al. The impact of cognitive stressors in the emergency department on physician implicit racial bias. *Academic Emergency Medicine*. 2016;23(3):297–305.

44. Gitlin JN, Cook LL, Linton OW, Garrett-Mayer, E. Comparison of 'B' readers' interpretations of chest radiographs for asbestos related changes. *Academic Radiology*. 2004;11:843–56.

45. Kempe CH, Silverman FN, Steele BF, Droegemueller W, Silver HK. The battered-child syndrome. *JAMA*. 1962;181 (1):17–24.

46. Leake HC, III, Holbrook RF. Medical testimony. In *Child abuse and neglect: A medical reference*. NS Ellerstein, ed. Wiley, 1981, pp. 327–43.

47. Duhaime AC, Christian CW. Abusive head trauma: Evidence, obfuscation, and informed management. *Journal of Neurosurgery: Pediatrics*. 2019;24(5):481–8.

48. Brown SD. Ethical challenges in child abuse: What is the harm of a misdiagnosis? *Pediatric Radiology*. 2021;51(6):1070–5.

49. Risinger DM, Saks MJ, Thompson WC, Rosenthal R. The Daubert/Kumho implications of observer effects in forensic science: Hidden problems of expectation and suggestion. *California Law Review*. 2002;90:1–56.

50. Stevenage SV, Bennett A. A biased opinion: Demonstration of cognitive bias on a fingerprint matching task through knowledge of DNA test results. *Forensic Science International*. 2017;276:93–106.

51. Dror IE, Peron AE, Hind S-L, Charlton D. When emotions get the better of us: The effect of contextual top-down processing on matching fingerprints. *Applied Cognitive Psychology*. 2005;19:799–809.

52. Kirschner RH, Stein RJ. The mistaken diagnosis of child abuse: A form of medical abuse? *American Journal of Diseases of Children*. 1985;139(9):873–5.

53. Hampton RL, Newberger EH. Child abuse incidence and reporting by hospitals: Significance of severity, class, and race. *American Journal of Public Health*. 1985;75 (1):56–60.

54. Lane WG, Rubin DM, Monteith R, Christian CW. Racial differences in the evaluation of pediatric fractures for physical abuse. *JAMA*. 2002;288 (13):1603–9.

55. Flaherty EG, Sege RD, Griffith J et al. From suspicion of physical child abuse to reporting: Primary care clinician

decision-making. *Pediatrics*. 2008;122 (3):611–19.

56. Hymel KP, Laskey AL, Crowell KR et al. Racial and ethnic disparities and bias in the evaluation and reporting of abusive head trauma. *Journal of Pediatrics*. 2018;198:137–43.

57. Jenny C, Hymel KP, Ritzen A, Reinert, SE, Hay TC. Analysis of missed cases of abusive head trauma. *JAMA*. 1999;281 (7):621–6.

58. Laskey AL, Stump TE, Perkins SM et al. Influence of race and socioeconomic status on the diagnosis of child abuse: A randomized study. *Journal of Pediatrics*. 2012;160(6):1003–8.

59. Loos MLH, Allema WM, Bakx R et al. Paediatric femur fractures: The value of contextual information on judgement in possible child abuse cases. Are we biased? *European Journal of Pediatrics*. 2021;180 (1):81–90.

60. Najdowski CJ, Bernstein KM, Wahrer, KS. Do racial stereotypes contribute to medical misdiagnosis of child abuse? Investigating tunnel vision in the emergency room. *Wrongful Convictions Law Review*. 2020;1 (2):153–80.

61. Fawver B, Thomas JL, Drew T et al. Seeing isn't necessarily believing: Misleading contextual information influences perceptual-cognitive bias in radiologists. *Journal of Experimental Psychology: Applied*. 2020;26:579–92.

62. Oliver WR. Effect of history and context on forensic pathologist interpretation of photographs of patterned injury of the skin. *Journal of Forensic Sciences*. 2017;62:1500–5.

63. Oliver WR. Comment on Kukucka et al. 'Cognitive bias and blindness: A global survey of forensic science examiners'. *Journal of Applied Research in Memory and Cognition*. 2018;7:161.

64. Oliver WR. Comment on Dror et al. 'When expert decision-making goes wrong'. *Journal of Applied Research in Memory and Cognition*. 2018;7:314–15.

65. Medscape. (2016, 23 January). Medscape lifestyle report 2016: Bias and burnout. www.medscape.com/slideshow/lifestyle-2016-overview-6007335.

66. Medscape. (2017, 11 January). Lifestyle report 2017: Race and ethnicity, bias and burnout. www.medscape.com/features/slideshow/lifestyle/2017/overview.

67. Dror IE, Melinek J, Arden JL et al. Cognitive bias in forensic pathology decisions. *Journal of Forensic Sciences*. 2021;66:1751–7.

68. Duflou J. Commentary on Dror et al. 'Cognitive bias in forensic pathology decisions'. *Journal of Forensic Sciences*. 2021. https://doi.org/10.1111/1556-4029.14836.

69. Graber ML. Commentary on Dror et al. 'Cognitive bias in forensic pathology decisions'. *Journal of Forensic Sciences*. 2021. https://doi.org/10.1111/1556-4029.14857.

70. Obenson K. Commentary on Dror et al. 'Cognitive bias in forensic pathology decisions'. *Journal of Forensic Sciences*. 2021. https://doi.org/10.1111/1556-4029.14855.

71. Gill JR, Pinneri K, Denton JS, Aiken SS. Commentary on Dror et al. 'Cognitive bias in forensic pathology decisions.' *Journal of Forensic Sciences*. 2021. https://doi.org/10.1111/1556-4029.14838.

72. Speth P, Avedschmidt S, Baeza JJ et al. Commentary on Dror et al. 'Cognitive bias in forensic pathology decisions'. *Journal of Forensic Sciences*. 2021. https://doi.org/10.1111/1556-4029.14835.

73. Dror IE. The paradox of human expertise: Why experts get it wrong. In *The paradoxical brain*. N. Kapur, ed. Cambridge University Press, 2011, pp. 177–88.

74. Van den Eeden CAJ, de Poot CJ, Van Koppen PJ. The forensic confirmation bias: A comparison between experts and novices. *Journal of Forensic Sciences*. 2019;64:120–6.

75. Pronin E, Lin DY, Ross L. The bias blind spot: Perceptions of bias in self versus

others. *Personality and Social Psychology Bulletin*. 2002;28:369–81.

76. Peterson BL, Arnall M, Avedschmidt S et al. Commentary on Dror et al. 'Cognitive bias in forensic pathology decisions'. *Journal of Forensic Sciences*. 2021. https://doi.org/10.1111/1556-4029.14843.

77. Kukucka J. People who live in ivory towers shouldn't throw stones: A refutation of Curley et al. *Forensic Science International: Synergy*. 2020;2:110–13.

78. Oliver WR. Commentary on Dror et al. 'Cognitive bias in forensic pathology decisions'. *Journal of Forensic Sciences*. 2021. https://doi.org/10.1111/1556-4029.14841.

79. Wilson TD, Brekke N. Mental contamination and mental correction: Unwanted influences on judgments and evaluations. *Psychological Bulletin*. 1994;116:117–42.

80. Sherman M, Ricco J, Nelson S, Nezhad S, Prasad S. Implicit bias training in a residency program: Aiming for enduring effects. *Family Medicine*. 2019;51(8):677–81.

81. Zeidan AJ, Khatri UG, Aysola, J et al. Implicit bias education and emergency medicine training: Step one? Awareness. *AEM Education and Training*. 2019;3(1):81–5.

82. Fitzgerald C, Martin A, Berner D, Hurst S. Interventions designed to reduce implicit prejudices and implicit stereotypes in real world contexts: A systematic review. *BMC Psychology*. 2019;7(1):1–12.

83. Forscher PS, Lai CK, Axt JR et al. A meta-analysis of procedures to change implicit measures. *Journal of Personality and Social Psychology*. 2019;117(3):522–59.

84. Simon D. Minimizing error and bias in death investigations. *Seton Hall Law Review*. 2018;49:255–305.

85. McRobert AP, Causer J, Vassiliadis J et al. Contextual information influences diagnosis accuracy and decision-making in simulated emergency medicine emergencies. *BMJ Quality and Safety*. 2013;22(6):478–84.

86. Dror IE, Kukucka J. Linear sequential unmasking–expanded (LSU-E): A general approach for improving decision-making as well as minimizing bias. *Forensic Science International: Synergy*. 2021;3:100161.

87. Quigley-McBride A, Dror IE, Roy T, Garrett BL, Kukucka J. A practical tool for information management in forensic decisions: Using linear sequential unmasking-expanded (LSU-E) in casework. *Forensic Science International: Synergy*. 2022;4:100216.

88. Findley KA, Strang DA. Ending manner of death testimony and other opinion evidence of crime. *Duquesne Law Review*. 2022;60:302–39.

Chapter 14 Biomechanical Forensic Analysis of Shaking and Short-Fall Head Injury Mechanisms in Infants and Young Children

Kirk Thibault

14.1 Introduction

Biomechanical forensic analysis (BFA) of paediatric head injury is inherently different from its clinical counterpart. The biomechanical engineer utilises traditional engineering methodologies (e.g., the laws of physics, experimental material and mechanical property data of the tissues that constitute the head, and knowledge of how these tissues fail mechanically) to evaluate the mechanical link between a particular loading scenario and the resulting trauma. A biomechanical analysis of an injury-producing event is necessarily evidence-based and relies not only on accurate and well-characterised quantitative analysis, but also on explicitly stated assumptions and limitations governing the analysis. Such an analysis should be reproducible by any qualified biomechanical engineer due to its objective, well-defined analytical and data-driven methodology.

This approach contrasts that which is often encountered in clinical forensic evaluation, where qualitative and subjective interpretation of clinical findings can often lead to diverse and vastly different conclusions amongst clinical experts. Such diversity of opinion can lead to contentious and confusing expert testimony in legal proceedings related to allegations of child abuse, often to the detriment of the court and the accused. This confusion may be clarified by an objective, quantitative biomechanical analysis of the documented fact pattern in the case.

This chapter will introduce the concepts of biomechanical analysis as they pertain to forensic investigation of paediatric head injury in the clinical setting of alleged abusive trauma. A brief discussion of the concepts of biomechanics and the engineering approach to forensic analysis will be presented to orient the reader who may not be familiar with engineering terminology and forensic engineering analysis.

The age-dependent biomechanical properties of the rapidly developing infant head and its constitutive tissues will be presented to give the reader a better understanding of the unique aspects of analysing head injury in the young paediatric population. The workflow used to perform a BFA will be explained, with emphasis on the necessary investigative evidence, experimental data, assumptions, and limitations governing such analysis.

Finally, the reader will be presented with an example case study demonstrating the application of these concepts. Specific attention will be focused on a case of a 'short fall' versus alleged 'shaking', two common scenarios encountered in cases of alleged abusive head trauma (AHT). This chapter is not intended to be an exhaustive review of the published experimental data related to the biomechanics of paediatric head injury – equipped with the basic information presented in this chapter, the reader is encouraged to expand their knowledge of the rapidly evolving field of paediatric head injury biomechanics by consulting the references cited throughout.

14.2 Human Injury Biomechanics and Biomechanical Forensic Analysis

Bioengineering is the application of traditional engineering concepts and methodologies to the study of biological systems such as the human body. Biomechanics is a discipline within the field of bioengineering that emphasises the application of mechanical engineering, structural mechanics, and the biological and natural sciences to living structures and systems. Human injury biomechanics is the study of failure of the human body (whole body, anatomical region, organ, tissue, and cell) – this failure may be structural (e.g., a broken bone or lacerated skin) or functional (e.g., temporary dysfunction of the brain due to concussion). Such failure is commonly known as 'injury' or 'trauma' in the clinical setting.

Biomechanical forensic analysis is based upon examining three essential aspects of an injury-producing event:

(1) The loading environment to which the injured subject was potentially exposed: what were the kinematics (movement) and kinetics (forces) acting on the subject as a result of the specific event?
(2) The mechanism of injury to the person's specific anatomical region, organ, tissue, or cell: how, from a mechanical and physiological point of view, does failure of those constitutive biological elements occur?
(3) The injury tolerance values, or injury tolerance criteria, associated with the various observed failure: what magnitude/direction/rate of critical physical parameters (e.g., force, acceleration, stress, strain, impact energy) is required to cause each observed failure?

Biomechanical forensic analysis attempts to answer the question: 'Did the loading environment present during the event provide the injury mechanism required to exceed the injury tolerance for the specific, observed failure?' In simpler terms, 'Were the forces applied to the subject during the event sufficient to produce the observed injuries?'

Biomechanical forensic analysis starts with a hypothesis related to the cause of the observed injuries and then attempts to verify or falsify (test) the hypothesis through analysis of the physical evidence collected during the investigation. It is essential to understand that the hypothesis must be based on the history of the initiating traumatic event, most often provided by an eyewitness or other documented evidence (video). Biomechanical forensic analysis cannot be conducted on a history that is not specific enough to provide a clear definition of the hypothesis.

For example, if the witness simply says, 'the baby fell', without providing any further details about the fall, then BFA of such a scenario is not possible unless further details and clarification can be provided. What is required is a sufficiently precise account such as 'The baby fell from the changing table onto the carpeted floor while I turned to retrieve a diaper. I saw the rear of her head strike the floor first.' Proper investigation of this account, including collection of evidence such as the flooring material and the changing table, would permit a clear statement of the hypothesis ('The infant's injuries are the result of occipital head impact following a fall from the changing table to the carpeted floor') and a quantitative test of this hypothesis using BFA.

Several simplifications, assumptions, and limitations are inherent in BFA of a past event. Understanding these assumptions and limitations is critical, not only for the engineer performing the analysis, but also for any person reviewing and evaluating such an analysis. Some of the important assumptions and limitations of BFA include the following:

(1) Biomechanical forensic analysis must test the worst-case scenario. Because the engineer was not present to witness the event, simplifications and assumptions about various physical parameters and interactions between the subject and their environment must be made. One assumption in the previous fall example is that the child sustained an unimpeded free fall to the floor. This assumption will maximise the impact velocity of the head with the floor, producing the worst-case scenario. In general, such simplifications and assumptions leading to the worst-case scenario permit the engineer to conclude that if BFA verifies the hypothesis, then the stated history must be considered a reasonable explanation for the observed findings. However, if BFA falsifies the hypothesis, then the stated history can be ruled out as an explanation for the observed findings.

(2) Biomechanical forensic analysis cannot 'detect intent'. It is not inherently able to discriminate intentional from accidental injury because the tissues of the human body are not sensitive to the intent of the force applied to them. For example, the skull will fracture when it is struck with a hammer if sufficient force is applied during the impact, regardless of whether the hammer was wielded accidentally or intentionally.

(3) Biomechanical forensic analysis is not applied abductively to reveal 'what happened'. Abductive reasoning (also known as retroduction) is often used in the investigation of child abuse. Abductive reasoning starts with a set of known observations (e.g., a collection of clinical findings of injury) and then seeks, ostensibly, the simplest and most likely conclusion from the observations (the cause of the injuries). This form of backward-looking ('retro') reasoning is inherently fraught with uncertainty – the reasoning may lead to a 'plausible' explanation for the findings, but even if the explanation is exactly correct, it is not positively verifiable. This reasoning is often used by child abuse paediatricians (CAPs) in their attempt to evaluate the mechanism of a child's injuries. In contrast, BFA is a forward-looking analytical approach, starting with the historical facts and physical evidence and testing that history quantitatively to determine if the end result is compatible with the history. The BFA methodology is based on taking the witness account at face value, which has its own uncertainties and is a subject outside the scope of this chapter. The importance of this distinction will become more evident in the following case study discussion.

14.3 Unique Biomechanical Aspects of Evaluating Paediatric Head Injuries

Infants and children younger than 2 years of age are biomechanically unique and are not simply miniature adults. At this age, the head and its constitutive tissues and structures are rapidly growing and evolving, both physiologically and mechanically. The developing infant skull is a compliant structure that includes the thin, flexible bony plates of the skull joined by membranous sutures and open fontanelles. During vaginal delivery, this compliant structure deforms quasi-statically (slowly) to accommodate passage through the birth canal; however, the same qualities that facilitate birth also make the head vulnerable to injury from impact loading. During impact, the compliant skull deforms dynamically, leading to deformation of the adherent dura, vasculature, and intracranial contents. Because the skull is flexible, it can deform significantly without fracture and fail at relatively low levels of force once its deformation limit is reached.

As the infant grows into the toddler and young child, the thin skull bones develop into thicker bones with an optimised layered structure similar to the adult's skull (inner table, diploe, outer table) and a stronger, more homogeneous mechanical response to loading. Similarly, the sutures between bones start to interdigitate, forming joints that are more capable of carrying force and absorbing energy. These changes are balanced with the need to accommodate the continued growth of the brain. In general, as an infant develops into a young child, the head becomes capable of tolerating more mechanical force prior to failure of the skull and its intracranial contents. The reader is directed to several references related to these topics for more detailed experimental studies and data characterising the age-dependent biomechanical properties of the developing infant head [1–23].

The infant and young child are often exposed to unique loading scenarios that must be considered in the investigation of paediatric head injuries. Infants who are not independently mobile are often carried in the arms of caregivers and placed on elevated surfaces. The orientation of the infant in these scenarios (horizontal lying position versus upright sitting or standing) and the relatively large mass of the infant head will influence the infant's movement during an injurious event such as a fall. The infant's head often becomes the primary point of contact with its environment and is tasked with absorbing the majority of the resulting impact energy. A mobile toddler or young child's fall scenarios will differ from the infant's – when they do fall, they may be able to protect themselves reflexively, distributing the impact energy across multiple body areas and parts. An analysis of an injury-producing event in the infant and young child must account for these unique mechanical properties and loading scenarios.

14.4 Biomechanical Forensic Analysis Workflow and Case Study

The following discussion will present the application of the previously discussed principles of BFA by working through a contrived case study. In this example, the history and investigative facts will be summarised along with the salient clinical presentation and medical findings for the patient. From these observations and data, the foundational hypothesis of the analysis will be proposed and tested with mathematical modelling and reference to published experimental testing utilising an anthropomorphic test device (ATD, or 'crash-test dummy') and post-mortem human surrogates (PMHS, or cadavers). The conclusions from the analysis will be presented and discussed in the context of the allegations of child abuse brought against the caregiver who witnessed the child's injury.

14.4.1 Example Case: Infant Falls from a Changing Table

A 6-month-old infant (X) was at home with the mother's boyfriend (B) while the mother (M) was at work. B was not the biological father of the child, but shared care for X with M based on their work schedules. B had no history of previous arrests or convictions related to violent behaviour.

According to statements made to the police and the hospital personnel, B and X were at home in the morning and played together after X had woken from a nap. X had been in good health and well-baby visits did not appear to indicate any underlying health concerns. Following lunch, B was preparing X for a nap. B took X into the bedroom and laid X on the changing table, removing X's soiled diaper and cleaning X. B stated that he turned to his right to retrieve a fresh diaper – he looked away from X momentarily and heard X make a noise. B turned to see X falling from the changing table, with the back of X's head striking the carpeted floor. B immediately picked up X, who appeared stunned and unresponsive. X then began crying and vomited. B called M and explained to her what happened. M rushed home from work while B called emergency to summon an ambulance.

Emergency personnel arrived and assessed X. X was lethargic and vomited again. Emergency personnel noted some swelling in the right parietal-occipital region. They immediately transported X to the local trauma centre. The child was evaluated in the emergency department, where the swelling was again noted, but no other obvious external trauma was found. Imaging studies were ordered, including the head and cervical spine. A CT scan of the head revealed an area of soft tissue swelling over the right parietal-occipital area with a skull fracture extending across the right parietal bone and into the right occipital bone. There was evidence of bilateral subdural haemorrhage (SDH), right greater than left, with midline shift from the right to the left and scattered areas of subarachnoid haemorrhage. Imaging of the cervical spine was normal. Medical records indicated that X was 26 in (66 cm) long and weighed 17 pounds (7.7 kg). The child's head circumference was 17.25 in (44 cm). The child was approximately 50th percentile for length and weight.

Ultimately, the staff child abuse paediatrician (CAP) was called to consult on the matter and ordered a skeletal survey and an ophthalmological consult. The skeletal survey noted the cranial fractures but was otherwise negative. The ophthalmological consult was conducted on the day following X's admission to the hospital and found evidence of bilateral retinal haemorrhages. The CAP noted the history of the fall, but concluded that the extensive and severe nature of the injuries was 'not consistent' with the history of a 'short fall'.

The CAP opined that the injuries were 'consistent with abusive head trauma', ultimately leading to charges against B of inflicting X's injuries. When asked to provide more details related to the hypothetical mechanism of AHT, the CAP noted that the child was likely shaken and its head was slammed on an unspecified surface. This proposed alternative history was based on the CAP's interpretation of the injuries as well as an interview of B, despite B's consistently providing the fall narrative previously described. Investigators inspected and documented the scene of the incident with photographs and measurements of the bedroom and took the changing table and a sample of the carpet flooring into evidence. As the investigation proceeded, B's account of the incident essentially remained unchanged.

14.4.2 Analysis

B's legal defence engaged a biomechanical engineer to assess the history provided by B. The engineer was provided with the police investigation file, the medical records, and the photographs and measurements of the scene. The engineer also requested an inspection of the changing table, flooring material, and the incident site, taking measurements and photographs during their inspection.

The first step in the BFA process was to state the hypothesis to be tested, based on the eyewitness history, physical evidence and clinical data:

For an infant of X's age and anthropometry, a fall from a horizontal orientation on the changing table ending with a head impact on the carpeted floor, focused on the right parietal-occipital region of the head, will produce impact loads that exceed the injury tolerance values for skull fracture and acute SDH.

The goal of BFA is to examine the loading environment, injury mechanism, and injury tolerance for the subject event and the observed injuries. The following discussion will provide an overview of how BFA was applied to achieve each step of the process in the context of this contrived case study.

14.4.2.1 Loading Environment

The goal of this portion of the analysis is to determine the 'kinematics' and the 'kinetics' of the head during the fall and subsequent impact with the carpeted floor. The head's velocity and acceleration are kinematic parameters, meaning physical values related to the motion of the head, irrespective of the force required to produce that motion. In contrast, impact force is a kinetic parameter, meaning a physical value related to the forces acting on a body to cause motion. Both kinematic and kinetic parameters are useful in defining the physics of the loading event and the injury tolerance of the head and its constitutive elements. These physical parameters will ultimately be compared to injury tolerance values for X's observed cranial and intracranial medical findings to assess the fall event's potential to produce these findings acutely and traumatically.

The loading environment was estimated based on the worst-case assumption that X sustained an unimpeded free fall from the changing table to the floor. The police measured the height of the changing table surface above the floor to be 40 inches (3.3 ft or 1.0 m), a value confirmed by the engineer during their inspection. The flooring was a thin woven carpet, measuring 0.25 in (0.64 cm) thick, overlying a concrete floor, data confirmed during the engineer's inspection of the incident site.

The physical principle of conservation of energy was applied to estimate the impact velocity of X's falling body as it travelled through a vertical fall distance of 40 inches to the floor. Conservation of energy dictates that the total energy of a physical system (here X's head) must remain constant. In this case, the potential energy (PE) (energy available to do work) that X gained as a result of being lifted up to the table height, against the influence of gravity, must equal the kinetic energy (KE) (energy due to motion) that X's body gained as a result of falling to the floor. Mathematically, kinetic energy is defined as:

$$KE = \frac{1}{2}mv^2$$

where m is the object mass and v is the object velocity. Potential energy is defined as:

$$PE = mgh$$

where m is the object mass, g is the acceleration on Earth due to gravity (32.2 ft/sec^2 or 9.81 m/sec^2), and h is the height of the object above a designated reference point (in this case, the floor).

During the fall, all of the PE X possessed while lying on the changing table was converted to KE as X fell to the floor. Thus, the initial (i) PE equalled the final (f) KE ($PE_i = KE_f$) and:

$$mgh = \frac{1}{2}mv^2$$

or:

$$v = \sqrt{2gh}.$$

The engineer estimated the impact velocity of X's head, v, for a 40-inch free fall to be 14.7 ft/sec (4.5 m/s).

With the head impact velocity established, the dynamics of the impact event itself were examined. The impact between X's head and the carpeted floor resulted in X's head changing its velocity from the impact velocity (14.7 ft/sec) to 0 ft/sec over the duration of the impact. That is, X's head came to a complete stop as a result of its contact with the ground. The time over which it came to a stop is called the 'impact duration' or 'pulse width'.

The head's change in velocity during the impact and the duration of the impact define the head's mean linear acceleration. Mathematically:

$$a = \frac{\Delta v}{\Delta t},$$

where a is the mean linear acceleration of the head, Δv is the head's velocity change due to the impact, and Δt is the duration of the impact (the Greek letter Δ denotes change). To estimate the linear acceleration of the head in this example, the engineer consulted experimental data of paediatric head impacts with a carpeted floor and similar surfaces. These data include controlled free fall drop tests of the Child Restraint Air Bag Interaction (CRABI) 6-month-old ATD and PMHS infant subjects ranging in age from 3 months to 6 months. The experimental results for drop heights ranging between 1 ft (0.3 m) and 5 ft (1.5 m) were modelled mathematically to determine the estimated velocity-time and acceleration-time histories of the head for a 14.7 ft/sec carpeted impact ([9, 19], author's own work).

Figure 14.1 depicts the modelled acceleration-time head impact histories for each 40-inch fall simulation, including the average response of the combined models. Figure 14.2 depicts the velocity-time and acceleration-time histories for the average model response to a 40-inch fall onto carpet for an infant of X's age. The analysis indicates that the peak linear head acceleration of X's head ranged between 94 g and 133 g, with an average (SD) value of 111 g (14 g). Here, the unit g is the traditional unit of acceleration and is the result of dividing the computed acceleration in ft/sec^2 or m/sec^2 by its corresponding value for g (32.2. ft/sec2 or 9.81 m/sec^2). The average acceleration pulse width was approximately 15 milliseconds (0.015 sec), ranging between 13 milliseconds and 18 milliseconds (0.013 sec and 0.018 sec).

The impact force generated on the head as a result of the acceleration was computed based on Newton's second law of motion, which describes the effect that a force has on an object's motion. Mathematically, the second law is:

$$F = ma,$$

where F is the force applied to an object, m is the object's mass, and a is the object's acceleration. When acceleration is expressed in units of g, the weight of the child's head is used – in this case, anthropometry data were consulted to estimate X's head weight as

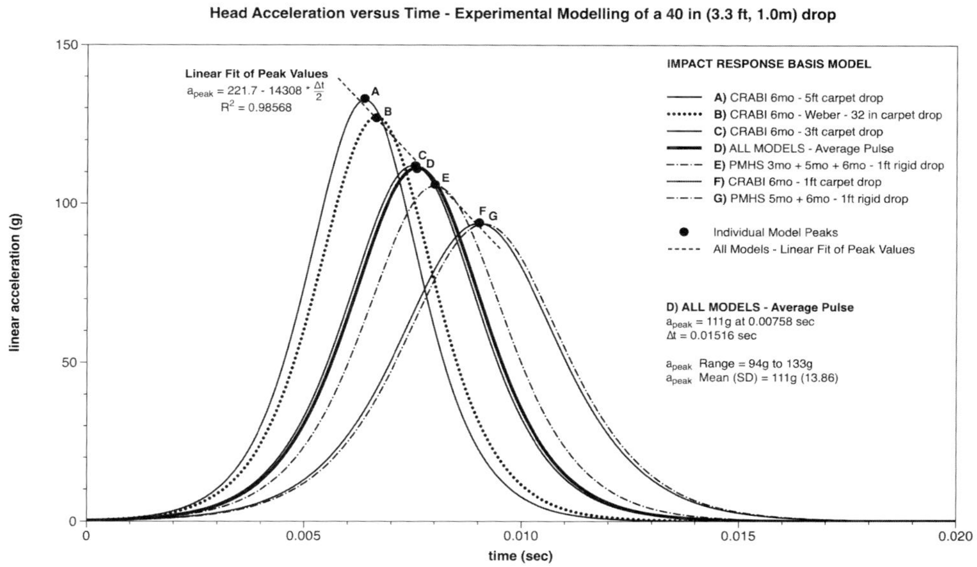

Figure 14.1 Mathematically estimated dynamic response of all experimental models for impact following a 40-in (3.3 ft, 1.0 m) fall, 6-month-old infant. Curves indicate each model's estimated acceleration-time history. Labelled points indicate each model's peak value. Plots are a composite of data from the author's testing using a CRABI 6-month ATD (curves A, C, and F), reconstruction of Weber's PMHS drop tests onto carpet [20, 21] using a CRABI 6-month ATD (B) [19], and Loyd's drop testing of PMHS 3-month, 5-month, and 6-month subjects (E, G) [9]. Curve fit of the peak values provides a linear relationship between pulse width and predicted peak linear head acceleration. The average model response (D) was generated from the average peak acceleration and pulse width of all of the models.

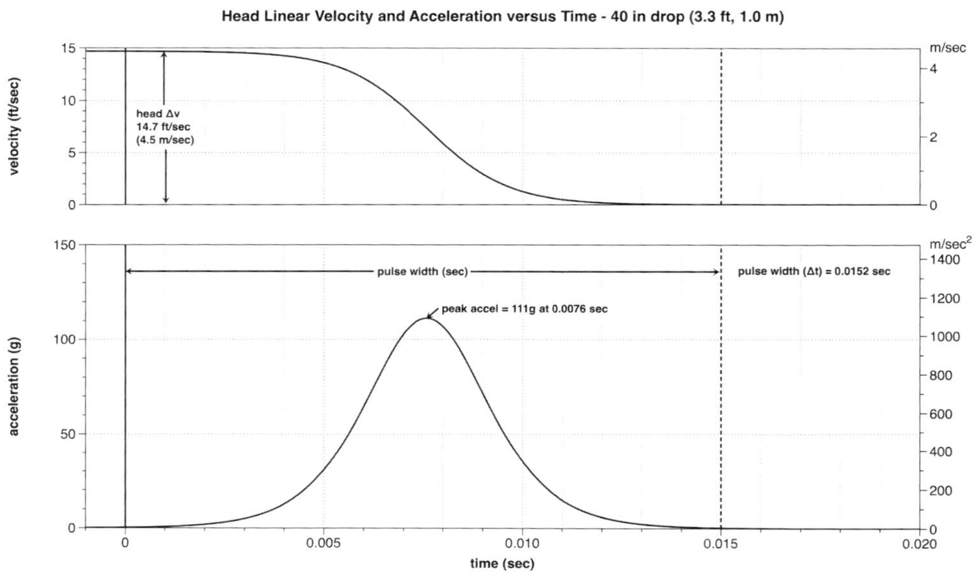

Figure 14.2 Estimated velocity and acceleration history for the head impact resulting from the modelled 40-in (3.3 ft, 1.0 m) fall, utilising the average response of all of the experimental data in the previous figure.

approximately 3 lb (1.4 kg). For a 111 g peak acceleration, the estimated contact force was 333 lb (1,480 N). The range of contact force corresponding to 94 g and 133 g peak head accelerations was 282 lb to 399 lb (1,254 N to 1,774 N).

Finally, the engineer estimated the angular acceleration of the head. The angular acceleration of the head is an important kinematic parameter related to specific types of brain injuries, particularly those related to inertial (acceleration) loading, including acute SDH and diffuse axonal injury (DAI). The physical relationship between linear acceleration and angular acceleration is:

$$\alpha = \frac{a}{r},$$

where α is the angular acceleration, a is the linear acceleration, and r is the distance between the centre of mass of the head and the point about which the head rotates. In this case, the centre of rotation was estimated to be in the mid-to-lower cervical spine, with a corresponding value of r of approximately 3 in (7.7 cm). For the 111 g impact, α was calculated to be 14,300 rad/sec^2 where 'rad' represents the unit of angular measure known as the radian. The range of peak linear acceleration (94 g to 133 g) corresponds to a range of peak angular acceleration between 12,110 rad/sec^2 and 17,130 rad/sec^2.

With the mathematical estimation of the loading environment complete, the engineer analysed the injury mechanism associated with X's medical findings and compared the loading environment results to the injury tolerance values associated with each of X's medical findings.

14.4.2.2 Injury Mechanism and Injury Tolerance

According to B, X became unresponsive immediately following the fall event, vomited, and then appeared to partially recover mental status over time. X's medical records indicate no sign of external trauma other than local swelling in the right parietal-occipital region. Imaging studies indicated SDH with midline shift and a right parietal skull fracture that crossed into the right occipital bone. The cervical spine was normal. X's trauma can generally be classified into 'contact' and 'inertial' injury mechanisms. Contact injury mechanisms involve trauma due to the direct application of force to the affected anatomy (e.g., during impact), in this case fracture of the skull and overlying soft tissue swelling. In contrast, inertial injury mechanisms involve failure of tissues due to the acceleration of the head, regardless of whether contact caused the acceleration. The acute SDH observed in X's records can result from both contact and inertial mechanisms that result in stretch and failure of the bridging vessels that drain blood away from the brain, causing blood to accumulate in the potential space below the dura (subdural).

The direct contact forces acting on X's head caused deformation of X's immature skull that exceeded its injury tolerance, resulting in fracture. The location and characteristics of the linear skull fracture in the right parietal region, across the entire bone and through the parietal eminence, are compatible with impact against a relatively flat, diffuse surface (the carpeted floor) versus an edge or corner of a stiff surface, where depressed and comminuted fractures would typically be produced. The fracture of the adjacent occipital bone suggests that the area of impact was near the lambdoid suture and adjacent occipital bone such that the occipital bone also sustained direct contact forces.

Experimental data related to infant skull fracture tolerance indicate a range of loading thresholds. Melvin [24] established a 50 g threshold for a 5% risk of skull fracture for the

CRABI 6-month ATD. Klinich et al. [25] reconstructed cases of airbag-induced injury in infants and proposed a threshold value of 85 g for a 50% fracture risk. Through reconstruction of PMHS infant skull fracture data published by Weber [20, 21], Van Ee et al. [19] proposed a threshold value of 82 g for a 50% fracture risk. The peak linear head acceleration estimated for X's head (111 g, range 94 g to 133 g) exceeds these thresholds for skull fracture in the 6-month infant. From a biomechanical perspective, it is reasonable to conclude that the subject incident provided the loading environment and injury mechanism to exceed the skull fracture threshold for an infant of X's age.

X's clinical findings also included acute SDH with observed midline shift from right to left. The inertial mechanism for acute SDH involves rotation of the head (angular acceleration) such that the mass of the brain causes it to lag behind the motion of the head. As a result, the blood vessels that originate on the brain's cortical surface and insert into the dural sinuses (the 'bridging vessels') can get stretched and leak or rupture. Angular acceleration thresholds for SDH have been proposed in the literature based on various experimental injury models. Ommaya et al. [13] and Ommaya [26] proposed a threshold for SDH of 4,500 rad/sec^2 for severe SDH, a finding in general agreement with the work of Gennarelli and Thibault [27]. Depreitere et al. [28] proposed a threshold of 4,500 rad/sec^2 for longer-duration impacts and 10,000 rad/sec^2 for shorter-duration impacts. Löwenhielm [29] proposed a threshold level at which SDH was unlikely at 4,500 rad/sec^2. All of these thresholds are for adult humans.

Scaling of adult angular acceleration brain injury tolerance data has been proposed based on a ratio of the brain masses [13, 30–32]. For the case of scaling adult data to an infant:

$$\alpha_{infant} = \alpha_{adult}\left[\frac{m_{adult}}{m_{infant}}\right]^{\frac{2}{3}},$$

where m is the mass of each brain and α is the angular acceleration tolerance of each brain. In this case, the brain masses used for scaling were 500 gm and 1,400 gm for the infant and adult brain, respectively. The scaled SDH threshold for X's brain ranged between 8,940 rad/sec^2 and 19,870 rad/sec^2 compared to the estimated angular acceleration of X's head, which ranged between 12,110 rad/sec^2 and 17,130 rad/sec^2. From a biomechanical perspective, it is reasonable to conclude that the subject incident provided the loading environment and injury mechanism to exceed the angular acceleration thresholds for SDH in an infant of X's age.

Although physical theory suggests that these adult values may be scaled to corresponding infant values based solely on brain mass, this theoretical conclusion assumes that the infant and adult brains are physically similar and fail at the same level of distortion. There is experimental evidence to suggest that infant brains are more fragile than adult brains, such that the scaled values based on brain mass alone would need to be decreased because of the infant brain's physical properties [16]. Brain mass scaling alone was used for this analysis because it generated conservatively high estimates of infant SDH tolerance.

Finally, the findings of retinal haemorrhage (RH) attributed by the CAP to AHT are clinically non-specific. Retinal haemorrhages are known to accompany intracranial pathology and can develop following short-fall events such as the subject incident. Consider the work of Aoki and Masuzawa [33] that details a series of 26 cases of acute SDH in infants ages 3 to 13 months who sustained head impact from short falls (mostly less than 2 feet), typically onto the floor or Japanese tatami mats. They found that most of the falls resulted in impacts to the occipital region of the head, and all of the patients had acute SDH of various severity

(2 cases were fatal). All 26 cases developed RH and pre-retinal haemorrhages. There were no reported skull fractures and Aoki and Masuzawa noted no external signs of head trauma (contusion, etc.). This clinical data set indicates that infants can sustain various levels of acute SDH and RH from impacts at even lower fall heights than X experienced, even in the absence of skull fracture.

To summarise, this BFA has verified the hypothesis posed at the beginning of this case study. The 'worst-case' 40-inch free fall with impact to the carpeted floor generated the loading environment required to produce the injury mechanisms and exceed the injury thresholds for X's observed acute trauma. In other words, the eyewitness account of a fall from the changing table is a biomechanically reasonable explanation for X's injuries. For a published example of BFA, see the reconstruction of a videotaped fatal fall of a toddler [18].

14.4.2.3 Comments in the Context of Allegations of Abusive Injury

The CAP in this case study provided three opinions that deserve comment:

(1) X's injuries were too severe to be explained by a 'short fall'.
(2) X's injuries were consistent with AHT.
(3) X's injuries were consistent with shaking and slamming X's head against an unspecified surface.

The CAP and similar clinical experts offered these opinions without any specificity – the basis for their opinions was their 'interpretation' of the particular 'constellation' or pattern of X's clinical findings. Abductive interpretation of the findings led the CAP to exclude all other causes or explanations, particularly the eyewitness account, and substitute their alternative, vague history of AHT as the most likely explanation for the clinical findings. The CAP's reasoning was not possible to test or validate and was not methodologically reproducible – it was speculative, not scientific. Further, the conclusions were based on published literature that is of low evidence-based quality, and subject to circular reasoning and confirmation bias. The reader is directed to two critical meta-analyses of this literature for further details [34, 35], as well as the one contained in Chapter 10 of this book.

The CAP rendered opinions related to the mechanism of injury without performing an analysis of the incident described in the history. The CAP generalised, referring to 'short falls' instead of considering the measured fall height, fall dynamics and consequences of X's actual fall event. Anecdote and 'experience' formed the basis for repeatedly rendering the same faulty opinion as in previous cases. Ultimately, the CAP's role in X's case took on legal significance as the CAP extended their 'diagnosis' from medical findings into the realm of prosecution. The CAP's interpretation of the clinical findings became the prosecution's only 'evidence' of wrongdoing. The CAP effectively bypassed the legal system by 'diagnosing' a criminal act and, as often occurs in these matters, placed the burden to 'prove' his innocence on B.

In the case study presented here, the CAP opined that the findings in X's medical records were consistent with shaking and slamming X's head into some non-specified surface. From a biomechanical perspective, it is not necessary to invoke 'shaking' at all – as shown previously, all of X's injuries can be explained by a parietal impact with concomitant angular head acceleration. The CAP's invocation of shaking as a mechanism to explain X's findings is arbitrary, a consequence of the CAP observing SDH and brain oedema accompanied by RH, a constellation of findings colloquially known as the 'triad'. There is no biomechanical evidence in the published literature that demonstrates that shaking produces any or all of these findings. Even if one accepts that shaking can produce the triad, the lack of findings one would expect with vigorous shaking of an infant (grip marks on the torso, fractured ribs, flail injuries to the extremities, cervical spine injury) were not observed for X and are typically not present in most cases labelled as AHT. Thus, in most cases of AHT where shaking is identified as a possible mechanism, the CAP's own definition of what should occur when a child is shaken can be used to demonstrate the internal inconsistency of the diagnosis. This observation highlights the arbitrary and speculative nature of the diagnosis.

For context, consider the quantitative comparison of shaking and head impact from a 'short fall' such as the case study incident. Biomechanical studies in which an ATD or similar physical model of an infant has been shaken have reported peak linear head accelerations ranging between 5 g and 15 g; compare this to the subject case study in which X sustained an estimated peak linear head acceleration of 111 g. In general, a 'short fall' produces peak head accelerations that are an order of magnitude (10 times) greater than

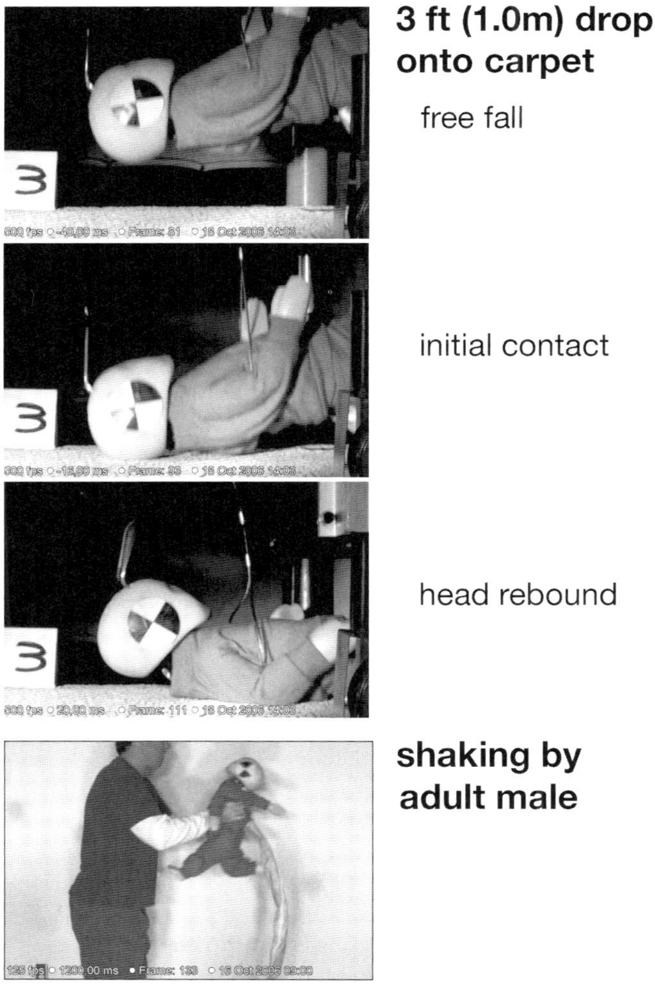

Figure 14.3 Still frames from high-speed video of testing conducted by the author utilising the CRABI 6-month ATD.

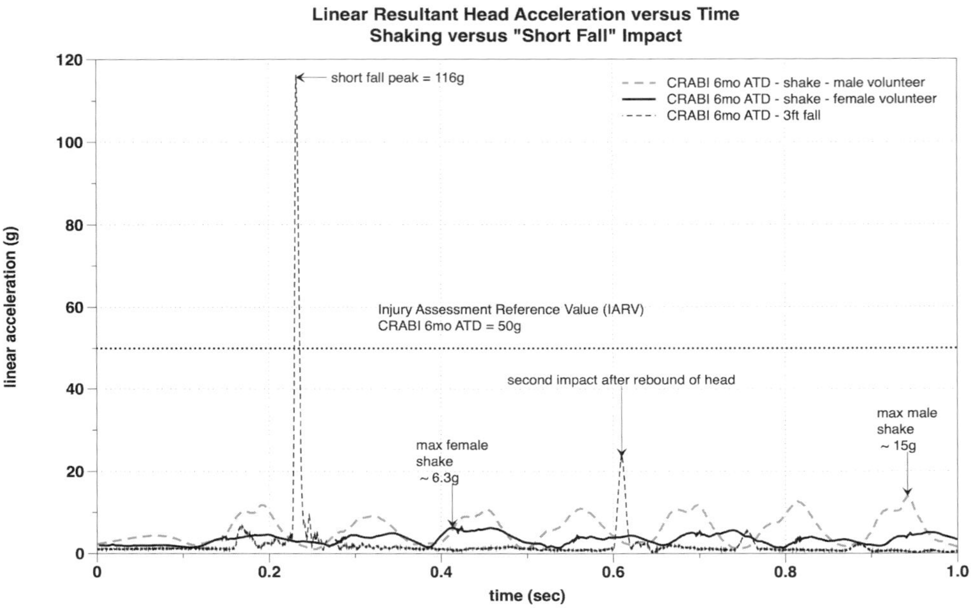

Figure 14.4 Head acceleration histories from the CRABI 6-month ATD testing conducted by the author. Compare the peak linear head acceleration from the 3 ft (1.0 m) 'short fall' onto carpet (116g) with the peak acceleration generated during maximal shaking (15g or less for typical male and female volunteers). The Injury Assessment Reference Value (IARV) for the CRABI 6 ATD of 50 g represents the linear head acceleration level at which there is a 5% risk of serious injury, based on the ATD response.

shaking. Figure 14.3 depicts still frames from high-speed video of a CRABI 6-month ATD undergoing a 3 ft (1.0 m) drop onto carpet and maximal effort shaking by an adult male (testing conducted by the author). Figure 14.4 depicts plots of the linear head accelerations measured during each test for quantitative comparison. This comparison is particularly important to consider because the CAP provided testimony that the forces generated during shaking are equivalent to a 'multi-story fall' or a 'high-speed car accident'. While this dramatic testimony is commonly offered in cases of AHT, it is simply false, incompatible with the laws of physics, and unsupported by experimental data.

14.4.3 General Comments Related to Short Falls, Injury Frequency, and Injury Severity

In theory, several factors influence the outcome of, for example, a fall of an infant off a changing table to the floor. These factors include fall height, anatomical location of impact, orientation of the head and the body at impact, the nature of the impact surface (surface compliance and conformation (flat surface versus an edge or corner)), and, of course, the age (developmental status) and biological and biomechanical variability of the child's head and its constitutive properties.

Children fall a lot as they develop, and it is not surprising that many of those falls result in no serious or fatal injuries, especially as children develop mobility and are able to protect themselves from falls, reflexively or otherwise. However, non-mobile infants in particular have the disadvantage of being put into positions that are mechanically unique to a certain extent – for example, elevated horizontal surfaces or carried within the arms of a caregiver. These scenarios can produce falls that have very different kinematics and subsequent impact characteristics when compared to what a clinician possibly believes must occur when an infant experiences a 'short fall'. The notion that clinicians are fixated on fall height alone as some determinant of outcome should bring pause to even the layperson in terms of a clinician's suspicion about falls in general.

There is likely not a single specific explanation for why the universe of all falls specifically results in a remarkably small number of serious or fatal injuries. The vagaries of the aforementioned factors can align to produce devastating injuries or none at all; however, some of the factors which may affect the variability and frequency of serious injuries in the context of falls may have nothing to do with the physics and biomechanics of falls, but may have to do with the way falls are coded, recorded, and statistically analysed. We know that falls are commonly 'disbelieved' as legitimate histories that explain a child's injuries, and these 'disbelieved' cases are usually the more serious and fatal cases ('Short falls don't cause serious injuries!'; see Chapter 15). Thus, there may be a not insignificant number of falls that have resulted in serious or fatal injury that have been discounted or recast as 'abuse' based on the belief that the fall cannot produce the observed outcome. This is one example of the circular reasoning built into the problem of 'diagnosing' abuse and directly affects the frequency of serious injury from short falls that some clinicians cite to reclassify a short fall injury as abuse.

In terms of differentiating between an impact that causes no fracture and one that causes fracture, the fall itself is a general descriptor of the loading event, but the assessment of, for example, skull fracture potential in the specific fall event has to do with the actual loading to the head. Thus, other factors such as load sharing across body segments, partial arrest of the fall trajectory due to interactions with other objects in the environment, anatomical points of contact and orientation of the body at impact, as well as the character of the impact surface(s) can all influence the outcome even for different falls from identical heights. Thus, each fall must be analysed in the context of the witness history, physical evidence, and the observed findings, instead of generalised epidemiological statistics based on potentially biased data. This is the essence of the difference between causation (a mechanistic explanation) and correlation (a statistical inference).

An analysis of a specific event requires adoption of a hypothesis (the witness account) and testing of that hypothesis through analysis of the incident's physical data. A worst case is assumed, with the acknowledgement that less-than-worst-case loading could affect the outcome, and biological variability and uncertainty are explicitly stated when reaching a conclusion in this regard. As is also noted, one cannot analyse the data pertaining to an event and determine what 'really' happened – one can only evaluate the history within the context of the physical evidence and test that history to verify or falsify it.

14.4.4 General Comments Regarding 'Shaking' As a Viable Biomechanical Explanation for Abusive Head Trauma

Shaking as a mechanism to explain the triad, or any constellation of findings associated with AHT, is a hypothetical construct thought to have originated with the work of Caffey [36, 37] and Guthkelch [38]. These clinicians reported the association of various clinical findings with explanations (reported or speculative) of a child's having been 'shaken' prior to injury. What exactly constitutes the findings associated with shaking has changed and evolved over time, making the definitive diagnosis of 'shaken baby syndrome' (SBS) or AHT a notoriously vague and variable one. As has been pointed out in various published work, the lack of scientific rigour and an evidence-based definition of SBS/AHT is a foundational weakness of the clinical entity. To this author's knowledge, there are no witnessed cases of shaking (e.g., incidents caught on video) that have produced the triad, while inversely there are witnessed and even videoed shaking episodes that have reportedly not produced the triad. Much of the purported evidence validating shaking as a mechanism of the triad, and related findings, relies on confessions from the accused, a source of data fraught with its own uncertainties (see Chapters 11 and 12).

From a biomechanical perspective, there are no definitive experimental studies of the proposed mechanism of SBS that demonstrate that shaking, in any form, can produce the intracranial findings associated with the triad, including acute SDH and RH. Further, shaking should cause precursor trauma to the torso and cervical spine that is typically not observed in cases of alleged SBS/AHT. Biomechanically, there is a lack of internal consistency between the hypothetical mechanism of intracranial injury thought to occur from shaking and the clinical observations noted in most cases of alleged SBS/AHT. In the context of SBS criminal proceedings, this author has not once encountered experts testifying in support of shaking who could describe any specifics as to how the child was shaken, for how long, in what direction, etc. Paradoxically, BFA is simply not possible in these cases – a biomechanical engineer would have to fabricate the unspecific circumstances of the alleged shaking event in order to test the alleged mechanism of shaking. In these cases, the vague notion of shaking cannot be tested forensically; however, an examination of the general biomechanical aspects of shaking is worthwhile to understand the lack of scientific support for the theoretical association between shaking and intracranial findings like the triad.

Laboratory biomechanical studies of SBS typically involve human volunteers shaking various ATDs (commercially produced or custom-made) to measure the resulting head kinematics and neck loads [39–42]. These studies generally demonstrate that shaking alone does not produce head accelerations that exceed the various tolerances for SDH, accepting that these tolerance values are still being determined and are largely based on scaling techniques. The studies that appear to report exceedingly large head accelerations from shaking typically suffer from limitations in their model that produce, for example, large spikes in head acceleration associated with non-physiological rigid contact between the rigid head and torso structures of the model.

With the rise in desktop computational power, computer models of SBS have appeared that purport to demonstrate a mechanistic link between shaking and injurious bridging vessel or retinal vessel loading [43–45]. The general computational modelling technique known as finite element modelling (FEM) is used in a wide variety of scientific and engineering disciplines and is a powerful analytical and visualisation tool for solving complex physical simulations. While FEM is typically a more accessible and less expensive alternative to experimental laboratory science, FEM itself is only as good as the basis for it, including the definition of the model, the physical data upon which it is based, the application of the specific loading conditions to the model, and the stability of the model itself.

The most critical aspect of FEM is the validation of the model results against reality – validation is a necessary part of FEM that is conspicuously absent in FEM studies of shaking. Unless FEM results are shown to predict reality, the model is typically just as speculative as anecdotal observation – and yet some of these articles are regularly cited in court as proof of shaking. As with any study, one should review the results and conclusions with healthy scepticism and within the context of the larger body of experimental data in the published literature. It is worth repeating here that our nascent understanding of the biomechanics of infant injury is a rapidly growing and developing field of investigation, and it behoves those interested in the topic to stay current with the state of the art in the published literature.

14.5 Conclusion

This chapter has introduced the reader to the concept of Biomechanical Forensic Analysis of injury and how it may be applied to aid one's understanding of infant injury mechanisms in the setting of alleged abusive trauma. Biomechanical forensic analysis seeks to evaluate the mechanism of observed clinical findings of injury in the context of a history, physical evidence, and the application of the laws of physics and experimental data. It utilises scientific methodologies that are reproducible and evidence-based, with explicitly stated assumptions and limitations. Biomechanical forensic analysis cannot inherently differentiate between 'accidental' and 'non-accidental' causes of injury because the tissues of the body and their failure mechanisms are not sensitive to the intent of the force applied to them.

Similarly, BFA cannot inherently determine 'what happened' solely from clinical findings of injury. It seeks to verify or falsify a history by reconstructing the loading environment present in that event through consideration of the eyewitness account, physical evidence, and clinical findings. The deliberate, scientific methodology inherent in BFA contrasts with that of the clinical expert who offers non-verifiable, abductive reasoning to speculate about the cause of an infant's injuries without analysing the initiating traumatic event, and without providing a high-quality, evidence-based rationale for their opinions. The reader is encouraged to explore the details of the experimental data and evidence base for the methodologies and techniques described in this brief introduction to BFA by consulting the references.

References

1. Coats B, Margulies SS. Material properties of human infant skull and suture at high rates. *Journal of Neurotrauma*. 2006;23:1222–32.
2. Ibrahim NG, Margulies SS. Biomechanics of the toddler head during low-height falls: An anthropomorphic dummy analysis. *Journal of Neurosurgery: Pediatrics*. 2010;6(1):57–68.
3. Ibrahim NG, Wood J, Margulies SS, Christian CW. Influence of age and fall type on head injuries in infants and toddlers. *International Journal of Developmental Neuroscience*. 2012;30(3):201–6.
4. Kriewall TJ, McPherson GK, Tsai AC. Bending properties and ash content of fetal cranial bone. *Journal of Biomechanics*. 1981;14:73–9.
5. Kriewall TJ. Structural, mechanical, and material properties of fetal cranial bone. *American Journal of Obstetrics and Gynecology*. 1982;143:707–14.
6. Leestma JE, Thibault KL. Physical injury to the nervous system. In *Forensic neuropathology*. 3rd ed. JE Leetsma, ed. CRC Press, 2014, pp. 417–594.
7. Loyd AM. Studies of the human head from neonate to adult: *An* inertial, geometrical and structural analysis with comparisons to the ATD head. Dissertation. Duke University, 2011.
8. Loyd AM, Nightingale RW, Luck JF et al. The compressive stiffness of human pediatric heads. *Journal of Biomechanics*. 2015;48:3766–75.
9. Loyd AM, Nightingale RW, Luck JF, Cutcliffe HC, Myers BS. The response of the pediatric head to impacts onto a rigid surface. *Journal of Biomechanics*. 2019;93:167–76.

10. Margulies SS, Thibault KL. Infant skull and suture properties: Measurements and implications for mechanisms of pediatric brain injury. *Journal of Biomechanical Engineering*. 2000;122:364–71.

11. McPherson GK, Kriewall TJ. The elastic modulus of fetal cranial bone: A first step towards an understanding of the biomechanics of fetal head molding. *Journal of Biomechanics*. 1980.

12. McPherson GK, Kriewall TJ. Fetal head molding: An investigation utilizing a finite element model of the fetal parietal bone. *Journal of Biomechanics*. 1980;13:17–26.

13. Ommaya AK, Goldsmith W, Thibault L. Biomechanics and neuropathology of adult and paediatric head injury. *British Journal of Neurosurgery*. 2002;16:220–42.

14. Prange MT, Margulies SS. Regional, directional, and age-dependent properties of the brain undergoing large deformation. *Journal of Biomechanical Engineering*. 2002;124(2):244–52.

15. San Cheong V, Karunaratne A, Amis AA, Bull AMJ. Strain rate dependency of fractures of immature bone. *Journal of the Mechanical Behavior of Biomedical Materials*. 2017;66:68–76.

16. Thibault KL, Margulies SS. Age-dependent material properties of the porcine cerebrum: effect on pediatric inertial head injury criteria. *Journal of Biomechanics*. 1998;31:1119–26.

17. Thibault LE, Gennarelli TA, Margulies SS, Marcus J, Eppinger R. The strain dependent pathophysiological consequences of inertial loading on central nervous system tissue. In *International conference on the biomechanics of impacts*. Bron. 1990.

18. Van Ee C, Raymond D, Thibault K, Hardy W, Plunkett J. Child ATD reconstruction of a fatal pediatric fall. IMECE2009-12994. *International Mechanical Engineering Congress and Exposition*. 2009.

19. Van Ee C, Morowski-Browne B, Raymond D et al. Evaluation and refinement of the CRABI-6 anthropomorphic test device injury criteria for skull fracture. IMECE2009-12973. *International Mechanical Engineering Congress and Exposition*. 2009.

20. Weber W. [Experimental studies of skull fractures in infants] (in German). *Zeitschrift fur Rechtsmedizin*. 1984;92:87–94.

21. Weber W. [Biomechanical fragility of the infant skull] (in German). *Zeitschrift fur Rechtsmedizin*. 1985;94:93–101.

22. Weber W. [Predilection sites of infantile skull fractures following blunt force] (in German). *Zeitschrift fur Rechtsmedizin*. 1987;98:81–93.

23. Yoganandan N, Kumaresan S, Pintar FA, Gennarelli TA. Pediatric biomechanics. *Accidental injury: Biomechanics and prevention*. AM Nahum, JW Melvin, eds. Springer, 2002, pp. 550–87.

24. Melvin JW. Injury assessment reference values for the CRABI 6-month infant dummy in a rear-facing infant restraint with airbag deployment. *SAE Transactions*. 1995.

25. Klinich K, Hulbert GM, Schneider LW. Estimating infant head injury criteria and impact response using crash reconstruction and finite element modeling. *Stapp Car Crash Journal*. 2002;46:165–94.

26. Ommaya AK. *Biomechanics of head injuries: Experimental aspects*. Appleton-Century-Crofts, 1984.

27. Gennarelli TA, Thibault LE. Biomechanics of acute subdural hematoma. *Journal of Trauma*. 1982;22:680–6.

28. Depreitere B, Van Lierde C, Vander Sloten J et al. Mechanics of acute subdural hematomas resulting from bridging vein rupture. *Journal of Neurosurgery*. 2006;104:950–6.

29. Löwenhielm P. Tolerance level for bridging vein disruption calculated with a mathematical model. *Journal of Bioengineering*. 1978;2:501–7.

30. Holbourn AHS. Mechanics of head injuries. *Lancet*. 1943;242:438–41.

31. Ommaya AK, Hirsch AE, Yarnell P, Harris EH. Scaling of experimental data on cerebral concussion in sub-human primates to concussion threshold for man. appsdticmil. 1967. https://apps.dtic.mil/sti/citations/AD0666837.

32. Meaney DF, Thibault KL, Gennarelli TA, Thibault LE. Experimental investigation of the relationship between head kinematics and intracranial tissue deformation. *Advances in Bioengineering*. 1993;24:8–11.

33. Aoki N, Masuzawa H. Infantile acute subdural hematoma: Clinical analysis of 26 cases. *Journal of Neurosurgery*. 1984;61:273–80.

34. Donohoe M. Evidence-based medicine and shaken baby syndrome. Part I: Literature review, 1966–1998. *American Journal of Forensic Medicine and Pathology*. 2003;24 (3):239–42.

35. Elinder G, Eriksson A, Hallberg B, Lynøe N. Traumatic shaking: The role of the triad in medical investigations of suspected traumatic shaking. *Acta Paediatrica*. 2018;107(Suppl 472):3–23.

36. Caffey J. On the theory and practice of shaking infants: Its potential residual effects of permanent brain damage and mental retardation. *American Journal of Diseases of Children*. 1972;124(2):161–9.

37. Caffey J. The whiplash shaken infant syndrome: Manual shaking by the extremities with whiplash-induced intracranial and intraocular bleedings, linked with residual permanent brain damage and mental retardation. *Pediatrics*. 1974;54(4):396–403.

38. Guthkelch AN. Infantile subdural haematoma and its relationship to whiplash injuries. *British Medical Journal*. 1971;2(5759):430–1.

39. Cory CZ, Jones MD. Can shaking alone cause fatal brain injury? A biomechanical assessment of the Duhaime shaken baby syndrome model. *Medicine, Science and the Law*. 2003;43(4):317–33.

40. Duhaime A-C, Gennarelli T, Thibault LE et al. The shaken baby syndrome: A clinical, pathological, and biomechanical study. *Journal of Neurosurgery*. 1987;66 (3):409–15.

41. Jenny CA. Biomechanical response of the infant head to shaking: An experimental investigation. *Journal of Neurotrauma*. 2017;34(8):1579–88.

42. Prange MT, Coats B, Duhaime AC, Margulies SS. Anthropomorphic simulations of falls, shakes, and inflicted impacts in infants. *Journal of Neurosurgery*. 2003;99(1):143–50.

43. Roth S, Raul JS, Ludes B, Willinger R. Finite element analysis of impact and shaking inflicted to a child. *International Journal of Legal Medicine*. 2007;121 (3):223–8.

44. Nadarasa J, Deck C, Meyer F et al. Development of a finite-element eye model to investigate retinal hemorrhages in shaken baby syndrome. *Biomechanics and Modeling in Mechanobiology*. 2007;17 (2):517–30.

45. Rangarajan N, Kamalakkannan SB, Hasija V et al. Finite element model of ocular injury in abusive head trauma. *Journal of the American Association for Pediatric Ophthalmology and Strabismus*. 2009;13(4):364–9.

Chapter 15

When Lack of Information Leads to Apparent Paradoxes and Wrong Conclusions

Analysis of a Seminal Article on Short Falls

Leila Schneps

The importance of the issue of short falls of less than 1.5 meters (5 feet) and the potential harm they can cause to small infants cannot be overstated. If parents or caretakers bring to the hospital a child presenting with certain types of brain lesions – most particularly subdural haematoma (SDH) with or without retinal haemorrhage (RH) – then most often the explanation of a short fall will be immediately deemed insufficient and incompatible with the injuries, the child will be diagnosed with shaken baby syndrome (SBS), and the parents will come under direct suspicion of child abuse.

This fact is based on the belief that short falls cannot produce this kind of harm in small infants, a belief that continues to be widely held in spite of the fact that it has repeatedly been proven false. Already in 1984 a Japanese study [1] found 26 infants in whom acute SDH followed a witnessed short fall; a 2018 American study by Atkinson et al. [2] described eight witnessed cases of short falls with SDH. Nearly all children in both studies had associated RH and both studies note that occipital impact is particularly dangerous. In between these two, numerous other case series and individual case reports have shown that short falls and accidental household trauma can indeed cause SDH (unilateral or bilateral), subarachnoid haemorrhage (unilateral or bilateral), and RH (unilateral or bilateral), including diffuse RH, perimacular folds, and retinoschisis (see [3–19] for many such cases).

The authors of a large-scale study [23] of short fall fatality observed several fatal cases, including two that took place in hospitals, both with SDH. The authors of this study warn that 'we do not argue with the statement that severe injuries are extremely uncommon after minor falls, yet while the risk is rare, they do happen' [24]. Even some of the strongest proponents of SBS and specialists of child abuse have recently acknowledged that short falls may be dangerous [20–22]; we read, for example, of 'the rare household fall that results in life-threatening injury or death' in a 2017 article [25]. One case of a fatal fall from a height of 2 feet, involving SDH and RH, is even accepted by the health authority in France, one of the countries which most rigorously rejects short falls as a possible explanation for SDH (see Chapter 22), thanks to the fact that this particular fall was caught on camera.

Altogether, there are multiple published cases of children presenting with SDH and RH after (sometimes fatal) witnessed short falls. Such cases do occur, although they are certainly rare. Yet the claim that a short fall must be rejected as an explanation for these lesions persists and is even regularly cited in court as proof that a parent or caretaker is lying about the history of a child's accident.

The danger of denying the potential harmfulness of short falls in children goes even beyond the miscarriages of justice caused by ignoring the explanations of parents or caretakers. As Hall et al., the authors of the study [23], point out in a letter to the editor of the *Journal of Trauma* [24], 'Delays in presentation were caused by both parents and emergency room personnel who felt that minor falls were benign and waited until late symptoms developed before becoming concerned', which may take time due to the fact that 'the first symptom appears only after gradual expansion of the clot has been sufficient to reach a significant pressure'.

Given all this, where does this belief in the non-harmfulness of short falls come from? It is the consequence of a number of studies purporting to have observed the extreme rarity or near non-existence of a fatal short fall. Unfortunately, these publications tend to be riddled with logical and numerical errors. The purpose of the present chapter is to examine one of them in detail; although there are many possibilities, we selected this particular one ([26]) because, on the one hand, its absolute conclusion that short falls cannot be harmful has made it into a powerful weapon in the hands of SBS proponents, and, on the other, examining its errors in detail appears to us like a more pedagogical approach than trying to examine many different articles in a short space. See, however [27], which examines a similar type of study by Williams [28], and also Chapter 17 of this book, which examines a different study using different methods. These articles claiming that short falls cannot cause serious harm are not only dangerous, but they are wrong.

15.1 Seminal 1991 Article by Chadwick et al.

One of the most frequently cited pieces of scientific research in the field of SBS is a 1991 article by Dr D. L. Chadwick et al. [26] entitled *Deaths from Falls in Children: How Far Is Fatal?*[1] It is difficult to overestimate the influence of this short but striking article, which has been cited countless times both in medical articles and in court and is referred to by all physicians who deal with head trauma in children.

The authors of the article present data observed over a 42-month period in the children's trauma centre serving San Diego County, California. During this time, a total of 317 children under 15 years old were brought into the trauma centre because of injuries attributed to falls. Thirty-four cases in which no information about the height of the fall was known were dropped from the study, which concentrated on 283 cases in which specific circumstances were provided by the person bringing the child to the centre. These 283 cases and the fatality outcomes were divided into categories as follows:

Table 15.1 Number of cases and fatalities as a function of fall height in Chadwick et al.'s study [26]

Fall height	Number of cases	Number of fatalities
1–4 feet	100	7
5–9 feet	65	0
> 9 feet	118	1

[1] For example, it is used by the French national guidelines on SBS to rule out short falls as a possible explanation for infantile SDH and RH. See Chapter 22.

Table 15.2 Observed injuries in Chadwick et al.'s study [26]

Injury type	Number observed
Old fractures	2
Bruises on trunk or extremities	3
Genital injury	2
Two head impact sites	2
No associated injury	2

The article describes the situations to which the short fall deaths are attributed as follows: one fall on stairs, two from the arms of an adult, and four from furniture. It gives a brief description of three of the seven cases (concerning infants aged 6 weeks, 13 months, and 11 months) as well as the single long fall fatality (11 months).

After providing this information, Dr Chadwick and his co-authors go on to discuss the possibility that the caretaker's description of a short fall to explain a child's injuries may not be truthful. They note that one can often reliably diagnose child abuse in cases where the victim presents multiple other injuries in different stages of healing, or multiple impact sites on the head observed in cases where the given explanation is a single short fall (not a fall on stairs, which is considered as a sequence of short falls). They observe that several such injuries were observed in the seven children whose deaths were attributed to short falls, detailed in Table 15.2.

This collection of additional data, obtained from examination and autopsy of the deceased children, adds great weight to the statement that many badly hurt children brought to the hospital by caregivers who attribute their injuries to a short fall are actually abused.

The next part of the article addresses the problem of children whose injuries strike the examining doctor as 'discrepant' or not compatible with the caretaker's account of what caused them. In such cases, 'inflicted injury is often diagnosed when the clinician can state with a high level of certainty that the single injury seen in a child could not possibly have been produced by the event described by the caretaker'.

This assertion may give one pause. How does a clinician reach a high level of certainty? In order to state that a given injury cannot have been produced by a certain cause, he or she needs to be certain that such a thing is not merely rare, but has actually never occurred. Such a claim must necessarily be based on large-scale studies, since studies of just a few individuals are unlikely to reveal rare events. If a clinician is certain that a short fall can never be fatal, then he or she will diagnose abuse any time a child dies after a claimed short fall; thus it is clearly of major importance to know whether it is possible for a short fall to be fatal or not. The remainder of Chadwick et al.'s three-page article focuses essentially on attempting to settle this question in the negative by citing a number of previous studies. Let us summarise his findings.

The vast database of the National Electronic Injury Study of the Consumer Product Safety Commission (NEISS) was investigated in a study by Sweeney [29] which concluded that children can die from falls from heights of as little as 1 foot. However, Chadwick et al. dismiss these results on the grounds that the NEISS database itself may not be reliable, in that unrecognised cases of inflicted injury may be included in the database as short falls.

A detailed study by Hall et al. [23] reviewing records in the medical examiner's office of Cook County, Illinois, which found 18 cases in which fatal head injury was attributed to a fall of 3 feet or less, is also dismissed by Chadwick et al. on the same grounds, namely that 'their work omits the detailed information necessary to exclude inflicted injury, and many of those cases might be in that category'.

Instead, Chadwick et al. rely on five studies of falls which occurred in public places (hospitals or outdoors) rather than relying solely on caretakers' stories. Two of these studies observed a total of 180 small children who fell from heights of less than 4 feet while in the hospital and found that they sustained only very minor injuries or were uninjured. Two more studied falls from buildings (one using cases from 10 years of experience and the other a set of 66 cases) and concluded that only falls from the fourth floor or higher resulted in death. The fifth study observed 100 falls of children and adults and, apart from one death in an apparent 10-foot fall of a child which was unobserved, found that life-threatening injury required at least a 15-foot fall.

In contrast, write Chadwick et al. of their own observations of the San Diego trauma centre records, 'the data in the present study show an astonishing concentration of risk of death in the group with the shortest falls'. It is this contrast with the five previously mentioned studies that leads them to their main conclusion:

> If the histories of short falls are accepted as correct, the conclusion would be reached that the risk of death is eight times greater in children who fall from 1 to 4 feet than for those who fall from 10 to 45 feet. Since this conclusion appears absurd, it is necessary to seek another explanation . . . The best explanation of the findings is that for the seven children who died following short falls the history was falsified.

15.2 Statistical Errors and Omissions in the Chadwick et al. Study

On first reading, Chadwick et al.'s conclusion seems straightforward. Experience and common sense tell us that child abuse exists, that short falls cannot cause more deaths than long ones, and that seven deaths out of 100 short falls seems like too many. Add in the other injuries seen on the children, and their conclusion can seem nothing short of inevitable. This is how it is taken by pretty much the entire body of medical professionals working in SBS. Nowadays, the diagnosis of inflicted injury arises automatically whenever a child presents serious injuries or dies following an event explained by the caretaker as a short fall. This diagnosis generally leads to arrest, investigation, and trial, most often with immediate separation of the suspected parents from all of their children.

On a second, more careful reading of Chadwick et al.'s paper, however, a number of problems arise. Each of these problems is based on the same key issue, namely the existence of invisible information left out of the analysis whose presence could make a major difference to the conclusions.

15.2.1 Number of Short Falls versus Long Falls in the General Population of Children

The first and main example of missing information concerns the frequency with which small children actually fall. As every parent knows, short falls are extremely common, whereas long falls are very rare. Indeed, Chadwick et al. clearly accept that every child who sustains a long fall will automatically be taken to the hospital, so that 118 represents the true number of long falls in the population of San Diego County, and the death rate from long falls can be taken to be about 1 in 118.

We first observe that an important piece of information has been missed in drawing this conclusion, namely the fact that children who died at the scene of a long fall would not have been transported to the hospital. A French study [30] of long falls in children from 2006 counted a total of 64 long falls (> 3 meters or about 10 feet) in the Île-de-France region, of which 61 were transported to hospital and 3 died at the scene. Four of the hospitalised children subsequently died, for a total fatality rate of 7 out of 64 or about 11%. If the in-hospital death rate had been used, as in Chadwick et al., the fatality rate would have been calculated as 4/61 or about 6%, around half of the true rate. For these reasons, it is legitimate to suppose that Chadwick et al.'s rate of 1 in 118 is likely too small and the true rate may be quite a bit larger.

But Chadwick et al.'s error concerning long falls is not nearly as significant as their error concerning short falls. When Chadwick et al. use 7 in 100 as the fatality rate of short falls, they are making the unspoken assumption that just as for long falls, the 100 children brought to hospital following short falls are all cases of children sustaining short falls. This is clearly nonsense; children take short tumbles all the time.

Let us attempt to correct this error by estimating a realistic fatality rate for short falls. We begin by summarising the results of several reference articles studying the incidence of traumatic brain injury (TBI) from any type of fall (ranging from light cases to death) in children aged 0–15, the same age range observed by Chadwick et al.

In the article [31] by Reid et al. studying paediatric traumatic brain injury in Minnesota, the following data are given: 209 children 0–15 brought in with TBI from falls out of a population of 1.07 million in one year (1993). This would mean that one could expect about 766 cases over a 44-month period as in Chadwick et al.'s study for a population of 1.07 million. Since they in fact saw 317 cases, we may assume that Chadwick et al.'s hospital served a population of roughly half a million children aged 0–15.

Since children up to 15 make up roughly 20% of the total population in the United States, this would correspond to a total population of 2.5 million people, which is in fact very close to the total population of San Diego County in 1991, the county served by Chadwick et al.'s hospital. The population of children aged 0–4 would then be about 120,000. According to Chadwick et al.'s article, about 175 of the 317 falls studied occurred in children 0–3 and 61 in children 4–6, from which we may estimate that about 195 out of 317 were children aged 0–4, around 60%, which is close to the 56% observed by Reid et al.

About one third of the falls studied by Chadwick et al. were short falls (they count 100 out of 317, but recall that there were quite a number of falls from 'unknown heights' of which at least some were surely short falls). Of these, nearly all the 30 falls in children aged < 1 were certainly short falls; it is rare for children under 1 to fall from windows, although the single long fall fatality in Chadwick et al.'s article was 11 months old. Therefore some 70 or 80 of the falls sustained by children aged 1–4 were also short falls that led to hospital.

An article by Kravitz et al. [32] interrogated families and discovered that about half of all babies fall off furniture in their first year of life. This estimate is probably low for toddlers, who likely take short falls and hit their heads several times a year. However, using Kravitz et al.'s 50% as a low estimate, we could expect a total of 60,000 short falls a year in the San Diego County population of 0–4 year olds of 120,000, making a total of 220,000 short falls in this age range over the 44-month period of the study. The fatality rate, as noted by Chadwick et al., was 7; though the ages are not specified, they are certainly all under 4 since the falls were from standing position, from arms, or from furniture with the single exception of a stairway fall in a child of 11 months. From all this, we may draw the conclusion that the fatality rate of short falls in children aged 0–4 observed by Chadwick et al., with their own data, should have been 7 in 220,000 and certainly not 7 in 100.

Since all the children whose ages are given were aged 0–13 months, it may make more sense to consider that age group only on the assumption that all 7 fatalities were babies. The population of babies aged 0–13 months would be about 32,500; the number of short falls according to Kravitz et al. about 16,250 per year, and over the 44-month period there would be around 60,000 short falls in that population; the fatality rate that Chadwick et al. should have given (if they had restricted their attention to the age group 0–13 months) would thus have been 7 in 60,000, or about 1 in 10,000.

The important point is that *this fatality rate is much, much lower than the fatality rate for long falls*. Even if we accept 1/118 as the fatality rate for long falls (and as we saw, it is almost certainly too low), we find the following corrected statement using Chadwick et al.'s own data: the fatality rate for long falls in children aged 0–15 is 100 times greater than the fatality rate for short falls in babies aged 0–13 months.

This is obviously completely different from Chadwick et al.'s absurd assertion that 'the risk of death is eight times greater in children who fall from 1 to 4 feet than in those who fall from 10 to 45 feet'. The error here is to calculate the fatality rate of short falls as though the 100 children who were brought to the trauma centre for short falls are all children in the entire population who experienced short falls, just as Chadwick et al. assume that the 118 children brought in for long falls are all children who experienced long falls. They are clearly not aware that, by ignoring the data of the number of short falls among children, they are implicitly making this assumption.

Clearly the number of children actually brought to the hospital for short falls is the wrong denominator when considering the risk of death from short falls, which is of course in reality the number of fatalities per total number of short falls in a population. Ignoring the statistical information 'how many short falls normally happen in a population of children' that is entirely absent from the article thus leads to absurdly wrong statements such as 'the risk of dying from a short fall is eight times higher than from a long fall'. The seeming paradox that led Chadwick et al. to conclude that all the short fall stories were falsified is nothing but an optical illusion.

15.2.2 Ages of the Victims

The second example of important missing information is the ages of the children who died. Generally speaking, babies are more fragile than toddlers, toddlers more fragile than schoolchildren, and children more fragile than most adults ('Despite similar injury severity scores, infants sustained more skull fractures than toddlers (71% v. 39%)'; cf. [33]). But children who fall from heights greater than 10 feet must be climbing; they cannot be tiny pre-mobile babies. Most of the detailed information on the ages of the children who fell from different heights in Chadwick et al.'s study is absent. We are told that, among the 317 children brought to the trauma centre, there were 30 babies less than 1 year old, 145 toddlers aged 1–3, 61 children aged 4–6, 65 aged 7–12, and 16 aged 13–15, but the table of ages of the children who had short falls or long falls or the ages of the children who died is not given apart from what can be gleaned from the brief description of a few cases mentioned earlier in this chapter (namely that three of the short fall victims were aged 6 weeks and 11 and 13 months, and the single long fall fatality was 11 months old). These data are insufficient to draw any conclusions or to refine those of the article. However, were the complete data available, they could possibly lead to quite different conclusions.

To illustrate this, let's invent a purely theoretical, hypothetical but perfectly plausible set of data giving the ages of the children who fell and those of all the fatalities. We naturally suppose the great majority of infants aged less than 1 year fell from low heights, with only a small proportion of these physically capable of climbing up to a dangerous place and furthermore unsupervised. We also assume that few of the older children aged 4–15 are in the group where the height of the fall could not be determined, as children of this age can explain precisely what occurred. Finally, we place more toddlers in the long fall group than in the medium fall group, reflecting the fact that the average age of children who fall out of windows is known to be around 4, whereas medium falls tend to take place more on playgrounds, where children are on average somewhat older. The following table of hypothetical data respects these plausible hypotheses.

Let us imagine that the 100 children brought to the trauma centre for short falls, with average age 18 months, were hypothetically grouped as follows:

28 babies under age 1 (5 0–3, 11 3–6, 7 6–9, 4 9–12 in months)

73 toddlers aged 1–3

and that the 65 children who fell from a height of 5–9 feet were hypothetically grouped as follows:

1 baby under age 1

15 toddlers aged 1–3

49 children aged 4–15

whereas the 118 children who sustained long falls, with average age 4, were hypothetically grouped as follows:

1 baby under age 1

29 toddlers aged 1–3

87 children aged 4–15.

These hypothetical data are entirely plausible according to the considerations listed earlier in this chapter. The remaining 34 children (28 toddlers and 6 older children) who fell from unknown heights are not listed.

Let us also assume that all eight deaths occurred in babies aged 0–13 months, as we already know is the case for four of them. If this hypothetical information were known to be true, what would be the most likely explanation for the short fall and long fall fatality rates observed by Chadwick et al.? The most natural conclusion would be:

> Whether short or long, falls are much more dangerous and likely to be fatal in babies than in older children. The reason there are so few fatalities in the long fall group is because most tiny babies are more supervised and also unable to climb. In particular, even though the average age of children who fall out of windows is 4 years old, the only fatality was a child of 11 months.

Let me immediately make clear that I am not suggesting that this is in fact the correct interpretation of Chadwick et al.'s observations. Indeed, I am as far as possible from denying that child abuse exists and must be detected and stopped whenever possible; furthermore, the existence of additional injuries on children is a key element, which we will discuss further later in this chapter. This scenario has been given to illustrate the fact that invisible information can have major significance and lead to very different but equally natural hypotheses explaining the data, just as we saw in the previous section, and that, in its absence, reliable conclusions cannot be drawn. A lot of pitfalls can be avoided by including all of the relevant statistics in any study. The sections that follow contain several more striking examples of invisible information.

15.2.3 The True Risk of Death from Short Falls

It seems that the importance of knowing the true risk of death from short falls eventually came to Chadwick et al.'s attention – in 2008, nearly two decades after the publication of the article we are analysing, Chadwick and another group of colleagues published another article, entitled *Risk of Death Resulting from Short Falls among Young Children: Less than 1 in 1 million* [34] that deals precisely with this question. The authors use the only approach that really makes sense, namely an examination of databases and of previous studies in order to determine the number of deaths in small children that can reliably be attributed to short falls without suspicion of abuse. The plan is a good one, but as we will see, this article suffers like previous one from multiple problems in the way it was carried out.

A study of the California Epidemiology and Prevention for Injury Control Branch (EPIC) database covering the whole state of California yielded the following information. Over the 5-year period 1999–2003, 34 deaths due to falls were recorded for a population of 2.5 million children aged 0 through 4 years, of which 13 were classified as short falls. Chadwick et al. obtained the 13 corresponding death certificates and examined the causes of death in more detail. They excluded 7 cases that are not considered real cases of short falls, leaving a total of 6 'ordinary' short falls that were considered legitimate causes of death according to the medical records and not attributed to any abuse or inflicted injury. In the 2008 article, Chadwick et al. use this data to conclude that, if 6 such falls were seen in 2.5 million children over a 5-year period, then the expected fatality rate is about 0.48 per million children per year; this is the 'less than 1 in a million' of the title.

However, there are numerous reasons to believe that this fatality rate of 0.48 per million children per year is somewhat too low. To begin with, it is unclear exactly why Chadwick et al. discarded 7 of the 13 deaths recorded in the EPIC database as short fall deaths. They gave valid reasons for some of the exclusions, such as cases that involved falling furniture rather than falling children, and one fall from a second-story window. They further excluded two deaths attributed to suffocation following a fall, an explanation that seems somewhat mysterious, and one further case in which the fall height was not specified, even though it was classified as a short fall in the EPIC database. This one may truly have been a short fall and excluding it may incorrectly lower the frequency. Finally, they excluded a case where a child fell from the arms of an adult onto rocks. This again seems like a legitimate short fall – why exclude it? Is it because the description of the fall history would not be considered 'discrepant' in this case? There seems to be a whiff of circular reasoning in the choice to discard this example.

The second, more important reason to believe that the 0.48 figure may be too low comes from the existence of other studies. Both of the Chadwick et al. papers cite two earlier large-scale database studies that give higher risk assessments; the NEISS study [29] and the work of J. Hall et al. [23]. Both of these studies, already dismissed by Chadwick et al. in the 1991 article, are mentioned and dismissed once again in 2008. Since they both produce risk rates that are markedly different from the final rate of 0.48 per million children per year accepted by Chadwick et al., it is worth having a closer look at their reasons for rejecting them.

The NEISS database is specifically concerned with deaths involving commercial products. Over a 12-year period, it lists 9 deaths from falling off playground equipment in a population of 400,000 children under 5. As 6 of these cases were either from heights greater than 4 feet or had no witnesses, Chadwick et al. retain only 3 and thus calculate the risk of deaths from short falls in children as 3 in 400,000 over 12 years, which comes to an average rate of 0.625 such deaths per million children per year.

This might not seem significantly different from the rate of 0.48 emerging from the EPIC database – except that these fatalities are from playground falls alone and therefore exclude all falls of pre-mobile babies! Chadwick et al. do actually point this out, noting specifically that the database 'captures almost all product-related injuries' but 'may fail to capture deaths resulting from short falls that are not involved with products'. However, instead of noting that what this limitation implies is that the true risk of death from short fall is likely greater than 0.625 per million children per year, they take it as a reason to discard the NEISS data altogether as unreliable.

As for the Hall et al. study, its authors examined the records of the medical examiner of Cook County, Illinois, over a 4-year period and identified no fewer than 18 deaths. In their 1991 article, Chadwick et al. dismissed this study with the brief sentence 'Their work omits the detailed information necessary to exclude inflicted injury, and many of those cases might be in that category.' In the 2008 article, Chadwick and his co-authors are even briefer; the article is dismissed with the comment 'Fall histories not validated'.

It so happens that, in terms of population, Cook County is the second largest county in the United States, with about 300,000 children under 5. San Diego County is ranked fifth, so Chadwick et al. are hardly fair in stating that the Hall et al. study 'did not involve a large population'. Similarly, it is a bit absurd to complain that 'the conclusions are not quantitative' in Hall et al.'s study, since the risk of death from short falls per million children per year can be calculated from their data simply noting that 18 deaths per 300,000 children in 4 years corresponds to 60 deaths per million children in 4 years, or 15 deaths per million children per year, a figure that is more than 30 times higher than Chadwick et al.'s rate of 0.48 per million children per year. Stating that the conclusion of the Hall et al. study is 'not quantitative', yet adding that it nevertheless 'indicated a low frequency of short-fall deaths', is, to say the least, ingenuous.

This impression is reinforced by an exchange of letters published in the *Journal of Trauma* shortly after the appearance of the Hall et al. study [23]. At least three different authors addressed letters to the editor raising the same doubts about Hall et al.'s work as Chadwick et al., essentially that his results contradict previous studies and that, in order to exclude inflicted injury, it was insufficient to use merely the medical examiner's records together with a police investigation, but not the hospital records. The three earlier studies cited as contradicting Hall et al.'s work were respectively: one of 246 children under 5 who fell out of bed, another of 363 children under 5 who fell down stairs, and one of 85 children who fell off beds, gurneys or changing tables in hospitals. None of the children in these studies sustained any serious injury at all.

Here is another fallacy: it is simply not true that Hall et al.'s results contradict those of the three smaller studies. Applying their fatality rate of 15 deaths per million children per year to a group of 246 children, the expectation of seeing a fatal case is just 0.000246, which means there is a chance of just 0.0246 % – less than 3/100ths of 1%! – of actually seeing a fatality in a group of 246 children using Hall's risk rate.[2] (The figure becomes 0.0363% and 0.085% in the groups of 363 and 85 children.) Thus we see that Hall et al.'s fatality rate is perfectly coherent with the lack of fatal cases in the small studies.

As for their use of the medical examiner's records and police investigation, Hall et al. responded to the letters to the editor with a letter of their own in which they explained that each of the patients in the study

> had a complete report prepared by an investigator from the medical examiner's office. This gave a detailed description of the cause of the accident and a summary of the [ambulance, pre-hospital, and hospital] records. These reports were thus of superior quality to hospital records. All children had not only a complete investigation by the local police department but also by an investigator from the medical examiner's office. All children had a complete post-mortem plus full body X-rays . . . We cannot conceive of a more independent nor complete investigation.

Given the fact that this published exchange of letters took place in 1990, just before the publication of Chadwick et al.'s 1991 article in which they claim that the work of Hall et al. 'omits the detailed information necessary to exclude inflicted injury, and many of those cases might be in that category', and his similar (but more summary) dismissal of the Hall et al. study in 2008 merely with the words 'Fall histories not verified', Chadwick et al.'s choice to dismiss this study and their description of their reasons for doing so do not appear justifiable.

Certainly the risk rate of 15 deaths per million children per year in Hall et al. seems very high. Hall et al. admit that, in spite of the best efforts of the police and the medical examiner, 'it may be impossible to rule out all cases of abuse'. At the same time, it is also the case that the risk can be different in demographically different areas; it is greater in urban areas with many buildings, in areas of greater poverty where children grow up with less supervision, and in places where natural dangers are associated with geographic elements. Cook County is very different from San Diego; it has a significantly lower median income, another type of urban landscape, and vastly different weather. Indeed, it is worth noting that at least 2 of the 18 victims in Hall's study fell out of the arms of parents who slipped on ice, an unlikely circumstance in San Diego County.

15.2.4 Fallacy in the Final Conclusion

Even if we consider Chadwick et al.'s risk figure of 0.48 acceptable, it seems to be used by the authors to reach an erroneous conclusion. Indeed, it is quite clear from their article that Chadwick et al. interpret the figure of 0.48 deaths per million children

---

[2] One could object here that the children in these studies did not form a general population since they were all victims of falls. However, there is no real need to differentiate between the population of children who have sustained short falls and the general population, since just about every child has sustained short falls. If we were considering long falls, this would be a legitimate point and we would need to distinguish carefully between the rate of deaths among children who sustain long falls, which is high (1/118, according to Chadwick et al.'s data) and the rate of deaths from long falls among the general population of children (1/2.5 million children/5 years, or 0.08/million children/year, again according to Chadwick's data). Given that Chadwick gives 0.48/million/year as the risk of death from short falls, this shows that a random child in the population runs a risk of short fall death that is six times greater than their risk of a long fall death. This may seem like another surprising and paradoxical conclusion, but it is perfectly true, quite simply because short falls are so frequent and long falls so rare. Both death rates in the general population are extremely low.

per year as so low and indicating an event so extremely rare that, faced with an actual case of fatality due to an alleged short fall, the attending physician should consider the story as false and assume that they are seeing a case of inflicted injury. In particular, they consider that the very low fatality rate of 0.48 per million children per year justifies their earlier conclusion that the seven fatalities observed in the 1991 study are all cases with falsified histories.

However, that reasoning is wrong. It is a simple matter to use the risk rate of fatal short falls in a probability calculation to see how many legitimate deaths of small children from short falls one would expect to see in San Diego County over a 44-month period. Given that Chadwick et al.'s calculated rate is artificially low due to the exclusion of legitimate cases, we will simply use the probability figure of 1 in a million given in their title. As mentioned earlier, the population of children under 5 in San Diego County in the 1990s was about 200,000 observed over 44 months, which is equivalent to observing a population of about 733,333 children over 1 year. Using these figures and the binomial formula, we find that the probability of seeing zero fatal short falls in this population is equal to about 48%, so there is about a 52% chance of seeing at least one legitimate short fall fatality in the period and population under study, and indeed a 16% chance of seeing two or more – probabilities that are certainly not vanishingly small.[3]

The fact that Chadwick et al.'s table listing the associated injuries among the seven fatalities observed in the 1991 study reveals exactly two cases with no associated injuries at all shows that it is absolutely unjustified to decree on statistical grounds that these two histories were falsified and that the parents are guilty of abuse. The error consists in assuming that it is incredibly unlikely to see an event that only occurs with a frequency of 1 per million children per year, forgetting that if one is actually observing a population containing a million children, it is actually quite likely that one will see one or two occurrences of the 'rare' event.

15.3 Conclusion

It is obvious from Chadwick et al.'s tone and that of their colleagues that, since the 1990s, they have been engaged in an admirable battle to make sure cases of child abuse are detected and children are saved from inflicted injuries and swiftly removed from dangerous situations. Hall et al., however, write equally passionately about the danger involved in persuading people that short falls are benign and cannot be fatal. Indeed, according to their study, several of the 18 children who died in Cook County did so because their caregivers delayed seeking treatment due to a general impression that short falls cannot be very harmful: 'Delays in presentation were caused by both parents and emergency room personnel who felt that minor falls were benign and waited until late symptoms developed before becoming concerned.' Hall et al. assert that this represents a major problem: 'The myth ... that all minor falls are benign must be expunged; some can be serious. Abuse does need to be ruled out, but falls regardless of height are potentially fatal.' Both sides are trying to protect children. There should be no controversy between them. If there is one, it is due to misunderstandings about what statistics really tell us and errors in using them properly. In a world where statistics

[3] Letting $f = 1$ in a million $= 0.000001$ be the probability of a fatal short fall per child per year, the probability of seeing no fatal short falls in a population of $p = 733{,}333$ children over 1 year is given by $(1-f)^p \approx 0.48$.

were well gathered, well understood, and well-interpreted, this controversy would not exist.

References

1. Aoki N, Masuzawa H. Infantile acute subdural hematoma. *Journal of Neurosurgery*. 1984;61(2):273–80.
2. Atkinson N, Van Rijn R, Starling S. Childhood falls with occipital impacts. *Pediatric Emergency Care*. 2018;34 (12):837–41.
3. Ikeda A, Sato O, Tsugane R et al. Infantile acute subdural hematoma. *Child's Nervous System*. 1987;3(1):19–22.
4. Duhaime AC, Christian C, Armonda R, Hunter J, Hertle R. Disappearing subdural hematomas in children. *Pediatric Neurosurgery*. 1996;25(3):116–22.
5. Christian CW, Taylor AA, Hertle RW, Duhaime AC. Retinal hemorrhages caused by accidental household trauma. *Journal of Pediatrics*. 1999;135(1):125–7.
6. Plunkett J. Fatal pediatric head injuries caused by short-distance falls. *American Journal of Forensic Medicine and Pathology*. 2001;22(1):1–12.
7. Denton S, Mileusnic D. Delayed sudden death in an infant following an accidental fall: A case report with review of the literature. *American Journal of Forensic Medicine and Pathology*. 2003;24(4):371–6.
8. Lantz PE, Sinal SH, Stanton CA, Weaver RG Jr. Perimacular retinal folds from childhood head trauma. *British Medical Journal*. 2004;328(7442):754–6.
9. Gardner HB. A witnessed short fall mimicking presumed shaken baby syndrome (inflicted childhood neurotrauma). *Pediatric Neurosurgery*. 2007;43(5):433–5.
10. Lueder GT, Turner JW, Paschall R. Perimacular retinal folds simulating nonaccidental injury in an infant. *Archives of Ophthalmology*. 2006;124(12):1782–3.
11. Lantz PE, Couture DE. Fatal acute intracranial injury, subdural hematoma, and retinal hemorrhages caused by stairway fall. *Journal of Forensic Sciences*. 2011;56(6):1648–53.
12. Ramdas S, O'Colmain U, George NDL, Kirkpatrick M. Retinal haemorrhage in an infant following an accidental fall: A case report. *European Journal of Pediatrics*. 2014;173(10):1395–7.
13. Scheller J, Huisman TAGM. Moderate bilateral retinal hemorrhages in an infant following a short fall. *Clinical Pediatrics*. 2015;54(10):999–1002.
14. Steinbok P, Singhal A, Poskitt K, Cochrane DD. Early hypodensity on computed tomographic scan of the brain in an accidental pediatric head injury. *Neurosurgery*. 2007;60(4):689–95.
15. Shuman MJ, Hutchins KD. Severe retinal hemorrhages with retinoschisis in infants are not pathognomonic for abusive head trauma. *Journal of Forensic Sciences*. 2017;62(3):807–11.
16. Aoki N. Infantile acute subdural hematoma with retinal hemorrhage caused by minor occipital impact witnessed by an ICU nurse: A case report. *Journal of Pediatric Neurology and Neuroscience*. 2020;4 (1):47–50.
17. Mulligan CS, Adams S, Tzioumi D, Brown J. Injury from falls in infants under one year. *Journal of Paediatrics and Child Health*. 2017;53(8):754–60.
18. Behera C, Rautji R, Dogra TD. Fatal accidental fall from height in infants and children: A study from South Delhi. *Medicine, Science and the Law*. 2010;50 (1):22–4.
19. Burrows P, Trefan L, Houston R et al. Head injury from falls in children younger than 6 years of age. *Archives of Disease in Childhood*. 2015;100(11):1032–7.
20. Hughes J, Maguire S, Jones M, Theobald P, Kemp A. Biomechanical characteristics of head injuries from falls in children younger than 48 months. *Archives of Disease in Childhood*. 2016;101(4):310–15.
21. Hajiaghamemar M, Lan IS, Christian CW, Coats B, Margulies SS. Infant skull fracture

risk for low height falls. *International Journal of Legal Medicine*. 2019;133 (3):847–62.

22. Chaudhary S, Figueroa J, Shaikh S et al. Pediatric falls ages 0–4: Understanding demographics, mechanisms, and injury severities. *Injury Epidemiology*. 2018;5 (1):77–87.
23. Hall JR, Reyes HM, Horvat M, Meller J, Stein R. The mortality of childhood falls. *Journal of Trauma*. 1989;29(9):1273–5.
24. Joffe M, Diamond P, Helfer R et al. Letters to the editor. *Journal of Trauma*. 1990;30 (11):1421–3.
25. Leventhal JM, Edwards GA. Flawed theories to explain child physical abuse: What are the medical-legal consequences? *JAMA*. 2017;318(14):1317–18.
26. Chadwick DL, Chin S, Salerno C, Landsverk J, Kitchen L. Deaths from falls in children: How far is fatal? *Journal of Trauma*. 1991;31(10):1353–5.
27. Schneps L, Rossant C. Chutes de faible hauteur et syndrome du bébé secoué, erreurs numériques et logiques. In *Hématomes sous-duraux et collections péri-cérébrales du petit nourrisson*. B. Échenne, A. Couture, G. Sébire, eds. Sauramps, 2020, pp. 299–328.
28. Williams RA. Injuries in infants and small children resulting from witnessed and corroborated free falls. *Journal of Trauma*. 1991;31:1350–2.
29. Sweeney TB. X-rated playgrounds? [Commentary]. *Pediatrics*. 1979;64:961.
30. Institut de Veille Sanitaire. *Les chutes accidentelles de grande hauteur d'enfants en Ile-de-France, Nord-Pas-de-Calais et Provence-Alpes-Côtes d'Azur*. Institut de Veille Sanitaire, 2006.
31. Reid SR, Roesler JS, Gaichas AM, Tsai AK. The epidemiology of pediatric traumatic brain injury in Minnesota. *Archives of Pediatric and Adolescent Medicine*. 2001;155(7):784–9.
32. Kravitz H, Driessen G, Gomberg R, Korach A. Accidental falls from elevated surfaces in infants from birth to one year of age. *Pediatrics*. 1969;44(5 suppl):869–76.
33. Ibrahim N, Wood J, Margulies S, Christian C. Influence of age and fall type on head injuries in infants and toddlers. *International Journal of Developmental Neuroscience*. 2012;30(3):201–6.
34. Chadwick DL, Bertocci G, Castillo E et al. Annual risk of death resulting from short falls among young children: Less than 1 in 1 million. *Pediatrics*. 2008;121:1213–24.

Chapter 16

Epidemiology of Findings Claimed to Be Highly Specific for Shaken Baby Syndrome/Abusive Head Trauma, a Prerequisite to Improve Diagnosis of Child Abuse

Ulf Högberg

'[...] ensure both that a minimum number of false-positive cases is included and that a minimum of true cases is missed.' [1]

16.1 Introduction

Epidemiological studies on the occurrence, distribution, and determinants of findings claimed to be highly specific for shaken baby syndrome/abusive head trauma (SBS/AHT) provide valuable data for improved/evidence-based diagnosis of child abuse. The World Health Organization (WHO) and the International Society for Prevention of Child Abuse and Neglect (ISPCAN) emphasise the importance of basic epidemiological information to achieve high predictive value of the diagnostic criteria, both sensitive and specific, for the diagnosis of child abuse, in order to 'ensure both that a minimum number of false-positive cases is included and that a minimum of true cases is missed' [1].

Already in 1978, it was considered that the predictive value of screening using a protocol for latent markers of child abuse might be low in unselected populations. In other words, there was (and is) a real possibility that misclassification can occur when diagnostic categories overlap, as in the case of abuse and accidents/diseases [2].

The diagnostic test is a cornerstone of healthcare. Hospital-based studies, case studies, and observational studies reporting certain diseases or syndromes may be misleading if the premises are based on erroneous beliefs regarding a condition that may have a variety of causes. Thus, medical mistakes and iatrogenesis continually challenge medical practice. The capacity of a diagnostic test to identify a disease or syndrome depends on a proper reference test based on population incidence rates of findings that may be part of the disease or syndrome. Otherwise, predictivity, sensitivity, and specificity can be misleading and indeed wrong.

A systematic review by Maguire et al. has estimated the predictive value of findings like retinal haemorrhage (RH) or rib fracture for diagnosing AHT to be around 60%, and for long bone fracture 35%, while for the combinations of two or more of these findings, such as both RH and rib fracture, or RH, rib fracture, and long bone fracture, the predictive value for AHT rises to nearly 100% [3]. This systematic review, among others, was assessed by the Swedish Agency for Health and Social Services Assessment (SBU) to be of low quality (high risk of bias) because of circular reasoning, lack of defined exposure – that is, shaking – and use of the general term AHT without a detailed description of specific findings [4] (see Chapter 10).

Circularity bias has been identified as a major flaw in current knowledge about SBS/AHT because so many publications are based on case series, case control, or observational studies, without any proper reference test. The critical issue in the diagnostic process of infant abuse is whether the findings assessed by physicians might have other, non-abuse causes such as disease or accidental trauma [4]. The SBU report has identified several evidence gaps in the diagnosis of SBS, leading to the major question: how can epidemiological research findings contribute to improved evidence-based diagnosis of child abuse?

Studies on occurrence – that is, incidence rates – by surveillance, observation, or screening can provide information of distribution by time, place, and population. Observational studies and clinical epidemiological case control studies can add new data about causal mechanisms (biological and injury), behavioural and social aspects (e.g., doctor-dependent factors in the diagnostic process of child abuse), and geographical aspects (e.g., differences that might reflect different degree of use of a SBS/AHT protocol in detection of child abuse in different areas).[1]

Sweden, which has a lower rate of diagnosed SBS/AHT than the United Kingdom or the United States (see Chapter 10), may contribute valuable information on these matters. Furthermore, epidemiological research, both population-based and clinical, can also provide evidence of causal inferences by applying the Bradford Hill criteria, though this is inherently probabilistic.[2] Clinical case control studies of hypothesis testing and analytical research could potentially also provide improved evidence of other causal chains explaining certain findings currently stated to be specific for SBS/AHT.

16.2 Swedish Population Data and Diagnostic Considerations of Infant Abuse

Swedish health registries offer a unique possibility to provide epidemiologic knowledge on findings said to indicate SBS/AHT. While for mainly symptomatic findings caused by disease or trauma, healthcare statistics should come rather close to true population incidence rates, for mainly asymptomatic and occult radiological findings, the true incidence and prevalence rates are not possible to determine without screening. Incidental cases can indicate underlying disease or trauma as well as the use of a screening protocol for abuse. Thus, for mainly invisible and occult radiological findings, incidences are uncertain and

---

1 The number of instances of illness/injuries commencing, or of persons falling ill, during a given period in a specified population. More generally, the number of new health-related events in a defined population within a specified period of time. It may be measured as a frequency count, a rate, or a proportion. (Porta M. A *Dictionary of epidemiology: International Epidemiological Association*. 6th ed. 2014)

2 Bradford Hill criteria, used to infer causation, are as follows. Associations that are strong, consistent, and specific are likely to be causal. Obviously the cause must precede the effect in time. A dose–response relationship is important: the severity of the cause should be positively correlated with the severity of the effect. The relationship between cause and effect should be biologically plausible and form part of a coherent biological theory. Ideally there should be experimental evidence confirming a cause-and-effect relationship. In some, cases argument by analogy can be useful to clarify complex relationships. Acres and Morris 2014 http://dx.doi.org/10.1016/j.mehy.2013.09.017e.

reported estimations vary depending on methodology, type of injuries, and geographic location. Short fall accidents can be classified as slight to moderate trauma and are reported by ICD10 codes (W00–W19): falls on the same level, falls involving beds, chairs, or furniture, falls from being carried, and falls from stairs and steps.

By linkage of information from the Swedish Patient Register (inpatient and outpatient specialised care), Death Cause Register, Medical Birth Register, and Register of Out-of-Home Care, we have analysed the epidemiology for infants aged less than 1 year born in Sweden in the period 1997–2014. We have shown that findings of subdural haemorrhage (SDH), RH, rib fractures, and long bone fractures were strongly associated with a diagnosis of abuse among Swedish infants [5].

In the remainder of this chapter, we will address the present state of knowledge from Swedish data (population epidemiology, and case control studies) of SDH [6, 7], RH [5, 7, 8], long bone [9–11] and rib fractures [5, 7, 9, 12], incidences, age and sex distributions, perinatal risk factors, proportion of fall accidents, proportion of abuse diagnoses, and hypothesis testing conducted up to now regarding their association with SBS/AHT. We note that our findings concern the period before the publication of the SBU report, when a steep increase in infant abuse diagnosis was observed (see Chapter 10).

16.3 Subdural Haemorrhage

16.3.1 Incidence, Age, and Sex Distribution

In national registers, categories of SDH are defined by ICD codes. We found that 18.0% had a birth injury (P10.0), 45.3% had traumatic SDH (S06.5), and 31.7% had non-traumatic SDH (I62.0), while 4.9% had both diagnoses (S06.5 and I62.0).

The overall Swedish incidence was 16.5 per 100,000 infants. Few comparable studies of national incidence rates have been published, although an incidence of 24.1 per 100,000 infants is reported from the British Isles [13]. The Swedish case fatality rate was 6.2%, while 19% for children aged 0–2 is reported from the British Isles [13].

We found a marked male preponderance, 64.7%, equal to that reported from the British Isles [13]. Most SDH cases are diagnosed during the first 6 months of life; only 17.2% were older at diagnosis. Mean and median age at diagnosis for all SDH cases was 3.3 and 2.5 months, respectively. This is comparable to figures reported from the British Isles [13].

Perinatal Risk Factors

When comparing all SDH cases with the general population, statistically significant increases were found for the following factors: preeclampsia, dystocic labour, non-normal mode of delivery, prematurity, multiple birth, small-for-gestational-age, birth asphyxia, cephalic haematoma, respiratory distress, neonatal sepsis, convulsions, and other cerebral disturbances of the newborn. For the maternal and perinatal risk factors, no statistically significant differences could be found between traumatic SDH and non-traumatic SDH, or between either of those two and the diagnosis of abuse.

Subdural haematoma (0–6 days) had distinct risk factors of dystocic labour, emergency caesarean delivery, assisted vaginal delivery, asphyxia, preterm birth, birth injury to the scalp or skeleton, and neonatal morbidity, especially convulsions and other cerebral disturbances of the newborn. Dystocic labour or mode of delivery had no association with SDH beyond 6 days of age. Male sex and preterm birth (32–36 weeks) had increased odds for traumatic SDH, but had no other risk increase.

Multiple birth, preterm birth, small-for-gestational-age (< 2.5 percentile), and neonatal convulsions showed increased odds for both non-traumatic SDH and abuse-diagnosed SDH. For abuse-diagnosed SDH, the odds were even higher than for non-traumatic SDH of being born before week 32 or being small for gestational age.

16.3.2 Accidental Falls

For Swedish cases of SDH in children aged < 1 year, 34% were due to alleged falls, while for the subgroup of SDH among cases diagnosed as abuse it was 16%. Comparable figures are available from the Hobbs study in the British Isles reporting 7 accidents out of 186 SDH cases (4%) in children < 2 years of age [13], but it was also reported that 'Carers provided a history of minor injury in 41/97 cases of NAHI and in 2/16 undetermined cases.' Whether accidental falls were among those with 'minor injury' cannot be ascertained from the British Isles study, but it is unlikely that the risk of exposure to falls differs substantially between the two settings. In the study by Hobbs et al., the proportion of carers reporting accidental falls was 28% (50/182), not much lower than in Sweden. These observations indicate that a different clinical understanding of whether slight or moderate trauma can cause traumatic SDH or re-bleeding from a chronic or subacute SDH/hygroma might be one explanation of the different proportions of abuse diagnoses among SDH cases between the British Isles and Sweden.

16.3.3 Proportion Having an Abuse Diagnosis

In the British Isles, 57% of SDH cases were diagnosed as non-accidental head injuries [13], while the proportion in Sweden was considerably lower, only 19%. There was a sixfold difference in incidences for SDH and abuse between the British Isles and Sweden, 14.2 and 2.3 per 100 000, respectively [6, 13].

16.3.4 Does Traumatic Shaking Cause Subdural Haematoma?

The SBU report [4] concluded as follows (see Chapter 10):

- There is limited scientific evidence that the triad and therefore its components can be associated with traumatic shaking (low-quality evidence).[3]
- There is insufficient scientific evidence on which to assess the diagnostic accuracy of the triad in identifying traumatic shaking (very low-quality evidence).

We have now further tested the hypothesis that shaking can cause SDH, RH, and encephalopathy, using a definition of physical abuse by shaking that is independent of medical findings or symptoms – that is, not compromised by circularity [7].

In order to accomplish this, we evaluated symptoms and medical findings in infants subjected to admitted or witnessed shaking, with or without blunt force head impact. To our knowledge, this is the first study assessing the association of SDH and RH from prior witnessed or admitted physical abuse by shaking. Hence, in this study no cases of confessions of shaking provided under certain conditions – for example, in a legal setting – or

[3] Three components of a whole. The triad associated with SBS usually comprises SDH, RH, and encephalopathy.

shaking in attempted resuscitation cases, were included, as they were in the systematic review of Edwards et al. [14].

We were able to retrieve medical records for 257 out of 337 infants with any diagnosis of maltreatment in Sweden during the period 1997–2014. Out of these 257, we found 36 satisfying our inclusion criteria. Witnessed shaking was defined as shaking that was either directly observed by a witness or filmed (e.g., by webcam or smartphone). Admitted shaking was narrowly defined as a spontaneously delivered history of shaking before or in direct connection with seeking care, taking place before any diagnostic procedures such as computed tomography (CT), magnetic resonance imaging (MRI), or fundoscopy were performed.

We found no cases of SDH or RH among 30 infants with no possibly predisposing factors who were subjected to shaking with or without blunt force trauma. Six infants had finding(s) suggestive of physical abuse; 2 of them had possible acute intracranial pathology. One of those, born preterm, had combined shaking and impact to the head, and the findings were SDH (acute and chronic/hygroma), subarachnoid haemorrhage, suspected cortical vein thrombosis, RH, and bruises. The other infant had subarachnoid haemorrhage (acute) and SDH (chronic).

These findings do not support the hypothesis that acute SDH or RH are caused by isolated shaking of a healthy infant. This is contrary to the study by Feldman et al. presenting five cases of independently witnessed shaking with SDH and RH [15]. However, in that study, the case descriptions are too sparse and the definition of an independent witness falls short of the usual child abuse standard (at least one adult, unrelated to and not involved in the care of, the child)

Indeed, our findings imply that SDH or RH have low sensitivity for AHT; believing these features have a high predictive value for abuse leads to a serious risk of false positive determinations of abuse. We conclude that the results of this study do not support the notion that certain medical findings are highly suggestive of shaking to the exclusion of other possible causes. Nevertheless, our results do indicate that isolated shaking may cause intracranial haemorrhage with or without RH in vulnerable infants having certain risk factors.

16.4 Retinal Haemorrhage

The overall incidence of RH in the Swedish health register was 7.9 per 100,000 (n = 147), of which 49% were more than 1 month of age. The overall proportion of abuse was 19% [6]. However, for infants beyond 1 month of age, the proportion of abuse was 36%. Of these, 85% had concomitant SDH.

There are conflicting hypotheses that non-birth-related RH in infants is independent of intracranial pathology – that is, caused by direct forces in the eye, vitreo-retinal traction forces versus RH being secondary to intracranial pathology associated with raised intracranial pressure (see Chapters 3 and 9). These hypotheses have now been tested in a Swedish national case control study [8]. We again used the 257 infants for whom medical records could be retrieved from the total of 337 infants with any maltreatment diagnosis in Sweden during the period 1997–2014. For this study, inclusion criteria were that the infant had to have been examined with both fundoscopy and neuroimaging by CT and/or MRI (n = 148). Medical findings and reported type of trauma in infants investigated for suspected physical abuse were compared with presence (n = 29) or absence of RH (n = 119).

We found a strong association between RH and intracranial pathology in infants with suspected SBS/AHT. Almost all (97%) infants with RH also had intracranial pathology (chronic and/or acute SDH with or without acute subarachnoid haemorrhage, non-specific white matter changes, suspected cortical venous thrombosis), whereas only a small proportion (13%) without RH did. Conversely, a large proportion (62%) of infants with intracranial pathology also had RH. Retinal haemorrhage without intracranial pathology was found in only two cases. In both, the RH was unilateral. In one of them, RH in a 3-week-old infant may have originated at birth. For infants harbouring bilateral RH, the association with intracranial pathology was absolute. Findings indicative of raised intracranial pressure were found in 59% in the RH group compared to 27% in the non-RH group. Neurological symptoms (vomiting, seizures, lowered level of consciousness, and apnoea) were found in 76% in the RH group as opposed to 10% in the non-RH group.

The conclusions from these findings are that non-birth-related RH in infants is secondary to intracranial pathology compatible with raised intracranial pressure, which may be of traumatic or non-traumatic origin, and not the result of traction forces between the retina and vitreous body acting directly on the retinal vessels. Further, the presence or absence of RH cannot be regarded as a reliable basis for determining the underlying aetiology of the intracranial pathology. Finally, we concluded that RH is likely to have low sensitivity for detecting head trauma, thus also for ruling out infant maltreatment, making RH of limited value in the investigation of suspected infant abuse.

16.5 Fractures

We analysed long bone and rib fractures during infancy by incidence, age and sex distributions, and trauma. We have moreover explored the metabolic bone disease hypothesis for fractures by analysing perinatal and infant risk factors [9–12, 18]. We plan to test the metabolic bone disease hypothesis in clinical case control studies using data of biochemical or radiological signs (other than classic metaphyseal lesions (CMLs)) of healing rickets or risk factors for intrauterine rickets.

16.5.1 Long Bone Fractures

16.5.1.1 Population Incidence, Age, and Sex Distributions

The Swedish population-based study shows an incidence of long bone fracture among infants aged < 1 year of 112.8 per 100,000 [9]. This is comparable to a multi-hospital-based study from England reporting an incidence of 94.5 per 100,000 [16]. Our study showed mean and median age of 8 and 9 months respectively. There was a male preponderance, 56%, for fractures of infants younger than 6 months, but not for 6–12 months.

The Swedish incidence of non-birth-related femur shaft fracture, 15.4 per 100,000, more prevalent in the 6–12 month age group, is higher than that reported from the United Kingdom [17]. The incidence of humerus shaft fractures, 7.3 per 100,000, more prevalent during the first 6 months, seems to be higher than that previously reported [11].

16.5.1.2 Perinatal and Infant Risk Factors

Metabolic bone disease risk factors for any long bone fracture were maternal obesity, male sex, prematurity, and rickets/vitamin D deficiency [9]. For femur shaft fracture before the age of 6 months, the risk factors were multiple births, prematurity, and small-for-gestational-age, while from 6–12 months only small-for-gestational-age prevailed [11]. Only a few cases had diagnoses of osteogenesis imperfecta or rickets/vitamin D deficiency. It should be noted that although not diagnosed as birth-related, early femur and humerus shaft fractures were associated with the risk factor of a difficult birth [11], which may indicate a delayed diagnosis of an unobserved birth-related fracture [18].

16.5.1.3 Proportion of Reported Accidental Falls

Accidental falls were reported in 72.0% cases of long bone fracture (all types), 76.7% for femur shaft fracture, and 58.4% for humerus shaft fracture. For both of these categories a lower proportion was observed during the first 6 months of life. No accidental fall was reported for one-third of these infants, which is comparable to the UK report for femur shaft fractures [15], but not compatible with previous Swedish hospital studies of fractures in children. One explanation for this could be that there were detailed clinical circumstances in the records, but not a registered ICD-code of an accidental fall. The proportion of fall accidents for humerus shaft fractures was considerably higher than that reported from the United States [11].

16.5.1.4 Proportion of Infants Having Any Abuse Diagnosis

For femur and humerus shaft fractures the proportions having any abuse diagnosis were 9% and 11% respectively [11]. However, out of all long bone fractures the proportion was 2.7% [9]. The proportion found in the multi-hospital study in England was 18.9%, seven times higher [19, 20]. By adding cases of long bone fractures without a concomitant abuse diagnosis but with out-of-home-care [21], the Swedish proportion increased to 3.8%. Still, the proportions in Sweden and England differ by a factor of five in spite of similar incidences of long bone fractures. The difference with the United States is even higher; the proportion of abuse-related fractures for radius/ulna, tibia/fibula, humerus, and femur are 62.1%, 58.0%, 43.1%, and 30.5% respectively [22].

16.5.2 Rib Fractures

Rib fractures are claimed as highly specific of SBS/AHT and are strongly associated with a diagnosis of abuse among infants in the Swedish setting [5]. The population incidence of rib fractures is not possible to estimate as the majority are asymptomatic, occult, and mostly in different stages of healing [12]. However, it should be noted that in some cases they may be found during clinical examination by a popping sound from the chest [12]. Incidental cases are mainly found when X-rays are performed for other reasons, such as abuse investigation protocol, health investigation after a fall, transport accidents, vomiting, infection, before a major operation, and any other reasons for chest X-ray, such as preterm or difficult birth [10, 12]. Rib fractures are mainly found in very young infants. Mean and median ages are 3.3 and 2.9 months [9]. The male preponderance is pronounced: 78% [12].

16.5.2.1 Perinatal and Infant Risk Factors

The most prominent risk factors for metabolic bone disease are preterm birth followed by maternal obesity, but small-for-gestational-age does not appear to be a risk factor [9]. In a few cases, rickets/vitamin D deficiency or osteogenesis imperfecta are diagnosed either concomitantly or subsequently to the observation of rib fractures [12].

16.5.2.2 Proportion with Abuse Diagnosis

In the Swedish setting, the proportion of infants with rib fractures also having a diagnosis of abuse is 42% (28/66) [12]. A systematic review reports a considerably higher proportion, 67% to 82% [22]; however, circular reasoning limits the reliability of such high percentages. A recent systematic review only using admitted, witnessed, or video-recorded cases as a reference test, with the purpose of avoiding circular reasoning and inclusion bias, concluded that 'there is insufficient scientific evidence that rib fractures can be caused by abuse, and therefore also insufficient scientific evidence on which to determine the diagnostic accuracy of rib fractures for abuse' [23].

16.6 Interpretation and Conclusions

Promotion of patient safety is an overarching consideration in preventing harm in healthcare. An estimated 10–20% of harm in Swedish healthcare is due to diagnostic and other errors, while the percentage for abuse diagnosis among Swedish infants has not yet been addressed. Correct diagnosis of infant abuse comprises the ethical principles of beneficence, non-maleficence, and justice. Misclassification, false positives, and false negatives can be extremely severe for afflicted children and their parents and should be minimised [1]. The consequences of false positives among alleged SBS cases were mentioned as early as 1997 by Dr Sunderland: 'In the absence of definitive physical signs we may need to profess fallibility. Humility avoids hubris. False diagnoses not only harm children and their families but also devalue the profession' [24].

We have explored Swedish parents' experiences of seeking healthcare and encountering allegations of SBS/AHT. The qualitative analysis showed the overarching theme of 'fighting for protection of their child after being trapped by doctors' with sub-themes of 'being accused of injuring the child', 'chaos and powerlessness', and 'wounded post-traumatic growth'. The study concluded that being wrongly accused of child abuse and alleged SBS/AHT evoked emotions of intense stress, which parents endured because they were fighting to regain custody of their child/ren. However, the trauma had a long-term impact on their life with residual post-traumatic stress symptoms and mistrust towards paediatric healthcare providers and authorities [25].

The geographical differences in findings associated with SBS/AHT might have several explanations, such as differences in socioeconomic settings, abuse exposure, and healthcare utilisation. However, a major driver contributing to the geographical differences in cases attributed to abuse is likely to be different interpretation and implementation of scientific evidence supporting an abuse diagnosis.

The similar incidences of SDH and long bone fractures in Sweden and the United Kingdom but with huge differences in those attributed to abuse indicate that this may well be the case. If the mechanism of accidental falls is not accepted as a possible cause of SDH, the low proportion of abuse diagnosed (14.1%) among Swedish infants must be due to missed abuse. If, on the other hand, accidental falls are plausible causes of SDH, then confirmation bias or selection error in clinical diagnosis [26], based on the belief that short falls cannot cause SDH, or rejecting carers' histories as unreliable, would explain the high proportion (52.2%) of British infants with SDH being diagnosed as abused.

It should be noted that neither of these situations excludes the other; both may be simultaneously true. However, it indicates that risk factors for SDH have been overlooked in the settings of perinatal vulnerability, prematurity, and small-for-gestational-age, whose rates were the same for infants with acute (non-traumatic) SDH and those with SDH attributed to abuse.

Similarly, the incidence of long bone fracture is similar in Sweden and the United Kingdom, but the proportion attributed to abuse differs by a factor of five. This huge geographical difference is unlikely to be due to a vast difference in exposure to abuse; it is much more likely to be due to differences in diagnostic considerations of the cause of the fracture, whether accidental or non-accidental, and the knowledge and significance of bone fragility disorders that may contribute to fractures as shown from our studies.

Certainly, the geographical differences indicate an implementation gap of evidence-based child protection, an evidence gap that calls for further research. What is the scientific evidence for the statements that SDH and fractures can be, or are always, caused by abuse? The SBU report identified several evidence gaps in the diagnosis of infant abuse (see Chapter 10), and WHO and ISPCAN emphasise the need for further research [1]. Further research on infant abuse, its circumstances, and specific findings that are indicative of abuse, is urgently needed in order to improve the practice of evidence-based child protection.

References

1. World Health Organization (WHO). *Preventing child maltreatment: A guide to taking action and generating evidence.* World Health Organization, 2006.
2. Daniel JH, Newberger EH, Reed RB, et al. Child abuse screening: Implications of the limited predictive power of abuse discriminants from a controlled family study of pediatric social illness. *Child Abuse and Neglect.* 1978;2:247–59.
3. Maguire SA, Kemp AM, Lumb RC, et al. Estimating the probability of abusive head trauma: A pooled analysis. *Pediatrics.* 2011;128(3):e550–64.
4. Elinder G, Eriksson A, Hallberg B et al. Traumatic shaking: The role of the triad in medical investigations of suspected traumatic shaking. *Acta Paediatrica.* 2018;107(Suppl 472):3–23.
5. Högberg U, Lampa E, Högberg G et al. Infant abuse diagnosis associated with abuse head trauma criteria: Incidence increase due to overdiagnosis? *European Journal of Public Health.* 2018;28(4):641–6.
6. Högberg U, Andersson J, Squier W et al. Epidemiology of subdural haemorrhage during infancy: A population-based register study. *PloS One.* 2018:1–17.
7. Thiblin I, Andersson J, Wester K et al. Medical findings and symptoms in infants exposed to witnessed or admitted abusive shaking: A nationwide registry study. *PLoS One.* 2020;15(10):e0240182.
8. Thiblin I, Andersson J, Wester K, et al. Retinal haemorrhage in infants investigated for suspected maltreatment is strongly correlated with intracranial pathology. *Acta Paediatrica.* 2021;111 (4):800–8.
9. Högberg U, Andersson J, Högberg G, et al. Metabolic bone disease risk strongly contributing to long bone and rib fractures during early infancy: A population register study. *PLoS One.* 2018;13(12):e0208033.
10. Högberg U, Fellman V, Thiblin I, et al. Difficult birth is the main contributor to birth-related fracture and accidents to other neonatal fractures. *Acta Paediatrica.* 2020;109(10):2040–8.
11. Von Heideken J, Thiblin I, Högberg U. The epidemiology of infant shaft fractures of femur or humerus by incidence, birth,

accidents, and other causes. *BMC Musculoskeletal Disorders*. 2020;21(1):840.

12. Högberg U, Thiblin I. Rib fractures in infancy, case-series and register case-control study from Sweden. *Journal of Pediatric Endocrinology and Metabolism*. 2021;34(3):363–72.
13. Hobbs C, Childs AM, Wynne J, et al. Subdural haematoma and effusion in infancy: An epidemiological study. *Archives of Disease in Childhood*. 2005;90 (9):952–5.
14. Edwards GA, Maguire SA, Gaither JR, et al. What do confessions reveal about abusive head trauma? A systematic review. *Child Abuse Review*. 2020;29(3):253–68.
15. Feldman KW, Melville JD, Johnson KL et al. Abusive head trauma follows witnessed infant shaking. *Child Abuse Review*. 2022:e2739.
16. Mitchell PD, Brown R, Wang T et al. Multicentre study of physical abuse and limb fractures in young children in the East Anglia region, UK. *Archives of Disease in Childhood*. 2019;104(10):956–61.
17. Talbot C, Davis N, Majid I et al. Fractures of the femoral shaft in children: National epidemiology and treatment trends in England following activation of major trauma networks. *Bone and Joint Journal*. 2018;100-B(1):109–18.
18. Högberg U, Winbo J, Fellman V. Population-based register study of children born in Sweden from 1997 to 2014 showed an increase in rickets during infancy. *Acta Paediatrica*. 2019;108(11):2034–40.
19. Högberg U, Andersson J, Högberg G, et al. Why is there a multi-fold difference in diagnosis of abuse among infants with long bone fracture in East Anglia compared with Sweden? *Archives of Disease in Childhood*. 2019;104(11):1122.
20. Mitchell P, Brown R, Wang T, et al. Challenges in comparing physical abuse, fractures and metabolic bone disease in young children in the UK and Sweden. *Archives of Disease in Childhood*. 2019;104 (11):1122–3.
21. Högberg U, Sennerstam R, Högberg G et al. Medical diagnoses among infants at entry in out-of-home care: A Swedish population-register study. *Health Science Report*. 2019;2(8):e133.
22. Paine CW, Fakeye O, Christian CW, et al. Prevalence of abuse among young children with rib fractures: A systematic review. *Pediatric Emergency Care*. 2019;35 (2):96–103.
23. Güvencel A. With what certainty can it be claimed that rib fractures or classical metaphyseal lesions in infants are attributed to physical abuse? A systematic literature review [MSc]. University of Dundee, 2019.
24. Sunderland R. Head injury: Abuse or accident. *Archives of Disease in Childhood*. 1997;76:393–7.
25. Högberg U, Eriksson G, Högberg G, et al. Parents' experiences of seeking health care and encountering allegations of shaken baby syndrome: A qualitative study. *PLoS One*. 2020;15(2):e0228911.
26. Groopman J. *How doctors think*. Mifflin, 2007.

Chapter 17

Shaken Baby Syndrome

Exploring Concerns about the 'Triad' Diagnosis and Its Statistical Validation Using a Causal Bayesian Network

Norman Fenton and Scott McLachlan

'It is said that for a scientific theory to be valid, it must be factually based. For a medical theory, all that is required is that doctors believe it.'
John Blatt [1]

17.1 Introduction

During the 1970s, radiologist John Caffey described battered baby syndrome and in particular that the component whiplash shaking need not be particularly violent to potentially result in permanent brain damage [2, 3].[1] Caffey catalogued apparently innocent, accepted, habitual practices that could whiplash the brain and lead to permanent brain damage.[2] While Caffey and Guthkelch [4] both asserted that shaking could cause intracranial and retinal injuries, neither ever suggested that those injuries are caused only by shaking or abuse. However, by the late 1970s, child abuse literature cited both authors in claiming that infants presenting with encephalopathy, thin subdural haemorrhages, and retinal haemorrhages – the triad – always or nearly always evidenced shaking and abuse.[3] One commentator later summarised: The mechanism of shaking and the so-named syndrome gained immediate acceptance and enormously widespread popularity, with no real investigation or even question as to its scientific validity (see [6]).

What is interesting about the largely unquestioned ascent of shaken baby syndrome (SBS) is that its key tenets contradicted pre-existing understandings and literature. Shaken baby syndrome relied on the premise that retinal haemorrhages (RH) are traumatic injuries typically caused by shaking, yet long-standing literature identified RH as merely a potential secondary complication of intracranial haemorrhage and raised pressure, regardless of the mechanism or cause (see also Chapters 3 and 9).[4] It also rejects such asymptomatic

[1] Caffey describes whiplash shaking as vigorous manual shaking of infants by the extremities or shoulders resulting in whiplash-induced intracranial and intraocular bleeding absent external signs of head trauma.

[2] These include 'such playful practices' as repeated vigorous tossing of a baby into the air, 'riding the horse, in which the infant faces the parent while sitting on his pendulant shin', and other similar activities.

[3] See page 65 of [5]: 'In an otherwise healthy child who is outside of the neonatal period, characteristics of intracranial and retinal haemorrhaging help distinguish between accidental and AHT.'

[4] See [7]: 'Retinal haemorrhages occur because elevated cerebral pressure increases central retinal venous pressure.'

occurrences as the routine observance of cerebral haemorrhage and RH in infants after normal vaginal birth.[5] Studies have established that RH is present in one quarter to one half of all vaginal deliveries – and may be evident on ophthalmic examination for as much as 8 weeks post-natally [9, 10].

Before 1987, the paediatric community made little effort to test or validate SBS.[6] A 1986 review of the SBS literature concluded little had been learned about whiplash shaken infant syndrome in the 12 years since Caffey's original report [12]. The first challenge to SBS was raised in 1987 by Ann-Christine Duhaime, a paediatric neurosurgeon, together with a team that included biomechanical engineers. They constructed models of infants with various neck and head properties to measure forces created by shaking and impact [13]. They retrospectively examined SBS cases, which revealed that many of the babies had impact trauma to their heads, including several who had skull fractures or contusions not identified until autopsy. They also observed that adult volunteers could not shake the models sufficiently hard to generate acceleration within the injury range believed necessary to cause intracranial injury.

By contrast, when models' heads were impacted against a padded surface, the accelerations generated reached estimated thresholds to cause subdural haemorrhage and brain injury. This study concluded that severe cases attributed to shaking could not have resulted from shaking alone (see [13] and Chapter 14). However, the Duhaime study did not cause the paediatric community to ask the obvious questions: If these babies' injuries were not caused by shaking, then what did cause them and how do we know they were abused?

Indeed, despite this challenge, the SBS narrative continued to gather momentum with the notorious case of Louise Woodward adding to the confusion (see this book's foreword) [14, 15]. Like Dr Guthkelch,[7] Dr Patrick Barnes, the paediatric radiologist whose expert testimony had been crucial to her successful prosecution, has maintained since 2011 that he would not give the same testimony today.[8] 'We started realising there were a number of medical conditions that can affect a baby's brain and look like the findings that we used to attribute to shaken baby syndrome or child abuse' [16, 17]. Several subsequent studies have confirmed that shaking generates accelerations well below those thought necessary to cause SBS [18–23].

17.2 The Current Challenges

The current state of affairs on the SBS debate is thus, as Randy Papetti puts it, contradictory: 'Critics now regularly challenge past convictions based on SBS' purported scientific collapse [24, 25, 31], yet prosecutors and child protection agencies continue to file SBS

5 See [8]: 'Asymptomatic brain and retinal haemorrhages were identifiable in up to 43% of all vaginally delivered children.'

6 See [11]: 'No one has yet marshalled an argument to support a conclusion that the estimated infant injury thresholds are off by such a significant magnitude as to overcome the conclusions of the research – that shaking alone cannot cause the injuries ascribed to it by the SBS hypothesis.'

7 Dr Guthkelch was interviewed by the *New York Times* in 2016, during which he was asked his feelings about prosecutors using his science as the basis to convict individuals. He replied that he was utterly shocked and desperately disappointed and entirely against defining this as a syndrome in the first place (Retro Report: The New York Times Video, 2015).

8 https://to.pbs.org/3NAwsXe. 'If you were called to testify in the Woodward case today, what would you say? I would say that this is most likely a traumatic impact injury, that I would not be considering shaking, that this could be accidental just as it could be non-accidental or abusive. And I would say that from the imaging findings, my area of expertise, you cannot select out, accuse, indict or convict any particular caretaker based on the medical evidence that we have.'

cases [26].[9] Critics argue that the science is so flawed that past convictions must be vacated [27, 28]; proponents insist the science is sufficiently sound that it can establish proof beyond a reasonable doubt [29, 30]. The debate itself is horribly polarized. Each side views the other as wholly lacking in scientific vigor and integrity' [31].

While courts around the world have allowed prosecutions relying upon SBS diagnoses and testimony, it is clear that, if SBS is not scientifically reliable,[10] then it should not be cited in the courtroom.[11] The precise number of SBS-based prosecutions is unknown. Even the most informed estimates are highly uncertain given that the diagnosis is referred to by different names and that, in many SBS cases, the court records are not accessible and those that are do not clearly or always reflect that the allegations are based on SBS. In 2013, the Medill Justice Project published a database that compiled more than 3,000 criminal accusations of SBS in the United States.[12] This figure did not include the almost certainly greater number of family and juvenile court actions based on SBS, many of which occur *in camera* and with broad reporting restrictions.[13]

One study from a group at Cardiff University (hereafter the Cardiff study) is seen as a confirmatory tool for identifying shaken infant abuse which 'could also assist clinicians offering medical testimony in civil or criminal proceedings' [29]. Not only is it often cited in texts and legal cases in support of the triad and SBS generally, but it has been accepted as part of the evidence base for the Child Protection Guidance of the Royal College of Paediatrics and Child Health (RCPCH). There are, however, some issues with the Cardiff study, and we are not the first to point them out (see [32]). The limitations and potential for bias our team contend exist in the methodology led us to consider alternative approaches for evaluating the probability that abuse led to a child's injuries or death.

Setting the tone for their work, the opening claim made in the Cardiff study is that abusive head trauma (AHT) remains the commonest form of fatal child abuse. This claim is attributed to another work, the Keenan study [33]. Considering the limitations of the very small number of cases analysed in the Keenan study, this claim is at best a gross generalisation and at worst an exaggeration based wholly on the Keenan study's self-classifying slightly more cases as 'inflicted' (80 cases) than 'noninflicted' (72 cases).

The Keenan study was limited to a small catchment in North Carolina and even in cases where no suggestion of inflicted abuse was ever made either by a treating clinician or by the medical examiner, inflicted abuse was determined post hoc by the Keenan study's authors reviewing an 'abstract of the case' prepared by the project coordinator of their own study.

---

9 See also Aberdeen WJ. Babysitter accused of putting girl's life in danger after 'shaking' the infant so hard she bled from her brain. *The Press and Journal*. 13 February 2019. https://bit.ly/3Ur5oM7.

10 The UK Supreme Court of Judicature Court of Appeal (Criminal Division) [2005] EWCA Crim 1980 at [69–70]. The Justices, when presented with a cluster of SBS and AHT cases (Case Nos.: 200403277, 200406902, 200405573, and 200402848) also questioned the validity of the triad of symptoms (i.e., encephalopathy, subdural haemorrhage, and retinal haemorrhage), commenting at [69] in their judgment that 'the unified hypothesis can no longer be regarded as a credible or alternative cause of the triad of injuries'.

11 The Court noted that the triad itself is a hypothesis and that it was not possible to find that it must automatically and necessarily lead to a diagnosis of non-accidental head injury.

12 US Shaken-Baby Syndrome Debate Database, last updated 20 May 2015. www.medilljusticeproject.org.u-s-shaken-baby-syndrome-database.

13 A term that describes proceedings held in a closed or private court absent members of the public.

No example of an anonymised medical record with the resulting 'abstract' was provided to enable us to ascertain the accuracy and fairness of the prepared abstract's contents.

In fact, where clinical staff failed to record that the parent offered an immediate explanation of the mechanism of their child's injury on presentation to hospital, this absence itself was used to directly infer inflicted injury. This inference more than any other was used to classify parental abuse in the Keenan study, representing 100% of all 'no explanation offered' cases identified in their cohort and accounting for almost 64% of all their abuse classifications. There appears to be no suggestion or recognition that medical records created in the heat of the moment could be incomplete, that parents may have been too anxious and emotionally upset about their sick child to stop and discuss the details of the mechanism of injury, that harried staff might have been too busy treating the child to make more than the necessary examination and treatment notes, or that one staff member might have assumed that another staff member would be responsible for recording the statements of the parents. Unfortunately, the Cardiff study reproduces and even expands several of the methodological errors observed in the Keenan study.

The Cardiff study's authors contend that an evidence-based calculation that assimilates the clinical data and contributes to determining the probability of AHT would be a valuable adjunct for the professionals concerned – and with this statement, we agree. However, the methodology used to provide the supporting evidence for such a probabilistic tool must be carefully considered. For this reason, we now turn to the methodology employed by the Cardiff study's authors for developing their cohort data set. The methodology proposed by the Cardiff study is summarised pictorially in Figure 17.1.

Their method begins with an already highly selective collection of cases reported in earlier SBS/AHT studies. It goes on to exclude: (1) those children who do not meet the age criteria (retaining only those under 3 years of age); (2) those children whose records do not describe the diagnostic (subdural, subarachnoid, or extradural haemorrhage, intra-parenchymal injury, cerebral contusion, diffuse axonal injury, and/or cerebral oedema) or symptom (RH, long bone fractures, seizures or apnoea and head/neck bruising) criteria established by the authors for SBS/AHT; and (3) those children whose cases had already been established as having a non-abuse traumatic or organic cause.

The Cardiff cohort then consisted of those cases the authors primarily self-identified as SBS/AHT, leaving aside the fact that they could not actually confirm the abuse except in those rare situations where it was independently witnessed. This process biased the data set to be representative of only what they believe *is* inflicted abuse, completely omitting any exemplars of what *is not*. This is the cohort data set they propose is suitable for use by professionals to support decisions of what is or is not SBS/AHT. Then, as shown by the loop numbered 5 in Figure 17.1, when 'multidisciplinary assessment' declares abuse based on the erroneous belief that a case is confirmed where there is no acceptable explanation of the triad and supported by the output of the Cardiff study's model, these clinical teams effectively self-reinforce their assumptions without any scientific basis to support the abuse finding [34].

Another concerning aspect of the Cardiff study's approach is that all granularity and any doubt regarding whether the child was or was not abused is removed. The Cardiff study reduces all cases to a binary choice, as shown in the outer band of Figure 17.2. We believe this is a mistake as it completely removes the potential (possibility or probability) that a given case may have a currently unknown or innocent cause. It is also one of several statistical factors in the study's methodology that would lead to a greatly exaggerated likelihood for

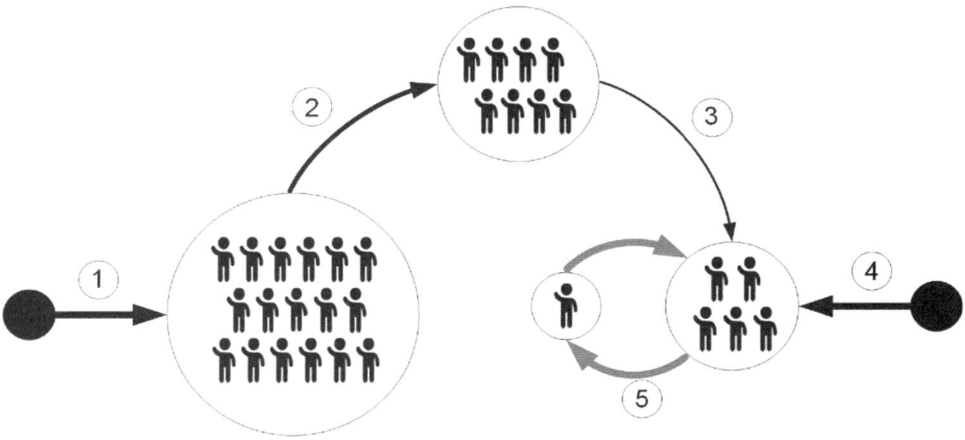

1. Limit starting dataset to cases from other Abusive Head Trauma studies
2. Exclude cases not meeting age, diagnostic and symptom criteria
3. Exclude cases with non-abuse traumatic or organic cause or where abuse is not the 'confirmed cause' (abuse ranking 1 & 2)
4. Impute values of missing data for one child from another similar child in the cohort
5. Use the resulting cohort to categorise future cases as non-AHT or AHT, with AHT-classified cases being included in the cohort.

Figure 17.1 Cardiff study: Methodology overview

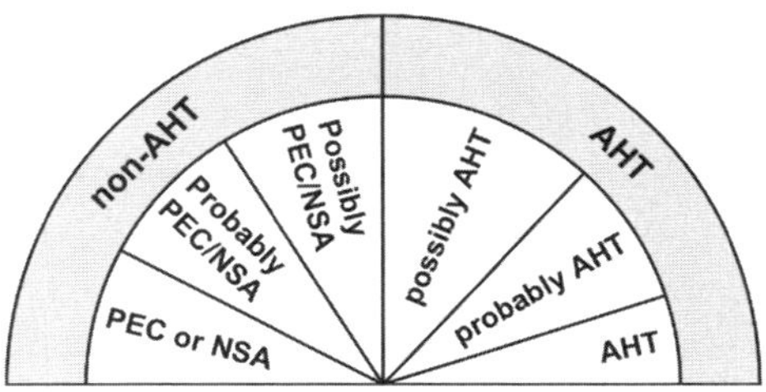

Figure 17.2 The scope of SBS/AHT cases (PEC – pre-existing condition, NSA – non-suspicious accident)

finding the outcome of interest, namely that a child has suffered inflicted abuse.[14] It limits the basis for decision-making to a collection of symptoms absent knowledge of the mechanism of injury, patient history, and any other potential causal information. Cuellar describes several issues that could result in important errors in the Cardiff Study's outcomes:

[14] Section 4 of [32] provides several examples of methodological components in the Cardiff study that could result in misleading or overestimated results and errors in the outcome variable.

i. The Cardiff study's authors cannot confirm the abuse.
ii. They use indirect analysis to determine abuse/non-abuse.
iii. Obtaining a legal decision determining abuse by the adult is one step removed from confirming abuse on the child.
iv. The court may have tried the wrong adult.
v. They make the assumption that the adult with the child when the child became ill must have caused the injuries.
vi. Any error in the physician's assumption regarding when an injury occurred could result in the wrong adult being blamed.
vii. Any cases decided by means of a confession and plea bargain may bias the confirmed-SBS cohort.

Finally, while the study's authors were aware of the potential for circularity arising from their dependence on symptoms alone, their use of indirect analysis by means of a ranking system to mitigate this circularity only served to introduce greater potential for error (see [32]) and further invalidated any resulting prediction.

17.3 A Causal Bayesian Network Model for SBS Decision-Making

A Bayesian network (BN) [35], also sometimes known as belief network or causal probabilistic network, is a graphical method for visualising risk that enables us to model the cause-and-effect relationships between risk factors and observed data. It combines causal knowledge and data to make predictions or diagnoses. With BNs we can incorporate causal knowledge and hence make better use of what are often only very limited amounts of relevant data. This means that, in contrast to purely machine-driven statistical methods, BNs enable us to reason about – and explain – interventions and counterfactuals. Because they address the fundamental limitations of purely data-driven approaches, BNs are increasingly used in a wide range of applications, including risk assessment in medical decision-making.

Specifically, a BN, such as the simple example shown in Figure 17.3, is a graph that describes the causal relationships between a set of variables. It consists of qualitative and quantitative parts. The qualitative part consists of nodes and directed arcs. The nodes represent random variables such as events or actions. In the example, there is a directed arc from node 'Driving over speed limit' to node 'Serious injury' since the former has a direct causal or statistical influence on the latter. The quantitative part of the BN consists of probability tables associated with each node.

For nodes like 'Driving over speed limit' and 'Seat belt worn' that have no parent nodes, the probability tables are simply the prior probabilities. So, in this case, the assumption is that, in 90% of car crashes, people were wearing seat belts and, in 20%, the car was driving over the speed limit. For nodes like 'Serious injury' that have parents, the probability table describes the strength of the relationship between a node and its parents. So, for example, in this case, it is assumed that, if seat belts were worn, then 30% of the crashes resulted in serious injury if the driver was over the speed limit, compared to just 10% if not over the speed limit.

By focusing only on direct dependencies between variables, the BN is a compact way of representing the full joint probability distribution for all the variables. Once the graph and probability tables are specified, a variety of probabilistic reasoning processes based on Bayes theorem can be performed as shown in Figure 17.4.

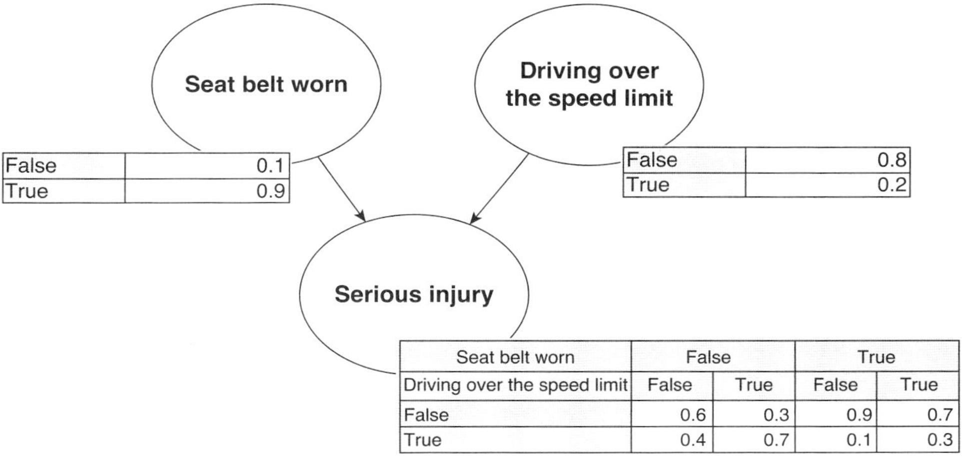

Figure 17.3 A simple Bayesian network for car crashes showing the nodes, arcs, and probability tables

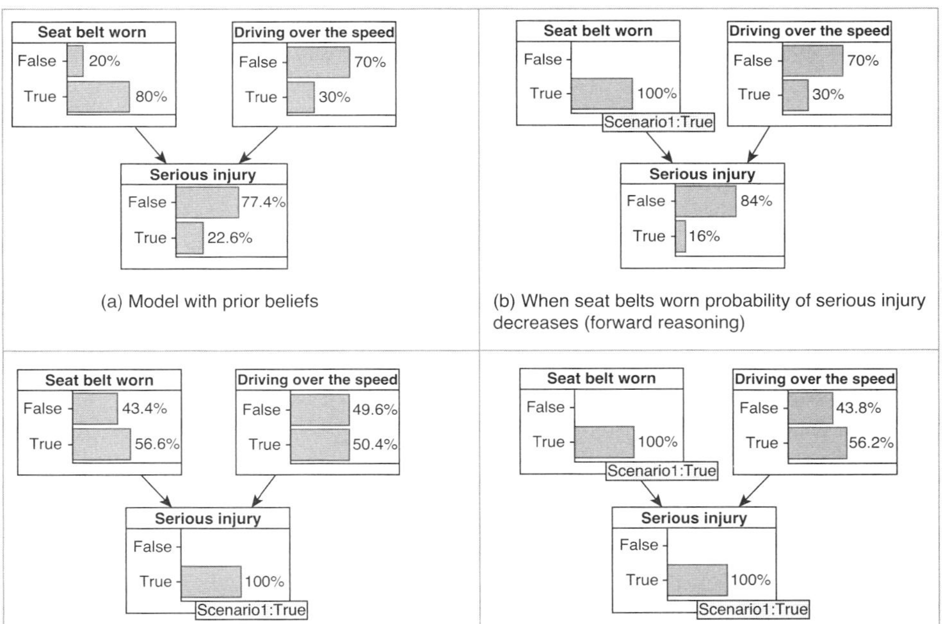

(a) Model with prior beliefs

(b) When seat belts worn probability of serious injury decreases (forward reasoning)

(c) If we know there was a serious injury then probability seats worn decreases and probability driving over the sped limit increases (backward reasoning)

(d) But if we discover seat belts were worn then the probability of driving over the speed limit increases further ('explaining away')

Figure 17.4 A simple Bayesian network for car crashes showing the nodes, arcs, and probability tables

Bayesian probabilistic reasoning is the process of updating our prior beliefs about the uncertain variables once we observe evidence. For example, in Figure 17.4b, once we observe the evidence that a seat belt was worn, the posterior probability of serious injury decreases from the prior 22.6% to the posterior 16%. This is an example of forward inference (also called prognostic reasoning) because the reasoning process follows the direction of the arc. Bayesian networks also enable us to perform backward inference (also called diagnostic reasoning) where the reasoning process is counter to the direction of the arc. For example, in Figure 17.4c, if we have observed a serious injury in a crash, then this updates our belief in both the probability a seat belt was worn (which decreases from the prior 80% to a posterior of 56.6%) and the probability of driving over the speed limit (which increases to 50.4% from a prior of 30%). One of the most powerful and unique features of BNs is the ability to perform 'explaining away' as shown in Figure 17.4d, whereby our further increased belief that driving over the speed limit was the cause of the serious injury is explained by the fact that we know seat belts were worn.

While it is feasible to do the necessary calculations manually using Bayes theorem for very small BNs like this example, such calculations are infeasible for larger models. Well-established propagation algorithms are implemented in widely used software to do the calculations automatically.

The idea of using causal models to better understand and explain SBS data and decision-making is not novel. Cuellar developed such a model [32] and the model we propose here extends those ideas and enables us to provide a full Bayesian probabilistic analysis of a range of scenarios which can replicate the statistical 'predictions' in the Cardiff studies while explaining why the underlying decision-making is flawed.

17.3.1 The Core Part of the Model

The model presented herein is not intended to be comprehensive, but rather provides a high-level explanation of the causal structure of the problem. In particular, since it is a BN with relevant prior probabilities, we are able to observe how these probabilities are revised as we get different types of evidence. The core part of the model is shown in Figure 17.5.

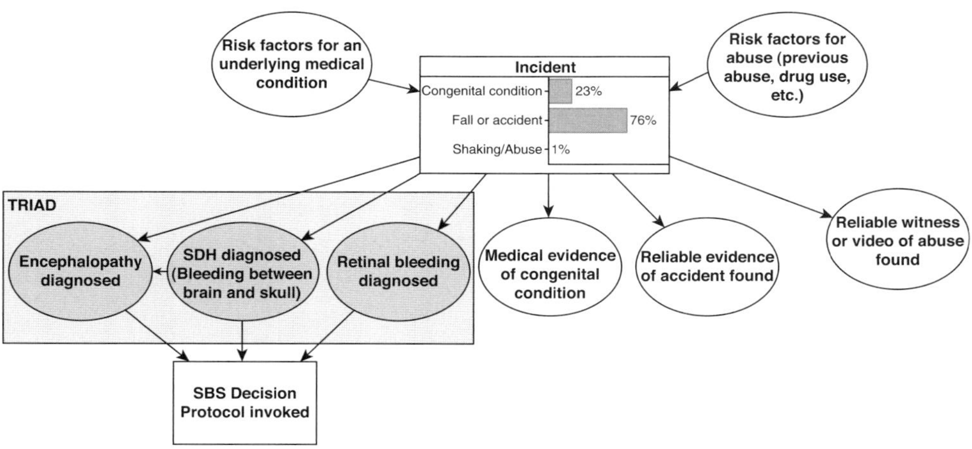

Figure 17.5 Core part of the causal model

The model and its prior probabilities are intended to represent the population of children under the age of 3 who are brought to a doctor or hospital with any kind of head injury or medical condition associated with the head (including seizures, apnoea, vomiting, irritability, etc.). The node 'Incident' represents the set of possible events (or causes) that give rise to the symptoms triggering the doctor/hospital visit. For simplicity, we assume these are mutually exclusive and exhaustive.

While the model uses the term 'Congenital condition', this is merely intended as a shorthand for any pre-existing or naturally acquired medical condition the child may have. Crucially, the true 'incident' in some cases may never be known; the primary objective of the model is indeed to see how the probabilities change as we gather evidence. Hence, even with the most comprehensive data sets, the prior probabilities can only ever be estimates. Here we make the following assumptions corresponding roughly to various published data sets: we assume that, in most cases (76%), the child has suffered a fall or accident while an underlying medical condition is the cause of most others. For deliberate shaking/abuse, we make two separate assumptions (1% of cases and 5% of cases), based on extrapolating information from recent studies [36]. While it is highly possible that 5% may actually be a large overestimate due to overdiagnosis of abuse, we nevertheless run it in the model to show that, even so, the Cardiff conclusions are not justified.

In many cases, there will exist underlying causal (or risk) factors that make a given incident more or less likely. For simplicity, we have grouped all such factors into two: those that can lead to an underlying medical condition (such as family history or defects at birth) and those that can lead to child abuse (such as a history of violence or drug abuse).

All of the nodes that are children of the 'Incident' node can be regarded as 'evidence' nodes. For example, retinal bleeding is considered one of the symptoms of shaking. Hence diagnosing this symptom is considered evidence of shaking. However, shaking can occur without this symptom being diagnosed and, inversely, this symptom can sometimes be diagnosed after a fall/accident or with a natural condition. Hence, we give the conditional probability table for the node 'Retinal bleeding diagnosed' shown in Figure 17.6.

This table tells us, for example, that there is a 30% chance of diagnosing retinal bleeding after a baby is shaken but only a 5% chance of diagnosing it if there is a natural condition. Retinal bleeding is one of the proposed triad of symptoms for SBS. The others are represented as the nodes 'SDH' and 'Encephalopathy'.

There is much debate about possible dependencies between these symptoms (see Chapter 3). While it was once (and by some pathologists, is still) believed that RH was pathognomonic for SDH [37] and more recently as a result of the SBS/AHT 'diagnosis' pathognomonic for abuse [38], here we have assumed that retinal bleeding and SDH are conditionally independent given the Incident cause. This means that, if we know, for example, that shaking is the cause, then diagnosing retinal bleeding does not impact the probability of diagnosing SDH and vice versa. However, we have assumed a direct dependency between SDH and encephalopathy. By definition, the node 'SBS decision protocol invoked' is true if and only if each of the triad factors is observed to be true.

Incident	Congenital condition	Fall or accident	Shaking/Abuse
False	0.95	0.9	0.7
True	0.05	0.1	0.3

Figure 17.6 Conditional probability table for the node 'Retinal bleeding diagnosed'

While the triad symptoms might be the most immediate forms of 'evidence' actually used to determine whether the incident should be classified as abuse, there may be (albeit sometime after the child is brought to the hospital) other, far more probative forms of evidence. Here, we include, for example:

- 'Medical evidence of a pre-existing condition': This might either be already recorded somewhere or be discovered by further tests.
- 'Reliable evidence of accident found': In the case where the injury was caused by an accident, the attending nurse or doctor may dismiss a carer's immediate claim of such an explanation (or the carer may themselves be unaware that this was the cause). However, it is possible that reliable evidence of such an accident may subsequently be found (such as via a video recording or a witness).
- 'Reliable evidence of abuse found': In the case where the injury was caused by abuse, it is unlikely that the carer admits to this in the immediate aftermath. However, it is possible that reliable evidence of abuse may subsequently be found (such as via a video recording or a witness).

17.3.2 Impact of Prior Assumptions and Evidence

To see the impact of the model assumptions we first look at the marginal (i.e., 'starting') values of all of the nodes in the model as shown in Figure 17.7.

If we diagnose retinal bleeding, then the model updates as shown Figure 17.8.

Although the probability of abuse increases significantly, the low prior probability means that it is still very unlikely to be the cause: the increase is from 1% to 3.2% (under the 5% prior for abuse the increase is from 5% to 14%). However, when SDH is also diagnosed, the probability increases to 9.7% (35% under the 5% prior assumption) as shown in Figure 17.9.

Note that, because of the dependency between SDH and encephalopathy, the latter diagnosis is now extremely likely: 90.5% (91.7% under the 5% prior assumption).

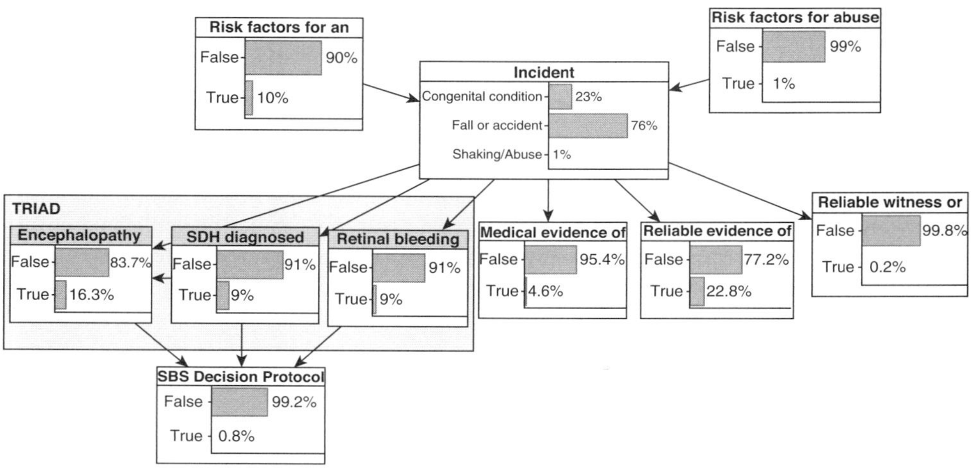

Figure 17.7 Core part of model with marginal probabilities shown

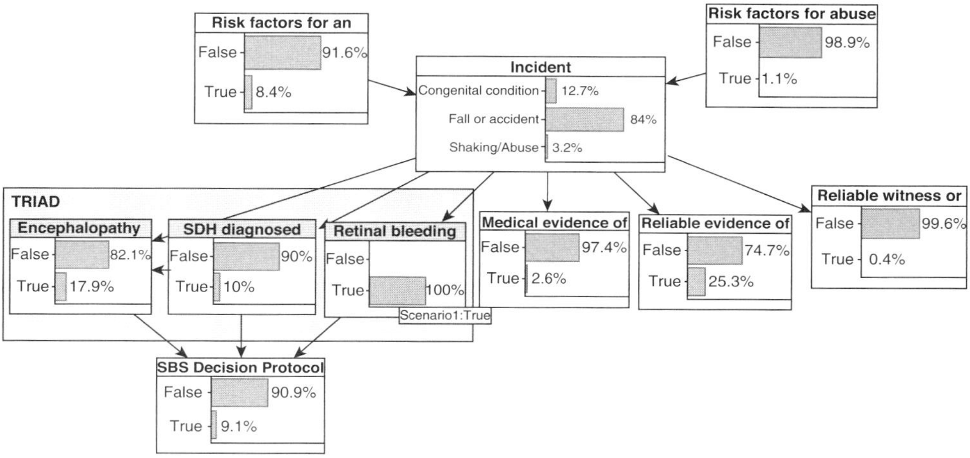

Figure 17.8 Retinal bleeding diagnosed

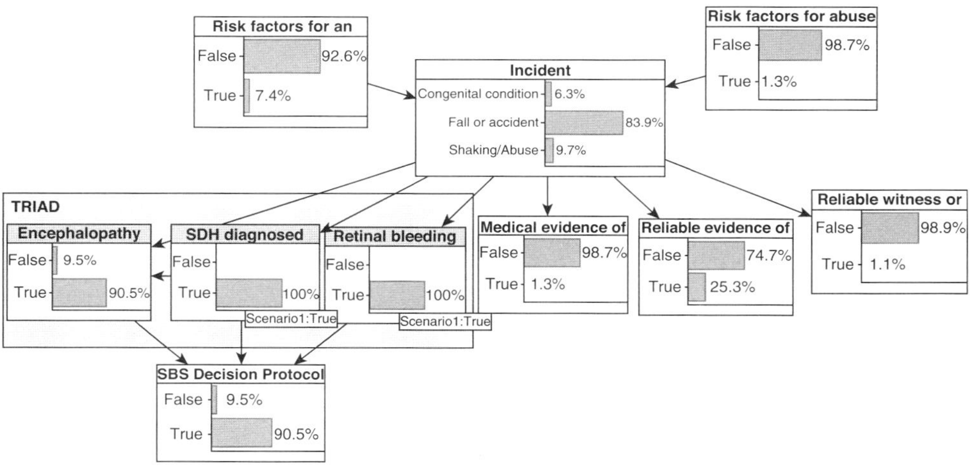

Figure 17.9 SDH diagnosed

Consequently, if such a diagnosis is made it has little impact overall – the probability of abuse increases from 9.7% to 10.2% (35% to 36% under the 5% prior assumption).

Note that diagnosis of the triad, in the absence of any other information, has led (in the model) to a greater than 10-fold increase in the posterior probability that the true incident cause is abuse. However, because the prior probability was low (1%), it is still unlikely that abuse is the true cause. In statistical terms, it can be shown that the likelihood ratio of the triad evidence (defined as the probability of observing the triad if abuse is the cause divided by the probability of observing the triad if abuse is not the cause) is quite high – in the model, it is just over 10. A common error of probabilistic reasoning is to assume that a high likelihood ratio for some evidence in favour of a hypothesis means that the hypothesis is very likely to be true if the evidence is observed (see [39]). But, in fact, this depends on the prior. Bayes tells us that the posterior odds of the hypothesis is simply the prior odds times the likelihood ratio. If the prior was 50%, then observing the triad would result in a posterior of about 91% for abuse. But the prior here is only 1%, which explains why the posterior is only 10.2%.

This high likelihood ratio in support of the abuse hypothesis replicates the kind of results reported in the Cardiff study, but, in the absence of other evidence, our model shows abuse is very unlikely to be the true cause. First, let us consider the impact of other 'hard' evidence that may be available:

- If there is reliable evidence of abuse (such as a witness or video), then, given the triad, the probability of SBS becomes close to 100%.
- If there is either reliable evidence of an accident or medical evidence of a pre-existing condition, then, as expected, the probability of SBS becomes close to zero.

However, in most cases, there will be no hard evidence of this type; because of this, the fact that we do not have such evidence (i.e., we enter 'false' for these 'Evidence found' nodes) has little impact in terms of updating the probabilities of the incident cause. We would be more likely to find evidence of risk factors for abuse (indeed, once the triad is observed it is common to look for such factors). If such factors are found, we have the scenario shown in Figure 17.10. The probability of abuse has now risen to 37% (under the 5% prior for abuse this would be 59%).

17.3.3 The Full Causal Model

In order to highlight the problems with the Cardiff study assumptions in such circumstances, we first reveal the more complete causal model in Figure 17.11.

The key points of the model are:

- Medical evidence of a pre-existing condition will only be found if appropriate tests are made. However, if the triad is diagnosed, the SBS protocol is invoked and this makes

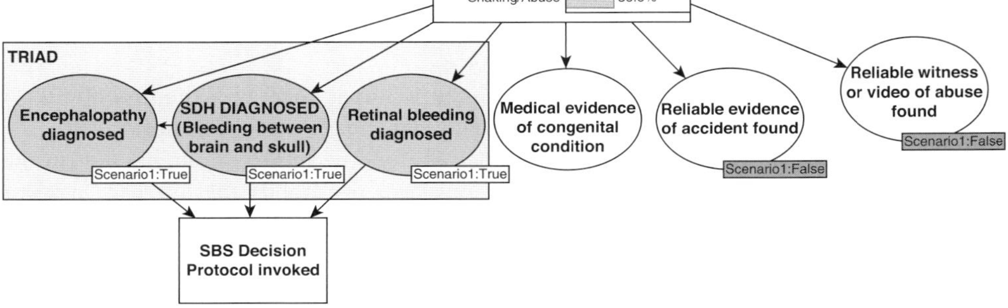

Figure 17.10 Impact of evidence of risk factors for abuse plus the triad

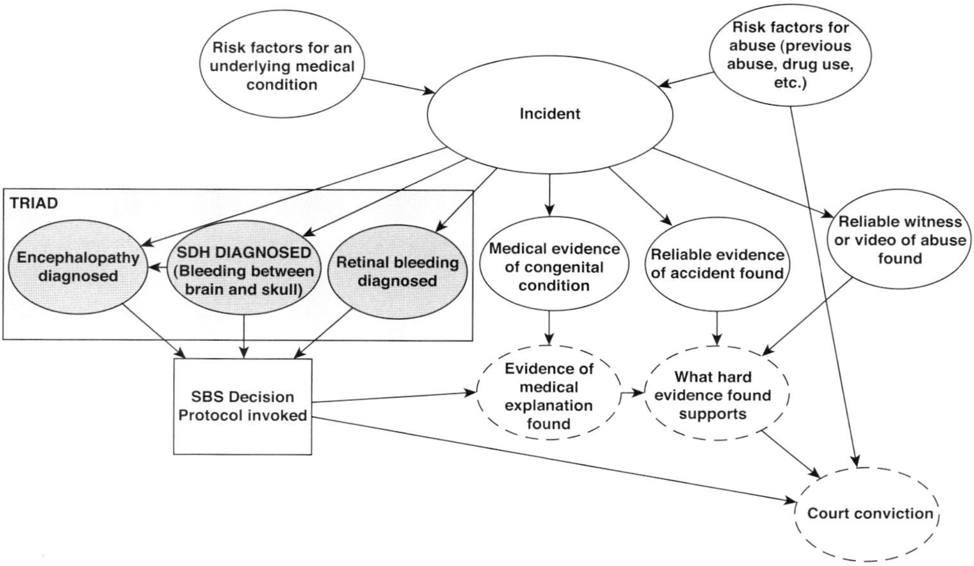

Figure 17.11 Full causal model

it less likely that such evidence will be found even when there is a pre-existing condition.

- If a case is brought to court (and here we include family courts as well as criminal courts), the evidence considered is: the triad diagnosis, other hard evidence found (namely medical evidence, evidence of accident, or evidence of abuse if any of these are available), and evidence of abuse. (Note that a court conviction can be true or false where false includes the possibility that no case is ever brought).

With the evidence scenario of Figure 17.10 we can now see the impact on the full model in Figure 17.12.

Because the court verdict takes account of the triad diagnosis and the abuse evidence, a conviction for abuse is highly likely (80%), even though the probability of abuse is only 37% (or 59% in the case where the prior probability of abuse is 5%). This mismatch between the probability that the 'true' cause of the incident is abuse and the probability of a conviction for abuse compromises the Cardiff analysis; in a case where the evidence is as presented in Figure 17.12, the Cardiff classification would very likely be 'abuse' even though non-abuse is the more probably true state. The full model described here is available at www.eecs.qmul.ac.uk/~norman/Models/shaken_baby4.cmpx and can be run using the free trial version of AgenaRisk. While the assumptions in the model are simply indicative, they are quite robust under sensitivity analysis. A version of the model that includes more comprehensive risk factors and symptoms is also available: www.eecs.qmul.ac.uk/~norman/Models/shaken_baby5.cmpx.

17.4 Conclusion

The causal model presented in this work considers risk factors and evidence both supporting and disproving of a potential SBS/AHT diagnosis. Our model provides a more reliable probability for whether the child may have been abused. Further, through addition of a node

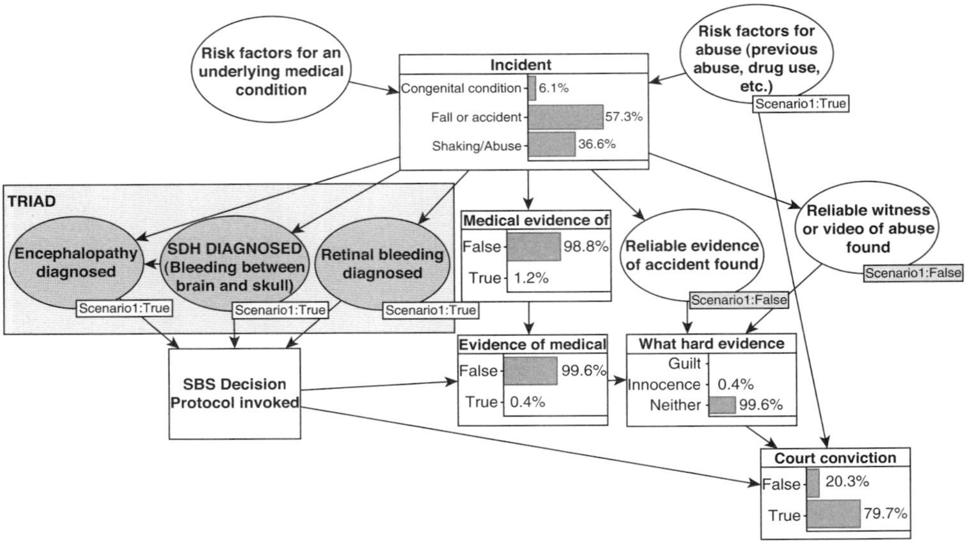

Figure 17.12 Impact of evidence: Full model

to consider how courts have previously decided SBS/AHT cases based on the assumptions of models like those found in the Keenan and Cardiff studies discussed in this work, we also demonstrate the strong biases and errors built into those models that result in overestimation and classification of abuse where such a finding may not otherwise be reasonable.

Cases of potential child abuse should never be ignored. However, the emotions they engender, both in the heat of the moment in the clinical setting or during adjudication – or indeed when researchers post hoc review the medical record, should lead us to take pause and temper our approach and responses. Prosecutions for SBS/AHT continue to be one of those rare case types that come before the court where legal and clinical commentators alike have noted a distinct disregard for innocent until proven guilty.

Acknowledgements

While this is not an exhaustive list, this work has benefitted from meetings involving Lina Kyrimi, David Lagnado, Sophia Langley, Martin Neil, and Maggie Wang.

References

1. Blatt J. *Stolen innocence: The Sally Clark story*. Ebury, 2004.
2. Caffey J. On the theory and practice of shaking infants: Its potential residual effects of permanent brain damage and mental retardation. *American Journal of Diseases of Children*. 1972; 124(2):161–9.
3. Caffey J. The whiplash shaken infant syndrome: Manual shaking by the extremities with whiplash-induced intracranial and intraocular bleedings, linked with residual permanent brain damage and mental retardation. *Paediatrics*. 1974;54 (4):396–403.

4. Guthkelch AN. Infantile subdural haematoma and its relationship to whiplash injuries. *British Medical Journal.* 1971;2(5759):430–1.

5. Hinds TS, Giardino AP. Clinical perspective. In *Child physical abuse: Current evidence, clinical practice, and policy directions.* Springer Briefs in Public Health. Springer, 2017. https://doi.org/10.1007/978-3-319-61103-7_2.

6. Uscinski R. Shaken baby syndrome: An odyssey. *Neurologia Medico-chirurgica (Tokyo).* 2006;46(2):57–61.

7. Stewart M, Hasan S, Collins C et al. Can baseline computerised tomography scans be used to identify patients at high risk of vision loss due to Terson syndrome? *American Journal of Ophthalmology.* 2019;211:217–28.

8. Ami O, Maran J, Gabor P et al. Three-dimensional magnetic resonance imaging of fetal head molding and brain shape changes during the second stage of labor. *PLoS One.* 2019;14(5):e0215721.

9. Watts P, Maguire S, Kwok T et al. Newborn retinal hemorrhages: A systematic review. *Journal of the American Association for Pediatric Ophthalmology and Strabismus.* 2013;17(1):70–8.

10. Hughes LA, May K, Talbot JF, Parsons MA. Incidence, distribution, and duration of birth-related retinal hemorrhages: A prospective study. *Journal of the American Association for Pediatric Ophthalmology and Strabismus.* 2006;10(2):102–6.

11. Findley K, Risinger M, Barnes M et al. Feigned consensus: Usurping the law in shaken baby syndrome/abusive head trauma prosecutions. *Wisconsin Law Review.* 2019:1211–67.

12. Dykes L. The whiplash shaken infant syndrome: What has been learned? *Child Abuse and Neglect.* 1986;10:211–21.

13. Duhaime AC, Gennarelli T, Thibault L et al. The shaken baby syndrome: A clinical pathological and biomechanical study. *Journal of Neurosurgery.* 1987;66(3):409–15.

14. Purkiss D. The children of Medea: Euripides, Louise Woodward, and Deborah Eappen. *Cardozo Studies in Law and Literature.* 1999;11(1):53–64.

15. Bower H. Woodward appeal rests on medical evidence. *Lancet.* 1998;351(9105):812.

16. Thompson AC, Shapiro J, Bartlett, S, Lee C. The child cases: Guilty until proved innocent. 2011. https://text.npr.org/s.php?sid=137454415.

17. Haberman C. Shaken baby syndrome: A diagnosis that divides the medical world. *New York Times.* 2015. https://nyti.ms/3WCSPPJ.

18. Goldsmith W, Plunkett J. A biomechanical analysis of the causes of traumatic brain injury in infants and children. *American Journal of Forensic Medicine and Pathology.* 2004;2(25):89–90.

19. Wolfson DR, McNally DS, Clifford MJ, Vloeberghs M. Rigid-body modelling of shaken baby syndrome. *Journal of Engineering in Medicine.* 2005;219(1):63–70.

20. Lloyd J, Willey E, Galaznik J, Lee W. Biomechanical evaluation of head kinematics during infant shaking versus paediatric activities of daily living. *Journal of Forensic Biomechanics.* 2011;2(9):1–9. https://doi.org/10.4303/jfb/F110601.

21. Jones M, Martin P, Williams J, Kemp A, Theobald P. Development of a computational biomechanical infant model for the investigation of infant head injury by shaking. *Medicine and the Law.* 2015;55(4):291–9.

22. Vester M, Bilo R, Loeve A, Rijn R, Van Zandwijk JP. Modelling of inflicted head injury by shaking trauma in children: What can we learn? *Forensic Science, Medicine and Pathology.* 2019;15(3):408–22.

23. Bonnier C, Mesples B, Carpentier S, Henin D, Gressens P. Delayed white matter injury in a murine model of shaken baby syndrome. *Brain Pathology.* 2022;12(3):320–8.

24. Gardner H. A witnessed short fall mimicking presumed shaken baby

syndrome (inflicted childhood neurotrauma). *Paediatric Neurosurgery.* 2007;43(5):433–5.

25. Lynøe N, Elinder G, Hallberg B et al. Insufficient evidence for 'shaken baby syndrome': A systematic review. *Acta Paediatrica.* 2017;106(7):1021–7.
26. Cormack L. Father charged after allegedly shaking baby, causing brain damage. *Sydney Morning Herald.* 14 November 2018. https://bit.ly/3sZZg1N.
27. Horan-Block J, Newman ET. Accidents happen: Exposing fallacies in child protection abuse cases and reuniting families through aggressive litigation. *CUNY Law Review.* 2019;22(2):382–425.
28. Tuerkheimer D. *Flawed convictions: 'Shaken baby syndrome' and the inertia of injustice.* Oxford University Press, 2015.
29. Maguire S, Kemp A, Lumb R, et al. Estimating the probability of abusive head trauma: A pooled analysis. *Paediatrics.* 2011;128(3):e550–e564.
30. Cowley L, Maguire S, Farewell D, Kemp A. Letter to the editor. *Law, Probability and Risk.* 2018;17(3):275–7.
31. Papetti R. *The forensic unreliability of the shaken baby syndrome.* Academic Forensic Pathology International. 2018.
32. Cuellar M. Causal reasoning and data analysis: problems with the abusive head trauma diagnosis. *Law, Probability and Risk.* 2017;16(4):223–39.
33. Keenan HT, Runyan DK, Marshall SW, Nocera MA, Merten DF. A population-based comparison of clinical and outcome characteristics of young children with serious inflicted and noninflicted traumatic brain injury. *Paediatrics.* 2004;114(3):633–9.
34. Lynøe N, Elinder G, Hallberg B et al. Easier to see the speck in your critical peers' eyes than the log in your own? Response to Debelle et al. *Archives of Disease in Childhood.* 2018;103(7):714.
35. Pearl J. *Probabilistic reasoning in intelligent systems: Networks of plausible inference.* Morgan Kaufmann, 1988.
36. Trefan L, Houston R, Pearson G et al. Epidemiology of children with head injury: A national overview. *Archives of Disease in Childhood.* 2016;101(6):527–32. https://doi.org/10.1136/archdischild-2015-308424.
37. Henderson JG. Subdural haematoma and 'battered baby'. *British Medical Journal.* 1968;3(5619):678.
38. Piatt JH. A pitfall in the diagnosis of child abuse: External hydrocephalus, subdural hematoma, and retinal haemorrhages. *Neurosurgical Focus.* 1999;7(4):1–8.
39. Fenton N, Neil M. Calculating the likelihood ratio for multiple pieces of evidence, 2021. http://arxiv.org/abs/2106.05328.

Chapter 18

Mandatory Reporting of Child Maltreatment

Felicity Goodyear-Smith

18.1 History of Child Protection and Mandatory Reporting

Recognition that children may be mistreated or neglected is not a new phenomenon, although there was little reference to this in the medical literature, apart from the occasional case story, until the late nineteenth century [1]. Throughout most of human history, children were considered small adults with no special rights. They were owned by their parents or guardians, who could exert absolute control. Initial consideration of children's rights centred around public concern about the plight of young children employed in inhumane conditions in mines and factories during the Industrial Revolution in the late eighteenth to the early nineteenth century, with calls to abolish exploitative child labour.

In 1860, French forensic pathologist Tardieu published 32 cases of physical abuse and neglect of children, generally severely badly beaten, sometimes fatally, by either or both parents [2]. However, his work failed to receive much attention. Gradually there was increasing social recognition of potential mistreatment of children within families. In 1874, the New York Society for the Prevention of Cruelty to Children was founded, followed by the Society for the Prevention of Cruelty to Children in Britain in 1883. The latter saw parents convicted for a number of crimes against their children, including physical assault and 'dangerous neglect'.

The first half of the twentieth century saw a growing literature regarding infantile subdural haematoma (SDH). In 1936, Ingalls recorded a strong association of SDH in infants with malnourishment and scurvy [3]. Ingraham and Matson reported 98 cases of SDH in 1944 which they postulated were always due to trauma [4]. In only about half the cases was there history of either birth or postnatal trauma including falls. Retinal haemorrhages (RH) were found in 21 and skull fractures in 11 of these children, and many also had systemic disease (infection, vitamin C or vitamin K deficiency, and other effects of malnutrition), which the authors considered as likely exacerbating factors increasing the risk of bleeding. In 1946, Caffey described six infants with SDH who also had fresh and healed fractures in long bones with no acknowledged history of trauma from caregivers [5].

During the 1940s and 1950s, there was debate as to whether skeletal lesions with the appearance of fractures (with or without the presence of SDH) where parents gave no history of trauma were due to abuse ('undesirable vectors of force') [6], or to natural phenomena ('underlying structural abnormality of the growing skeleton') [7]. In 1962, Kempe et al. published their seminal paper in which they coined the term 'battered-child syndrome' [8]. They argued that this should always 'be considered in any child exhibiting evidence of fracture of any bone, subdural hematoma, failure to thrive, soft tissue swellings or skin bruising, in any child who dies suddenly, or where the degree and type of injury is at variance with the history given regarding the occurrence of the trauma'. Kempe et al. declared that physicians must overcome their reluctance and believe that 'parents were guilty of abuse'.

Guthkelch described cases of SDH in 1971 where there were no external signs of injury, and hypothesised that this may be due to the infant having been shaken [9]. This was followed up in 1972 by Caffey, who described how the 'whiplash' shaking of babies can cause 'grave permanent damage to infantile brains and eyes' as well as 'skeletal lesions' and was a common cause of death [10]. He extended this discussion in 1974 where he identified the presence of SDH and RH, with or without lesions to the long bones, usually where there is 'no history of trauma of any kind', as 'whiplash shaken infant syndrome' [11]. The term 'shaken baby syndrome' (SBS) subsequently came into common usage, diagnosed by the presence of SDH, RH, and cerebral oedema/encephalopathy. By the turn of the century, the term SBS was being replaced by non-accidental head injury (NAHI) [12] or abusive head trauma (AHT), which might include trauma caused by direct impact to the head. The Committee on Child Abuse and Neglect described SBS as 'a subset of AHT' [13].

Where the 'triad' of SDH, RH and encephalopathy was present, there was a general assumption that an infant must have been violently shaken, often resulting in children removed from their homes and parents prosecuted. However, as this book attests, the 'triad' has been described as occurring from both trauma and natural causes: 'after delivery and in association with such conditions as various convulsive states, certain haemorrhagic diseases, infectious diseases, metabolic disorders, immunological diseases, skeletal diseases and vascular malformations' [14] (see Chapters 3–9). The biomechanics of shaking actually causing such findings is also in question [15] (see Chapter 14).

Kempe's diagnosis of battered child syndrome and the spotlight on child abuse led to major developments to address maltreated children in the United States, Britain, and other nations, particularly in the developed world. Child protection agencies were set up in many countries, with laws, policies, regulations, and services developed to prevent and address the abuse, neglect, and exploitation of children. In 1974, the Child Abuse Prevention and Treatment Act was passed in the United States to fund Child Protective Services and hotlines to protect children from maltreatment [16]. Britain passed the Children Act 1989 and a large number of other countries soon followed suit [17].

There was a rapid proliferation of research into child maltreatment. Kempe was the founding editor of the peer-reviewed journal *Child Abuse and Neglect*, dedicated to the topic of child protection. The sub-specialty of child abuse paediatrics was established for the evaluation of children who may be victims of abuse or neglect. The definition of child abuse expanded to include sexual and psychological maltreatment and exposure to family violence. In 2006, the World Health Organization defined child abuse and neglect as 'All forms of physical and/or emotional ill-treatment, sexual abuse, neglect or negligent treatment or commercial or other exploitation, resulting in actual or potential harm to the child's health, survival, development or dignity in the context of a relationship of responsibility, trust or power' [18]. In many countries, professionals working in health, educational, or social settings are now mandated to report to authorities whenever they encounter a child whom they suspect might be abused or neglected.

There is a potential cognitive bias when doctors are specialised as child abuse paediatricians, invoking the law of the hammer ('if all you have is a hammer, everything looks like a nail'). In the desire to keep children safe, there may be a reluctance to accept possible non-abuse causes for medical findings. When SDH and RH are defined as signs of head injury, the assumption is that some trauma must have occurred. However, when erring on the side of safety and mandating reports of suspicions, the potential harmful effects of such actions are rarely considered (see also Chapter 19). Parents facing such accusations may be bewildered, frightened, or angry, and the investigative process may be stressful to the family even when no abuse has occurred. The massive increase in reporting, particularly as the definition of abuse progressively broadened, has overloaded the child protection services, which may be unable to adequately respond and investigate all these cases [19]. Huge numbers of cases are unsubstantiated, but often the media equate the number of referrals as actual child maltreatment cases, making the problem seem much larger than it is. Families may be stigmatised. 'Once an agency . . . labels a parent as abusive, other agencies tend to accept this label and treat the family accordingly' [20]. They may be subjected to statutory child protection assessments before they can receive any support services, which may reduce their willingness to access these. Children may be removed from their families and placed in care, sometimes permanently, because authorities fear that abuse might have occurred despite absence of proof. Children raised in foster homes have significantly worse physical and mental health than those not placed in care, and such action should not be taken lightly [21].

There are examples where overzealous paediatricians have wrongly equated physical findings as evidence of child abuse with devastating consequences. In 1983, US paediatrician Hendrika Cantwell published a paper claiming that a hymenal opening in pre-pubertal girls greater than 4 mm was an indicator of sexual molestation [22]. For a number of years, sexual abuse was diagnosed on the basis of this sign, with children removed from families and fathers facing criminal charges. This sign was subsequently discredited and paediatricians stopped measuring the diameter of the vaginal opening.

In 1986, paediatricians Marietta Hobbs and Geoffrey Wyatt described the sign of reflex anal dilatation as an indicator that a child had been victim of buggery [23]. More than 120 children were removed from their parents in the English county of Cleveland alone on the basis of this diagnostic test. Following public outcry, the Butler-Sloss inquiry concluded that most of the diagnoses were incorrect and this test is also now discredited. Further, there is overwhelming evidence that, as well as sexual transmission, vulvovaginal gonorrhoea in pre-pubertal girls may be acquired non-sexually via contaminated fingers, bathing in contaminated water, or via fomites such as washcloths and towels [24]. Despite this, international guidelines assert that gonorrhoea in children is definitive, or nearly always definitive, evidence of sexual abuse, leading to children placed in care and alleged perpetrators prosecuted.

18.2 Case History from New Zealand

I present a case history on the diagnosis of SBS/AHT and the operation of child protection services in my own country, New Zealand (NZ). Child abuse is defined in the NZ Children, Young Persons and their Families Act 1989, now the Children, Young Persons, and Their Families (Oranga Tamariki) Legislation Act 2017, as 'the harming (whether physically, emotionally, or sexually), ill-treatment, abuse, neglect or deprivation of any child or young person'. Reporting of child abuse is not mandated in NZ.

Because of the broad range of types and severity of activities that might be included in this definition (e.g., from smacking a child to inflicting fatal trauma), it is difficult to give figures for the prevalence of non-fatal abuse. New Zealand was reported as having an average 1.2 deaths from maltreatment of children under 15 years per 100,000 children over a 5-year period in the 1990s (fifth highest in the Organisation for Economic Co-operation and Development (OECD)) [25]. In the 5-year period from 2015 to 2019, 11 children aged under 1 year, 19 aged 1–4 years, < 6 aged 5–14 years, and 45 aged 15–24 years were reported to have died from assault, an overall rate of 1.01/100,000 population. The majority were young people, not pre-school children. This figure is therefore less than that reported from the 1990s [26].

In many countries, there are a few key professionals who drive the call to identify and address cases of child abuse. In NZ, the leading advocate is paediatrician Dr Patrick Kelly, clinical director of the Starship Child Protection Team based in a multi-agency child advocacy centre. The Starship is the paediatric hospital in Auckland and the site of the country's only paediatric intensive care unit. Kelly has been a key member of the Paediatric Society of New Zealand and was its chair from 2000 to 2012. He frequently appears as an expert witness in child abuse and homicide court cases. He received a NZ Order of Merit in 2016 and was cited as NZ's 'foremost expert witness on child protection' and the driving force behind establishing NZ's first multi-agency child protection service [27].

Since the 1990s, Kelly has repeatedly called for mandatory reporting of suspected child abuse by general practitioners and other health professionals. Despite this, reporting is not mandated, although people are encouraged to report any suspicions of abuse to a statutory agency, the police, or the Ministry for Children (Oranga Tamariki) [28]. However, effectively there is mandatory reporting from hospitals. In 2011, the Clinical Network for Child Protection, a group under the Paediatric Society of New Zealand led by Kelly and contracted by the Ministry of Health, arranged for all of the country's District Health Boards (DHBs) to sign a memorandum of understanding (MoU) with Oranga Tamariki and the police [29]. The DHBs run all of NZ's public hospitals. The MoU includes a guideline for the management of children and young people admitted to hospital with actual or suspected child abuse and/or neglect. The DHBs must report their concerns to Oranga Tamariki, who in general also notify the police. The Child Protection Protocol between the police and Oranga Tamariki 'creates a process whereby when either party is advised of serious child abuse, they will immediately consult with each other, agree [on] an investigation plan, implement the plan, and advise each other of the outcomes'.

When abuse is suspected, there will be a meeting of the clinical team, Oranga Tamariki social workers, and the police within 24 hours of a receipt of concern to develop a Multi-agency Management Plan to address safety issues for the child, as well as for siblings and other children living in the home [29]. This may lead to a Place of Safety Warrant, or a declaration that children, and sometimes their siblings, are in need of care and protection and hence removed from their families and placed into care under the Children, Young Persons, and Their Families (Oranga Tamariki) Legislation Act 2017.

Kelly started diagnosing SBS in the 1990s. In 2004, he published a NZ case review of children aged under 2 years with SDH and RH between 1988 and 1998 [30], and, in 2008, a NZ case report of SBS, to which he also referred as NAHI, between 2000 and 2002 [12]. Kelly et al. conducted a 20-year (1991 to 2020) review of 345 children referred to the Child Protection Team for suspected accidental head injury (AHI). They found that the numbers had escalated from 88 in the first decade to 257 in the second [31]. Children under the age of 2 years were likely to be diagnosed as AHI where there was SDH and hypoxic-ischaemic injury with no history of trauma. The actual incidence of AHI was expected to be much higher because 'children who may be shaken in a manner that does not lead to symptoms may never be counted' [32].

In their public educational material, Kelly et al. still refer to SBS rather than AHT or NAHI. The Paediatric Society of New Zealand and the Starship Foundation, supported and funded by the Ministry of Health, run KidsHealth, a public-facing website. This aims to provide 'parents and whānau [family] with accurate and reliable information about the health and wellbeing of tamariki [children] and rangatahi [young people] in Aotearoa [New Zealand]' [33]. Shaken baby syndrome is said to be 'the single most preventable cause of serious head injury in babies under one year of age in New Zealand. It is a combination of serious injuries that can occur when someone violently shakes an infant or young toddler'. The public are told:

> [I]t may only take one or two hard shakes to seriously injure a small child. This is because babies and toddlers have relatively big, heavy heads and weak neck muscles. When they are shaken, the brain slams back and forth inside the skull, resulting in bleeding around the brain and damage to the brain itself. Some babies may even stop breathing, which can cause further brain damage. The shaking can also cause bleeding into the back of the eyes. Many babies who are shaken also have broken ribs because they are held forcibly around the chest and squeezed when they are shaken. They may also suffer other broken bones during the shaking.

The site states that, '[O]verall, in babies diagnosed with shaken baby syndrome, approximately 20% will die and 30–60% will suffer moderate to severe injuries.'

Kelly et al. emphasise that there should be a high suspicion of NAHI where SDH is detected but parents deny any history of trauma. In a 10-year review of 519 children aged under 3 years with 'structural head injury', they found that many aged under 6 months had SDH with no history of trauma and no natural conditions that might cause SDH, and hence 'it must be seriously considered that the history is false' [34]. In an opinion piece on the diagnosis of AHT in the United States and other selected countries/regions 'where child abuse physicians are actively involved in the evaluation of AHT', they claim that the legal system does not serve children well, with defence lawyers contesting that SBS or AHT may not have occurred. They complain that 'highly paid defence experts, mostly from the US and the UK, travel internationally to refute and challenge a diagnosis that has a strong history and evolution of research to support its basis' [32]. In an article giving advice to ophthalmologists giving evidence to the court, they claim that RH 'are exceedingly rare in accidental head trauma' but commonly occur in SBS 'from a direct mechanical effect at the vitreoretinal interface with resulting traction from (possibly repeated) acceleration–deceleration' [35]. They caution that using the term 'consistent with' NAHI is problematic and, where there is no other evidence, ophthalmology expert witnesses should 'explain why, in your view, alternative diagnoses are not consistent with the findings you observed'. In other words, the experts should be unequivocal that RH indicates NAHI.

A further study by Kelly et al. looked at fatal head injuries in children under 15 years seen by the Auckland coroner's office from 1991 to 2020 [36]. They found 12 children aged under 2 years with SDH and RH who were diagnosed with AHT. In their retrospective case review of the outcome of referrals to statutory authorities from 1988 to 1998 [37], 39 infants out of 64 cases of infantile SDH were deemed to have an NAHI, with the rest assigned as accidental injury. Of these 39 children, 6 had died, 15 were placed with other family members, 9 were placed permanently away from home, and charges were laid in 18 cases, resulting in 15 cases going to trial and 14 convictions (11 fathers, 3 mothers, 1 stepfather).

18.3 Child Protection and Mandated Reporting in a Selection of Other Countries

Abuse reporting laws were enacted in every US state by 1967 [38]. Initially, mandatory reporting applied only to physicians reporting serious non-accidental physical injuries [20]. Amendments to the federal Child Abuse Prevention and Treatment Act subsequently included nurses, teachers, social workers, mental health workers, and other professionals as mandated reporters, with criminal penalties for those who failed to report. Rather than investigate themselves or wait for proof, professionals are mandated to report any suspicions of abuse to Child Protective Services, who then conduct the investigations. Rapid action is advocated to prevent the suspected victim undergoing further harm. In 20 states, everyone, even strangers, is legally required to report their suspicions using the hotlines and they have immunity from civil and criminal liability for their 'good faith' reporting [38]. The laws now cover all forms of suspected child maltreatment (physical, emotional, and sexual).

Mandatory reporting has been introduced in many other countries (see also Chapters 21–26). Israel followed the US lead and introduced a law to mandate reporting of child abuse in 1980 [39]. Doctors, teachers, social workers, psychologists, and other professionals are obligated by law to report any suspicion of child abuse, with failure to report being a criminal offence. Israeli common law has recognised SBS/AHT since the early 2000s. Medical protocols in hospitals specify that signs of the 'triad' are grounds for suspecting abuse and sufficient for a medical diagnosis of SBS/AHT. Doctors are ordered to report to the police or social services about cases with observed 'triad' signs for which there are no other explanations, such as traffic accidents. However, SBS may be diagnosed solely on the basis of RH and cerebral oedema in the absence of SDH [40].

Anglo-American countries generally follow a similar model to the United States. England has had a strong child protection focus although no mandatory reporting. While only social workers and police are obliged to report child abuse suspicions, health professionals and teachers have often been expected to do so. Central government lays out detailed guidance for both professionals and citizens to refer to local-authority statutory child-welfare agencies when they have any concerns that a child might be at risk of harm [41]. Volunteer counsellors at the National Society for the Prevention of Cruelty to Children receive thousands of calls daily from both children and adults on their free phone lines. Local authorities also have their own detailed procedures for child protection work, with severe consequences for professionals and organisations where the guidance has not been followed, if things go wrong. Penalties may include job dismissal, removal from a professional register, or being pilloried in the press.

The 1970s through the 1990s saw growing public concern about the failures of UK health and welfare professionals to protect certain children from death or serious injury in high-profile cases. On the other hand, the forensic approach to child protection gave rise to concerns about over-intervention, with children inappropriately removed from their parents [41]. In the mid-2000s, child welfare departments were established, and the Every Child Matters: Change for Children programme was launched, aiming for a 'shift to prevention whilst strengthening protection'. All children, at some point in their lives, might be vulnerable to some form of risk, and the idea was to identify problems and provide early help.

In 2007, the death of a baby reignited public criticism of the failure of the system to protect children, and, since 2009, the UK government has reverted to framing policy in terms of child protection rather than safeguarding and promoting the welfare of the child. The system is not coping with demand. More than one in five children born in 2009 and 2010 were referred to children's services before the age of five [42]. A quarter of these were formally investigated and a high proportion were not offered support. Suspicion of child abuse is concentrated on families living in poorer communities [43], which can create a climate of fear and distrust [44].

In Canada, provincial and territorial laws mandate the reporting of suspicions of child abuse or neglect [45]. There is a long list of professional groups considered mandated reporters, including medical, mental health, and educational personnel and anyone else working with children or youth. In 1998, 45% of 135,573 reported cases were said to be substantiated, which included physical, emotional, and sexual maltreatment and neglect [46]. Shaken baby syndrome was substantiated in 200 cases. The use of standardised risk assessment is said to have led to social workers giving high-risk scores for fear of making a mistake, with increasing numbers of children placed in care [47].

All Australian states and territories have legislation requiring doctors and other professionals to report suspicion of child abuse to statutory child protection services, although in Western Australia this is only for child sexual abuse [48] (see Chapter 25). During 2019 to 2020, investigations of reported abuse/neglect were conducted for 117,900 children, with 48,900 cases (42%) substantiated [49]. One in 23 (14,300) of these were Aboriginal and Torres Strait Islander children, almost seven times the rate of non-Indigenous children. Approximately 46,000 children were in out-of-home care, 30,600 for 2 years or more, with 42% long-term placements for Indigenous children. Physical abuse accounted for 14% of cases said to be substantiated, but specific diagnoses were not reported. In 2012, the rate of AHT requiring hospital admission in Queensland was an estimated 29.6 per 100,000 children under the age of 2 years [50].

Other countries with mandated reporting include Brazil, where child maltreatment was added to the compulsory notification of diseases ordinance [51]. Notification should be enforced by the health and educational systems, although significant underreporting appears likely [52]. In South Korea, mandatory reporting obligations are imposed on medical personnel, teachers, facility workers of specialised child protection institutions, and public officials under the Child Welfare Act [53]. In Taiwan, a series of legislative acts since 1993 stipulates that doctors, nurses, social workers, clinical psychology workers, educational and day-care personnel, police, and other providers of children and youth welfare services must report all suspected cases of child abuse to the authorities [54]. In the best interests of the children, the authorities may place children and youth in foster families or turn them over to relatives, third parties, or children and youth welfare or other placement institutions.

Although there is no special law against child abuse in China, people have been subject to criminal punishment under the Law of the People's Republic of China on the Protection of Minors. Mandatory reporting is just being introduced in China, with the Supreme People's Procuratorate in conjunction with a number of government agencies issuing an 'Opinion on establishing a system for compulsory reporting of cases against minors' for trial implementation [55]. Under this Opinion, organisations in close contact with minors are obliged to immediately report suspected child abuse, sexual assault, injury, abandonment, and abduction (see Chapter 26).

18.4 Family-Support Focus

Some countries have a family-support rather than a child protection focus [19]. This could be considered to be in line with the Convention on the Rights of the Child, ratified by the General Assembly of the United Nations in 1989. The Convention states that every child has basic rights, including the right to be raised by their parents within a family or cultural grouping and to have a relationship with both parents, even if they are separated. While the child-protection-focused system focuses on managing risk of abuse and neglect, the priority of the family-support model is to respond to family needs and address child abuse prevention, protection, and support in a holistic manner [19]. Such a system looks to work with family dysfunction before problems escalate [56]. It provides supportive or therapeutic responses to help resolve issues facing children and families, rather than legalistic and investigative processes formulating child-safety plans. These flexible services are often embedded within and normalised by broad child welfare and public health services, in comparison to the adversarial, standardised 'standalone' child protection orientation. Removal of children from their families is a last resort and mainly voluntary [19].

Nordic countries, with their social democratic welfare state regimes, have family support-oriented child welfare systems, with or without a mandatory reporting component. When a referral is made in Sweden by a mandated reporter, the object of the investigation is not to determine whether an allegation is correct (see Chapter 23). Rather, family functioning is examined, including parent–child interactions, and support is offered to address issues rather than impose intrusive state interventions [56]. Family centres are universally provided resources focused on parents and children, with integration of antenatal and child healthcare, pre-school education, and social welfare activities. A range of different professional groups work together with families including midwives, paediatric nurses, paediatricians, pre-school teachers, social workers, and psychologists, providing health and social services, ongoing education, and support on good parenting practices [57]. In Finland, there is a similar orientation, with a strength-based approach assessing notified cases as to what service might be provided, rather than focusing on problems or risks [58]. Social workers assess in relation to what might be expected to be a 'good enough' childhood or family life, rather than against a gold standard of parenting. Open-care measures are prioritised, with provision of a wide range of psychosocial, financial, and practical supportive services. Placing a child into care is a last resort.

Continental European countries generally also orientate towards a family support approach, with different policies on mandatory reporting. In the Netherlands, the Department for Youth and Family generally focuses more broadly on reducing poverty and promoting safety and health, rather than specifically on child abuse. Reporting child maltreatment is not mandatory although it is being increasingly encouraged [59]. Families are seen to malfunction frequently and introduction of the Electronic Child Dossier provides monitoring of every family in the country, facilitating intervention when young people at risk are identified. Mostly these interventions seek to support the family's autonomy instead of undermining it. Belgium also does not have mandatory reporting, although it is considered the moral responsibility of all to provide or facilitate help if confronted with a situation of suspected child abuse and neglect [60].[1] The Belgian system operates on the continuum between caring for children and their families and criminalising parents deemed abusive [60]. The majority of services are aimed at preventing abuse and contributing to the welfare of children, with a small group of cases dealt with by services tasked to improve the safety and well-being of abused and neglected children. The focus is on easily accessible help and care, not forensic evaluation, aiming to restore safe relationships between children and parents and safe parenting.

18.5 Conclusion

The way child abuse is framed may influence what happens to children and their families to a greater extent than whether there is mandatory reporting. Child protection-oriented services are adversarial, demanding that children are protected from harm that might be inflicted by parents and other relatives. Removal of children from their homes is seen to be warranted, as it is better to be safe than sorry. In contrast, the family-support-orientated approach views abuse as a problem of family conflict or dysfunction arising from social and psychological difficulties, which will respond to support and assistance. The system operates in partnership with parents. The state's focus on safeguarding children is with policies that emphasise participation, prevention, and family support rather than a forensic approach.

The implications of this are of particular concern where authorities believe that the presence of SDH, RH, and/or the 'triad' is diagnostic of SBS/AHT. The fact that the parents deny the occurrence of any traumatic event is interpreted as giving a false history and confirms that they cannot be trusted with the care of their children. Their denial means that they present an ongoing risk. Removal of children from their care is justified to keep them safe from dangerous parents. Where the children have died, those deemed responsible are to be held criminally liable [34].

However, SBS is not a medical diagnosis; it is the diagnosis of a crime, a statement that an illegal act has taken place. In countries where there is a child protection orientation, a diagnosis of SBS is likely to lead to loss of child custody and parental incarceration. Likewise the term 'abusive head trauma' presupposes an action with malicious intent. This emotive label should have no place in a medical diagnosis.

References

1. Lynch MA. Child abuse before Kempe: An historical literature review. *Child Abuse and Neglect*. 1985;9(1):7–15.
2. Roche AJ, Fortin G, Labbé J, Brown J, Chadwick D. The work of Ambroise Tardieu: The first definitive description of child abuse. *Child Abuse and Neglect*. 2005;29(4):325–34.
3. Ingalls TH. The role of scurvy in the etiology of chronic subdural hematoma. *New England Journal of Medicine*. 1936;215(27):1279–81.
4. Ingraham FD, Matson DD. Subdural hematoma in infancy. *Journal of Pediatrics*. 1944;24(1):1–37.
5. Caffey J. Multiple fractures in the long bones of infants suffering from chronic subdural hematoma. *American Journal of Roentgenology Radium Therapy and Nuclear Medicine*. 1946;56(2):163–73.
6. Woolley PV, Evans WA. Significance of skeletal lesions in infants resembling those of traumatic origin. *JAMA*. 1955;158 (7):539–43.

[1] See Chapter 22 for an overview of the situation in France.

7. Astley R. Multiple metaphyseal fractures in small children (metaphyseal fragility of bone). *British Journal of Radiology*. 1953;26 (311):577–83.
8. Kempe CH, Silverman FN, Steele BF, Droegemueller W, Silver HK. The battered child syndrome. *JAMA*. 1962;181(1):17–24.
9. Guthkelch AN. Infantile subdural haematoma and its relationship to whiplash injuries. *British Medical Journal*. 1971;2(5759):430–1.
10. Caffey J. On the theory and practice of shaking infants: Its potential residual effects of permanent brain damage and mental retardation. *American Journal of Diseases of Children*. 1972;124(2):161–9.
11. Caffey J. The whiplash shaken infant syndrome: Manual shaking by the extremities with whiplash-induced intracranial and intraocular bleedings, linked with residual permanent brain damage and mental retardation. *Pediatrics*. 1974;54(4):396–403.
12. Kelly P, Farrant B. Shaken baby syndrome in New Zealand, 2000–2002. *Journal of Paediatrics and Child Health*. 2008;44 (3):99–107.
13. Christian CW, Block R. Abusive head trauma in infants and children. *Pediatrics*. 2009;123(5):1409–11.
14. Elinder G, Eriksson A, Hallberg B et al. Traumatic shaking: The role of the triad in medical investigations of suspected traumatic shaking. *Acta Paediatrica*. 2018;107:3–23.
15. Squier W. The triad of retinal haemorrhage, subdural haemorrhage and encephalopathy in an infant unassociated with evidence of physical injury is not the result of shaking, but is most likely to have been caused by a natural disease: Yes. *Journal of Primary Health Care*. 2011;3 (2):159–61.
16. US Congress. Child Abuse Prevention and Treatment Act (CAPTA). PL 93-247, 1974.
17. UK Government. The Children Act 1989. House of Commons Vol. C41. London, 1989.
18. World Health Organization. *Preventing child maltreatment: A guide to taking action and generating evidence*. World Health Organization, 2006.
19. Price-Robertson R, Bromfield L, Lamont A. International approaches to child protection: What can Australia learn? CFCA paper. *Australian Institute of Family Studies*. 2014;23:1–11.
20. Besharov DJ. Responding to child sexual abuse: The need for a balanced approach. *Future Child*. 1994;4(2):135–55.
21. Turney K, Wildeman C. Mental and physical health of children in foster care. *Pediatrics*. 2016;138(5):1–11.
22. Cantwell HB. Vaginal inspection as it relates to child sexual abuse in girls under thirteen. *Child Abuse and Neglect*. 1983;7 (2):171–6.
23. Hobbs C, Wynne J. Buggery in childhood: A common syndrome of child abuse. *Lancet*. 1986;2:792–6.
24. Goodyear-Smith F. What is the evidence for non-sexual transmission of gonorrhoea in children after the neonatal period? A systematic review. *Journal of Forensic and Legal Medicine*. 2007;14 (8):489–502.
25. United Nations International Children's Emergency Fund (UNICEF). *A league table of child maltreatment deaths in rich countries*. Innocenti Research Centre, 2003.
26. Child and Youth Mortality Review Committee. *15th data report Te pūrongo raraunga 15 2015–19*. Wellington Health Quality & Safety Commission, 2021.
27. SM. Influential Auckland pediatrician recognised with ONZM. *Stuff*. 2016, 5 June.
28. Ministry of Health. Family violence questions and answers: Is it mandatory to report abuse? www.health.govt.nz/our-work/preventative-health-wellness/family-violence/family-violence-questions-and-answers.
29. Clinical Network for Child Protection. *Schedule 1: Children admitted to hospital with suspected or confirmed abuse or neglect*. Clinical Network for Child Protection, 2011.
30. Kelly P, Hayes I. Infantile subdural haematoma in Auckland, New

Zealand: 1988–1998. *New Zealand Medical Journal*. 2004;117(1201):U1047.

31. Kelly P, John S, Vincent AL, Reed P. Abusive head trauma and accidental head injury: A 20-year comparative study of referrals to a hospital child protection team. *Archives of Disease in Childhood*. 2015;100(12):1123–30.
32. Frasier LD, Kelly P, al-Eissa M, Otterman GJ. International issues in abusive head trauma. *Pediatric Radiology*. 2014;44(Suppl 4):S647–53.
33. KidsHealth. What is shaken baby syndrome? www.kidshealth.org.nz/never-ever-shake-baby.
34. John SM, Kelly P, Vincent A. Patterns of structural head injury in children younger than 3 years: A ten-year review of 519 patients. *Journal of Trauma and Acute Care Surgery*. 2013;74(1):276–81.
35. Vincent AL, Kelly P. Retinal haemorrhages in inflicted traumatic brain injury: The ophthalmologist in court. *Clinical and Experimental Ophthalmology*. 2010;38 (5):521–32.
36. John SM, Jones P, Kelly P, Vincent A. Fatal pediatric head injuries: A 20-year review of cases through the Auckland coroner's office. *American Journal of Forensic Medicine and Pathology*. 2013;34 (3):277–82.
37. Kelly P, MacCormick J, Strange R. Non-accidental head injury in New Zealand: The outcome of referral to statutory authorities. *Child Abuse and Neglect*. 2009;33 (6):393–401.
38. Pence DM, Wilson CA. Reporting and investigating child sexual abuse. *Future Child*. 1994;4(2):70–83.
39. Oz S, Balshan D. Mandatory reporting of childhood sexual abuse in Israel: What happens after the report? International research. *Journal of Child Sex Abuse*. 2007;16(4):1–22.
40. Morad Y, Avni I, Capra L et al. Shaken baby syndrome without intracranial hemorrhage on initial computed tomography. *Journal of Pediatric Ophthalmology and Strabismus*. 2004;8 (6):521–7.
41. Parton N, Berridge D. Child protection in England. In *Child protection systems: International trends and orientations*. N Gilbert, N Parton, M Skivenes, eds. Oxford University Press, 2011, pp. 60–85.
42. Bilson A, Martin KEC. Referrals and child protection in England: One in five children referred to children's services and one in nineteen investigated before the age of five. *British Journal of Social Work*. 2016;47 (3):793–811.
43. Bywaters P, Brady G, Sparks T, Bos E. Inequalities in child welfare intervention rates: The intersection of deprivation and identity. *Child and Family Social Work*. 2016;21(4):452–63.
44. Hooper C, Gorin S, Cabral C, Dyson C. *Living with hardship 24/7: The diverse experiences of families in poverty in England*. Frank Buttle Trust, 2007.
45. Tufford L. *Child abuse and neglect in Canada: A guide for mandatory reporters*. Oxford University Press, 2019.
46. Trocmé NM, Tourigny M, MacLaurin B, Fallon B. Major findings from the Canadian incidence study of reported child abuse and neglect. *Child Abuse and Neglect*. 2003;27(12):1427–39.
47. Swift K. Canadian child welfare. In *Child protection systems: International trends and orientations*. N Gilbert, N Parton, M Skivenes, eds. Oxford University Press, 2011, pp. 36–59.
48. Bird S. Child abuse: Mandatory reporting requirements. *Australian Family Physician*. 2011;40(11):921–6.
49. Australian Institute of Health and Welfare. *Child protection Australia 2019–20*. Australian Institute of Health and Welfare, 2021.
50. Liley W, Stephens A, Kaltner M et al. Infant abusive head trauma incidence, outcomes and awareness. *Australian Family Physician*. 2012;41 (10):823–6.

51. Ministry of Health Brazil. *Annex 1 Ordinance No 104 Federative Republic of Brazil*. Brasilia, 2011.

52. Cardia N, Lagatta P, Affonso C. *Assessment of child maltreatment prevention readiness: Country report*. University of São Paulo, 2012.

53. Republic of Korea. Child Welfare Act. In Welfare PS. 12361. Seoul 2014.

54. Ministry of Health and Welfare. *The protection of children and youths welfare and rights act*. Republic of China, 2003.

55. Supreme People's Procuratorate, National Supervision Commission, Ministry of Education et al. *Opinions on establishing a mandatory reporting system for cases of violations against juveniles (provisional) in procuratorate SPs*. Supreme People's Procuratorate, 2020.

56. Wiklund S. Signs of child maltreatment. The extent and nature of referrals to Swedish child welfare agencies Barnavårdsanmälningar i Sverige: omfattning, källor och problembilder. *European Journal of Social Work*. 2006;9 (1):39–58.

57. Ångman I, Gustafsson M. *Combating child abuse and neglect in Sweden*. 2011.

58. Pösö T. Combatting child abuse in Finland. In *Child protection systems: International trends and orientations*. N Gilbert, N Parton, M Skivenes, eds. Oxford University Press, 2011, pp. 112–30.

59. Knijn T, Van Nijnatten C. Child welfare in the Netherlands. In *Child protection systems: International trends and orientations*. N Gilbert, N Parton, M Skivenes, eds. Oxford University Press, 2011, pp. 223–40.

60. Desair K, Adriaenssens P. Policy toward child abuse and neglect in Belgium. In *Child protection systems: International trends and orientations*. N Gilbert, N Parton, M Skivenes, eds. Oxford University Press, 2011, pp. 204–22.

Chapter 19

Shaken Baby Syndrome/Abusive Head Trauma Opinion Evidence in American Courts

Kathleen Pakes

In the healthcare setting, the shaken baby syndrome/abusive head trauma (SBS/AHT) label is assigned by child protection teams (CPTs). Despite protests to the contrary, the CPT classification of SBS/AHT is not a medical diagnosis and carries no medical significance. Unlike a patient's treatment team, the CPT is not involved in stabilising a patient, writing orders, performing surgeries, or prescribing medications and therapy. Members of CPTs are mandatory reporters and advocates for children; their diagnostic process favours child protection and errs on the side of child safety. 'Treatment' consists of reporting to and working with law enforcement and Child Protective Services, removing children from their homes [1], and advocating for children to make sure they receive necessary follow-up services such as mental health treatment and family counselling [2]. Once cases labelled 'abuse' are introduced to the legal system, prosecutors and child protection workers rely upon members of the CPT, generally child abuse paediatricians, to provide an 'expert' opinion that the child was abused.

This chapter discusses the crossroads of child protection medicine and legal proceedings. Clinical decision-making errs on the side of child safety. The law does not. In the courtroom, the law presumes innocence; reliability, not advocacy, drives the use of expert opinion. In the courtroom, a *clinically* 'valid' opinion may be inadmissible because it lacks the scientific foundation the law demands. Although many US courts have admitted SBS/AHT medical opinion evidence, a consistent application of governing legal principles would exclude opinion evidence purporting to 'diagnose' SBS/AHT.

19.1 *Daubert* and Expert Opinion Admissibility Standards

In legal proceedings, expert opinion evidence is often necessary to assist the trier of fact to understand or determine a fact in issue. Experts are therefore afforded greater testimonial leeway than ordinary witnesses whose testimony is limited to statements of historical fact. Because expert testimony can be both powerful and misleading due to the difficulty in evaluating it, the courts act as gatekeepers to its admissibility.

Special rules govern the admission of expert testimony. In the US federal court system and in the majority of states, admissibility is governed by the principles described in *Daubert v Merrell Dow Pharmaceuticals, Inc.* [3]. In *Daubert*, the plaintiff's expert opined that prenatal drug exposure caused birth defects [4]. Referring to this subject matter as scientific testimony, the Court noted that admissibility depended upon relevance and reliability. Relevance is an expansive test, generally defined as 'any tendency to make the existence of any fact that is of consequence to the determination of the action more probable or less probable than it would be without the evidence' [5].

Reliability of expert opinion depends upon (1) whether the reasoning or methodology underlying such opinion is scientifically valid, and (2) whether reasoning or methodology was properly applied to the facts in issue [4, 6]. In *Daubert*, the Court identified non-exclusive factors that judges could consider in determining admissibility: whether a theory or technique has been tested, whether a theory or technique is subjected to peer review and publication, whether the technique has a known rate of error, and whether there is general acceptance within the relevant scientific community. In *Kumho Tire Co., Ltd. v Carmichael*, the Court held that the judiciary's gatekeeping role extends to expert opinions involving technical or specialised knowledge as well as scientific knowledge, and that the admissibility test is flexible and should consider the particular circumstances of each particular case [6].

If reliable and relevant to an issue in the case, testimony must also be helpful to the jury. In this context, helpfulness means expert opinions are admissible only if they draw on expertise or knowledge beyond common knowledge and beyond the jury's capacity to evaluate the facts on its own. If medical causation relies on consideration of evidence that is within the jury's common experiences and knowledge, such as the meaning or veracity of statements by a witness or the accused, then expert testimony is neither helpful nor necessary [7].

In a minority of states that do not follow *Daubert*, admissibility is generally governed by the *Frye* standard [8]. Under *Frye*, expert opinion based on a scientific technique is inadmissible unless the technique is 'generally accepted' as reliable in the *relevant* scientific community.

19.2 Admissibility and Medical Expert Testimony

19.2.1 The Differential Diagnosis and Specific Causation Opinion

In clinical medicine, the differential diagnosis is the methodology for identifying and treating disease [9]. In conducting a differential diagnosis on a patient, a physician considers the history of present illness, objective medical findings, laboratory tests, and past medical history. The physician then rules in, or compiles, a list of all conditions or diseases that could underlie that patient's medical findings and symptoms. After ruling in potential illnesses or conditions, the physician systematically eliminates identified possibilities, usually as the result of specific tests, and selects the most probable that remains – also referred to as specific causation opinion [9]. Once arriving at specific causation opinion, the physician may prescribe a procedure, treatment, or therapy to remedy the illness or medical condition. Feedback from the patient informs the physician whether to consider another diagnosis or treatment, order more tests, or consult with specialists.

19.2.2 Differential Aetiology

When a physician strays beyond assessing and treating medical conditions and divines what external actions, toxins, or insults *might* have *caused* the medical condition leading to symptoms, the clinician is speculating about aetiology. Aetiology speculation is often irrelevant for treatment purposes. For example, a physician who identifies and diagnoses a patient with HIV treats that patient with drugs. The aetiology of the HIV – for example, whether the patient acquired the virus through drug use or sexual contact – does not affect the treatment. Likewise, whether a patient's lung cancer is from smoking or other environmental toxins does not change the treatment for the cancer. Because aetiology speculation, even if wrong, may be accompanied by generally good and harmless 'treatment' advice, such as don't smoke or engage in illicit drug use, there is no downside to 'overdiagnosing' aetiology [10].

Courts have excluded aetiology opinions, finding the process used to arrive at such opinions is less reliable than the process used to identify medical conditions for treatment. For example, one court allowed a physician to diagnose the type and extent of a patient's back injuries causing pain, but prohibited the physician from offering opinion testimony that the back injuries were *caused* by the vibrations the patient experienced while working as an engineer on a train locomotive. The court noted that this opinion (vibrations caused the back injury) was the product of a differential aetiology, not a differential diagnosis, and that the former lacked the assurances of reliability that might be present with the latter [11]. Other courts have likewise found that aetiology opinion is unreliable and inadmissible when there is a lack of scientific evidence establishing that the ruled-in external causation could actually cause the patient's condition [12, 13].

As problematic as external causation (aetiology) determination can be in tort cases, that determination is even more challenging and *less scientifically reliable* in SBS/AHT cases. In the typical tort case, such as the back injury case, exposure is undisputed. The issue is whether the *undisputed exposure* (e.g., experiencing the vibrations on the locomotive) is capable of causing and did in fact cause a known injury or outcome (e.g., the back injury). In SBS/AHT cases, exposure *and* causation are disputed. The clinician assumes an exposure occurred, despite the fact the exposure has not been observed or otherwise proven [14]. The clinician *further assumes* the *assumed* exposure is capable of causing and did in fact cause the identified medical conditions (see sections 2.3 and 2.4).

Such methodology is a form of 'negative corpus diagnosis' – eliminating obvious causes of medical conditions and, in the absence of an acceptable clinical history, defaulting to crime as an explanation [15]. Negative corpus methodology – which is the methodology employed by child protection physicians – was once the standard in arson investigation, but is no longer accepted in that field due to unreliability [16]. In Canada, the Goudge inquiry into paediatric death investigation criticised methodology that defaults to abuse. The Goudge report emphasised that, '[i]f, on examination of all the evidence in an infant death case, every possible known cause has been excluded, the cause of death remains unknown' [17].

19.2.3 Specific Causation Opinion Can Be Reliable

Specific causation opinion, reached via a differential methodology, *can* satisfy *Daubert* reliability standards [9]. For specific causation opinion to be admissible the expert must have executed the differential diagnosis (or aetiology) in a reliable manner [18, 19]. This means the differential must be based on scientifically valid decisions as to which potential causes to rule in [18]. Causes are reliably ruled in if general causation has been established – that is, if it has been shown that the cause (exposure) *is actually capable of producing the medical symptoms* for which a patient suffers. Federal courts have therefore held that a plaintiff must establish the reliability of the general causation assumptions before evidence of specific causation can be admitted [20, 21]. Once general causation has been reliably established, the plaintiff must then prove that the general causation theory selected actually caused the specific condition. Whether the process used produced a reliable opinion is a case-by-case determination [18].

19.2.4 Clinical Decision-Making Is Not a Scientifically Valid Methodology for Establishing General Causation

Clinicians are not bench researchers. Built into every doctor's differential process is the *assumption* that general causation has been previously proven [22] – that is, that the final 'cause' is actually capable of producing the condition [20].

Because the differential diagnosis (or differential aetiology) methodology *assumes* the validity of general causation assumptions (which may be wrong), courts have held that *the differential diagnosis is not a scientific method* by which a physician can reliably determine whether a specific exposure is capable of causing symptoms in humans [22]. In other words, a clinician's 'ability to diagnose medical conditions is not remotely the same ... as the ability to deduce, delineate, and describe, in a scientifically reliable manner, the causes of those medical conditions' [23]. Legal scholars have also emphasised this principle – that is, clinicians are not trained and lack the ability to exercise 'background' causal analysis [24].

Thus, for admissibility purposes, a clinician's specific causation opinion, derived through a differential process, satisfies *Daubert* only if general causation has been established for the causes ruled in, including the final diagnosis. For example, in *McClain v Metabolife International, Inc.*, the plaintiff's expert, a clinical neurologist, purported to employ a differential process to reach the opinion that exposure (use of diet supplement) caused strokes [25]. The court found this opinion failed to meet *Daubert* admissibility standards because there was insufficient scientific proof that the ruled-in cause (diet supplement) was actually capable of causing strokes. The court emphasised that, while the differential diagnosis may, under circumstances that ensure reliability, produce an admissible opinion, use of the differential diagnosis was not enough to overcome the fundamental failure of laying a scientific groundwork for general causation [25].

The National Academy of Sciences, as *Amici* to the *Daubert* litigation, underscored that a court's reliability analysis must specifically address whether underlying general causation assumptions are supported by sound science [26]. Courts have acknowledged this principle and cautioned that allowing a party to rely on a specific causation opinion to establish general causation theory amounts to an impermissible end run around the general causation requirement [21]. Accordingly, causal assumptions also implicate relevance. Courts have held that testimony regarding specific causation in a given patient is irrelevant unless general causation is established for that opinion [20].

19.3 The Unproven Shaken Baby Syndrome General Causation Assumptions and the Problem of Circular Reasoning

19.3.1 Syndrome Diagnosis Lacks General Causation Foundation

A syndrome is a complex of non-specific symptoms and physical findings which indicate a condition for which a direct cause is not necessarily understood [27]. Most syndromes are not well defined and their definition may change over time [28]. Shaken baby syndrome is generally described as a constellation of symptoms and medical findings that include subdural bleeding, retinal haemorrhages (RH), and encephalopathy [29]. Underlying the SBS/AHT clinical diagnostic paradigm is the assumed but unproven general causation belief that shaking (exposure) is capable of causing such medical findings and symptoms.

These SBS/AHT general causation assumptions stem from biomechanical studies of primates subjected to rear-end collisions producing whiplash. In the early 1970s, such studies led a British neurosurgeon, Norman Guthkelch, and an American radiologist, John Caffey, to hypothesise an external biomechanical cause (whiplash) of unexplained subdural bleeding, neurological compromise, and RH in infants [138, 30, 31] (see Chapter 2). Despite the lack of scientific methodology establishing general causation (that human shaking could generate the force necessary to cause such injuries), Caffey's whiplash shaking theory became entrenched in American clinical belief and practice [32–35]. By the late 1990s, Caffey's unvalidated general causation theories were the practice standard. The child protection community accepted that from the presence of subdural haemorrhage, RH, and encephalopathy a clinician could 'diagnose' shaking in the absence of another explanation [36].

At the same time, concerns over clinical use of these unproven general-causation theories were growing. Biomechanical and medical researchers criticised clinical extrapolation from adult primate studies to support unproven general causation assumptions in infants [37] (see Chapter 14). In 2002, the US Department of Health and Human Services convened a conference to address the growing contention over the SBS diagnosis [38]. Organisers acknowledged that very little scientific experimental or descriptive work supported the SBS diagnosis, that the pathophysiology of medical findings remained obscure, and that the relationship to biomechanics was even cloudier [38].

Conference contributors also recognised that compounding the poorly understood pathophysiology and the lack of reliable scientific research was a clinical methodology that relied on circular reasoning [39]. In SBS/AHT cases, circular reasoning starts with a clinician's general causation belief – that shaking infants can directly cause certain symptoms or conditions such as subdural bleeding, RH, and encephalopathy. Then, when clinicians observe these symptoms in the absence of a known medical cause or clinically acceptable explanation, they refer back to their belief system and *assume* both exposure (shaking) and causation [36, 39].

In civil litigation, methodology based on circular reasoning has been soundly rejected as unreliable by the courts [40–43]. For example, expert opinion was held inadmissible where the expert engaged in circular reasoning by presuming that plaintiff's cataracts 'were radiation induced, and then presumed that the plaintiff must have somehow been exposed to a high enough dose to exceed the threshold in order to have caused the cataracts, thereby justifying his initial diagnosis' [44]. Likewise, a court found an expert's methodology in diagnosing 'mold illness' unreliable because, among other things, 'he used circular reasoning to work backwards from diagnosis to proof of exposure' [41].

19.3.2 Unreliable Processes Lead to Unreliable Data

Because SBS/AHT general-causation assumptions have never been scientifically validated and because the child abuse diagnostic process relies upon circular reasoning, clinical decision-making produces unreliable data. This unreliable data problem is well known and acknowledged in the child abuse field. As one researcher noted, '[h]aving worked on this topic [child abuse] for over 10 years, we have always been amazed by the lack of reliable data and of proper scientific reasoning on matters which are the cornerstone of judgments which can either send innocent caretakers to jail or allow a child molester to roam free', and that, '[a]mong the flawed scientific logic, circular reasoning (e.g., evaluating the incidence of retinal hemorrhages in child abuse while using the presence of retinal hemorrhage as a criterion of abuse) appeared the most obvious' [45].

19.4 Parallel Process: The Reliability of Treating Medical Conditions versus the Unreliability of Social-Value Decision-Making

How is it that a general causation theory (shaking) with little to no scientific foundation continues to be a 'ruled-in' bedrock of clinical practice? To understand, one must consider that, instead of treating medical conditions and disease, the abuse classification system is designed to trigger social services and law enforcement involvement and to advocate for those cases in the legal system.

19.4.1 Mandatory Reporting and Erring on the Side of Safety: Anything Suspicious Must Be Labelled Abuse

In the late 1960s, US states began adopting child protection laws. By 1970, all US states required mandatory physician reporting of suspected abuse [46]. Implicit in the child protection legislation was the assumption that the balance between children's rights and parental rights was to be weighed in favour of protecting children from abuse [47]. The standard for reporting suspected abuse is low: 'cause to suspect', 'believes', or 'reasonable suspicion' have been deemed sufficient for reporting [47, 2]. Other laws provide criminal penalties and civil liability for failing to report but guarantee immunity for healthcare providers who erroneously report abuse [47, 2]. Such system design maximises child protection but encourages over-reporting (see Chapter 18). Indeed, Australian researchers recognised an overload of the child protection system due to reporters making 'reports, not because they are concerned about child abuse, but because they are concerned about criminal charges if they do not report even the slightest incident' [48].

Alongside the mandatory reporting obligations and penalties for failing to report, child abuse physicians are motivated by a moral duty to protect children. In 2019, 12 nationally known child protection advocates underscored that 'in pediatric medicine where the patient is invariably unable to advocate for his or her own interests, the safety of the patient takes precedence over all other concerns' [49]. In 2020, Duhaime and Christian advised that, if sufficient suspicions of abuse are raised, then protection of the child is prioritised 'even if the determination cannot be made definitively' [50]. In 2021, Brown noted that overdiagnosis of child abuse is a reality and that, when clinicians prioritise saving lives over the risks of overdiagnosis, they 'are adhering to ... strongly held values – not empirical truth' [51].

Such sentiments are not novel. In 1962, Kempe instructed that 'bias should be in favor of the child's safety' and 'the physician should not be satisfied to return the child to an environment where even a moderate risk of repetition exists' [52]. Guthkelch advised 'all cases of infantile subdural haematoma are best assumed to be traumatic unless proved otherwise' [138]. Helfer said that any perceived inconsistency between the history and physical findings *must be diagnosed* as a suspected case of child abuse [53].

19.4.2 Human Interpretation Bias: Social Risk Factors

Methodologies that incorporate human judgement are 'especially vulnerable to human error, inconsistency across examiners, and cognitive bias' [54] (see Chapter 13).

The child abuse diagnostic methodology has been historically influenced by human judgment about social risk factors believed to be associated with abuse, including minority status, poverty, perceived delay in seeking care [55], reporting to the hospital at odd hours [56], or whether the caretaker was disliked, for unknown reasons' by the physician [53]. While the American Academy of Pediatrics (AAP) diagnostic guidelines indicate that social risk factors should be used for anticipatory guidance rather than indicators of abuse [2, 57], researchers acknowledge that social pathology influences clinical decision making [55]. One clinical paper claimed the combination of an inconsistent history with parental risk factors 'was 100% predictive of inflicted head injury' [58]. Upon finding that children of immigrants were four times as likely to be 'diagnosed' as abused, Norwegian researchers questioned whether social stigma played a factor [59].

Not only does subjective assessment of social risk factors influence clinical decision-making, it leads to incorrect diagnoses [60]. Anderst found that clinician assessment of social risk factors is one of the main causes of overdiagnosing abuse [61]. Keenan reported that, when presented with a reversal of social risk factors, child abuse physicians changed their diagnosis from abuse to not abuse in 40% of cases [55]. They also found that the higher the clinician's risk perception of social indicators, the higher the clinician's diagnostic certainty of abuse, but that such certainty was not consistent with diagnostic accuracy, and has been linked to common cognitive errors [55]. Other consequences of relying on subjective social risk factors is that child abuse classifications reflect pronounced biases against and differential consequences for minority and low-income families [59].

19.4.3 The Child Protection Methodology Lacks a Reliability Mechanism: The Feedback Loop

In the treatment of disease or medical conditions, the differential diagnosis is part of a long-term process that gathers feedback and information from the patient with the goal of eventually returning the patient's health to baseline. If a patient does not improve, or the doctor is unsure about the original diagnosis, the physician may order more tests, refer to specialists, rethink the working diagnosis, or order different treatment. Through a constant information-gathering process, physicians learn from mistakes, leading to improved reliability in decision-making [62].

Child advocacy classifications, on the other hand, have no feedback loop. The 'diagnosis' is a one-time assessment, often urgently performed in an emergency setting, and designed to ensure child protection by triggering *immediate* social service and law enforcement intervention [35, 63]. Treatment (complying with mandatory reporting and ensuring child protection) is largely complete as soon as investigative and social-service agencies are notified.

Within this context, 'child abuse' may be simultaneously a 'valid diagnosis' and an incorrect 'diagnosis' – 'valid' because clinicians are professionally trained and morally obligated to assume exposure and include a final discharge determination that complies with mandatory reporting and errs on the side of child safety. But because there is no gold-standard or reference test to 'confirm' a suspicion of abuse, 'diagnostic for abuse' does not mean 'is' abuse. 'Diagnostic for abuse' simply means the clinician feels he or she is required to 'diagnose' abuse and refer to the proper authorities. At the same time, abuse may be an incorrect label, as it may not be the actual cause of the infant's condition. For such reasons, Guthkelch, who introduced the SBS hypothesis [138], emphasised that, when the SBS/AHT 'diagnosis' is exported to the courts, the uncertainty in the diagnosis should be acknowledged [64].

19.4.4 Child Advocacy Bias Encourages Over-Classification of Abuse

Largely driven by social values and lacking a gold standard, there is an inherent uncertainty in child protection determinations. Hobbs urged restraint, arguing 'the diagnosis of abuse demands absolute certainty to avoid conviction of innocent parents and unwarranted removal of children' [65]. The AAP opposed Hobbs's position and recommended a far lower standard for 'diagnosing' abuse. According to AAP publications, reasonable suspicion of abuse was sufficient to determine abuse for reporting to investigative agencies [34].

Researchers recognise that prioritising child safety encourages incorrect classifications. Because CPTs 'have a strong moral sense of protecting children . . . the criteria with which they identify child abuse might come to be oriented to prove guilt, rather than being medically or scientifically motivated' [66]. Accordingly, 'the task is not primarily to classify shaken baby cases correctly, but rather to protect the child from future risk of abuse, even if it involves a risk of convicting an innocent parent or guardian' [66].

In Sweden, epidemiologists cautioned that an increase in child abuse diagnoses was related to an increase in the use of CPTs, not an increase in violence [67] (see also Chapter 23). American researchers noted a similar trend. An increased number of infant deaths labelled homicide coincided with an increase in the focus on child protection, not an increase in the rate of death [68].

19.5 Scientifically Unvalidated General Causation Theories

At the core of the SBS/AHT *Daubert* analysis is whether sound science supports the general-causation assumptions. In SBS/AHT classification, general-causation assumptions are as follows. In the absence of a known biological cause or clinically acceptable evidence of trauma, (1) SDH is an assumed marker of exposure (an acceleration deceleration event) by which one can infer (2) manual shaking and (3) that this assumed exposure (shaking) also produced assumed microscopic (clinically invisible) damage to axons in the brain (traumatic axonal injury), (4) explaining clinical neurological symptoms such as lethargy or vomiting [69]. It is further assumed that symptoms caused by this inferred process would appear immediately and that the last person with the child 'did it' [70]. If RH are present, clinicians can also assume they were caused by the same assumed exposure (shaking) [71]. The reliability of opinions resting on a chain of causal assumptions is seriously undermined if any of those assumptions lack reliability.

19.5.1 Subdural Haematoma Is Not a Reliable Marker of Trauma or Shaking

Biomechanical studies have not validated the general-causation assumption that manual shaking of infants can cause subdural haematoma (SDH) (see Chapter 14). Clinical studies demonstrate that SDH, without signs of impact, is not a reliable marker of trauma. The differential for SDH is extensive and includes biological causes [71, 72] (see Chapters 3–9). Disrupted bridging veins, or non-traumatic oozing from the inner dural plexus, may create SDH [139]. Matschke found that, in infants who died with subdural bleeding, most bleeding was not traumatic in origin [73]. In 2013, Scheimberg reported cases of infants and children with non-traumatic intradural and subdural bleeding associated with hypoxia [74]. Research into the origins of SDH lacks homogeneous studies controlling for confounding factors and SDH can be clinically silent. When medical conditions can be occult in the background population, the prevalence, and therefore the predictive value, of such findings is unknown [75].

19.5.2 Neurological Symptoms Are Not a Reliable Marker of Trauma or Shaking

Like SDH, neurological symptoms have a wide differential diagnosis. Neurological symptoms develop in response to other non-specific conditions (such as seizures or raised intracranial pressure (RICP)), including conditions with non-traumatic origins [76]. For 30 years, the clinical assumption that unexplained neurological symptoms could be attributed to shaking-induced traumatic axonal damage went unchallenged.

Then, in 2001, Geddes published the first peer-reviewed studies [77, 78] demonstrating that the clinical belief that one could infer shaking from neurological symptoms was wrong (see Chapter 3). Geddes, a neuropathologist, recognised that children 'diagnosed' as abused often presented with swollen brains and hypoxic changes, but that there was little scientific evidence to conclude this abnormal pathology was *traumatic* in origin [78]. With the use of improved staining techniques, Geddes and other researchers examined the brains of children previously labelled 'abused'. The overwhelming majority of children did not have traumatic axonal injury [73]. Instead, these children had non-specific hypoxic brain damage from which one could *not* infer trauma. Accordingly, Geddes advised that clinicians could not extrapolate general causation assumptions (shaking) or an amount of force, and that 'it is possible that the severe acceleration-deceleration injury that is so often cited does not in fact occur in shaken-baby syndrome' [78]. Later neuropathology research confirmed Geddes's findings [79, 80].

19.5.3 All Clinical Shaken Baby Syndrome/Abusive Head Trauma Assumptions Are, for These Reasons, Unvalidated and Unreliable

Upon discovering that the assumed biological cause (traumatic axonal damage) of neurological symptoms did not exist and that the proximate cause of such encephalopathy was non-specific (hypoxic), Geddes questioned the assumptions underlying the SBS 'diagnosis' [81]. Based on the non-traumatic hypoxic origin of brain damage, Geddes hypothesised that a combination of severe hypoxia, brain swelling, and raised central venous pressure might also cause vessels to leak into the subdural space, and that a similar mechanism might explain RH. Harshly criticised by the child protection community for this hypothesis, Geddes acknowledged that this was a hypothesis, but countered that the traditional 'shaking' theory, while preferred by clinicians, was also a hypothesis and may be wrong [82] (see Chapter 1).

19.5.4 The Retinal Haemorrhage Bogeyman

19.5.4.1 Retinal Haemorrhages Are Non-specific

Retinal haemorrhages are a non-specific finding that develop as a secondary response to intracranial pathology caused by disease, medical conditions, or trauma [83, 71] (see Chapters 2, 3, 9). They rarely develop in neurologically normal patients [84], and the severity of intracranial pathology, no matter the cause, correlates with the severity of the RH that develop [85]. There is no type, size, distribution, or appearance of RH that is unique to abuse [86]. Because of the various contexts in which RH develop, researchers have cautioned that their presence is not a reliable marker of abuse [87, 84].

19.5.4.2 The Pathophysiology of Retinal Haemorrhages Is Elusive

While the child protection community has historically associated the presence of RH with abuse, a 2007 study noted that '[t]he mechanism of retinal hemorrhage formation in child abuse has been the subject of great speculation and little agreement' [88]. In 2014, Forbes, an ophthalmologist, testified for the prosecution and acknowledged that doctors cannot identify the precise mechanism in the body that causes RH and that medicine has not established a causative relationship between AHT and RH [89].

19.5.4.3 The Child Protection Theory of Retinal Haemorrhage Development

19.5.4.3.1 Vitreo-retinal Traction and 'Severe' Retinal Haemorrhage

The child protection diagnostic process assumes the vitreo-retinal traction (VT) theory of general causation for RH development. This biomechanical theory is twofold, speculating (1) that a repetitive acceleration-deceleration mechanism (human shaking) is capable of causing the vitreous body to pull on its retinal attachments, thus disrupting the layers of the retina and causing bleeding, and (2) that 'severe' RH are highly suggestive of shaking [85].

Undermining the reliability of these child protection theories are studies documenting that severe RH develop in contexts unrelated to abuse and are a secondary response to other biological processes such as birth [90], subarachnoid haemorrhage (SAH) [91, 92], bleeding disorders and natural disease [93], and raised intracranial pressure (RICP) from any cause, especially hyper-acute spikes [94, 85]. Because RH, including severe RH, develop in non-abusive contexts, critics point out there is no need to invoke a speculative mechanism such as shaking [95, 96]. Vinchon recognised the clinical assumption that severe RH are a marker of SBS/AHT creates data influenced by selection bias and circular reasoning, undermining the reliability of clinical studies [97].

19.5.4.3.2 The 'Evidence Base' for the Retinal Haemorrhage General Causation Assumption (Shaking) Is the Fact Clinicians Are Trained to Believe It Is True

Biomechanical studies, including those involving humans shaking animals, have not established the VT theory [98, 99] (see Chapter 14). Computer modelling (finite-element modelling (FEM)) is unreliable because it lacks known injury threshold data. In a study reporting 36 cases of witnessed and/or confessed violent shaking (where confession was spontaneous and not tainted by CPT or police questioning), only two infants developed any RH [100].

The support base for the general-causation VT theory is that it has been favoured by child protection clinicians and repeatedly referenced in the clinical literature. Levin argued that the 'theoretical role of vitreotraction supports what we know about RH in SBS' [101] and that 'the body of literature *suggests*' shaking causes shearing injury and is the primary factor generating RH [102]. Tagioka reasoned that 'the sheer number of articles with consistent [clinical] findings supports using RH as a physical examination finding consistent with SBS' [103]. The 2010 [104] and 2018 [85] AAP statements emphasise that the *clinical association* of RH with AHT had been demonstrated repeatedly in clinical studies and clinical experience, and that 'extensive literature' supports the theory. One need not point out that if the AAP and clinical literature train clinicians to associate RH with abuse, then clinical data and clinical literature will reflect that training and association. Kahneman described the repetition of belief as a form of cognitive ease that creates illusions of truth [105].

From a legal perspective, preferred clinical beliefs, clinical experience applying those preferred beliefs, and studies relying on data generated by those preferred clinical beliefs are not scientific proof of general-causation principles and are not sufficient to bridge the general-causation gap [22, 106]. Accordingly, courts have held that studies 'suggesting' a causal effect based on clinical observations are insufficient to establish a scientific foundation for general-causation theory [107].

19.5.4.3.3 Lack of Confounding Factors Research Renders the Vitreo-retinal Traction Theory Inadmissible

Further undermining the reliability and admissibility of the VT theory is a failure to account for confounding factors. A confounding variable is an unmeasured factor that influences both supposed cause and supposed effect. Therefore, lack of understanding of confounding factors is a major hurdle to the legal admissibility of any scientific theory or medical diagnosis [106]. This is because medical cause-and-effect testimony is reliable and admissible only where 'medical science understands the physiological process by which a particular disease or syndrome develops and knows what factors cause the process to occur' [108].

Infants are known to develop severe RH in complicated clinical pictures, unrelated to trauma, involving confounding factors [93]. In 2018, the AAP acknowledged that confounding factors such as hypoxia, anaemia, reperfusion injury, vascular dysregulation, coagulopathies, and raised intracranial pressure may play a role in RH development and appearance and more study was needed [85]. Forensic pathologists, with the benefit of their specialty training and autopsy experience, recognise that natural disease process and biological sequelae unrelated to abuse can cause severe RH [98, 109].

Because the VT RH theory is scientifically unsupported, and because clinicians cannot exclude biological confounding factors and sequelae as the cause of RH development, the clinical assumptions that one can infer (1) exposure (shaking) and (2) general causation from the presence of 'severe' RH are unreliable rendering opinion inadmissible under *Daubert* [98].

19.6 The Relevant Scientific Community Includes Those with the Education, Training, and Experience to Critically Appraise the Child Protection General-Causation Theories

Under *Daubert*, 'general acceptance' in the relevant scientific community remains a factor in the admissibility analysis, although no longer a dispositive factor, as it was under *Frye*. A closely related factor is whether the discipline or theory is published and peer reviewed.

For this part of the admissibility analysis, it is necessary to distinguish between clinical (specific causation) and general-causation peer review. Peer review and/or publication by a group or journal that assumes the validity of general-causation theories are not relevant or helpful to an analysis of whether there is a reliable scientific basis supporting those general-causation theories.

Under the *Daubert* and *Frye* admissibility analysis, peer review is meaningful if the theory or technique has been critiqued or accepted by the *relevant* scientific community. What is the relevant scientific community to assess SBS/AHT general-causation theory? Narang argues that the relevant scientific community is limited to the paediatric clinical providers trained in the 'differential diagnosis' and familiar with the clinical literature [71]. This position conflates specific and general-causation principles and does not address the relevant issues for *Daubert* analysis.

As discussed, for *Daubert* (and *Frye*) purposes, clinical assumptions are irrelevant. The relevant issues are whether the ruled-in general-causation assumptions are scientifically supported and whether the process for establishing general causation and for moving from general to specific causation is reliable. Thus, disciplines with the training, education, and experience to critically evaluate general-causation assumptions are the relevant scientific community [110].

19.6.1 Forensic Pathology, Neuropathology, and Biomechanical Engineering Critique of Shaken Baby Syndrome/Abusive Head Trauma Theories

Child protection teams operate in a hospital setting with live patients. Thus, not only are their opinions (and data they generate) influenced by mandatory reporting, advocacy bias, and a lack of patient feedback, their opinions and data are based on limited information. They do not at that point have the benefit or experience of information that can only be learned at autopsy and which may demonstrate their clinical assumptions were wrong.

For example, Duhaime identified cases with no *clinical* evidence of impact, classified by clinicians as 'shaking', but for which autopsy revealed evidence of impact [111]. In a series of cases labelled abuse by clinicians, Kirschner identified causes, other than abuse, at autopsy [60]. Forensic pathologists' experiences are that RH, including severe RH, appear in conditions unrelated to abuse [83, 98, 110, 112]. In a survey study, 60% of forensic pathologists responding indicated they did not consider SBS a valid diagnosis [113]. Neuropathologists disproved the clinical beliefs that one could reliably infer (1) traumatic axonal injury from clinical symptoms and (2) that 'shaking' caused such inferred symptoms [77–79] (see Chapter 3).

What's more, clinicians do not have the education and training of biomechanical engineers. Clinicians are not experts in the laws of physics, mechanics, and materials' properties; they do not conduct experiments studying the application of force to the human body and the consequences of that force. Clinicians do not design safety-belt systems, car seats, playground equipment, or helmets. Biomechanical engineers, perhaps the most relevant scientific community in assessing general-causation principles of force applied to the human body, underscore that the child-advocacy belief a person can violently shake an infant and cause subdural bleeding, RH, or axonal damage, and the belief it can be done without damaging the neck is not proven and scientifically improbable (see Chapter 14).

19.6.2 Peer Review of the Literature for Evidence of Sound Scientific Foundation

Where peer review has *critically* assessed the literature for scientific studies supporting the validity of SBS/AHT general-causation theory, such review has found insufficient scientific evidence to support those theories. Donohoe was the first to attempt such review [114]. Searching the pre-2000 SBS literature, he was unable to identify sound *scientific* research supporting the shaking mechanism theories. Critics of Donohoe's paper argue the research parameters were under-inclusive, but such critics have failed to identify any specific studies from that time frame that undermine Donohoe's ultimate conclusion that the scientific evidence base for SBS/AHT was poor [1, 71]. In 2001, a major forensic pathology treatise examined the SBS literature and echoed Donohoe's observations, concluding, '[t]here is just no conclusive evidence that this entity exists' [115].

In 2002, the National Institutes of Health convened a conference specific to SBS for precisely the reasons Donohoe observed – a scientific basis for SBS theory was lacking [38]. In 2011, a prominent child abuse text mirrored these observations, noting that no one had 'yet marshaled a coherent and comprehensive argument in support of shaking as a causal mechanism for abusive head injury' [116]. In Sweden, dispute over whether a 'scientifically robust body of knowledge' supported SBS/AHT general causation assumptions led to a systematic assessment (peer review) of the SBS literature [117, 118]. Researchers combed thousands of publications and concluded there was insufficient (very low-quality) scientific evidence on which to assess the diagnostic accuracy of the triad as proof of shaking, and low-quality evidence that any or all components of the triad could be associated with shaking at all (see Chapter 10).

Thus, biomechanical studies, neuropathological studies, forensic pathology studies, and systematic review of the literature for scientific studies validating the SBS/AHT theory are consistent – the SBS/AHT general-causation hypotheses have not been scientifically validated. This lack of scientific support renders general-causation expert opinion testimony inadmissible under *Daubert*.

Lacking scientific support for general-causation theories, clinicians argue that the legal system, via the child protection process, gives their theories scientific legitimacy. That is, once the CPTs identify what they believe to be SBS/AHT cases, they provide their theory of abuse to the police. Because the police (who accept the theories as true) are sometimes able to extract 'confessions' or statements purportedly matching the child protection theories, those theories must be correct. For this reason, 'confessed shaking' has been touted as 'the evidentiary basis for shaking' [116]. Social protection and legal process is not a scientific method for validating pathophysiologic and biomechanical hypotheses. For further discussion, including the unreliability of police generated statements and guilty pleas, and the reasons (other than guilt) that innocent people 'confess', see Chapters 11, 12, 20, and 22.

19.7 Clinical Consensus Is Not Science

In *General Elec. Co. v Joiner*, the US Supreme Court considered the admissibility of expert opinion that exposure to PCBs caused lung cancer [119]. The Court found the testimony inadmissible, noting too great an analytical gap between the data and the expert's opinion.

The Court held that *Daubert* did not require a court to admit expert opinion evidence that was connected to existing data only by the *ipse dixit* of the expert.

In SBS/AHT cases, there is an especially wide analytical divide between the medical findings and the clinical opinion that assumes both exposure and general causation. While the child protection community may be united in consistently applying preferred but scientifically unsupported general-causation assumptions to bridge this gap, such methodology is nothing more than a guild test that trades the *ipse dixit* of the individual for the *ipse dixit* of the group [110].

In response to criticisms of the adherence to unvalidated SBS/AHT theories, members of the child protection community, via a non-transparent and hastily conducted process [120], orchestrated the publication of a so-called consensus statement proclaiming that SBS is a valid evidence-based diagnosis [121]. Science, of course, does not derive reliability from consensus, and group consensus that a 'diagnosis' is 'valid' does not satisfy the *Daubert* analytical gap. 'Abuse' may very well be a 'valid' classification for child protection purposes and compliance with mandatory reporting. But the fact a group proclaims a diagnostic label 'valid' does not mean the label is correct in a given case or that the general causation assumptions upon which the 'valid diagnosis' relies are scientifically sound. Likewise, an expert's expression of *confidence* based on expressions of group consensus about the purported accuracy of their field is no substitute for sound statistics [54, 122].

19.8 Diagnostic Consistency Is Not Scientific Proof of General Causation Assumptions

In contrast to the SBU finding that the overwhelming majority of the child abuse literature is methodologically flawed and of insufficient quality to support general-causation assumptions, Narang claims the child abuse literature is robust – reaching evidence-based medicine (EBM) levels 1(b) and 2(a) and providing a future foundation for the highest level of evidence based medicine available – level 1(a) [71]. One problem with such questionable claims is that clinical consistency in applying unproven general-causation theories, and reliable study *designs* are not substitutes for a scientifically sound foundation for general causation theories. A high-quality study *design* may comprise unreliable data and conclusions, and well-designed systematic reviews (SRs) may simply magnify and replicate flaws in original studies [123]. Where Narang et al. argue child abuse SRs are high quality, the SBU ranked the child abuse systematic reviews as low quality due to the significant methodology limitations of the underlying studies (see Chapter 10).

The SBU assessment that child abuse SRs are low quality is consistent with the acknowledged limitations of those publications. The child abuse systematic-review researchers recognise that clinical data unreliability is a significant limitation of their studies. Bhardwaj noted that 75% of clinical studies were compromised by circular reasoning and that, in more than half of the studies, it was unclear whether the child abuse cases were correctly identified [124]. Likewise, other systematic reviews acknowledge the confidence of their conclusions are undermined by circular reasoning, selection bias, confounding bias, and the inclusion criteria of the underlying clinical studies [125–128].

19.9 Lack of False Positives Renders Child Protection Clinical Data and Methodology Unreliable for *Daubert* Purposes

In syndrome diagnosis, there is no gold-standard or reference test to confirm the diagnosis. Therefore, in SBS/AHT cases, clinical preferences – not reference tests – influence data and control statistics. If clinicians are trained to make the abuse 'diagnosis' when certain factors are present and to exclude the 'diagnosis' when those factors are absent, then the diagnostic specificity and sensitivity of those factors will be high [28]. The clinical literature reflects this point. Vinchon's triad supposedly provides for 100% specificity [129]. Greeley boasts he can diagnose child abuse with 100% certainty [130]. Maguire suggests clinicians can 'identify' abuse with up to 100% certainty [126].

Researchers have pointed out that, while the child abuse data assumes 100% accuracy, nothing in science is 100% accurate and a lack of false positives renders the child abuse data unreliable. Aspelin noted,

> They have no false positive cases. But then you can't calculate positive predictive values. That is scientifically wrong. There is not one single false positive case in these meta-analyses and statistics. And that makes all these epidemiology predictive values worthless. At least, you cannot use it as a proof. So the mechanical theory is not proven; it's not evidence-based. The epidemiology outcome is not proven; it's not evidence-based [131].

When Lynøe et al. expressed concern that 'both the specificity and positive predictive value of the "Vinchon triad" was 100%' [132], Vinchon acknowledged that his team was 'a bit disturbed to find a 100% positive predictive value' for the clinical association of medical findings with SBS because the figure did not look like a scientific result. Nonetheless, Vinchon argued that, from a legal perspective, 'we think this is precisely what a judge hopes for' [133]. Lynøe pointed out that 'relying solely on a theory that makes judges and child protection teams happy will – if used in scientific studies – bring about diagnostic tests that are biased and inaccurate when diagnosing SBS/AHT' and that such a system risks generating false confessions [134].

Thus, while some in the child protection community claim low p-values support the reliability of clinical diagnosis, such claims are misleading. At their core, p-values rely on probabilities [71]. Syndrome diagnosis cannot be objectively evaluated by calculation of probabilities, since clinicians assume (and therefore determine) diagnostic accuracy [28, 122] (see Chapter 17).

19.10 Conclusion

For medical expert opinion to be admissible in the legal system, such expert opinion must be the product of methodology that is (1) reliable and (2) reliably applied. The child abuse diagnostic process fails on both counts. The methodology is fraught with advocacy bias and the general-causation beliefs upon which it relies have not been scientifically validated.

Federal courts recognise that one of the most 'troubling aspects of trying to apply *Daubert* to forensic evidence is that very few defense counsel are equipped to take on this challenge' [3]. Criminal defence counsel lack the training and resources to educate judges on these complex issues [3, 135]. Where criminal defence counsel have had the training and resources to present a well-developed challenge, courts have indeed recognised the unreliability of SBS/AHT diagnostic process [136, 137] (see Chapter 20).

In 2022, after five days of hearings, a New Jersey court summed SBS/AHT as 'more conjecture than' diagnosis [137]. The court found SBS a 'flawed diagnosis because *it originates from a theory based upon speculation and extrapolation* instead of being anchored in facts developed through reliable testing. There is no proof provided that AHT is, in fact, a valid diagnosis explaining an inflicted trauma which causes a pathology. Instead, what the literature and testimony have clearly shown is that *AHT is an assumption packaged as a medical diagnosis, unsupported by any medical or scientific testing*' (emphasis added) [137].

Expert testimony must be consistent with evidentiary and constitutional principles. Thus, depending on the facts of a specific case, testimony that a finding could be or is consistent with abuse may be admissible but, in SBS/AHT cases, testimony assuming exposure to a specific mechanism, and assuming the scientific validity of general causation principles, can only be unreliable.

References

1. Narang SK, Melville JD, Greeley CS et al. A Daubert analysis of abusive head trauma/ shaken baby syndrome. Part II: An examination of the differential diagnosis. *Journal of Health Law and Policy*. 2013;203–327.
2. Christian CW. Committee on Child Abuse and Neglect clinical report: The evaluation of suspected child physical abuse. *Pediatrics*. 2015;135(5):e1337–e1354.
3. Berger MA. The admissibility of expert testimony, the federal judicial center and National Research Council. In *Reference manual on scientific evidence*. 3rd ed. Committee on the Development of the Third Edition of the Reference Manual on Scientific Evidence, ed. National Academies Press, 2011, p. 12.
4. *Daubert v Merrell Dow Pharmaceuticals, Inc.*, 509 U.S. 579 (1993).
5. Fed. R. Evid. 401.
6. *Kumho Tire Co., Ltd. v Carmichael*, 526 U.S. 137 (1999).
7. Findley KA, Strang DA. Ending manner-of-death testimony and other opinion determinations of crime. *Duquesne Law Review*. 2022;60:302–38.
8. *Frye v United States*, 293 F. 1013(D.C. Cir. 1923).
9. Wong JB, Gostin LO, Cabrera OA. Reference guide on medical testimony: The Federal Judicial Center and National Research Council. In *Reference manual on scientific evidence*. 3rd ed. National Academies Press, 2011, p. 690.
10. Lynøe N, Eriksson A. A diagnostic test can prove anything if you use incorrect assumptions and circular reasoning. *Acta Paediatrica*. 2018;107:2051–3.
11. *Bowers v Norfolk S. Corp.*, 537 F. Supp. 2d 1343, 1360-61 (M.D. Ga. 2007), *aff'd*, 300 F. App'x 700 (11th Cir. 2008).
12. *C.W. ex rel. Wood v Textron, Inc.*, 807 F.3d 827 (7th Cir. 2015).
13. *Tamraz v Lincoln Elec. Co.*, 620 F.3d 665, 673 (6th Cir. 2010).
14. Findley KA, Risinger DM, Barnes PD et al. Feigned consensus: Usurping the law in shaken baby syndrome/ abusive head trauma prosecutions. *Wisconsin Law Review*. 2019:1211–67.
15. Findley KA, Barnes PD, Moran DA, Sperling C. Examining SBS convictions in light of new medical scientific research. *Oklahoma City University Law Review*. 2012;37:219–50.
16. Smith DW. The death of negative corpus. *Proceedings of the 5th International Symposium on Fire Investigation Science and Technology*. National Association of Fire Investigators International, 2012.
17. Goudge Report. P. 520 Inquiry into Pediatric Forensic Pathology in Ontario. Volume 3. www.fixcas.com/news/2008/Vol_3_Eng.pdf.
18. *Ervin v Johnson & Johnson, Inc.*, 492 F.3d 901 (7th Cir. 2007).

19. *Hendrix v Evenflo Co., Inc.*, 609 F.3d 1183 (11th Cir. 2010).
20. *Hall v Baxter Healthcare Corp.*, 947. F. Supp. 1387 (D. Oregon 1996).
21. *In re Bausch & Lomb Inc. Contact lens Solution Products Liability Litigation*, 2010 WL 1627807 (D.S.C., 2010).
22. *In re Breast Implant Litigation* 11 F.Supp.2d 1217 (D. Colorado 1998).
23. *Wynacht v Beckman Instruments, Inc.*, 113 F.Supp.2d 1205, 1209 (E.D. Tenn. 2000).
24. Sanders J, Faigman DL, Imrey PB, Dawid P. Differential etiology: Inferring specific causation in the law from group data in science. *Arizona Law Review*. 2021;63:851–921.
25. *McClain v Metabolife Int'l, Inc.*, 401 F3d 1233, 1253 (11th Cir. 2005).
26. Brief for the American Association for the Advancement of Science and the National Academy of Sciences as Amici Curiae, *Daubert v Merrell Dow Pharmaceuticals, Inc.*, 509 U.S. 579 (1993).
27. Calvo F, Karras, BT, Phillips R et al. Diagnoses, syndromes, and diseases: A knowledge representation problem. *In AMIA 2003 annual symposium proceedings*, vol. 2003. American Medical Informatics Association, 2003, p. 802.
28. Wulff, HR. *Rational diagnosis and treatment: An introduction to clinical decision-making*. 2nd ed. Blackwell Scientific, 1981. Diagnosis As a Matter of Opinion, p. 109.
29. Brooks W, Weathers L. Overview of shaken baby syndrome. In *The shaken baby syndrome: A multidisciplinary approach*. S Lazoritz, VJ Palusci, eds. Haworth Press, 2001.
30. Caffey J. On the theory and practice of shaking infants. *American Journal of Diseases of Children*. 1972;124:161–9.
31. Caffey J. The whiplash shaken infant syndrome. *Pediatrics*. 1974;54(4):396–403.
32. Dykes LJ. The whiplash shaken infant syndrome: What has been learned? *Child Abuse and Neglect*. 1986;10:211–21.
33. Ludwig S, Warman M. SBS: A review of 20 cases. *Annals of Emergency Medicine*. 1984;13(2):104–7.
34. Billmire E, Myers P. Serious head injury in infants: Accident or abuse? *Pediatrics*. 1985;75(2):340–2.
35. American Academy of Pediatrics Committee on Child Abuse and Neglect. Shaken baby syndrome: Inflicted cerebral trauma. *Pediatrics*. 1993;92(6):872–5.
36. Chadwick DL, Kirschner RH, Reece RM et al. Shaken baby syndrome: A forensic pediatric response. *Pediatrics*. 1998;101:321–3.
37. Ommaya AK, Goldsmith W, Thibault L. Biomechanics and neuropathology of adult and paediatric head injury. *British Journal of Neurosurgery*. 2002;16(3):220–42.
38. Reece RM, Nicholson, CE, eds. *Inflicted childhood neurotrauma: Proceedings of a conference sponsored by Department of Health and Human Services, National Institutes of Health, National Institute of Child Health and Human Development, Office of Rare Diseases, National Center for Medical Rehabilitation Research*. American Academy of Pediatrics, 2002.
39. Jenny C. Modes of presentation of inflicted childhood neurotrauma. In *Inflicted childhood neurotrauma: Proceedings of a conference sponsored by Department of Health and Human Services, National Institutes of Health, National Institute of Child Health and Human Development, Office of Rare Diseases, National Center for Medical Rehabilitation Research*. RM Reece, CE Nicholson, eds. American Academy of Pediatrics, 2002, pp. 49–63.
40. *Nelson v Tennessee Gas Pipeline Co.*, 243 F.3d 244, 254 (6th Cir. 2001).
41. *Young v Burton*, 567 F. Supp.2d 121, 137 (D. D.C. 2008).
42. *Mancuso v Consol. Edison Co. of N.Y.*, 967 F. Supp. 1437, 1450 (S.D.N.Y. 1997).
43. *Durden v Sec'y of Dep't of Health & Human Servs.*, No. 05-163V, 2007 WL 4962000, at *13 (Fed. Cl. 26 September 2007).

44. *O'Conner v Commonwealth Edison Co.*, 807 F. Supp. 1376, 1396 (C.D. Ill. 1992).
45. Vinchon M. Reply to Professor Charles Hyman: The scientific controversy over AHT in infants. *Child's Nervous System*. 2011;27:203–4.
46. Rowe DS, Leonard MF, Seashore MR et al. A hospital program for the detection and registration of abused and neglected children. *New England Journal of Medicine*. 1970;282:950–2.
47. Besharov DJ. What physicians should know about child abuse reporting laws. In *Child abuse and neglect: A medical reference*. NS Ellersetin, ed. Wiley, 1981, pp. 21–50.
48. Hansen P, Ainsworth F. Examining child protection practice in New South Wales: Non-accidental injury and the principle of strict liability. *Children Australia*. 2020;45:8–13.
49. Choudhary AK, Narang SK, Moreno JA et al. A consensus response on the complete picture: Reply to Lynøe and Eriksson. *Pediatric Radiology*. 2019;49:424–8.
50. Duhaime AC, Christian CW. Abusive head trauma: Evidence, obfuscation, and informed management. *Journal of Neurosurgery: Pediatrics*. 2019;24:481–8.
51. Brown SD. Ethical challenges in child abuse: What is the harm of a misdiagnosis? *Pediatric Radiology*. 2021;51:1070–5.
52. Kempe CH, Silverman FN, Steele BF et al. The battered child syndrome. *JAMA*. 1962;181:17–24. Reprinted in Journal of the American Medical Association. 1984;251(24):3294.
53. Helfer RE, Kempe CH. The child's need for early recognition, immediate care and protection. In *Helping the battered child and family*. CH Kempe, ed. Lippincott, 1972, pp. 69–78.
54. Report to the President Forensic Science in Criminal Courts. Ensuring Scientific Validity of Feature-Comparison Methods, Executive Office of the President, President's Council of Advisors on Science and Technology, 2016, pp. 1–160.
55. Keenan HT, Campbell KA, Page K et al. Perceived social risk in medical decision-making for physical child abuse: A mixed-methods study. *BMC Pediatrics*. 2017;17(214):1–10.
56. Rivara FP, Kamitsuka MD, Quan L. Injuries to children younger than 1 year of age. *Pediatrics*. 1988;81(1):93–7.
57. Kellogg ND. Evaluation of suspected child physical abuse. *Pediatrics*. 2007;119 (6):1232–41.
58. Goldstein B, Kelly MM, Bruton D et al. Inflicted versus accidental head injury in critically injured children. *Critical Care Medicine*. 1993;21(9):1328–32.
59. Wester K, Stridbeck U, Syse A, Wikstrom, J. Re-evaluation of medical findings in alleged shaken baby syndrome and abusive head trauma in Norwegian courts fails to support abuse diagnoses. *Acta Paediatrica*. 2022;111(4):779–92. https://doi.org/10.1111/apa.15956.
60. Kirschner RH, Stein RJ. The mistaken diagnosis of child abuse: A form of medical abuse? *American Journal of Diseases of Children*. 1985;139:873–5.
61. Anderst J, Nielsen-Parker M, Moffatt M et al. Using simulation to identify sources of medical diagnostic error in child physical abuse. *Child Abuse and Neglect*. 2016;52:62–9.
62. Schiff GD. Minimizing diagnostic error: The importance of follow-up and feedback. *American Journal of Medicine*. 2008;121 (5A):S38–S42.
63. American Academy of Pediatrics Committee on Child Abuse and Neglect. Shaken baby syndrome: Rotational cranial injuries. Technical report. *Pediatrics*. 2001;108(1):206–10.
64. Guthkelch AN. Problems of infant retino-dural hemorrhage with minimal external injury. *Houston Journal of Health Law and Policy*. 2012;12:201–8.
65. Hobbs CJ. Skull fracture and the diagnosis of abuse. *Archives of Disease in Childhood*. 1984;59:246–52.
66. Lynøe N, Juth N, Eriksson A. From child protection to paradigm protection: The

genesis development and defense of a scientific paradigm. *Journal of Medicine and Philosophy*. 2018:1–13. https://doi.org/10.1093/jmp/jhy015.

67. Högberg U, Lampa E, Högberg G et al. Infant abuse diagnosis associated with abusive head trauma criteria: Incidence increase due to overdiagnosis? *European Journal of Public Health*. 2018;28 (4):641–6.

68. Riggs JE, Hobbs GR. Infant homicide and accidental death in the United States, 1940–2005: Ethics and epidemiological classification. *Journal of Medical Ethics*. 2011;37:445–8.

69. Case ME, Graham MA, Handy TC et al. Position paper on fatal abusive head injuries in infants and young children. *American Journal of Forensic Medicine and Pathology*. 2001;22(2):112–22.

70. Tuerkheimer D. Science-dependent prosecution and the problem of epistemic contingency: A study of shaken baby syndrome. *Alabama Law Review*. 2011;62:513–69.

71. Narang SK. A Daubert analysis of abusive head trauma/shaken baby syndrome. *Houston Journal of Health Law and Policy*. 2011;11:505–635.

72. Hymel KP, Jenny C, Block RW. Intracranial hemorrhage and rebleeding in suspected victims of abusive head trauma: Addressing the forensic controversies. *Child Maltreatment*. 2002;7(4):329–48.

73. Matschke J, Voss J, Obi N et al. Nonaccidental head injury is the most common cause of subdural bleeding in infants < 1 year of age. *Pediatrics*. 2009;124 (6):1587–94.

74. Scheimberg I, Cohen MC, Zapata RE et al. Nontraumatic intradural and subdural hemorrhage and hypoxic ischemic encephalopathy in fetuses, infants, and children up to three years of age: Analysis of two audits of 636 cases from two referral centers in the United Kingdom. *Pediatric and Developmental Pathology*. 2013;16:149–59.

75. Hogberg G, Colville-Ebeling B, Hogberg U et al. Circularity bias in abusive head trauma studies could be diminished with a new ranking scale. *Egyptian Journal of Forensic Sciences*. 2016;6:6–10.

76. Blumbergs P, Reilly P, Vink R. Trauma. In *Greenfield's neuropathology: Volume I*. 8th ed. S Love, DN Louis, DW Ellison, eds. Edward Arnold, 2008, pp. 733–831.

77. Geddes JF, Hacksaw AK, Vowels GH et al. Neuropathology of inflicted head injury in children I. Patterns of brain damage. *Brain*. 2001;124:1290–8.

78. Geddes JF, Vowels GH, Hacksaw AK et al. Neuropathology of inflicted head injury in children II. Microscopic brain injury in infants. *Brain*. 2001;124:1299–1306.

79. Oehmichen M, Schleiss D, Pedal I. Shaken baby syndrome: Re-examination of diffuse axonal injury as cause of death. *Acta Neuropathologica*. 2008;116:317–29.

80. Matschke J, Buttner A, Bergman M et al. Encephalopathy and death in infants with abusive head trauma is due to hypoxic-ischemic injury following local brain trauma to vital brainstem centers. *International Journal of Legal Medicine*. 2015;129:105–14.

81. Geddes JF, Tasker RC, Hacksaw AK et al. Dural haemorrhage in non-traumatic infant deaths: Does it explain the bleeding in 'shaken baby syndrome'? *Neuropathology and Applied Neurobiology*. 2003;29:14–22.

82. Geddes JF. Nonaccidental trauma: Clinical aspects and epidemiology of child abuse. *Pediatric Radiology*. 2009;39(7):759–61.

83. Lantz PE, Stanton CA. Postmortem detection & evaluation of retinal hemorrhages. *Proceedings of the National Academy of Sciences of the United States of America*. 2006;271:12 (retinal haemorrhages present at autopsy in infants who died from meningitis, asphyxia/suffocation, prematurity/congenital conditions, heart disease, in utero haemorrhage, blunt force trauma, sudden infant death syndrome/resuscitation, apnoea/gastro-oesophageal reflux, and birth-related causes).

84. Thiblin I, Andersson J, Wester K et al. Retinal hemorrhage in infants investigated

for suspected maltreatment is strongly correlated with intracranial pathology. *Acta Pediatrica*. 2021;00:1–9.

85. Christian CW, Levin AV. The eye examination in the evaluation of child abuse. *Pediatrics*. 2018;142(2):1–8.
86. Mattheij M, Venstermans C, de Veuster I et al. Retinal haemorrhages in a university hospital: Not always abusive head injury. *Acta Neurologica Belgica*. 2017;117:515–22.
87. Duhaime AC, Alario AJ, Lewander WJ. Head injury in very young children: Mechanisms, injuries, and ophthalmologic findings in 100 hospitalized patients younger than 2 years of age. *Pediatrics*. 1992;90(2):179–85.
88. Emerson MV, Jacobs E, Green, WR. Ocular autopsy and histopathologic features of child abuse. *Ophthalmology*. 2007;114:1384–94.
89. *Del Prete v Thompson*, 10 F.Supp.3d 907, 931-2 (N.D.Ill. 2014).
90. Callaway NF, Ludwig CA, Blumenkranz MS et al. Retinal and optic nerve hemorrhages in the newborn infant: One-year results of the Newborn Eye Screen Test (NEST) study. *Ophthalmology*. 2016;123(5):1043–52.
91. Mena OJ, Paul I, Reichard RR. Ocular findings in raised intracranial pressure. *American Journal of Forensic Medicine and Pathology*. 2011;32:55–7.
92. Bhardwaj G, Jacobs MB, Moran KT et al. Terson syndrome with ipsilateral severe hemorrhagic retinopathy in a 7-month-old child. *Journal of the American Association for Pediatric Ophthalmology and Strabismus*. 2010;14:5;441–3.
93. Agrawal S, Peters MJ, Adams GW et al. Prevalence of retinal hemorrhages in critically ill children. *Pediatrics*. 2012;129 (6):e1388–e1396.
94. Minns RA, Jones PA, Tandon A et al. Raised intracranial pressure and retinal haemorrhages in childhood encephalopathies. *Developmental Medicine and Child Neurology*. 2017;59:597–604.
95. Gardner HB. Letter to editor. *Archives of Pediatrics*. (16 April 2012).
96. Galaznik J. Response to 'Retinal Hemorrhages in Children' by Ms Shiau and Dr. Levin. (16 April 2012).
97. Vinchon M, Delestret I, Defoort-Dhellemmes S et al. Subdural hematoma in infants: Can it occur spontaneously? Data from a prospective series and critical review of the literature. *Child's Nervous System*. 2010;26:119501205.
98. Shuman MJ, Hutchins KD. Severe retinal hemorrhages with retinoschisis in infants are not pathognomonic for abusive head trauma. *Journal of Forensic Science*. 2017;62(3):807–11.
99. Coats B, Binenbaum G, Smith C et al. Cyclic head rotations produce modest brain injury in infant piglets. *Journal of Neurotrauma*. 2016;33:1–13.
100. Thiblin I, Anderson J, Wester K et al. Medical findings and symptoms in infants exposed to witnessed or admitted abusive shaking: A nationwide registry study. *PLoS One*. 2020;15(10):1–14. https://doi.org/10.1371/journal.pone.0240182.
101. Levin AV. Retinal hemorrhages of crush head injury: Learning from outliers. *Archives of Ophthalmology*. 2006;124:1773–4.
102. Levin AV. Ophthalmic manifestations of inflicted childhood neurotrauma. In *Inflicted childhood neurotrauma: Proceedings of a conference sponsored by Department of Health and Human Services, National Institutes of Health, National Institute of Child Health and Human Development, Office of Rare Diseases, National Center for Medical Rehabilitation Research*. RM Reece, CE Nicholson, eds. American Academy of Pediatrics, 2002, pp. 127–64.
103. Togioka BM, Arnold MA, Bathurst MA et al. Retinal hemorrhages and shaken baby syndrome: An evidence-based review. *Journal of Emergency Medicine*. 2009;37(1):98–106.
104. Levin AV, Christian CW, Committee on Child Abuse and Neglect, Section on Ophthalmology. The eye examination in the evaluation of child abuse. *Pediatrics*. 2010;126;376.

105. Kahneman D. *Thinking fast and slow.* Farrar, Straus and Giroux, 2011, p. 62.

106. Kaye DH, Freedman DA . Reference guide on statistics. *In Reference manual on scientific evidence.* 3rd ed. National Academies Press, 2011, pp. 218–19.

107. *Meister v Medical Engineering Corp.*, 267 F.3d 1123, 1129, 347 U.S.App.D.C. 361, 367 (C.A.D.C.,2001).

108. *Black v Food Lion, Inc.*, 171 F.3d 308, 314 (5th Cir.1999).

109. Levinson JD, Pasquale MA, Lambert SR. Diffuse bilateral retinal hemorrhages in an infant with a coagulopathy and prolonged cardiopulmonary resuscitation. *Journal of the American Association for Pediatric Ophthalmology and Strabismus.* 2016;20(2):166–8.

110. Risinger DM. Defining the task at hand: Non-science forensic science after *Kumho Tire Co. v Carmichael. Washington and Lee Law Review.* 2000;57:767, 776–7.

111. Duhaime AC, Gennarelli RA, Thibault LE et al. The shaken baby syndrome: A clinical, pathological, and biomechanical study. *Journal of Neurosurgery.* 1987;66:409–15.

112. Matshes, EW. Retinal and optic nerve sheath hemorrhages are not pathognomonic of abusive head injury. *Proceedings of the American Academy of Forensic Sciences.* 2010. www.aafs.org/sites/default/files/media/documents/AAFS-2010-G1.pdf.

113. Narang SK, Estrada C, Greenberg S et al. Acceptance of shaken baby syndrome and abusive head trauma as medical diagnoses. *Journal of Pediatrics.* 2016;177:273–8.

114. Donohoe M. Evidence-based medicine and shaken baby syndrome. Part I: Literature review, 1966–1998. *American Journal of Forensic and Medical Pathology.* 2003;24:239–42.

115. DiMaio VJ, DiMaio D. *Forensic pathology.* CRC Press, 2001, p. 362.

116. Dias MS. The case for shaking. In *Child abuse and neglect.* C. Jenny, ed. Saunders, 2011, pp. 364–72.

117. SBU Assessment Report 255E/2016 Traumatic Shaking. The role of the triad in medical investigations of suspected traumatic shaking: A systematic review. Swedish Agency for Health Technology Assessment and Assessment of Social Services.

118. Lynøe N, Elinder G, Hallberg B et al. Insufficient evidence for 'shaken baby syndrome': A systematic review. *Acta Paediatrica.* 2017;106:1021–7.

119. *101 General Elec. Co. v Joiner*, 522 *R.C.* U.S. 136 (1997).

120. Findley KA, Risinger DM, Barnes PD et al. Feigned consensus: Usurping the law in shaken baby syndrome/abusive head trauma prosecutions. *Wisconsin Law Review.* 2019;1211:1238–45.

121. Choudhary AK, Servaes S, Slovis T et al. Consensus statement on abusive head trauma in infants and young children. *Pediatric Radiology.* 2018;48(8):1048–65.

122. Findley KA, Barnes PD, Moran DA, Squier W. Shaken baby syndrome, abusive head trauma, and actual innocence: Getting it right. *Houston Journal of Health Law and Policy.* 2012;12:209–312.

123. Greenhalgh T. *How to read a paper: The basics of evidence-based medicine and healthcare.* 6th ed. Wiley Blackwell, 2019.

124. Bhardwaj G, Chowdhury V, Jacobs MB et al. A systematic review of the *Diagnostic Accuracy of Ocular Signs in Pediatric Abusive Head Trauma. Ophthalmology.* 2010;117:983–92.

125. Maguire S, Pickerd N, Farewell D et al. Which clinical features distinguish inflicted from non-inflicted brain injury? A systematic review. *Archives of Disease in Childhood.* 2009:94:860–7.

126. Maguire SA, Kemp AM, Lumb RC et al. Estimating the probability of abusive head trauma: A pooled analysis. *Pediatrics.* 2011;128;e550.

127. Piteau SJ, Ward MGK, Barrowman NJ et al. Clinical and radiographic characteristics associated with abusive and nonabusive head trauma: A systematic review *Pediatrics*. 2012;130 (2):315–23.

128. Kemp AM, Jaspan T, Griffiths J et al. Neuroimaging: What neuroradiological features distinguish abusive from non-abusive head trauma? A systematic review. *Archives of Disease in Childhood*. 2011;96(12):1103–12. https://doi.org/10.1136/archdischild-2011-300630.

129. Vinchon M, Deefoort-Dhellemmes S, Desuromont M et al. Accidental and nonaccidental head injuries in infants: A prospective study. *Journal of Neurosurgery (Pediatrics 4)*. 2005;102:380–4.

130. Greeley C. Justice for Rehma. Science under attack: 'I can say with 100% medical certainty that abusive head trauma is what a child has and then I stop [.]' https://edition.cnn.com/interactive/2021/12/health/shaken-baby-syhndrome-legal-battle/chapter-2.html.

131. Aspelin P. Keynote address: Can a sign or occult finding predict a causal relationship? How to reason about possible child abuse. *University of Michigan Journal of Law Reform*. 2017;50 (3):757.

132. Lynøe N, Rosen M, Eriksson A. Questions about isolated traumatic shaking and confessions. *Child's Nervous System*. 2017;33:731–2.

133. Vinchon M. Response to Lynøe: Questions about isolated trauma shaking and confessions. *Child's Nervous System*. 2017;33(9):1423–4.

134. Lynøe N, Rosen M, Eriksson A. Vinchon's responses raise additional questions about the shaken baby-study. *Child's Nervous System*. 2018;34:11–13.

135. Damon-Moore SL. Trial judges and the forensic science problem. *New York University Law Review*. 2017;92:1532–70.

136. *State v Jacoby*, 2018 WL 5098763(N.J. Super.L.)(Trial Order).

137. *State v Darryl Nieves*, Decision issued 7 January 2022 (Indictment No. 17- 06-00785)(N.J.Super.Court).

138. Guthkelch AN. Infantile subdural haematoma and its relationship to whiplash injuries. *British Medical Journal*. 1971;2:430–1.

139. Shapiro M, Walker M, Carroll KT et al. Neuroanatomy of cranial dural vessels: Implications for subdural hematoma embolization. *Journal of Neurointerventional Surgery*. 2021;13:471–7.

Chapter 20

Undoing Wrongful Convictions

Exonerating the Innocent in Shaken Baby Syndrome/Abusive Head Trauma Cases

Keith Findley

20.1 The Science–Law Interface

A tension is often observed at the interface of law and science that arises because of the very different objectives and methods of the two disciplines (see Chapter 1). Science moves slowly, deliberately, seeking answers to universal truths, and is never settled; it continually evolves, adding to existing knowledge or replacing old truths with new, better-informed truths. The law seeks not universal truths, but truth in individual cases, and it demands swift and definitive answers; it places an enormous premium on finality, on settling the matter between adversaries once and for all, without much room for developing or incorporating new knowledge or understandings. In shaken baby syndrome and abusive head trauma (SBS/AHT), that tension is starkly evident.

Indeed, that tension is almost uniquely evident in SBS/AHT cases because of the singular role the medical hypothesis plays in many SBS/AHT cases. Virtually alone among criminal cases, SBS/AHT cases often turn entirely or almost entirely on the opinion evidence of the medical expert. Child abuse physicians frequently offer testimony that alone satisfies all required elements of the criminal case: what happened (known in the law as *actus reus*), with what mental state (known in the law as *mens rea*), and who did it (identity).[1] In the classic SBS/AHT case, the expert opines that *what happened* had to have been violent shaking or shaking with impact; that the person who did it had to have done it with the requisite *mental state* – knowingly, intentionally, recklessly, or whatever mental state is required under the particular charges – because it would require such massive force it could not be inflicted accidentally; and that, because the child would have become immediately comatose and unresponsive, the last person with the child before collapse had to be the perpetrator.[2] No other case turns so completely on a medical hypothesis; these are indeed the starkest form of a science-dependent prosecution. They entail what former child abuse prosecutor and now law professor Deborah Tuerkheimer has aptly described as 'a medical diagnosis of murder' [2–4].

This stark interface between law and science in SBS/AHT cases has consequences for both the law and science. For the law, the near-total dependence on the science means that the law must find ways to adapt as the scientific foundations shift. Yet the law is notoriously

[1] It is important to note that this discussion does not apply to the more ordinary cases that turn on other evidence, such as eyewitness accounts of beatings, or other medical and physical evidence, such as burn marks or extensive bruising, but rather is directed to the classic SBS/AHT case that for so long has confounded the medical community – the case with extensive intracranial lesions but no serious external signs of injury.

[2] This last claim is based on the old belief that a child so injured would not maintain lucidity after injury (i.e. would not experience a 'lucid interval'). That belief has now been thoroughly debunked [1], but the claim is still made quite often today by child abuse physicians.

slow to respond to such changes; it has what Professor Jennifer Laurin calls a 'science lag' [5]. But without adequately adapting to changing science, science-dependent cases run the risk of locking in not just scientific error about universal truths, but also injustice in individual cases.

For medicine, the interconnection to law has other unfortunate consequences. The *only* significance of a medical determination of SBS/AHT is legal – there are no medical treatments for SBS/AHT, only legal consequences (removal of the child, prosecution of the caregiver). The science in these cases therefore inevitably bends to pressures imposed by the law in ways that most sciences do not. As law is by nature adversarial (even in inquisitorial systems, such as on the European Continent, the law pits the state against the individual; see Chapter 22), it imposes adversarial pressures on the science.

The result is an advocacy bias by child abuse specialists, who in their more candid moments make no pretence of being neutral scientists and instead expressly advocate for erring on the side of the child, or placing protection of the child above the interests of protecting family integrity or protecting the liberty of accused parents (see Chapter 19). An additional consequence is a strong, almost reflexive resistance to any challenges to the validity of their scientific and medical hypotheses, borne of a concern that acknowledging flaws in the hypothesis might make it harder to prosecute such cases in court and thereby, in their estimation, put children at risk. The resistance is seen in the extreme efforts child abuse physicians make to dismiss and even demonise scientific critics rather than engage in real scientific debate and inquiry (see Chapter 1).

But, as this book demonstrates, the science is changing, and both law and science must find a way to adapt. In the law, that means prosecutors and defence lawyers must learn the new science and must be prepared to address it appropriately and fully at trial. It means courts must overcome their resistance to revisiting old cases – their almost blind fealty to finality – and must be willing to reopen old cases that are dependent on the old science.

Despite the law's 'science lag', such changes are beginning. Slowly but noticeably, defence lawyers are learning about the weaknesses in the SBS/AHT hypothesis and are marshalling the scientific evidence to challenge SBS/AHT allegations at trial. And while caregivers continue to be convicted (sometimes appropriately so, based on other types of evidence, but often still on little more than the child abuse physician's opinion evidence), acquittals are noticeably on the rise. Likewise, courts are now beginning in a few cases to exclude some expert opinion evidence as scientifically unreliable under *Daubert v Merrell Dow Pharmaceuticals, Inc.* [6] (see Chapter 19).

Moreover, a growing number of courts are considering the new scientific challenges to the SBS/AHT hypothesis and are vacating old, flawed convictions. Litigating a post-conviction challenge to an SBS/AHT conviction is no simple matter. It requires massive resources (which imprisoned people rarely have) and the availability of legal avenues for relief in a system filled with procedural and substantive barriers to post-conviction relief [7–9]. It requires a court that is willing to listen to and learn the complex science and to then buck the massive pressures of the prosecution and child protection communities to grant relief. When courts do take the time to hear fully litigated post-conviction claims, in which top experts on both sides of these debates testify extensively, they are granting relief, and doing so with increasing frequency.

20.2 The Breakthrough Cases

The first case in which a court vacated a conviction on the basis of the shifted science involved a woman named Audrey Edmunds in the state of Wisconsin in the United States.[3] This was a classic, triad-based prosecution in which the entire case turned on medical opinions that the child in question had to have been shaken, or perhaps shaken and then slammed.[4] In post-conviction proceedings, the court heard detailed testimony on the science from 10 prominent medical experts from a variety of specialties – 6 by the defence and 4 by the prosecution. The defence experts challenged the prosecution's experts on every one of the legal elements of the crime, offering research that challenged shaking as the only possible mechanism (the *actus reus* element), the claims that the force applied had to have been so massive it could not have been accidental (the *mens rea* element), and the claim that the child could not have experienced a lucid interval (the identity element). On this record, the Wisconsin Court of Appeals vacated Edmunds's conviction, concluding that a new trial was required because she had presented newly discovered evidence (the new medical research) that created a reasonable probability of a different result at a retrial [10]. The Court held:

> Edmunds presented evidence that was not discovered until after her conviction, in the form of expert medical testimony, that a significant and legitimate debate in the medical community has developed in the past ten years over whether infants can be fatally injured through shaking alone, whether an infant may suffer head trauma and yet experience a significant lucid interval prior to death, and whether other causes may mimic the symptoms traditionally viewed as indicating shaken baby or shaken impact syndrome.

The state subsequently dismissed all charges against Edmunds.

Other courts began to follow suit. In 2005, Jennifer Del Prete was convicted in Illinois of first-degree murder for shaking to death a 3-month-old child in her care. Del Prete subsequently sought federal habeas corpus review of her conviction. Because she had failed to raise her constitutional claim properly in state court, however, she could not raise it in federal habeas corpus review unless she could make a sufficient showing that she was 'actually innocent', which would permit the federal court to overlook her procedural error.

After a lengthy hearing in federal court, conducted on multiple dates between 2012 and 2014, in which numerous top experts from both sides of the SBS/AHT debates again testified, federal district court judge Matthew Kennelly found that Del Prete had sufficiently established her actual innocence to permit her to proceed on her defaulted claims. Judge Kennelly wrote, 'the Court finds that Del Prete has established by a preponderance of the evidence that based on all of the relevant evidence, no reasonable jury would find her guilty beyond a reasonable doubt' [11]. Judge Kennelly added, in an important footnote, that the 'recent developments in this area ... arguably suggest[] that a claim of shaken baby syndrome is more an article of faith than a proposition of science'. Del Prete's conviction was ultimately overturned, after she had spent almost 10 years in prison, and all charges were subsequently dismissed.

---

3 Full disclosure: I was Audrey Edmunds's attorney in those post-conviction proceedings.

4 As noted throughout this book, the classic triad of findings historically used to 'diagnose' SBS/AHT include subdural haematoma, retinal haemorrhages, and encephalopathy or cerebral oedema (or sometimes bone fractures).

Today, although there is no official list of such cases, and no good way to find and count them all (since most exonerations occur at the trial court level in proceedings that produce no publishable or centrally searchable records), dozens or more cases have been overturned on the basis of new scientific developments.

20.3 Bases for Post-conviction Relief

The bases for reopening old convictions, including old SBS/AHT convictions, vary from country to country and even from state to state within a country. In the United States, all 50 states and the federal courts have procedures for reviewing convictions by appellate courts directly after conviction, and also for re-examining older convictions when new issues or facts arise or are discovered after the time for direct appeal elapses [12]. While those procedures exist, they are notoriously difficult to invoke, both because they are littered with procedural obstacles and because the substantive standards for relief are quite high [8, 9, 12]. The reversal rate is low (anywhere from about 4% to 20%) on direct appeal (when new scientific evidence is least likely to be available or serve as the basis for the reversal) [12]. Indeed, even in cases in which subsequent DNA testing proved the convicted person was *actually innocent*, only 14% of those innocent individuals succeeded in winning a reversal on direct appeal, and even fewer – just 9% – when death penalty cases are excluded [13]. The reversal rate is even lower in post-conviction proceedings outside the short time limits for direct appeal, ranging from 3% to 8% in state court in the relevant case categories and less than 1% for all cases in federal habeas corpus [14]. When relief is granted, it can be on the basis of a variety of legal principles.

Some SBS/AHT convictions have been overturned due to procedural or constitutional trial errors unrelated to the shifting science. Among those are cases like *State v Debelbot*, in which the Georgia Supreme Court in the United States reversed the convictions of a married couple because of the ineffective assistance of trial counsel for failure to object to the prosecutor's improper closing argument [15]. Such cases do not necessarily implicate the shifting science (although in *Debelbot* challenges to the science were indeed an important part of the case, although not ultimately the expressed basis for reversal). Of more relevance to this chapter are those cases in which the new science has formed the basis for overturning an old conviction. Most often, this happens not during the direct appeal, but later, during post-conviction proceedings, after new scientific evidence has emerged. In those cases, courts have granted new trials under several distinct legal theories.

First, as the *Edmunds* case demonstrates, courts have granted new trials directly on the basis that the science has shifted and the shift constitutes newly discovered evidence. These courts reason that, in a science-dependent case, a jury verdict premised on the old science should not stand; in such cases, to assess guilt fairly and reliably, the jury must have the opportunity to consider both the prosecution's and the defence's expert evidence, based on the new science. Other suspects whose cases were overturned under this principle include Rene Bailey in New York in 2014 [16], Armando Castillo in Arizona in 2011 [17], Elizabeth Ann Cicogni in Arizona in 2020 [18], Derick Epps in Massachusetts in 2016 [19], Heidi Fero in Washington in 2016 [20], Michael Hansen in Minnesota in 2011 [21], Cathy Lynn Henderson in Texas in 2012 [22], Kim Hoover-Moore in Ohio in 2021 [23], Zavion Johnson in California in 2018 [24], Clarence Jones III in Maryland in 2021 [25], Quentin Louis in Wisconsin in 2009 [26], Kenneth Marsh in California in 2004 [27], Maria Mendez in California in 2018 [28], Tonia Miller in Michigan in 2021 [29], Moussa Sissoko in Maryland in 2015 [30], Drayton Witt in Arizona in 2012 [31], and others.

Second, where the new evidence was already available at the time of trial, but defence counsel failed to find or present it (or to consult appropriate experts who could produce this evidence), some courts have found that the error is so significant as to constitute a deprivation of the constitutional right to the effective assistance of counsel. Again, these courts have reasoned that this new science is so important to a fair assessment of guilt that counsel's failure to present it to the jury rendered the conviction unsafe. Suspects whose cases in courts have vacated convictions on this basis include Leo Duwayne Ackley in Michigan in 2015 [32], Julie Baumer in Michigan in 2010 [33], Shiloh Brafford in Oklahoma in 2017 [34], Brandy Briggs in Texas in 2006 [35], Shawn Delano Brown in Michigan in 2019 [36], Armando Castillo in Arizona in 2011 [17], Terry Ceasor in Michigan in 2021 [37], Ronal Anthony Di Mambro in Michigan in 2016 [38], Gail Pinder Dobson in Maryland in 2014 [39], Derick Epps in Massachusetts in 2016 [19], Warren Hales in Utah in 2007 [40], Shawntee Shuree Jones in Arizona in 2020 [41], Kenneth Marsh in California in 2004 [27], Oswelt Millien in Massachusetts in 2016 [42], Jeremiah Mongold in West Virginia in 2016 [43], Nicholas Newbold in California in 2021 [44], Ronald Pheils in Ohio in 2015 [45], Brian Keith Roberts in Michigan in 2017 [46], Jake Schoonmaker in New Mexico in 2008 [47], Stephanie Spurgeon in Florida in 2020 [48], Krystal Voss in Colorado in 2017 [49], Melanie Ware in Georgia in 2009 [50], and others.

Third, under US constitutional law, in cases where expert testimony is necessary to present a defence but the defendant lacks the resources to retain experts, the court is obligated to provide funds for such expert assistance. In some cases where courts have failed to provide funds needed for experts in SBS/AHT, courts have vacated the convictions. Again, courts have reasoned that the science is so controverted that the resources must be provided for experts who will present the new science. For example, in the LeeVester Brown case in Mississippi in 2014 [51] and again in the Jason Isham case in 2015 [52], the Supreme Court of Mississippi vacated SBS/AHT convictions because the trial courts erroneously denied the defendants' requests for expert assistance. Likewise, in *State v Gallaway* in Delaware in 2015, the Superior Court vacated an SBS/AHT conviction because the failure to provide funds left the court with 'no confidence in the outcome of the trial given the absence of defense experts' [53]. Relatedly, in the Terry Ceasor case in Michigan, the court found that defence counsel was ineffective for failing to ask for court assistance in securing an expert [37].

Fourth, in some cases, courts have vacated convictions where the prosecution has violated its constitutional duty to disclose to the defence material exculpatory evidence, including medical evidence of an alternative aetiology for the injuries or death. This obligation arises as a requirement of due process under the Supreme Court's seminal decision in *Brady v Maryland* [54]. In *People v Di Mambro*, for example, the medical examiner withheld from the defence a disk containing 33 pictures from the autopsy [38]. The withheld photos were important to fair resolution of the case because the chief medical examiner had testified at trial that he found bruising on the head and brain that he said had to have been the result of blunt force trauma from two separate and discrete contacts. The additional photographs, however, demonstrated that the bruising on the brain resulted instead from medical intervention after the child was brought to the hospital. Similarly, in *State v Hansen* in Minnesota in 2011, the court found that newly discovered evidence warranted a new trial, and that the prosecutor arguably committed a *Brady* violation by withholding exculpatory medical findings [21].

20.4 Pushback from Child Abuse Physicians

Because the field is so contentious, it is not surprising that the pushback against post-conviction litigation from child abuse physicians and prosecutors has been fierce. Child abuse physicians publicly protest that there have been no shifts in the science, even while acknowledging that the pathophysiology of abuse is poorly understood and that new research emerges regularly, and while modifying their own position papers and testimony on SBS/AHT to accommodate some of the new science (see Chapters 1 and 2).

In 1993, for example, the official position paper of the American Academy of Pediatrics (AAP) recognised a 'presumption that the shaking alone is the sole source of the traumas' (also noting, however, that a biomechanical study by then had posed some challenge to that presumption) [55]. As new research emerged undermining those understandings, however, the AAP was forced to modify its official position.

As of 2001, for example, the AAP dropped its claim that shaking was the sole cause of such injuries and instead modified its presumed diagnosis to a 'presumption of *child abuse* when a child less than 1 year has suffered an intracranial injury' (emphasis added) [56]. The AAP also added a bald declaration that '[t]he constellation of these injuries does not occur with short falls' and asserted that '[s]ubdural hemorrhage [is] caused by the disruption of small bridging veins'.

In its next iteration, as more research emerged, the AAP policy statement backed off again from some of its stronger claims. By 2009, the AAP acknowledged that 'advances in the understanding of the mechanisms and clinical spectrum of injury associated with abusive head trauma compel us to modify our terminology to keep pace with our understanding of pathologic mechanisms. Although shaking an infant has the potential to cause neurologic injury, blunt impact or a combination of shaking and blunt impact cause injury as well' [57]. Accordingly, the AAP recommended changing the name from shaken baby syndrome (SBS) to the broader, less-specific term abusive head trauma (AHT). Also by 2009, the AAP explicitly acknowledged that research was adding to medical understandings about AHT, but that 'controversy remains' and that '[f]ew pediatric diagnoses engender as much debate as AHT'. Importantly, in 2009, the AAP abandoned altogether any presumption of abuse and instead acknowledged that '[p]ediatricians ... have a responsibility to consider alternative hypotheses when presented with a patient with findings suggestive of AHT. A medical diagnosis of AHT is made only after consideration of all the clinical data'. Significantly, the AAP also dropped its claim that short falls do not cause the constellation of injuries found in these cases, or any claim that subdural haematomas are caused by bridging vein rupture.

Finally, by 2020, while continuing to acknowledge the significant accumulation of research over the previous decade, the AAP conceded that 'there is not a particular pattern of cranial injury unique to AHT' and that short-fall events can indeed be fatal, albeit rarely [58]. The AAP also for the first time acknowledged the role that hypoxia/ischemia plays in brain damage and again made no mention of bridging vein rupture as the hypothesised source of subdural haematomas.

Court testimony followed a similar arc over this time. For example, in a case in Rochester, New York, that arose in 2001, childcare provider Rene Bailey was convicted of shaking to death a 2.5-year-old toddler, despite evidence that the child collapsed after she jumped off a chair and hit her head on a door frame.[5] At Bailey's 2001–2 trial, physicians for the prosecution relied explicitly on the 'triad' to determine that Bailey had shaken the child to death (reflecting not only the 'presumption of abuse' advanced by the AAP, but a near conclusive determination of abuse based on the triad). A prosecution physician specifically recited the triad as the basis for the determination:

> In the medical literature the three findings that are usually present are subdural hemorrhage which is the blood underneath the dura or subarachnoid hemorrhage or both, a regular [*sic* retinal] hemorrhage, and cerebral edema which is swelling of the brain [16].

Multiple prosecution experts also dismissed the defence claim that the child had died from her fall from the chair, proclaiming without reservation or limitation that 'short falls don't kill'.

Thirteen years later, in 2014, Bailey brought a post-conviction motion seeking to overturn her conviction because of the shifted SBS science. No longer did the prosecution's experts insist that the triad was alone virtually diagnostic of abuse, or that short falls can't kill. To the contrary, they eschewed reliance on the triad and even insisted that the triad was a 'straw man' constructed by defence attorneys (a bit of revisionist history frequently espoused by SBS-hypothesis advocates [59, 60]), despite the prosecution's own reliance on the triad at trial. And they conceded that short falls can indeed kill, albeit rarely. On cross-examination, for example, a prominent child abuse paediatrician called by the state testified:

> [DEFENCE COUNSEL]: So, again, if the doctors at this trial testified that short falls cannot cause this, that's just wrong, isn't it?
>
> [PROSECUTION EXPERT]: If they testified to that, yes, sir.

Despite admissions such as these, the prosecution continued to insist that the science had not shifted in any meaningful ways since trial. The court rejected the prosecution's claims and vacated the conviction. The court held:

> The credible and persuasive evidence presented by the Defense established, by a preponderance of the evidence, a significant change in medical science relating to head injuries in children, generally, and the Shaken Baby Syndrome hypothesis, in particular, since the time of the Trial in this matter. New research into the biomechanics of head injury reveals that the doctors who testified on behalf of the Prosecution at Trial misinterpreted the medical evidence to conclude that shaking, or shaking with impact, was the only mechanism capable of causing Brittney's injuries.

Expressly rejecting the prosecution's claim that the potential fatality of short falls was fully recognised in 2001, the court added: 'The Court determines, however, that the Defense established that the mainstream belief in 2001–2002, espoused by the Prosecution's expert witnesses at Trial, that children did not die from short falls, has been proven to be false.' The court added, 'the credible evidence adduced at the Hearing, which was supported by expert testimony from different disciplines and specialties – pediatrics, radiology, pathology, ophthalmology, and biomechanical engineering – established by a preponderance of the

[5] Full disclosure: I was co-counsel for Rene Bailey in the post-conviction proceedings, along with Adele Bernhard (lead counsel) and Kate Judson.

evidence that key medical propositions relied upon by the Prosecution at Trial were either demonstrably wrong, or are now subject to new debate'.

20.5 The New Attack: Minimising the Reversals

Apparently perceiving a threat from such court decisions, Dr Sandeep Narang, a vocal and prominent defender of the SBS/AHT hypothesis and frequent prosecution witness, and his colleagues have sought to demonstrate empirically that only a miniscule proportion of SBS/AHT convictions have been reversed based on the new science. In a paper published in 2020, Narang et al. reported that their search of a legal database for SBS/AHT cases from 2008 to 2018 revealed that, of the 1,431 unique AHT/SBS criminal convictions they found that had appellate rulings, only 49 convictions (3%) were overturned, and 1,382 (97%) were affirmed/upheld. Moreover, they claimed, of those overturned, only 20 cases (1% overall) were overturned on medical-evidence-related grounds [61].

In part, Narang's point is well taken – undoubtedly most SBS/AHT convictions have not been revisited by courts. Given all the obstacles to overturning 'final' convictions, the lack of resources available to convicted individuals, and the 'science lag' in the law, that reality is unsurprising. The movement to apply new science to old convictions has hardly claimed mission accomplished; to the contrary, the effort is just beginning.

Nonetheless, Narang's attempt to marginalise the judicial reversals as an empirical matter is methodologically invalid. To begin, it is unfortunate that his analysis begins in 2008, when the new science was just beginning to get judicial attention and very few cases were at that time being challenged, and ends in 2018, because the pace of SBS/AHT reversals has hastened in the years since 2018 (as a review of the dates of the cases listed earlier in this chapter reveals).

Even within the time period his study covers, Narang's methodology is inadequate for doing what he purports to do – quantitatively defining the extent to which SBS/AHT convictions have been overturned and qualitatively describing the world of such cases. Narang searched the Westlaw legal database for cases involving SBS/AHT and then counted the number of new-science-based reversals he found.

Searching the Westlaw legal database, however, is the wrong way to answer the question Narang has posed; it is a method that virtually guarantees a gross undercount. Westlaw is limited primarily to appellate decisions, not trial court decisions (especially in state courts, where most criminal cases arise). Yet, if new medical evidence is used to overturn a conviction, that will almost never occur on direct appeal. Not only does the direct appeal follow immediately after conviction, which affords little time for development of new science in the interval, but new medical information legally cannot be introduced for the first time in appellate courts in the United States. In most cases, the convicted person must file a post-conviction motion in the trial court, and many such cases are resolved at the trial court level, without an appeal or published opinion. Only if one of the parties appeals the trial court decision might an appellate opinion show up in Westlaw. Some of Narang's cases fall into that category, but that is no way to count all new-science reversals.

To understand the inadequacy of Narang's approach, consider that even a quick, non-systematic review of publicised trial-court reversals effortlessly produces numerous reversals that otherwise fit Narang's inclusion criteria, but that are absent from his 20-case tally. Cases not included by Narang, but that were overturned by trial courts in post-conviction proceedings between 2008 and 2018, include at least the following 11 cases, and likely many others: Shiloh Brafford (Oklahoma 2017) [34], Armando Castillo (Arizona 2011) [17], Julie Baumer (Michigan 2010) [33], Gail Pinder Dobson (Maryland 2014) [39], Michael Hansen (Minnesota 2011) [21], Zavion Johnson (California 2018) [24], Maria Mendez (California 2018) [28], Moussa Sissoko (Maryland 2015) [30], Krystal Voss (Colorado 2017) [49], Melonie Ware (Georgia 2009) [50], and Drayton Witt (Arizona 2012) [31].

Even (inappropriately) limiting the search as Narang did to appellate opinions in Westlaw, another quick, non-systematic review utilising Westlaw to search for 'shaken baby syndrome' finds at least two other cases that fully fit Narang's inclusion criteria but inexplicably are left off his list: *People v Ackley* (Michigan 2015) [31], and *State v Quentin Louis* (Wisconsin 2009) [25]. Given Narang's small sample size – he claims only 20 such cases over 10 years – missing at least 13 cases exposes the invalidity of his statistical claims.

Making matters worse, at least six of the overlooked cases – Baumer, Hansen, Johnson, Voss, Ware, and Witt – are easily discoverable in the National Registry of Exonerations – the very registry Narang himself cites. These cases are included in the National Registry of Exonerations because in each case the defendant was never re-convicted, either because the prosecution dismissed the charges or a retrial ended in an acquittal. These six easily discoverable exonerations alone demonstrate that Narang's tallies – including his claim that most cases resulted in re-conviction – are so off the mark as to be useless.

Narang et al. also pointedly note that some of the defendants whose SBS/AHT convictions were reversed ultimately pled guilty or no contest to reduced charges or a reduced sentence. That, however, says little about the reliability of those re-convictions. False guilty or no contest pleas are increasingly prominent features of the wrongful conviction landscape, comprising more than 20% of known exonerations in recent years [62]. New research shows that, when innocence advocacy organisations obtain reversals of convictions based on new evidence of actual innocence, prosecutors often respond by trying to preserve the convictions by making plea offers that are so generous they are hard for even innocent people to reject – typically plea offers to time served, which guarantee these likely innocent people that they will not have to spend another day behind bars if they will just accept entry of a judgment of conviction [63].

Indeed, in nearly 90% of such cases, when prosecutors plea bargained with innocence organisations, they offered time served, and they made these generous offers in serious cases. Moreover, despite vigorous and well-supported claims of innocence, 59% of these innocence-claiming defendants took the deals, choosing not to trust their fate to a legal system that they believed had betrayed them once already. Many of the pleas in SBS/AHT cases have followed this pattern. It is therefore a mistake to assume that re-conviction, including by plea bargain, proves much about the debated SBS/AHT hypothesis.

No claim is made here that the case citations in this chapter are exhaustive of all cases of overturned SBS/AHT convictions. Rather, the point is that these cases show that Narang also has not found all such cases, and to the extent he asserts statistical claims about the frequency and nature of overturned SBS/AHT cases, those statistical claims are meaningless.

Narang calls out the Innocence Network (of which I was president from 2009 to 2014) for allegedly overstating the rate at which SBS/AHT cases are overturned. But Narang mischaracterises the Innocence Network's statement on SBS. The Network's claim is that the innocent are still in prison, not that they are out [64]. Narang's data are at least consistent with that claim.

References

1. Gilliland MGF. Interval duration between injury and severe symptoms in non-accidental head trauma in infants and young children. *Journal of Forensic Science.* 1998;43:723–5.
2. Tuerkheimer D. The next innocence project: Shaken baby syndrome and the criminal courts. *Washington University Law Review.* 2011;87:1–58.
3. Tuerkheimer D. Science-dependent prosecution and the problem of epistemic contingency: A study of shaken baby syndrome. *Alabama Law Review.* 2011;62:513–69.
4. Tuerkheimer D. *Flawed convictions: Shaken baby syndrome and the inertia of injustice.* Oxford University Press, 2014.
5. Laurin JE. Criminal law's science lag: How criminal justice meets changed scientific understanding. *Texas Law Review.* 2015;93:1751–82.
6. *Daubert v Merrell Dow Pharmaceuticals, Inc.*, 509 U.S. 579 (1993).
7. Findley KA, Risinger DM. The science and law underlying post-conviction challenges to shaken baby syndrome convictions: A response to Professor Imwinkelried. *Seton Hall Law Review.* 2018;48:1209–27.
8. Hack P. The roads less traveled: Post conviction relief alternatives and the Antiterrorism and Effective Death Penalty Act of 1996. *American Journal of Criminal Law.* 2003;30:171–223.
9. Medwed DS. Up the river without a procedure: Innocent prisoners and newly discovered non-DNA evidence. *Arizona Law Review.* 2005;47:655–718.
10. *State v Edmunds*, 746 N.W.2d 590 (Wis. App. 2008).
11. *Del Prete v Thompson*, 10 F.Supp.3d 907 (N. D. Ill. 2014).
12. Findley KA. Innocence protection in the appellate process. *Marquette Law Review.* 2009;93:591–638.
13. Garrett B. *Convicting the innocent: Where criminal prosecutions go wrong.* Harvard University Press, 2011.
14. Flango VE. *Habeas corpus in state and federal court.* State Justice Institute, 1994.
15. *Debelbot v State*, 826 S.E.2d 129 (Ga. 2019).
16. *People v Bailey*, 47 Misc. 3d 355, 370 (N.Y. Co. Ct. 2014), *affirmed*, 144 A.D.3d 1562 (N.Y. App. Div. 2016).
17. Castillo A. https://bit.ly/3hl6iMc.
18. *State v Cicogni*, 2020 WL 5290709 (Ariz. Super. 2020).
19. *Commonwealth v Epps*, 553 N.E.2d 1247 (Mass. 2016).
20. In re Personal Restraint of Fero, 367 P.3d 588 (Wash. App. 2016).
21. *State v Hansen*, 805 N.W.2d 915 (Minn. 2011).
22. Ex Parte Henderson, 384 S.W.3d 833 (Tex. 2012).
23. Hoover-Moore K. National Registry of Exonerations. https://bit.ly/3UlGIVs.
24. Johnson Z. National Registry of Exonerations. https://bit.ly/3t5mOlQ.
25. Jones C , III. National Registry of Exonerations. https://bit.ly/3UjlWWu.
26. *State v Quentin Louis*, 2011 WL 867677 (Wis. Ct. App. 2011).
27. Marsh K. https://bit.ly/3fCUcNT.
28. Gerber M. Judge orders release of woman who served 11 years behind bars in grandson's death. *Los Angeles Times.* 2018. https://lat.ms/3T75zv3.
29. *People v Miller*, 2021 WL 1326733 (Mich. Ct. App. 2021).
30. Maryland appellate court cites subsequent scientific and medical literature in granting relief to a man convicted in 1999 of the shaken baby syndrome death of his infant son. https://bit.ly/3NHc1Ib.
31. *State v Witt*, 2012 WL 5991566 (Ariz. 2012).
32. *People v Ackley*, 870 N.W.2d 858 (Mich. 2015).
33. *People v Baumer*, 781 N.W.2d 309 (Mich. 2010).

34. Payne S. Woman sentenced to life after stepson's death released, may see new trial. *Tulsa World*. 2019. https://bit.ly/3UteKaq.
35. Ex Parte Briggs, 187 S.W.3d 458 (Tex. Cr. App. 2005).
36. *People v Brown*, 2019 WL 3386459 (Mich Ct, App. 2019).
37. *Ceasor v Ocwieja*, 655 Fed. Appx. 263 (6th Cir. 2016), and *People v Ceasor*, 954 N. W.2d 830 (Mich. 2021).
38. *People v Di Mambro*, 897 N.W.2d 233 (Mich. 2016).
39. Cenziper D. Shaken science: A disputed diagnosis imprisons parents. *Washington Post*. 2015. https://wapo.st/3zJPTHp.
40. *State v Hales*, 152 P.3d 321 (Utah 2007).
41. *State v Jones*, Superior Court of Arizona, Maricopa County, CR2004-036702-001, order entered 22 June 2020.
42. *Commonwealth v Millien*, 50 N.E.2d 808 (Mass. 2016).
43. WVU College of Law client freed from prison. 2016. https://bit.ly/3UcYM4l.
44. Newbold N. https://bit.ly/3E5Krkx.
45. *State v Pheils*, 2015 WL 5306548 (Ct. App. Ohio 2015).
46. *People v Roberts*, 892 N.W.2d 353 (Mich. 2017).
47. *State v Schoonmaker*, 176 P.3d 1105 (N. Mex. 2008).
48. *Spurgeon v State*, 298 So.3d 726 (Dist. Ct. App. Fla. 2020).
49. Voss, K. National Registry of Exonerations. https://bit.ly/3TbzYZ9.
50. *State v Ware*, 679 S.E.2d 797 (Ga. 2009).
51. *Brown v State*, 152 So.3d 1146 (Miss. 2014).
52. *Isham v State*, 161 So.3d 1076 (Miss. 2015).
53. *State v Gallaway*, 2105 WL 4460992 (Del. Sup. Ct. 2015).
54. *Brady v Maryland*, 373 U.S. 83 (1963).
55. American Academy of Pediatrics Committee on Child Abuse and Neglect. Shaken baby syndrome: Inflicted cerebral trauma. *Pediatrics*. 1993;92:872–5.
56. American Academy of Pediatrics Committee on Child Abuse and Neglect. Shaken baby syndrome: Rotational cranial injuries. Technical report. *Pediatrics*. 2001;108:206–10.
57. Christian CW, Block R, Committee on Child Abuse and Neglect. Abusive head trauma in infants and children. *Pediatrics*. 2009;123:1409–11.
58. Narang S, Fingarson A, Lukefar J, Council on Child Abuse and Neglect. Abusive head trauma in infants and children. *Pediatrics*. 2020;145:1–7.
59. Choudhary K, Servaes S, Slovis TL et al. Consensus statement on abusive head trauma in infants and young children. *Pediatric Radiology*. 2018;48:1048–65.
60. Findley KA, Risinger DM, Barnes PD et al. Feigned consensus: Usurping the law in shaken baby syndrome/abusive head trauma prosecutions. *Wisconsin Law Review*. 2019:1211–67.
61. Narang SK, Sachdev KK, Bertocci K et al. Overturned abusive head trauma and shaken baby syndrome convictions in the United States: Prevalence, legal basis, and medical evidence. *Child Abuse and Neglect*. 2021;122:105380. https://doi.org/10.1016/j.chiabu.2021.105380.
62. National Registry of Exonerations. https://bit.ly/3UqiKZ4.
63. Findley KA, Angulo Amaya MC, Hatch G, Smith JP. Plea bargaining in the shadow of a retrial: Bargaining away innocence. *Wisconsin Law Review*. 2022:533–618. https://papers.ssrn.com/sol3/papers.cfm?abstract_id=3944845.
64. Statement of the Innocence Network on Shaken Baby Syndrome/Abusive Head Trauma. https://bit.ly/3t6eUIU.

Chapter 21

Ptolemy Rather Than Copernicus

The State of Shaken Baby Syndrome in the British Legal System

Clive Stafford Smith

In 1542, Nicolaus Copernicus finally decided to publish his seminal work, *De Revolutionibus Orbium Coelestium* (*On the Revolutions of the Celestial Spheres*). In it, he relied on science to challenge the Ptolemaic 'truths' promoted by the Catholic Church: the sun does not, he said, revolve around the Earth, and the Earth is not the stationary centre of the universe.

Copernicus feared publication and, sure enough, his critics came from all sides. 'There is talk of a new astrologer who wants to prove that the earth moves and goes around instead of the sky, the sun, the moon, just as if somebody were moving in a carriage or ship might hold that he was sitting still and at rest while the earth and the trees walked and moved', Martin Luther had recently written in *Table Talk* (1539). 'But that is how things are nowadays: when a man wishes to be clever he must . . . invent something special, and the way he does it must needs be the best! The fool wants to turn the whole art of astronomy upside-down. However, as Holy Scripture tells us, so did Joshua bid the sun to stand still and not the earth.'

Copernicus was perhaps fortunate that he died in 1543 before he could be prosecuted for blasphemy. That privilege was reserved to those such as Galileo Galilei, who was deemed heretical in 1633 for 'following the position of Copernicus, which is contrary to the true sense and authority of Holy Scripture'. He was placed under house arrest for the final years of his life. Were the clerics not clearly correct? After all, in 1 Chronicles 16:30, the Bible makes clear that 'the world is firmly established; it shall never be moved'.

Indeed, the Catholic Church had a hard time coming to grips with the real world. It was not until 1979 that Pope John Paul II conceded that Galileo had to 'suffer a great deal – we cannot conceal the fact – at the hands of men and organisms of the Church' [1]. He also set up a committee to study the Galileo case more deeply. It still took another 13 years for the Church to admit Copernicus had been right: a mere 450 years late. 'The error of the theologians of the time, when they maintained the centrality of the Earth, was to think that our understanding of the physical world's structure was, in some way, imposed by the literal sense of Sacred Scripture' [2].

So we come to the British attitude to shaken baby syndrome (SBS). The sacred scripture of SBS derived from an article by Norman Guthkelch, who proposed a hypothesis in 1971 that shaking might be a cause of subdural haematoma (SDH). This became viewed as an important indication of abuse when seen in the 'triad' of observed injuries – SDH, cerebral oedema, and retinal haemorrhages (RH) [3].[1] In truth, it was just a theory, no more scientifically proven than Ptolemy's, but there was a church of believers ready to accept

[1] From the very beginning, there was disagreement as to what truly comprised the 'triad', and often the third element is identified as 'bone lesions'. This was not, however, the way it was normally presented in early criminal cases in the United States and firmly entrenched by Chadwick et al.

this theory too: the world had finally been waking up to the epidemic of child abuse and this seemed to provide a camera into the hidden nightmare of an abusive household.

When SBS emerged upon an unsuspecting world, it was almost unique – one of only two medical 'diagnoses' that have essentially no relevance to the treatment of the patient; the other, predictably, is battered child syndrome (BCS). When an infant presents at hospital, the doctors do not treat SBS; they treat what is actually wrong with the child – the subdural hematoma, for example. Both SBS and BCS are diagnoses of a *crime*, not an illness. The genesis of SBS is therefore best understood in the context of the criminal courtroom, even though it regularly raises its metaphorical head in family court as well.

There was an astoundingly rapid and unquestioning adoption of the SBS hypothesis. The scientific observer might be surprised: after all, until the COVID-19 crisis, no novel medical treatment would expect to be adopted without years of study. Furthermore, nothing about Guthkelch's hypothesis met the requirement of the scientific method. Beyond Guthkelch's fairly random observation that the injuries might be explained by shaking, there was *no evidence* that SBS was caused by shaking. Indeed, 40 years after propounding his hypothesis, Guthkelch himself observed that there was *still no evidence* for the hypothesis, as he expressed horror that it had been used as established science to imprison parents [4]. Yet an understanding of forensic science reveals that this rush to injustice is no stranger in the courtroom.

The scientific method, developed over many hundreds of years, is designed to test whether a particular hypothesis truly reflects the operations of Nature: whether the observer has happened upon a theory that can honestly be replicated, or whether it is just an alluring but random happenstance. The true scientist comes up with a hypothesis and then tests it; the scientist does randomised, controlled, double-blind studies. The scientist then publishes both the methods and data so others can attempt to reproduce the result, level criticism, and help establish the truth.

In order for the scientific method to operate, there must be others in the field who have an incentive to cast a critical eye over this work, otherwise it can never truly be deemed reliable. If the other experts come from within the same company, they may be keen to ensure that the expensive development of a new medicine will not go to waste. Those from a rival company may have a different partiality, hoping to demonstrate that the new pill is an expensive fraud. Ideally, then, the peer review comes from an independent body whose only motive is to establish the efficacy of a medication before another drug such as thalidomide is unleashed on the market.

When it comes to the courtroom, there is often no scientist with an incentive to question the proposed hypothesis (see Chapter 1). Take forensic hair analysis as a fairly typical example. Every day, a 'trace evidence expert' looks down her binocular microscope, where she can see two hairs at the same time, side by side. She compares a hair found at the crime scene with one belonging to the suspect. She runs her eye along the two hairs until she comes to the point where the two look most similar, and then she starts identifying an array of characteristics – the hair's colour, to be sure, but also its 'buckling', 'cortex', 'medulla', and so forth, a series of terms no layperson has ever previously encountered. She then reaches an opinion as to whether the two are microscopically similar, sometimes loosely referred to as a 'match'.

The forensic hair analyst then appears in court and takes the oath. The prosecutor has her list her qualifications and the hundreds of cases where her view has been deemed important. When the jury hears her opine with her impenetrable verbiage, who are they to disagree?

There is a fundamental flaw in all this, however: there is no use for 'forensic hair analysis' except to put someone in prison. Nobody spends their days looking down a binocular microscope wondering whether it is actual science, agonising that they might be wasting her time. In other words, there is nobody who questions whether what they see down the microscope actually tells them anything of consequence. Everyone trained as a forensic hair analyst believes that the work is valid, yet there has been no independent study that meaningfully validates it [5].[2]

This came into sharp focus for me in the 1995 case of Randy Bevill, who was on death row in Mississippi. The crime lab technician, Joe Andrews, compared the hundreds of hairs from the scene to those taken from Randy and found two pubic hair 'matches', one in the victim's pubic combing and one on her clothes. Since Randy denied committing the crime, the hair evidence took on huge significance: if it was to be believed, it proved that Randy was a liar and that he had been with the victim.

There were two key questions. First, was there any scientific evidence showing that a 'match' between hairs meant anything at all? Second, how likely was a false 'match'? Without statistical proof, this might range from one in two (no more probative than tossing a coin) to one in a billion (highly relevant).

Forensic hair analysis has been used in criminal trials since the 1850s. According to the Mississippi Supreme Court in Randy's original appeal, hair analysis is a '*very useful tool in criminology*' [6]. It has been used as the basis for innumerable death sentences, right up to recent times. Astoundingly, in the first 150 years it was used, only two studies were carried out in an effort to determine what a 'match' might mean. Both had been done by the same person – Barry Gaudette of the Royal Canadian Mounted Police [7, 8]. Gaudette made his living at the time as a forensic hair expert and was therefore hardly impartial: if he were to conclude that his expertise meant nothing, not only would he put himself out of a job, but he would also be saddled with a Himalayan sense of guilt for all the people he had sent to prison over the years.

According to Gaudette's study, the probability of a false match with respect to pubic hair was 1 in 800. In other words, according to him, there was a 99.875% chance that a single pubic hair found at the murder scene matched the sample removed from Randy Bevill. As there was no innocent explanation for Randy's hair being at the scene, then the prosecution might argue that this evidence alone was proof beyond a reasonable doubt.

I telephoned Gaudette to ask to see his raw data. He wanted to know who I was and, when I said I am a defence lawyer, he – a police officer – refused to share his materials. So much for scientific impartiality: he was only willing to share data with those who were committed to upholding his technique. I was reduced to using the figures he had published, which were incomplete but essentially sufficient for my purposes. Suffice it to say that Gaudette had made various assumptions that might be suited to a clean laboratory, but not to a grubby crime scene; he had also used an erroneous statistical method. By plugging the real-life numbers into Gaudette's equations, the odds dropped dramatically: we would expect to see between one and two *false* matches, and Andrews only claimed to see two valid ones. Thus, the evidence meant nothing.

---

2 With an apology, I refer those with more than a passing interest to a lengthy article I co-authored on the issue.

Some years after the Bevill case, we were able to begin cross-checking 'forensic hair analysis' with mitochondrial DNA. In one notorious case where the hair had placed Ron Williamson on death row, the DNA proved it was entirely wrong – as related in John Grisham's first nonfiction book, *The Innocent Man: Murder and Injustice in a Small Town* (2006). Subsequently, 'in April 2015, the US Department of Justice (DOJ) and the Federal Bureau of Investigation (FBI) stunned the criminal justice community by acknowledging that in the two-decade period before 2000, nearly every examiner in the FBI's microscopic hair comparison unit gave scientifically flawed testimony in criminal cases' [9].[3] In other words, they admitted that they had got it wrong in countless capital cases including scores where the prisoner has already been executed.

The same criticism can be levelled at a number of 'forensic sciences' that frequently bedazzle the audiences on television: they were dreamt up to put people in prison, without any other application. This is true for firearms and tool marks (popularly known as ballistics), fibre analysis, fingerprints, and, ultimately, SBS: there is no meaningful empirical evidence that any of these theories is valid. They all – like SBS – have never been scientifically validated through rigorous testing, they rely extensively on subjective judgements that render them vulnerable to cognitive biases (see Chapter 13), and they produce conclusions that are statistically meaningless, given that they have no data to inform them of the uniqueness of the features they observe and hence the statistical power of a 'match'. Shaken baby syndrome is, in a way, more dangerous: often the 'expert' who comes to court is a neurosurgeon (a 'brain surgeon', a common euphemism for the smartest person in the room), someone more likely than anyone else to sway a jury towards guilt.

Neither the British courts nor their American counterparts are immune from this danger. The main distinction is that, in the United States, there is a well-established method to challenge false or unsubstantiated science, which 'entails a preliminary assessment of whether the reasoning or methodology underlying the testimony is scientifically valid and of whether that reasoning or methodology properly can be applied to the facts in issue' [10]. This can be raised at any time in the proceeding, including prior to trial, where extensive evidentiary hearings are held and every plausible challenge to a particular expertise must be considered (see Chapter 19):

> The subject of an expert's testimony must be 'scientific knowledge'. The adjective 'scientific' implies a grounding in the methods and procedures of science. Similarly, the word 'knowledge' connotes more than subjective belief or unsupported speculation ... [I]n order to qualify as 'scientific knowledge', an inference or assertion must be derived by the scientific method. Proposed testimony must be supported by appropriate validation. [10]

One 'pertinent consideration is whether the theory or technique has been subjected to peer review and publication ... [S]ubmission to the scrutiny of the scientific community is a component of "good science", in part because it increased the likelihood that substantive flaws in methodology will be detected' [10]. 'Additionally, in the case of a particular scientific technique, the court ordinarily should consider the known or potential rate of error ... and the existence and maintenance of standards controlling the technique's operation' [10].

3 While it was admirable that the FBI took this belated step, in my view, they were more wrong than they admitted – without true scientific validation, their testimony should not be admitted into court at all.

The Supreme Court emphasised that the controlling principle must be to keep evidence from the jury if there is any doubt:

> It is true that open debate is an essential part of both legal and scientific analyses. Yet there are important differences between the quest for truth in the courtroom and the quest for truth in the laboratory. Scientific conclusions are subject to perpetual revision. Law, on the other hand, must resolve disputes finally and quickly. The scientific project is advanced by broad and wide-ranging consideration of a multitude of hypotheses, for those that are incorrect will eventually be shown to be so, and that in itself is an advance. Conjectures that are probably wrong are of little use, however, in the project of reaching a quick, final, and binding legal judgment – often of great consequence – about a particular set of events in the past. We recognize that in practice, a gatekeeping role for the judge, no matter how flexible, inevitably on occasion will prevent the jury from learning of authentic insights and innovations. That, nevertheless, is the balance that is struck by Rules of Evidence designed not for the exhaustive search for cosmic understanding but for the particularized resolution of legal disputes. [10]

Daubert is not without its limitations. It is often difficult to challenge a bogus science since it is, by definition, only practiced by bogus scientists. Thus, if 'general acceptance' in the relevant scientific community has a bearing on the inquiry, are the only people in the 'community' those who believe it to be valid? Who are the experts who can give testimony for the other side? The most important area in a *Daubert* challenge is therefore the absence of any demonstrable evidence that a hypothesis is actually proven.

When I first encountered SBS in a capital trial in the United States, we tried to challenge the 'science' – this was 1995, and there were, at the time, few doctors who were interested in questioning it. After all, there are plenty of reasonable doctors who wish to expose child abuse, but very few who make a cause out of doubting that the allegations are true – that role is usually left to the defence lawyers. Yet we in the defence bar have historically allowed far too much scientific drivel to enter the courthouse.

The voice in the wilderness at that point was Dr John Plunkett, who came to Mississippi to testify for my client. Dr Plunkett was drawn to the issue because of his own experience in a 1986 case and he eventually assembled 18 instances where he could prove that the supposedly impossible had occurred – a child developed the 'triad' and died resulting from a short fall (see Chapter 15) [11].

However, over the past quarter of a century, an ever-increasing number of American experts have questioned SBS and it has become a central area of challenges to wrongful convictions (see Chapter 20) [12]. The circular debate does continue in the United States. For example, as recently as 2016, faced with doubt expressed in the media and court judgments, an overwhelming majority of American paediatricians who took a survey still clung to SBS (or its more recent clone, abusive head trauma (AHT)) as the cause of injuries (88% of respondents diagnosed with SBS and 93% with AHT).

> Our empirical data confirm that SBS and AHT are still generally accepted by physicians who frequently encounter suspected child abuse cases, and are considered likely sources of subdural hematoma, severe retinal hemorrhages, and coma or death in young children. Other than a high-velocity motor vehicle collision, no alternative theories of causation for these findings are generally accepted [88% of respondents diagnosed SBS and 93% AHT]. [13]

The first problem faced by the British legal system is that it does not have nearly as meaningful a means of challenging pseudo-science in the courtroom as *Daubert* offers in the

United States. In 2005, the House of Commons Science and Technology Committee recommended the creation of a Forensic Science Advisory Council to regulate forensic evidence in the United Kingdom and observed:

> The absence of an agreed protocol for the validation of scientific techniques prior to their being admitted in court is entirely unsatisfactory. Judges are not well-placed to determine scientific validity without input from scientists. We recommend that one of the first tasks of the Forensic Science Advisory Council be to develop a 'gate-keeping' test for expert evidence. This should be done in partnership with judges, scientists and other key players in the criminal justice system, and should build on the US Daubert test. [14]

British experts have waffled back and forth on a rather central issue: what to call the supposed 'diagnosis'. 'We tend to call it something else, as calling it [shaken baby syndrome] presumes that you know the cause of the problem, that a baby has been shaken', Dr Geoff Debelle, child protection officer at the Royal College of Paediatrics and Child Health, told *The Guardian* in 2016. 'We call it abusive head trauma, though often the courts don't like that term, because it presumes that you know that [the injury] was abusive' [15]. That seems a fairly illogical response to criticism since all the doctors were doing was making their assertions stronger (it is now actively 'abusive') while the nature of the mistreatment is less specific (SBS assumed the particular form of the abuse).

In 2018, the Crown Prosecution Service published its position regarding SBS – focused on a change of terminology to non-accidental head injury (NAHI) [16]. They borrowed from the artist Prince, calling it the diagnosis 'formerly referred to as Shaken Baby Syndrome'. The Crown Prosecution Service opined that 'the use of the term Shaken Baby Syndrome should now be avoided as it can be considered to have emotive connotations, and more importantly, does not adequately describe the range of causes of head injuries'.

The Crown Prosecution Service announced that the presence of the triad generally should result in an allegation of NAHI, even if we do not know how this comes about. 'Whilst not entirely understood, the mechanism for these injuries is thought to be shaking of the infant, with or without impact on a solid surface . . . [D]espite medical uncertainty surrounding the mechanism, the triad of injuries is a strong medical pointer to the infliction of NAHI' [16].

This change is no change. This 'medical diagnosis' still purports to identify what the defendant did' it merely takes a highly dubious hypothesis and makes it so vague as to protect the witness from specific challenge. Dr John Plunkett could show that a short fall could kill a child, but now the Crown Prosecution Service would still want to say that the triad was caused by another NAHI – now unspecified.

The Crown Prosecution Service suggests that those who doubt the SBS/NAHI should bear the burden of proof:

> Those challenging the triad on occasions have also invited consideration of bio-mechanical evidence. There is, however, little data relating to the distance an infant would have to fall to suffer such injury to the head. Most experts also accept the difficulty for any biomechanical model to simulate the complex anatomy of an infant's brain.

In *A Local Authority v S [2009] EWHC 2115 (Fam)* the court essentially repeated this line:

> All agree that much remains unknown about SBS and the triad. It is essential, however that [defence expert] Dr. Squier and others engaged on such research avoid becoming zealots with the consequence that scientific rigor is lost or sacrificed.

This is perhaps ironic when we note that there has been no scientific rigour in the promotion of the SBS hypothesis. It is not the defendant's burden to prove that a supposed expertise is reliable. If the prosecution is seeking to present it, they must adduce peer-reviewed and replicable data that consider the complex variables that would demonstrate what distance a child would have to fall to suffer such an injury. This comes to the nub of the whole SBS debate because, at least since the Nuremburg tribunals, it has been illegal to experiment on children. In Britain, meanwhile, the General Medical Council (GMC), the courts and the police have worked closely together to vilify and neutralise experts who began to question the received orthodoxy (see Chapter 1).

Dr Plunkett did encounter harassment for his views in the United States, but the one time an aggrieved prosecutor (who had lost an SBS case) brought charges of perjury against him in 2005, he was acquitted [17]. Even this imbalance should give us pause when it comes to objective science: as a defence lawyer, I have no power to prosecute a state witness whose testimony I do not like, even when it puts my client on death row. But at least no US medical council sought to sanction Dr Plunkett and he went on to publish widely on the subject, persuading many of his peers to look much more closely at the SBS theory.

Meanwhile, in the United Kingdom, a number of experts took steps that might normally be considered laudatory: they kept an open mind and were willing to reconsider that which had been drummed into them in medical school. Dr Jennian Geddes and her colleagues researched a number of paediatric cases without head injury and suggested that the same triad of injuries could be caused by severe hypoxia (lack of oxygen in the tissues) which in turn might lead to brain swelling. Their hypothesis was that brain swelling combined with raised intracranial pressure (ICP) could cause both subdural haemorrhages and retinal haemorrhages – cardinal components of 'the triad' (see Chapters 1 and 3) [18].

When Dr Waney Squier relied on this work in the Lorraine Harris appeal, the prosecution announced that she had 'lost objectivity' – apparently because 'objectivity' demanded that the explanation should be SBS [19]. Yet Dr Squier and others who have questioned SBS do not pose their alternatives as the gospel truth. They are merely plausible possibilities. Since human experimentation is illegal, this is the most that an 'objective' expert can do.

On the other hand, the Crown Prosecution Service again turned the burden of proof on its head and announced that Dr Geddes's questions were not a 'credible challenge' to the SBS theory:

> In *R v Harris: R v Rock* [2006]1 Cr App R 5, Dr Geddes accepted that the hypothesis in this paper was not a credible challenge to the triad and was intended only to promote discussion. Attempts to rely on the unified hypothesis as a challenge to the triad are now rarely encountered and should always be subject to thorough testing. [16]

To the extent that Dr Geddes did want to promote discussion, hers was a healthy scientific challenge. But when Dr Squier and Dr Marta Cohen took this challenge up, they were both criticised for it by judges who – it must be recalled – know very little about the science [20]:

> Dr. Squier and Dr. Cohen, I find with regret, have each fallen into that category of expert identified by Butler-Sloss P. in *Re LU & LB*, namely the expert who has developed a scientific prejudice.

At one level this is folly: clearly any expert (or judge) who simply accepts the unproven SBS theory has a 'scientific prejudice'. But such prejudice is far more dangerous since it results in sending people to prison.

Part of the problem stems from language. Judges got upset when a witness (particularly Dr Squier) did not accept a diagnosis [21].[4] A diagnosis is not the truth (beyond reasonable doubt), however; it is sometimes referred to as a 'best guess' – and mistakes are often made when a professional fails to consider a different view [22]. Thus, the judges and the doctors are speaking a different language, yet they do not recognise it. If there is a plausible differential diagnosis, that is called a 'reasonable doubt'.

Indeed, meetings at which doctors were meant to confer and reach some kind of consensus illustrated how far the proponents of SBS have strayed from the vaunted 'objectivity'. In the *O'Toole* experts meeting, where Dr Squier agreed on a point with Dr Philip Anslow, a defence expert, one of the prosecution doctors on the call was – anonymously – heard to exclaim, 'Oh Christ, stupid c**t!' Later in the same conversation, an unidentified doctor (perhaps the same one) used another expletive when Dr Anslow suggested, entirely reasonably, that an expert in biomechanics would be more appropriate for calculating impact forces.

If some experts are themselves biased in favour of SBS, the police are worse. One officer gave a PowerPoint presentation in Florida bragging about their plan to go after Dr Squier to stop her from undermining their prosecutions. Then, in 2010, the police referred Dr Squier to the GMC, who held a lengthy hearing, and wrote a scathing report striking her off. Given that the proponents of SBS have long taken a blinkered approach without meaningful evidence, the GMC's position was ironic: 'Dr Squier failed to be objective because of her "preconceived and blinkered approach" and her conduct at various civil and criminal proceedings was irresponsible, deliberately misleading and dishonest' [23].

This was overturned on appeal, and, on 3 November 2016, the court published a judgment which concluded that 'the determination of the MPT is in many significant respects flawed' as she clearly had not been dishonest [24]. Yet Dr Squier was still barred from testifying for 3 years.

The chilling impact of this on others was manifest. In her GMC hearing, Dr Squier conceded that she held 'a minority view on shaken baby syndrome' but said 'that "many more" clinicians privately agree with her' [23]. I am aware of two experts who have declined to give evidence for fear of risking their careers. More to the point, in May 2016, I gave a talk to a large audience of forensic medical professionals in London. They were generally responsive to questions but when I asked anyone to put a hand up who believed SBS was an established medical diagnosis, nobody did. I asked who would be willing to say this in a courtroom, nobody replied. I do not pretend this to be a scientific experiment – any more than the SBS hypothesis is – but it is nevertheless telling. Just as the Inquisition penalised those who expressed doubts regarding Ptolemy's theory, so the GMC and the courts have intimidated medical experts.

In common with almost any scientific – or social – issue, the first port of call is often data. There are other areas where the United Kingdom makes it difficult for a full assessment of SBS in the system. A primary problem that advocates of the scientific method face in the

4 For example, in *Oyediran*, the judge complained that '[s]he repeated that HIV had not been excluded and referred to the fact that Femi's father came from a country where it was endemic. Dr. Squier should not have persisted in that suggestion'.

United Kingdom is the lack of a meaningful public record of who is saying what – in short, a lack of transparency. For example, the defence has had the right to a complete and public transcript of a trial in the United States for at least half a century [25]. It is difficult for the American advocate to comprehend this, but, in the United Kingdom, there is no such right, so collecting and evaluating the evidence of experts is not easy. To what extent have the prosecution witnesses morphed from SBS to AHT to NAHI? Where have they relied on dubious studies?

It is not easy even to understand where we are in terms of the judges. In the United States, it would be nearly impossible for a criminal appeal to be kept secret, save in cases of significant national security. In the United Kingdom, few SBS cases get posted on the British and Irish Legal Information Institute (BAILII), the site where published decisions appear.

Here, along with two students, I have been conducting a very preliminary study of such data as does appear [26]. It would be hypocritical to present this study as anything like the final word on the subject – it is not. Indeed, its purpose is to provoke disclosure, transparency, and a more thorough evaluation of the data. However, the preliminary indications should prompt considerable concern.

The study identified of a total of 94 publicly reported decisions from UK family and criminal courts between 1994 and 2018 (92 since 2001), involving 114 children. Only one of the children was identified as over the age of 3, with half under 3 months. All had either died or suffered significant injury ascribed to 'shaken baby syndrome', 'non-accidental head Injury', or 'abusive head trauma'. There are roughly 100 such cases in the United Kingdom each year. This, and estimates by experts, makes it possible that these published cases represent only around 5% of the total cases – with some 95% remaining sealed.

The 94 cases include 167 suspects of whom 73 were female (average age 24.88 years) and 94 male (average age 27.19). The cases discuss (but reject) possible alternative causes of death or ill health in 52 cases, including a genetic disorder or other disease (15), an issue surrounding birth (14), an accident (10), and something such as possible sudden infant death syndrome (5). Effort to resuscitate the child was offered as potential explanation for injuries in five cases.

Possible prior health issues were identified as a factor in 41 cases, the issues ranging from vomiting (9 cases) respiratory problems (7), colds (6), and abnormal faeces (5). 'Birth abnormalities' were identified in 39 cases, of which 19 babies were premature, 16 were C-section, 2 had a 'difficult' birth, and in 2 cases a mother's illness during pregnancy had been identified. That such an issue was not mentioned in the decision does not, of course, mean there was none.

While the 'triad' continues to be deemed relevant, the focus of medical testimony has now shifted. The medical witnesses have been moving towards the use of abusive head injury (AHI) or non-accidental head injury (NAHI) rather than SBS. In our study, only 82 of the 114 cases reported the existence of triad elements, and all three were only noted in 24 of the cases. One was missing in 36 cases, two in 13 and all three in 9.

One of the main facts that leaps out as they are known to date is the tiny pool of the experts who are presenting evidence to a group of judges and lawyers who are without apparent experience in the area. Just four medical experts appear 81 times in the decisions (providing 48.5% of all the expert testimony referenced); one of these testified in support of the GMC effort to have Dr Waney Squier struck off, potentially evincing a bias in favour of the SBS theory.

Meanwhile, an overwhelming majority of the legal players appear to have little significant expertise in SBS: 69% of the named judges, 86% of the defence barristers, and 88% of the prosecution barristers appear in just one case covered by the study. Equally relevant, the Sutton Trust found that the judiciary was the most 'elitist' of any professional body, and two thirds of judges were privately educated: of the 61 SBS case judges where the information is available online, an even higher percentage (88.9%) attended private school [27]. This is not intended as a class-divisive commentary, but rather a sense of the culture: there are a number of statements made by the authors of the judgments that stand out, some of which might appear classist – that going to a good university makes a particular individual less likely to abuse, or that living in a council house is somehow relevant. There are five cases where the judge saw fit to mention that the parents were born outside the United Kingdom, one judge describing an 'arranged marriage', one where the marriage is described as reflecting 'traditional religious home life'. None of these factors is demonstrably related to abuse, and again might better be seen in light of the judge's own culture.

The preliminary recommendations of the study are perhaps its most important contribution, since clearly there must be more data before any reliable conclusions may be drawn:

1. That this preliminary study be followed up with a properly funded one that is much more comprehensive.
2. That the authorities should cooperate with full transparency, providing copies of all SBS/NAHI/AHT judgments since 2000, redacted where necessary to protect the privacy interests of non-professionals.
3. That the government should establish an official inquiry into the science behind SBS/NAHI/AHT.
4. That a regime should be established to encourage the appearance of experts in criminal and family court trials, from the United Kingdom and abroad, who honestly and legitimately question current SBS/NAHI/AHT theories.
5. That training should urgently be offered to all judges, barristers, solicitors, and medical experts on questions that have been raised in other countries concerning SBS/NAHI/AHT theories.

Looking to the future, in the United States, a far greater openness to change has resulted in case after SBS case being thrown out. Typical of the trend was the appeal of Zavion Johnson, in prison for 16 years for the death of his daughter [28]. By 2017, two of the three doctors had reconsidered their emphatic testimony at trial, and the Sacramento district attorney supported Johnson's release. In the United States, 'an automatic determination of abuse based on the presence of the so-called triad has been discredited by the medical community. Anyone convicted based upon the triad and in prison today should reach out to an innocence project, conviction integrity unit, or similar resource. In light of the medical and legal communities' current understanding of shaken baby syndrome/abusive head trauma, people are listening and working to right the wrongs of the past' [29].

There was once hope that the same could happen in the United Kingdom. In 2015, with the intimidation of doctors in Britain already on the rise, a number of experts – including Norman Guthkelch – signed an open letter:

> Although those propounding the SBS construct tend to represent their views as the mainstream scientific view, SBS has never been proved as anything more than an hypothesis. Too

> often, specialists are unaware of, or may disagree with, the alternative explanations that may be provided by other specialisms, or even from other viewpoints within the same specialism. Moreover, there is an increasing body of entirely respectable science, published in peer-reviewed literature, which challenges the whole concept. Noticeably, the requirement for scientifically based evidence is far more rigorous in medical negligence cases than in the family or criminal courts where believing something to be true appears to have achieved sufficient evidential value to sway the determinations of the court. [30]

It is 'high time every case of a parent in [prison] for this had his or her case reviewed', Dr Guthkelch said. 'We went badly off the rails . . . on this matter' [28, 4].

For the victims of the British justice system, 2015 is now a long time ago. Dr Guthkelch has died, unable to stem the zealotry of those who have transformed his hypothesis into scientific fact without pausing for proof. Those who were willing to insist on the scientific method have been threatened and intimated.

Human folly normally only lasts for its season, but many people can suffer during that time. Eventually, the proponents of heliocentrism won the battle because they were scientists and they were demonstrably correct. We can only hope that the British legal system will learn to bow to Dr John Plunkett and Dr Waney Squier more quickly than the Catholic Church did to Copernicus and Galileo.

References

1. Wojtyla, KJ. Address by Pope John Paul II for the commemoration of Albert Einstein. 1979. https://bit.ly/3NDyfeb.
2. Wojtyla, KJ. Pope John Paul II on the Galileo Affair. 1992. https://bit.ly/3Td3wFP.
3. Chadwick DL, Kirschner RH, Reece RM et al. Shaken baby syndrome: A forensic pediatric response. *Pediatrics*. 1998;101 (2):321–3. https://bit.ly/3UylRhx.
4. Guthkelch AN. Problems of infant retino-dural hemorrhage with minimal external injury. *Houston Journal of Health Law and Policy*. 2012;12(2):201–8.
5. Stafford Smith CA, Goldman PD. Forensic hair comparison analysis: Nineteenth century science or twentieth century snake oil? *Columbia Human Rights Law Review*. 1996;27:227–91.
6. *Bevill v State*, 556 So. 2d 699, 707 (Miss. 1990).
7. Gaudette B, Keeping ES. An attempt at determining probabilities in human scalp hair comparison. *Journal of Forensic Science*. 1974;19(3):599–606.
8. Gaudette B. Probabilities and human pubic hair comparisons. *Journal of Forensic Science*. 1976;21:514–17.
9. Fries T. In the know: FBI admits flaws in microscopy testimony. 2016. https://bit.ly/3DK73FN.
10. *Daubert v Merrill Dow Pharmaceuticals, Inc.*, 113 S.Ct. 2786, 2796 (1993).
11. Plunkett J. Fatal pediatric head injuries caused by short-distance falls. *American Journal of forensic Medicine and Pathology*. 2001;22(1):1–12. https://doi.org/10.1097/00000433-200103000-00001.PMID:11444653.
12. Findley KA, Risinger DM, Barnes PD et al. Feigned consensus: Usurping the law in shaken baby syndrome/abusive head trauma prosecutions. *Wisconsin Law Review*. 2019;1211–67. https://papers.ssrn.com/sol3/papers.cfm?abstract_id=3328996.
13. Narang SK, Estrada C, Greenberg S, Lindberg D. Acceptance of shaken baby syndrome and abusive head trauma as medical diagnoses. *Journal of Pediatrics*. 2016;177:273–8.
14. House of Commons Science and Technology Committee. Forensic Science on Trial Seventh Report of Session 2004-5. 2005. https://bit.ly/3zObYES.

15. Campbell D. Battlelines drawn as shaken baby syndrome controversy set to run. *The Guardian*. 2016. https://bit.ly/3zRJcDg.
16. Crown Prosecution Service. Non Accidental Head Injury Cases (NAHI, formerly referred to as Shaken Baby Syndrome [SBS]) – Prosecution Approach. 2018. https://bit.ly/3E7k0Lo.
17. Luttner S. Dr John Plunkett, champion of justice, 1947–2018. 2018. https://bit.ly/3E6Jt7S.
18. Geddes J. Neuropathology of inflicted head injury in children. *Brain*. 2001;124:1290–8, 1299–1306.
19. *R. v Harris* [2005] EWCA Crim. 1980 (Lord Gage).
20. *A Local Authority v S* [2009] EWHC 2115 (Fam) (King J.).
21. *Oyediran* [2010] EWCA Crim. 1269 (Moses, L.J.).
22. Hayes A. Understanding medical diagnosis: Why it's all 'best guesses'. 2020. https://bit.ly/3t1IGib.
23. French A. GMC in John Radcliffe consultant Dr Waney Squier accused of bias. 2015. https://bit.ly/3NDSXdM.
24. *Squier v General Medical Council* [2016] EWHC 2739 (Admin).
25. *Hardy v United States*, 375 U.S. 277 (1964) (the accused has the right to 'a transcript of the testimony and evidence presented by the defendant and also the court's charge to the jury, as well as the testimony and evidence presented by the prosecution').
26. Girvan-Dutton E, Parrett A, Stafford Smith C. A preliminary study on shaken baby syndrome in the UK: Must Galileo wait another 377 years? 3D Centre (7 January 2022). https://bit.ly/3t1PgoM.
27. McKinney CJ. *Social mobility fail: two thirds of top judges went to private schools* (25 June 2019). https://bit.ly/3zNY71b.
28. Beiser V. Discredited shaken baby science sent this father to jail for 15 years. His ordeal could end this week. 2017. https://bit.ly/3E2uagh.
29. Clarke M. 'Shaken baby syndrome' diagnoses discredited, convictions questioned. 2018. https://bit.ly/3FKBXRg.
30. Wrennall L, Bache B, Pragnell C et al. Open letter on shaken baby syndrome and courts: A false and flawed premise. Argument and critique. January 2015. https://bit.ly/3TewuoK.

Chapter 22

Shaken Baby Syndrome in France

Cyrille Rossant and Grégoire Etrillard

22.1 Introduction

It took some 15 years after the birth of the notion of shaken baby syndrome (SBS) for the first scientific critiques to appear. In 1987, an American study used biomechanical analysis to question the possibility that shaking alone, without impact, could cause traumatic rupture of bridging veins and subdural haematoma (SDH) in infants (see Chapter 14) [1]. Ten years later, in 1997, the widely publicised Boston trial of the British au pair Louise Woodward spread the concept of SBS to the entire world (see the Foreword); the public discovered that in fact a vigorous medical debate surrounded the diagnosis. Since that time, the English-speaking press regularly discusses the latest developments on the question, whether medical, scientific, or judicial.

In France, surprisingly, the existence of a controversy around the diagnosis was almost never mentioned anywhere, at least not until 2017, a year which was in some sense a turning point, as we shall see. The single exception was a student who, in 2004, first identified some specifically French problems [2]. Unlike the raging controversy in the United Kingdom and the United States, France merely established a wall of silence: 'Our study shows that for the moment, in France, research on SBS is unanimous and originates from a single professor [Dr Dominique Renier] who incarnates scientific legitimacy. Consequently, everything in France functions as though no controversy existed; the public repeats the views of the scientific experts who all agree with each other, as though knowledge was factually established.' Indeed, during an interview conducted by this student researching SBS, one of these experts, the director of a paediatrics department in a large hospital, declared: 'There is no controversy. I really don't see what your thesis will even talk about.'

Since then, this idea that there is no serious controversy around SBS has been perpetuated by the majority of French specialists in the subject. This attitude has then propagated to all sources of information on the subject, including hospitals, clinics, researchers, governmental health authorities, and the press and other media. Concomitantly, while 20 years ago the diagnosis of SBS was treated with at least a certain amount of humility and an admission of uncertainty [3] today medical experts (who also are the experts generally called by the courts) consider it 'certain'.

While the French population is not aware of a scientific controversy, it is largely aware of the existence and danger of shaking. France has established an active programme to prevent shaking, including information in the Child Health Record provided to all parents at the birth of their child. A massive national prevention campaign was launched in 2022 on social media.[1]

1 www.gouvernement.fr/secouer-un-bebe-une-maltraitance-qui-peut-etre-mortelle.

In this chapter, we will briefly review the history of SBS in France. We will focus on the SBS and abusive head trauma (AHT) diagnostic guidelines of the French governmental National Health Authority (Haute Autorité de Santé (HAS)). First published in 2011 and revised in 2017, these guidelines form the cornerstone of all medical diagnoses and judicial procedures in every case of alleged SBS in France. They go well beyond the standards in other countries in terms of claiming 'certainty' on the sole basis of one or two components of the 'triad'. This diagnostic process contradicts the recent international 'consensus statement' denying the existence of 'near-mechanical determination based on the "triad"' [4].

The organising committee of these guidelines is constituted of a small group of physicians who claim to specialise in SBS. As forensic doctors and radiologists, they have no expertise in clinical paediatric neurology, genetics, haematology, neuropathology, biomechanics, any discipline actually involved with paediatric intracranial haemorrhage. They are also judicial experts in many SBS trials and teach in regular classes and conferences training physicians, judges, lawyers, police officers, and social workers about SBS. They unanimously insist that no controversy exists and publicly label every challenger of any aspect whatsoever of the science with the simple term 'denialist', a word whose main overtone in France indicates Holocaust denial.

22.2 From the First Shaken Baby Syndrome Diagnosis in France to the Haute Autorité de Santé Guidelines

It is difficult to find much information about the way in which SBS, first raised in the United States between 1971 and 1974, made its way to France.

In 1987, paediatrician Dr Michel Roussey published the first French study on 'shaken babies' in a paediatric journal [5]. Not until the 1990s did awareness of SBS become widespread in France, largely due to the work of a leading department located in Necker Children's Hospital which received international recognition. Even today, this department receives a quarter of all French children with any neurosurgical condition, and the majority of SBS cases in the Paris region.[2] It was in this hospital that the first team comprising paediatricians, paediatric neurosurgeons, psychologists, social workers, and nurses was constituted with the express purpose of dealing with SBS cases. This team met once a week to jointly discuss all cases of SBS in the hospital and develop a protocol for dealing with them. Such teams are present today in all children's hospitals and charged specifically with the task of detecting child abuse.

The Necker team was involved in 2005 in a major doctoral thesis on SBS; the thesis jury contained three members of a small and tight-knit group of doctors who are still major players in the French SBS arena today [6]. Dr Anne Laurent-Vannier presided over the HAS task force working on SBS. Along with the other members of her task force, such as Dr Adamsbaum and Dr Rey-Salmon, she organised and continues to organise frequent conferences and training courses on the subject for medical and legal professionals.

The HAS, a governmental health authority, was created in 2005 to evaluate the relevance and efficacy of every type of medical care and to write up general guidelines and recommendations. The HAS is the French analogue of the Swedish Agency for Health Technology Assessment (SBU) (see Chapter 10), and its president is chosen directly by the President of the Republic.[3] The organising committee of the HAS task force on SBS, constituted in 2008,

[2] Le Guide de l'Association Tête en l'air, page 16. https://teteenlair.asso.fr.

[3] The president of the HAS in 2017, when the latest guidelines on SBS were published, was Agnès Buzyn, who served as the minister of health in Emmanuel Macron's government from 2017 to 2020.

consisted of 17 members from various medical, social, and legal organisations and institutions, with Dr Laurent-Vannier as president. Under her leadership, the committee organised a public hearing on SBS. The reason for this hearing, organised and financed by the HAS at a cost of some €150,000, was to foster a 'public debate with experts and patients on the subject of a controversial health problem . . . where there is controversy or uncertainty on a specific theme with important repercussions in public health' [7].

Between 2009 and 2011, a committee of 21 members organised the hearing. The first meeting, attended by 400 professionals, took place in October 2009. Two people were charged with performing a literature review while 12 experts wrote papers describing their experiences and views. The public hearing then took place in 2011, followed by release in September 2011 of the HAS guidelines constituting recommendations for all professionals faced with cases of SBS.

The guidelines were updated in 2017; the eight authors included one lawyer, one judge, one member of the HAS, Dr Laurent-Vannier, and four other doctors (Drs Rambaud, Rey-Salmon, Adamsbaum, and Raul). These five doctors form a tight and unanimous group that has come to play a determining role in every aspect of SBS in France.

22.3 The Haute Autorité de Santé Guidelines for Shaken Baby Syndrome

The first version of the report, published in May 2011, comprised three parts: the process for diagnosing shaking, the mechanisms causing the observed lesions, and the judicial consequences.

22.3.1 The Diagnostic Process

The diagnostic process details the initial symptoms associated with SBS (essentially linked to encephalopathy), the risk factors (sex, age, socioeconomic background), and the list of medical findings frequently found: SDH and retinal haemorrhage (RH), as well as lesions of the skin, the bones, the neck, and the general clinical picture.

The guidelines also list certain differential (alternative) diagnoses for the findings associated with shaking. Accidental cranial trauma is the 'main differential diagnosis'; the other rare diagnoses that must be eliminated before arriving at a conclusion of shaking are:

- Coagulation disorders (congenital coagulation problems and severe thrombocytopenia).
- Arteriovenous malformations, said to be 'exceptional before the age of 1 year', are mentioned as possible causes of intracranial haemorrhage, but not SDH.
- Metabolic disorders: glutaric aciduria type 1 (25 cases/year in France) and Menkes disease (3 cases/year in France), both of which can cause SDH and RH.
- Osteogenesis imperfecta is presented as an alternative cause of fractures but not SDH.

Finally, this section of the report presents a decision-making algorithm for how to arrive at a diagnosis of shaking. In particular, the report states that:

> [F]or a child under one year, and after eliminating the above differential diagnoses, the diagnosis of shaking is *highly probable or even certain*, in the following case:
>
> - extra-axial multifocal intracranial haemorrhage (subdural or subarachnoid haemorrhage);

- and profuse RH, or RH extending to the periphery of the retina;
- and a trauma history that is absent, fluctuating or incompatible with the observed lesions or the age of the child.

Eventually, the report instructs that every bilateral SDH not explained to the satisfaction of the examining physician by the caretaker and not caused by one of the few differential diagnoses listed above should be interpreted to mean that shaking is at least probable or highly probable.

22.3.2 The Causal Mechanism

The authors of the report accept as proven the statement that shaking can cause SDH; this statement is explicitly qualified as 'data that cannot be put into question'. They did not assess the quality of the scientific proof of this causal relation. In contrast, the systematic literature review by the SBU (see Chapter 10), based on a similar methodology, concluded that the publications supporting this statement are of low quality, methodologically defective, and scientifically insufficient.

The authors note other frequently mentioned potential causes: short falls, shaking of a baby by another child, shaking during play, childbirth, hypoxia, resuscitation, coughing, and vomiting. However, each and every one of these mechanisms is categorically rejected as a possible cause for SDH and RH. For example, the report asserts that 'there is no case anywhere in the literature of a child of less than 1 year presenting with subdural haematoma and retinal haemorrhage following a short fall', which is incorrect as shown in Chapter 15. This statement leads many cases of short falls associated with SDH to be reported to authorities as cases of maltreatment in France.

The HAS report further states that all lesions such as SDH and RH that are caused during childbirth disappear after a period of at most 1 month. This is false, as shown, for example, by a study proving the persistence of perinatal RH for up to 58 days [8]. The report goes on to consider the question of the injury mechanism as a function of the different types of injuries, the tests performed, and the history. 'The symptoms following shaking generally appear immediately after the traumatic episode' and 'it seems that in the large majority of cases, if not in all cases of SBS, shaking causes immediate symptoms'.

Concerning the condition known as benign external hydrocephalus (BEH), the authors reject the series of published cases reporting SDH in children with this condition on the grounds that abuse can never be really ruled out. They also cite two biomechanical studies, which actually contradict each other, and conclude 'altogether, there are no arguments in the literature supporting the hypothesis that BEH is a predisposing factor for SDH in infants' [9, 10]. Chapters 5 and 6 in this book provide ample evidence against this claim.

22.3.3 Judicial Consequences

The final section of the report concerns the judicial responses to alleged SBS/AHT. It contains recommendations about mandatory reporting and the judicial processes following a diagnosis of shaking.

The authors indicate that in the case of a probable or highly probable determination of shaking, the case must be reported to the public prosecutor: 'the medical team is confronted with a double duty, both legal and ethical, to protect the infant from possible future violence'.

The reporting itself should not, however, include identification of the presumed abuser because that is the task of the judicial system. The guidelines emphasise the necessity of a consultation with the hospital's multidisciplinary team before the decision to report is made.

According to the guidelines, if the team decides to report, then the report should take place as quickly as possible: 'it is necessary to make the report with the least possible delay in order to protect the child if necessary, and not to hinder the investigation. The closer the report is to the alleged act, the more the criminal investigation can be performed efficiently'.

This part of the guidelines also details the risks that medical personnel run if they choose not to report – or if they make a report when it is not justified. In the first case, the repercussions are far more severe, including both criminal and disciplinary sanctions. Indeed, 'in the case of a death following a highly probable or certain shaking, a doctor who signs a death certificate attesting "death from natural causes" not associated with any medico-legal implications is guilty of the offence of forgery punishable by three years of imprisonment, a 45,000 euro fine and the prohibition of practising his or her profession'.

Conversely, if a doctor makes an unjustified report, 'any report made to the competent authorities under the conditions described in these guidelines cannot be the object of any disciplinary sanction'. In particular, 'such a report cannot lead to any judicial consequences harmful to the medical professionals, who are bound by professional secrecy, apart from the exceptional situation in which the report corresponds to a slanderous allegation'.

Each mandatory report leads immediately to two separate, almost always simultaneous judicial procedures:

1. A civil procedure with the goal of protecting the child. A juvenile court judge may place the child in a foster family, with limited to no parental rights, and, through successive decisions for periods of up to 2 years, may extend the duration of placement at his or her discretion.
2. A criminal procedure which aims to identify and decide whether to prosecute the alleged perpetrator of the reported criminal act. The criminal investigation, performed by a team of police investigators supervised by the public prosecutor and/or an investigating judge, is further tasked with determining the exact nature of the criminal act together with its circumstances and causes, and estimating the risk of recidivism.

The HAS guidelines also explicitly define shaking as criminal in nature, including by defining the mental state of the alleged perpetrator: 'The gesture itself is always described as "a voluntary act of violence"'. Financial compensation for the child victim of shaking is also mentioned.

22.3.4 The Updating of the Haute Autorité de Santé Guidelines in 2017

The main changes introduced in 2017 increase the rigidity of the diagnostic process and the dating of the criminal act. For example, the descriptive 'highly probable or certain' was changed to simply 'certain'. The report now reads:

> [I]n the case of an infant where the caretaker provides a history that is fluctuating or absent or incompatible with the observed lesions or the age of the child, after elimination of the differential diagnostics, the diagnosis of non-accidental head trauma by shaking is certain in the following cases:
>
> - multifocal SDH with clots at the convexity (vertex), indicating rupture of the bridging veins;

- or multifocal SDH and RH of any type;
- or unifocal SDH and cervical or medullar lesions.

Therefore, the HAS guidelines assert that every infant with multifocal SDH and RH, or multifocal SDH with bridging vein thrombosis, that is not explained by the listed differential diagnoses or by an 'adequate' story given by the caregiver must lead to a 'certain' determination of shaking.[4] The guidelines even state that the differential diagnosis should merely 'be noted, but does not exclude the possibility of abuse'. In other words, the accusation of abuse may be maintained even when one of the alternative causes of the observed symptoms is established.

The 2017 guidelines also eliminate any remaining doubt concerning the timing of the shaking: 'in every single case, the symptoms arise immediately following the shaking'. The 'loss of nuance' in the guidelines between 2011 and 2017 has been deplored by French paediatric neurologists [11].

22.3.5 The Problems Raised by the Haute Autorité de Santé Guidelines

22.3.5.1 Scientific Validity of the Articles Cited in the Guidelines

Chapter 10 of this book explores a Swedish report issued by the SBU which concluded that the SBS literature is of low quality due to serious methodological problems, including circular reasoning. The HAS also tasked a paediatrician and an anthropologist to perform a (non-systematic) review of the literature [7]. Grades were assigned to publications according to Table 22.1.

The two reviewers selected 139 studies, which were classified as indicated in Table 22.2. In particular, only 3 were assigned grade B [12–14] and none grade A. The remaining studies were assigned grade C or described as 'survey articles' and assigned no grade as they did not provide new research. Overall, 98% either had a 'weak level of scientific proof' or 'provided no scientific proof'.

The reviewers explained the difficulty of obtaining high-level scientific proof for SBS as follows:

> Concerning SBS, bibliographical research reveals a large number of references, but a major part of them cannot easily be graded according to the grading system by scientific level of proof as required by evidence-based medicine. Given the diagnostic, ethical and judicial stakes, it is obvious that no randomised trial can ever take place . . . The literature consists essentially of case histories, with data collected retrospectively. Numerous publications concern single or very small numbers of cases, which are of very little value as scientific proofs according to the requirements of evidence-based medicine, but which the public and the medical and judicial personnel involved may be tempted to use in order to support their decisions.

These findings, which fully align with the large-scale Swedish review discussed in Chapter 10 of this book, raise the question of whether a 'highly probable or certain' diagnosis of shaking is justified when 98% of the selected SBS publications on which this designation is based have a 'weak level of scientific proof' and *none* reaches a high level. While SBS cannot be studied according to the requirements of evidence-based medicine, the same is true for many other medical diagnoses (e.g., we can hardly inoculate human beings

[4] The lack of scientific evidence related to the diagnostic value of bridging vein thrombosis is tackled in Chapters 3 and 4.

Table 22.1 Table from the Haute Autorité de Santé literature review, September 2011 (p. 6)

Type of study	Level of scientific proof
Level 1 - Large-sized randomised comparative trials - Meta-analysis of randomised comparative trials - Decision analysis based on high-quality studies	**Grade A** **High-level scientific proof**
Level 2 - Small-sized randomised comparative trials - Non-randomised well-conducted studies - Cohort studies	**Grade B** **Medium-level scientific proof**
Level 3 - Case history studies **Level 4** - Comparative studies with serious biases - Retrospective studies - Case series - Descriptive epidemiological studies (cross-sectional or longitudinal)	**Grade C** **Low-level scientific proof**

Each study was evaluated by the authors of the literature review according to its methodological quality. Grade A corresponds to established scientific evidence, grade B to scientific presumption, and grade C to a 'low level of scientific evidence'.

Table 22.2 Grading of publications according to the Haute Autorité de Santé literature review from 2011 and 2017

Level	Count (2011)	Count (2017)
Level 1	0	1
Level 2	3	20
Level 3	5	57
Level 4	58	76
Comment	39	-
No grading	34	103
Total	139	257

with dangerous organisms or induce serious illnesses). This limitation does not provide any justification for qualifying shaking diagnoses as 'certain'.

The situation following the 2017 updating of the HAS guidelines is not significantly better (see Table 22.2). Of 257 publications analysed and graded, 1 was graded A and 20 were graded B. A total of 92% of the examined publications failed to reach even a medium level of scientific proof. Furthermore, the single article receiving the grade A did not even concern the diagnosis of shaking at all but rather the efficacy of prevention programmes in helping mothers to learn best practices when faced with an inconsolably crying baby (ask for advice, leave the room) [15]. The authors only evaluated whether mothers who had received information on these practices were better informed on such practices than mothers who had not – and, unsurprisingly, they were. That finding is the only 'high-level scientific proof' (Grade A) regarding SBS the HAS found in its review.

Note that this study only evaluated the mothers' knowledge – not whether the prevention programme had any impact on the number of diagnoses of shaking. This question has never been studied in France to this day. On the contrary, while there were fewer than 200 cases each year in the early 2000s, there may be up to 500 yearly cases nowadays despite numerous shaking-prevention campaigns [6].[5]

22.3.5.2 Validity of the Medical, Biomechanical, and Statistical Assertions in the Guidelines

This section offers only an outline of the problems concerned with the HAS guidelines since this book contains other chapters specifically devoted to these problems. Numerous statements made in the HAS guidelines have been criticised and even refuted in various publications (see Chapters 3–9).

A recent study challenged the notion that thrombosis/rupture of bridging veins can be taken as evidence of shaking at all, let alone a 'certain' proof of shaking as asserted in the guidelines (see also Chapters 3 and 4) [16]. Studies supporting this idea that are cited by the HAS literature review are *all* graded with level 4, the lowest quality.

A collaborative medical book in French has put into question several other major assertions in the guidelines, including:

- The rejection of a possible lucid interval between a traumatic incident and the appearance of symptoms.
- The statement that the cause of thrombosis/rupture of the bridging veins is unique and known to be due to shaking.
- The assertion that SDH localised at the falx cerebri and tentorium cerebelli are indicative of shaking.
- The claim that intraspinal SDH are strongly correlated with non-accidental trauma; according to Échenne et al., they are instead strongly correlated with 'intracranial hypertension and cerebral oedema, young age and rapid intraspinal spread of haemorrhage from the foramen magnum'.
- The assertion that RH are strongly correlated to non-accidental head trauma.
- The list of differential diagnoses, which, according to Échenne et al., should be completely revised, as it contains a number of errors and also a significant number of missing differential diagnoses. They also criticise the fact that the guidelines ignore developments in biochemistry and genetics of the past 40 years [17].

Échenne et al. also point out nearly 50 serious errors of mathematics, physics, and logic in the arguments cited in the HAS guidelines (and correspondingly in French courts) related to short falls (see Chapters 14 and 15) and external hydrocephalus (see Chapters 5 and 6). For

5 www.leparisien.fr/societe/ca-fait-encore-peur-de-parler-de-bebes-morts-de-maltraitance-une-campagne-pour-briser-le-tabou-de-lenfant-secoue-17-01-2022-PXXZGRHG6JFTHKNLK6D2YKW5Q4.php.

example, one study cited to justify the implausibility of fall-related deaths relies on flawed statistics, as detailed in Chapter 15 [18].

The HAS authors refute almost all alternative causes to the medical findings associated with SBS. For instance, the many witnessed cases of short falls causing SDH and RH are dismissed on the grounds that sometimes the witnesses are family members and therefore 'not independent'; sometimes a fall took place in a staircase and therefore 'doesn't count'; sometimes the fall was not vertical or – as in one case of a filmed short fall of a 23-month-old girl followed by fatal SDH – because the case gives no information about children aged less than 1 year. The rejection of the many published challenges to their assertions has serious consequences since it allows removal of all obstacles to major controversial conclusions of the HAS report, among which are:

- Shaking without impact can cause SDH (see Chapters 3, 4, 14).
- Short falls cannot cause SDH (see Chapters 14 and 15).
- Benign external hydrocephalus is not a predisposing factor for SDH (see Chapters 5 and 6).
- Major neurological symptoms appear immediately after the shaking (no lucid interval).

22.4 The Dysfunctions of the Judicial System in Shaken Baby Syndrome Cases

22.4.1 Foster Placement

The effect of the errors contained in the HAS guidelines go far beyond the purely medical or academic framework. The medical 'diagnosis' of abuse results in mandatory reporting, which then leads to judicial procedures in which the medical opinion plays a determining role. Thus, when the medical opinion is based on poor-quality science, it can produce diagnostic errors which lead directly to miscarriages of justice.

The French judicial process contains two distinct parts: a civil procedure (protecting the child) and a criminal procedure (prosecuting the perpetrator). The average length of judicial procedure in these cases is around 4 years, but cases can sometimes last as long as 8, 10, or more years.

Mandatory reporting almost always leads to placement of the child into foster care (very rarely in extended family such as grandparents) via a 'precautionary principle' (see Chapter 18). Risk avoidance in child-related matters is arguably extreme in France. Past cases of children who died when they were not removed from abusive parents have left a lasting impression on the French public that the justice system is eager to erase [27].

Child protection services are independently handled by each administrative region. Parents may see their child in foster care for an hour every week, sometimes less, rarely more. Social workers constantly supervise the visits. Parental rights are extremely limited and procedures requesting increased visitation rights may take many months. Children are generally put in foster care for a year, sometimes several years. Long-lasting negative consequences on children of prolonged separation from their parents [28] are rarely, if ever, considered in risk assessments and judicial decisions, even if 'the higher interest of the child' is frequently mentioned.

Although the civil and criminal procedures are supposedly independent, some juvenile court judges prevent parents from seeing their children or refuse to increase visitation rights until the parents are cleared in the criminal procedure (which lasts many years) or, even if they are, until they confess. One juvenile judge expressed it as follows:

> In cases of abuse, I never hesitate to create a time period of some weeks during which the child will not have to meet the person who abused or did not protect it. The attitude of the parents, first during the hearing and subsequently during interviews with the social worker, will be the measure of their capacity to question their own behaviour and comprehend the gravity of their actions and their effect on the child. If they continue to deny wrongdoing and trivialise the suffering of their child, then the initial decision to place the child in a foster home is unlikely to change. However, if the parents are able to progress in comprehension, then we will progressively increase their communication with their child even before the end of the foster placement. [19]

As we will see later in this chapter, such behaviours have major implications on the validity of confessions of shaking in French cases (see also Chapters 11 and 12).

22.4.2 The Criminal Process

The French criminal process concerning those suspected of SBS is also rife with major problems that have dramatic consequences. The French criminal system is inquisitorial, not adversarial as in the common law world (United States, United Kingdom, Australia, New Zealand, and other former British Commonwealth nations). In the adversarial system, two parties are face to face, each side bringing in medical experts who debate in front of a judge or a jury on an equal level (although this equality is sometimes compromised by the ability of one side to pay significantly more than the other). In the inquisitorial system, each case is initially handled by an investigating judge whose role is to 'find out the truth' with the help of police (who may conduct investigations, question family members, perform searches, tap telephones, etc.) and medical experts.

Once the investigation is complete, the investigating judge decides whether there is sufficient evidence for the accused to stand trial. The amount of time between the baby becoming ill and the first trial typically ranges from 3 to 5 years, a period during which the accused may be jailed awaiting trial.

22.4.3 The Role of the Judicial Experts

In SBS cases in France, judicial experts play a fundamental role. There is a central list of judicial experts in each of France's 36 appellate courts. Any professional can address a request to the public prosecutor to be added to the list in the jurisdiction in which they reside, and in the precise domain of his or her speciality. The Administrative Supreme Court (Cour de Cassation) also maintains a national list of experts. Judicial experts testify under oath.

The investigating judge may call upon any judicial experts from the list to obtain a professional evaluation of a technical fact upon which he or she is not competent to make a reliable judgment. In the inquisitorial system, these experts are not expected to work for one side or the other, but to be entirely independent. As one of them wrote, 'judicial experts have no conflict of interest since by law they are independent of any side, and judges choose which ones to call upon independently from an established public list' [20].

In principle, this neutrality should guarantee an expert evaluation that is as objective as possible. Indeed, these judicial experts regularly claim that the payment of judicial experts in the adversarial system is not in the interests of justice. In practice, however, this supposed neutrality is dubious.

To start with, all five of the doctors who participated in the writing of the 2017 HAS guidelines are also judicial experts and they are called upon in many 'shaken baby' cases; it is not surprising that their evaluations are systematically in line with the flawed HAS guidelines. Since those guidelines contain extensive errors as explained earlier in this chapter, the unanimous decisions made by these experts are open to question. Indeed, the constant recourse to this same group of five people who invariably rely on the same erroneous set of principles that they themselves established has led to a system of extreme centralisation, a near monopoly, on a subject of tremendous scientific complexity and worldwide debate.

While they might be neutral in the limited sense that they owe no fealty to either party, they are not at all neutral in the sense that they have staked out and owe great fealty to an extreme version of one side of the divide in the medical and scientific debates about SBS/AHT. And yet, unlike the adversarial system, the French criminal system makes it quite difficult to challenge an judicial expert's opinion if the defence believes it to be erroneous.

After starting as a public defender, criminal defence lawyer Grégoire Etrillard (co-author of this chapter) took his first shaken baby case in 2013, which led him to discover many of the problems we have described. Today, his firm is dealing with more than 130 shaken baby cases, which gives him an overall view of the legal process in France concerning SBS. At least one of the aforementioned five judicial experts is involved in nearly half of the firm's SBS cases, with this proportion increased to more than 60% of the firm's criminal cases. He was also able to determine that three of the five doctors perform on average two or more expert evaluations per month. Given that each of these physicians relies on their own published SBS theory, and that each one is paid a standard fee of at least €1,000, the absence of any conflict of interest is called into question.

Because they follow their own guidelines, these experts conclude a 'certain' diagnosis of shaking which occurred precisely when symptoms appeared. The perpetrator is therefore identified beyond doubt as the person who was with the baby at that moment. Thus, these experts determine altogether the existence of the criminal act, its nature, its perpetrator, its motivation (exasperation by the baby's crying). Alternative medical causes are almost never seriously considered.

Faced with these arguments within the inquisitorial system, the defence has few options. To start with, the defence lawyer can request a second opinion from another judicial expert. However, this other expert is highly likely to follow the HAS guidelines, either because he or she is another of its authors, or because medical experts are expected to follow HAS guidelines.

The second option open to the defence is to call on independent medical professionals as witnesses for the defence, although this is not common practice in French criminal procedure. These doctors are not necessarily on the official lists of judicial experts; however, they are certainly experts in their own specialities – for example, clinical paediatric neurology, genetics, or haematology; HAS judicial experts are not specialists in any of these disciplines.

Few doctors agree to testify against the HAS mainstream view due to professional repercussions. Those who do are frequently retired. Although they are generally allowed to testify, their testimony is considered by French courts as less probative than that of judicially mandated medical experts. Furthermore, these medical witnesses have difficulty in accessing the child's medical file. Although French law allows parents to obtain their child's medical files, it is virtually impossible to access them once they have been seized by the justice system. For the court, medical experts are the sole professionals allowed to investigate medical records. The main exception occurs when families manage to get a copy of the medical file before it is seized within days of mandatory reporting.

On the contrary, court-appointed judicial experts have access not only to the full medical files, but to the full judicial files too, including police interrogation transcripts and other non-medical facts surrounding the case. Despite the almost inevitable contextual biases (see Chapter 13), this information allows the judicial experts to determine based on the criminal case file and police statements the exact moment when they think the symptoms appeared, when the perpetrator was alone with the child. Indeed, it is suggested that timing of intracranial injuries should be based on legal reports rather than clinical protocols. Adamsbaum said, 'Assessing the time of the injury based on neuroimaging is difficult and it is based on models of accidental trauma' and advised that 'Determining the most likely timing of intracranial injuries is important for the legal proceeding and requires the full legal inquiries. Thus, it should not be given at the time of the medical diagnosis' [29].

In other words the normal clinical protocols for timing should be abandoned in favour of relying on police and judicial reports. In one recent study, some of these experts claimed that SBS never occurs in day care centres [20]. Since these authors, who believe that SBS always occurs at home, are the ones who determine the time and location of shaking, this result is likely an obvious consequence of circular reasoning [21].

A final disadvantage of the judicial expert system in France is that expert evaluations are shrouded in secrecy and can never be examined objectively by any outsider. Yet these evaluations are systematically collected and used as case studies in medical publications. These cases cannot be independently verified and their scientific validity is therefore fragile.

22.4.4 Adikia

Starting in 2015, accused families began to contact each other via social media. In 2017, they joined together to form the French association Adikia.[6] Between 150 and 250 new families contact Adikia each year.

Many of these families eventually saw their cases dismissed or end in acquittals, even after having been prosecuted for crimes described in the expert evaluations. Perhaps unsurprisingly, the main group of French judicial experts maintain that their evaluations are correct regardless of judicial outcomes. An acquittal will not change their database: in their publications, 'shaken babies' are the ones they decided were shaken. This dramatically increases the risk of circular reasoning since their own publications inform the HAS guidelines.

Many parents and caretakers have been declared innocent of wrongdoing in cases of children suffering from BEH. Yet this medical condition is not recognised by the HAS guidelines. Other caretakers have been acquitted in cases where the child suffered from medical conditions not even mentioned in the list of HAS-provided differential diagnoses, such as Ehlers–Danlos syndrome, bone disease, abetalipoproteinemia, congenital coagulation

6 One of the authors of this chapter, C. R., is the president of this association at the time of writing. His childminder was wrongly indicted for purportedly shaking his child before being cleared of all charges.

problems, meningitis, or Silver–Russell syndrome. Since these errors are not officially recognised, they are constantly repeated.

One highly publicised case (although not SBS) concerned a child with bruises on her face who was finally found to suffer from a rare genetic disorder shared with her mother – hereditary angioedema. This child spent 4 years in a foster home. The judicial experts who declared she was a victim of child abuse never retracted their statements [22]. These experts were eventually ordered to pay damages to the parents they had wrongly accused, an outcome almost unheard of in France. The experts appealed and the procedure is ongoing.[7]

An anonymous questionnaire sent to Adikia families in the winter of 2021 provides valuable information about the experiences of accused families. About 87% of the 136 families who responded were accused of shaking, with the remaining 13% accused of other types of abuse. For 79% of these families, the judicial process was still ongoing. About 11% of the respondents were not parents but nannies.

The psychological impact on families is enormous: 97% of respondents said this event was the single hardest event of their lives, 35% had to take sick leave, 68% suffered from depression, and 75% had major weight gain or loss. They reported frequent suicide attempts, hospital stays, break-ups, and loss of employment.

Of 77 SBS cases that were the subject of an expert evaluation, 33 were signed by at least one of the five authors of the HAS guidelines. In the 44 cases where none of these authors was involved, 19 (43%) of the expert evaluations excluded abuse, attributing the observed lesions to other causes. In the 33 cases in which the expert evaluation was signed by at least one of the HAS authors, abuse was diagnosed in *every single case (100%).*

Judicial experts collect all the cases they examine in a database, relying on their own final determination as to the diagnosis. For this reason, their databases are filled with cases marked as SBS, even the cases in which alternative diagnoses were made, the cases were dismissed, or the accused parents or caretakers were acquitted. These published studies are therefore fundamentally flawed since they include an unknown number of false positives. Even when these studies rely on confessions, their quality remains low because of the major issue of false confessions in France.

22.5 False Confessions

The occult inclusion of false positives in French experts' data sets highlights the persistent problem of circularity in the research, which is widespread throughout the SBS literature in every country (see Chapter 10). In France, circular reasoning arises when an expert decides a child was shaken based on the HAS guidelines, then uses this diagnosis as the basis for published research on shaking, and then in turn uses the research to confirm the conclusions of the HAS guidelines.

In order to appear to be minimising this circularity, certain researchers in France tend to rely on confessions to determine cases of SBS. They argue that, for SBS cases in France, the accused do not negotiate their sentences to enter into a plea bargain with the prosecutor. They contend that this removes all incentive for caretakers to make false confessions [23]. This question is critical as the only two articles qualified as 'medium quality' by the Swedish literature review (Chapter 10) were French articles based on confessions [24, 25].

7 www.leparisien.fr/faits-divers/parents-accuses-a-tort-de-maltraitance-deux-medecins-experts-condamnes-dans-laffaire-louna-03-04-2021-CGUJNITFAJEXVEJVMY3K236LVM.php.

As we will show, even without plea bargaining, innocent parents and caregivers have many reasons to falsely confess to shaking (see also Chapters 11 and 12). First, we have seen earlier that juvenile court judges may refuse to let parents see their children until they confess, which is a strong incentive for false confessions.

Second, many defendants 'confess' to gestures that do not fit the description of violent shaking, but instead refer to trivial gestures (playing with the child or scooping the child up quickly without supporting the head). Although these statements are incompatible with the SBS theory (only the most violent shaking can cause elements of the triad), they are nevertheless considered as 'confessions'.

Of note is the fact that neither of these two articles assessed as 'medium quality' for the Swedish national body gives specific details of the 'confessions' they claim to have received. This cannot allow scientific review as to whether those 'confessions' really fit with the SBS thesis at all. For instance, the confessed shakes could have been mild gestures not strong enough to cause intracranial bleeding under the SBS theory (an act 'so violent that individuals observing it would recognize it as dangerous and likely to kill the child' [30]).

The Adikia questionnaire reveals some interesting facts with respect to French judicial confessions under the premise that some of the respondents are potentially included in the two 'medium-quality' articles' database. Of the 136 families who responded, 97 had one or more family members who were taken into custody and questioned by police in an SBS case for which they denied any violence. While we obviously don't have access to the ground truth, these data remain valuable as they describe the experience of parents and caregivers who question the diagnosis of abuse and who deny any wrongdoing. Of these 97 respondents, 79% had spent at least one night in a holding cell, where they averaged about 4 hours of sleep. Lack of sleep is a well-known factor contributing to false confessions [26].

In 95% of these cases, the child was deceased, hospitalised, or placed in foster care at the time of the interrogation, another major emotional stress factor contributing to false confessions. In 80% of the cases, the police presented the fact of abuse as 'absolutely certain', often leading the interrogated caretaker to believe it must have occurred and to seek an explanation in a gesture performed by their spouse or themselves (playing, scooping up, etc.), unaware it could be dangerous.

In 44% of these cases, the interrogated caretaker was told that, if they confessed, their spouse would be allowed to take the child home, which elicited (purportedly false) confessions in 12% of cases. Also, 47% were told that, if they confessed, their sentence would be less harsh. This is akin to an informal form of plea bargaining. In 45% of cases, false information was fed to the suspect, such as that 'there was a famous case where a tall mother picked up her child too quickly from the floor and it died' or that various trivial gestures could cause serious harm to a small infant. This type of false information elicited 'confessions' of similar trivial gestures in 44% of cases. In 12% of cases, the parent admitted to having used rough gestures or gentle shaking when trying to resuscitate an unconscious child; this is invariably taken as a confession of violent shaking even though it could not have been the cause of the child's collapse if it occurred *after* the child collapsed.

Altogether, nearly half of all statements qualified as 'confessions' have been made by parents and caregivers who deny any wrongdoing and who would therefore qualify them as 'false confessions'. This proportion rises to two-thirds in cases where the child is deceased.

22.6 The Demand for the Repeal and Reform of the Haute Autorité de Santé Guidelines

On 2 December 2019, Grégoire Etrillard wrote to the HAS asking for the withdrawal of the HAS guidelines on SBS. In his letter, he detailed the many points raised in this chapter that question the legitimacy and validity of the 2011 and 2017 HAS guidelines on SBS/AHT. His request received a great deal of national press coverage.

Two weeks later, the HAS published a short answer to the letter, which did not respond to a single one of the points Mr Etrillard had raised, but merely reasserted 'the great importance of the guidelines for diagnosing SBS'. Signed by the HAS and 25 societies, national professional councils, federations, and associations, the answer reaffirmed 'the quality of the guidelines, in spite of the fact the competence and even the scientific probity of the authors are being subjected to unacceptable contestation'.

Mr Etrillard, representing Adikia and 137 families, brought a suit to the Administrative Supreme Court (Conseil d'État) that was refused in July 2021. In October 2021, Mr Etrillard brought this affair to the attention of the European Council for Human Rights. In 2022, the HAS announced the creation of a working group to publish a new revision of the SBS guidelines. Adikia made a request to participate in the working group. The procedure is ongoing at the time of writing.

22.7 Conclusion

France is characterised by its explicit reliance on an outdated theory – with few exceptions, all infants with unexplained RH and SDH and/or bridging vein thrombosis have been violently shaken – from which most other countries have distanced themselves for years already. While the Swedish national health agency reports insufficient scientific evidence for this theory (see Chapter 10), its French counterpart promotes the 'certainty' of that same theory in all hospitals and courts across the country. This theory is used as a basis for child removals, criminal prosecutions and convictions, while any physician and scientist challenging the situation is publicly labelled as a 'child abuse denialist'.

French national guidelines for the detection of child abuse must urgently be revisited. They should rely on up-to-date scientific data. They should be developed by medical professionals with clinical experience in relevant fields: paediatric neurology and neurosurgery, neuropathology, haematology, genetics, obstetrics, biomechanics, statistics, epidemiology, and psychology, rather than only forensic medicine and radiology. Child protection and criminal procedures (most notably the rules on medical expertise) should be reformed in order to reduce a high rate of wrongful allegations of shaking in France.

References

1. Duhaime AC, Gennarelli TA, Thibault LE et al. The shaken baby syndrome: A clinical, pathological, and biomechanical study. *Journal of Neurosurgery*. 1987;66(3):409–15.
2. Labrune M. *Le syndrome du bébé secoué: La controverse sur l'ambiguïté des symptômes*. 2004. https://controverses.minesparis.psl.eu//prive/promo03/C03B8/accueil/jeuaccueil.htm.
3. Renier D. *Le bébé secoué: Traumatisme crânien du nourrisson*. Karthala, 2001.
4. Choudhary AK, Servaes S, Slovis TL et al. Consensus statement on abusive head trauma in infants and young children. *Pediatric Radiology*. 2018;48(8):1048–65.

5. Roussey M, Dabadie A, Betrémieux P et al. Des sévices pas toujours évidents: l'enfant secoué. *Archives of French Pediatrics.* 1987;44:441–4.
6. Mireau E. Syndrome du bébé secoué: *Hématome* sous-dural du nourrisson et maltraitance, à propos d'une série de 404 cas. Thèse de médecine. Université de Paris V, 2005.
7. Haute Autorité de Santé. *Syndrome du bébé secoué. Synthèse bibliographique.* Haute Autorité de Santé, 2011.
8. Hughes LA, May K, Talbot JF, Parsons MA. Incidence, distribution, and duration of birth-related retinal hemorrhages: A prospective study. *Journal of the American Association for Pediatric Ophthalmology and Strabismus.* 2006;10 (2):102–6.
9. Papasian NC, Frim DM. A theoretical model of benign external hydrocephalus that predicts a predisposition towards extra-axial hemorrhage after minor head trauma. *Pediatric Neurosurgery.* 2000;33:188–93.
10. Raul JS, Roth S, Ludes B, Willinger R. Influence of the benign enlargement of the subarachnoid space on the bridging veins strain during a shaking event: A finite element study. *International Journal of Legal Medicine.* 2008;122:337–40.
11. Tardy-Joubert S. Contre-enquête sur les bébés secoués. *Revue XXI.* 2022; (58):84–101.
12. Bechtel K, Stoessel K, Leventhal JM. Characteristics that distinguish accidental from abusive injury in hospitalized young children with head trauma. *Pediatrics.* 2004;114(1):165–8.
13. Hymel KP, Makoroff KL, Laskey AL, Conaway MR, Blackman JA. Mechanisms, clinical presentations, injuries, and outcomes from inflicted versus noninflicted head trauma during infancy: Results of a prospective, multicentered, comparative study. *Pediatrics.* 2007;119 (5):922–9S.
14. Roth S, Raul JS, Ludes B, Willinger R. Finite element analysis of impact and shaking inflicted to a child. *International Journal of Legal Medicine.* 2007;121 (3):223–8.
15. Fujiwara T, Yamada F, Okuyama M et al. Effectiveness of educational materials designed to change knowledge and behavior about crying and shaken baby syndrome: A replication of a randomized controlled trial in Japan. *Child Abuse and Neglect.* 2012;36(9):613–20.
16. Zahl SM, Mack JA, Rossant C, et al. Thrombosis is not a marker of bridging vein rupture in infants with alleged abusive head trauma. *Acta Paediatrica.* 2021;110 (10):2686–94. https://doi.org/10.1111/apa.15908.
17. Échenne B, Couture A, Sébire G. Le syndrome du bébé secoué: Hématomes sous-duraux et collections péri-cérébrales du petit nourrisson. Sauramps Médical, 2020.
18. Chadwick DL, Chin S, Salerno C, Landsverk J, Kitchen L. Deaths from falls in children: How far is fatal? *Journal of Trauma.* 1991;31(10):1353–5.
19. Sanchez M. Le rôle du juge des enfants face au SBS. *Gazette du Palais.* 2018;6 (329):71–5.
20. Rey-Salmon C, de Boissieu P, Teglas JP, Adamsbaum C. Abusive head trauma in day care centers. *Pediatrics.* 2020;146(6): e2020013771.
21. Schneps L, Rossant C. Response to abusive head trauma in daycare centers, Rey-Salmon. 2020. https://pubpeer.com/publications/5981C32FF7BFD42A2C28C5CC3BF33B.
22. Bombarde S, Bombarde Y. *Plus jamais sans toi, Louna.* Michel Lafon, 2018.
23. Vinchon M et al. Confessed versus denied inflicted head injuries in infants: Similarities and differences. *Child's Nervous System.* 2022;38(1):147–52.
24. Adamsbaum C, Grabar S, Mejean N, Rey-Salmon C. Abusive head trauma: Judicial admissions highlight violent and repetitive shaking. *Pediatrics.* 2010;126(3):546–55.
25. Vinchon M, de Foort-Dhellemmes S, Desurmont M, Delestret I. Confessed abuse versus witnessed accidents in infants:

Comparison of clinical, radiological, and ophthalmological data in corroborated cases. *Child's Nervous System*. 2010;26 (5):637–45.

26. Blagrove M. Effects of length of sleep deprivation on interrogative suggestibility. *Journal of Experimental Psychology: Applied*. 1996;2(1):48–59.

27. Capelier F. L'affaire Marina, un cas d'école pour étudier la protection de l'enfance. *Journal du droit des jeunes*. 2012;8 (318):13–21. https://doi.org/10.3917/jdj.318.0013.

28. Gueguen, C. *Vivre heureux avec son enfant: un nouveau regard sur l'éducation au quotidien grâce aux neurosciences affectives*. Robert Laffont, 2015.

29. Mannes I, Drissi C, Adamsbaum C. Imaging findings in abusive head trauma (AHT). *Child's Nervous System*. 2022;1–10.

30. American Academy of Pediatrics Committee on Child Abuse and Neglect. Shaken baby syndrome: Rotational cranial injuries-technical report. *Pediatrics*. 2001;108(1):206–10.

Chapter 23

Shaken Baby Syndrome/Abusive Head Trauma in Sweden

Ulf Högberg and Göran Högberg

23.1 Swedish Child Protection before the Shaken Baby Syndrome/Abusive Head Trauma Paradigm

Sweden has long promoted child health and prevention of childhood morbidity and mortality. From the 1950s, national coverage of well-baby clinics was achieved in collaboration with antenatal clinics and, subsequently, with social services. Detection of child abuse and neglect came into focus from the late 1950s through case reports, government reports, media attention, and petitions to the parliament. Mandatory reporting of suspected child abuse to social services has been in place since then.

In 1979, Sweden became the first country to ban corporal punishment and emotional humiliation of children. Based on emerging knowledge of battered-child syndrome, child abuse was described by paediatricians based mainly on signs of external injuries, multiple fractures, and – more rarely – subdural haemorrhage (SDH). Most cases were reported in metropolitan areas; an increasing trend was seen and false negatives were considered plausible. The incidence was estimated to be substantially lower than in the United States and the United Kingdom. Actions recommended for prevention and early detection had an ecological framing describing individual, family, and societal risk factors as parental social or psychiatric adversities were commonly associated with abuse.

The first edition of the Swedish book *Emergency Paediatrics*, a manual of recommendations for diagnostics and treatment, was published in 1976. One chapter addressed child abuse and the text remained more or less unchanged from the second to the fourth edition (1981, 1984, 1990). The text underscored the importance of mandatory reporting when abuse was suspected because of: (i) the story told by the injuries and the parents' stated cause being inconsistent; (ii) multiple injuries such as widespread bruises or skin injuries, fractures, or internal injuries (pleural haematoma, injuries of the spleen, liver, kidneys, or intestines); (iii) previous healthcare provided to the child or a sibling for injuries that could have been caused by abuse; (iv) signs of neglect; or (v) delay in seeking care or parents giving vague and/or contradictory explanations or showing adverse feelings and animosity towards the child. Battered-child syndrome was not mentioned in any edition [1, 2].

23.2 Implementation of the Shaken Baby Syndrome/Abusive Head Trauma Paradigm into Swedish Healthcare

An extensive dissemination of knowledge supporting shaken baby syndrome/abusive head trauma (SBS/AHT) and the dangers of shaking took place in Sweden from the late 1990s. The intervention was led by paediatricians and neuroradiologists, mainly directed at healthcare, and supported by government agencies, the parliament, and regional councils.

Knowledge on SBS/AHT was based mainly on the work and publications of US and UK scholars. Members of the section Child Abuse and Neglect of the American Academy of Pediatrics and the Ray E. Helfer Society actively supported the implementation in Sweden. The implementation started without any previous research in the Swedish setting. However, an organisational readiness resulting from previously implemented knowledge on child abuse and a positive managerial attitude towards child protection may have facilitated the rapid process that followed. Champions played a major role in the implementation.

23.2.1 The First Years of Implementation

The first mention of SBS in Sweden came in 1994 in a short overview published in the *Swedish Medical Journal*. In 1997, the fifth edition of *Emergency Paediatrics* mentioned fundoscopy in case of 'intracerebral injury and head injury' [3]. In 1999, SBS was fully described in a chapter on child abuse in a Swedish textbook on paediatrics [4].

In 1999/2000, the work to create the first child protection team in Sweden started. Child protection team (Mio), at the Karolinska University Hospital, was established by a neuroradiologist and presented guidelines on diagnosing SBS/AHT which could be disseminated nationally upon request. These were later adopted as official guidelines for the Stockholm healthcare region [5, 6]. A paediatrician trained in child abuse paediatrics in the United States was also instrumental to the team at the Karolinska University Hospital, joining it in 2003 and becoming the founder of the task force for child protection of the Swedish Paediatric Society in 2009 and co-chair of the International Special Interest Group of the Roy E. Helfer Society [7].

In 2002, the government proposed strengthened legal protection for abused children through mandatory collaboration between social services, the police, forensic medicine, healthcare, nursery care, and schools under the leadership of social services, headed by the so-called Children's Houses. The proposal referred to the responsibility of the healthcare sector to detect children in at-risk environments and to give parental support through antenatal and well-baby clinics, and to the function of the Mio at the Karolinska University Hospital as a role model in detection of SBS [8].

In 2005, the sixth edition of *Emergency Paediatrics* was updated with information on SBS, referring to guidelines from the Karolinska University Hospital and adding computed tomography/magnetic resonance imaging to the guidelines [9]. In 2006, a national specialist training course on child maltreatment was established [10], and the neuroradiologist stated '[t]he radiologist and the ophthalmologist must be prepared to propose in plain text the diagnosis abuse, even though from a clinical view it may seem unlikely' [11].

23.2.2 Accelerated Implementation

In 2007, the ophthalmology chapter in the paediatrics textbook was updated to state that acceleration/deceleration/rotation of the eye due to shaking caused retinal haemorrhage (RH). In the same year, a symposium on child abuse entitled The Irresponsible Expert Testimony was organised at the Karolinska Institute with participation by Americans Robert M. Reece, author of *Child Abuse Medical Diagnosis & Management*, and District Attorney General Brian Holmgren [12].

Also in 2007, the official guidelines of the Karolinska Institute and the Stockholm healthcare region were published as regional clinical guidelines: *When physical abuse of infants and toddlers is suspected.* The guidelines stated that, through findings of the triad (SDH, RH, and encephalopathy), 'The medical diagnosis of abuse is confirmed. In practice there are no other alternatives than that the child has been shaken if a traffic accident or high fall can be excluded.' The guidelines referred to US and UK studies stating that close to 100 infants were physically abused in Sweden each year and that half of them would have no external signs of abuse, with one third abused through shaking, which carries the greatest risk of going undetected [6].

During the years 2008–10, a project on mental vaccination against SBS was implemented in parts of the Stockholm region. An information package on how to cope with parental stress when a baby cries inconsolably and the dangers of shaking, with a special focus on SBS, was handed out to (future) parents late in pregnancy, at birth, and at well-baby clinics. Most of the parents described the information as important and a considerable number reported benefitting from the project, which was supported by the Ministry of Social Affairs and the Stockholm region [13]. This effort was later expanded to the general public in Sweden, with information provided about the dangers of violent shaking, the risk of causing SBS/AHT, and advice to parents for prevention [14]. Reports suggested a positive response regarding shaking, and a national survey showed that none of the parents (n = 1,358) of infants admitted that they had 'pushed, grabbed and shook the child'. In 2017, one particular finding was commented on: 'The studies also suggested that Swedish parents have largely ceased to shake small children, particularly infants. It can be hoped that this is the result of national information campaigns that have been implemented over the last 10 years to inform the public of the danger of harming small children by shaking them' [15, 16].

In 2009, a task force for child protection was established by the Swedish Paediatric Society, later transformed into a sub-association of the society in 2015 [7]. Creation of child protection teams was the primary objective during the first years. These were initially implemented within local healthcare but were soon granted extra resources through regional parliamentary decisions and were subsequently established officially, in Stockholm (2011), Uppsala (2012), Gothenburg (2014), Region South (2018), and Region South-West (2018). Only the northernmost university health region has not established a child protection team.

In 2010, a PhD thesis entitled *Child abuse: Clinical investigation, management and nursing approach* [17] was published, based upon two published papers [18, 19] and two that remained unpublished as of 2021: 'Children diagnosed as abused: A retrospective study of reporting to social services and the police', concluding that further educational efforts were required, and 'Neuroradiology of intracranial haemorrhage and associated findings in children younger than 2 years who may be victims of child abuse', concluding that the neuroradiologist should give not only a description of the findings, but also an interpretation for further investigations of abuse.

In 2012, Internetmedicin.se (www.internetmedicin.se), an online manual for health professionals, published a section entitled *Clinical management overview of child physical abuse*. The first edition in 2012 had information to healthcare professionals providing an overview of child abuse, specifically addressing SBS/AHT (updated in 2015) [20]. In 2013, the electronic *National Handbook for Child Health Services* stated in the section *Signs of children being abused* that

> Infants who are exposed to severe shaking, pounding against a hard surface or a combination of the two are at risk of intracranial haemorrhage, brain damage and retinal bleedings. The child may become unconscious, have seizures and stop breathing . . . Often,

the child also has fractures of the ribs and long bone fractures as a result of the shaking. The risk for permanent brain damage or fatal outcome is great. [21]

Shaken baby syndrome/abusive head trauma was repeatedly addressed at conferences organised by the Swedish professional societies of paediatrics, neuroradiology, and ophthalmology, all sub-sections of the Swedish Society of Medicine. In 2013, a symposium entitled *Physical abuse of the young child, medical and legal challenges: What does the science tell us?* was held. The conference was supported by the Swedish Crime Victim's Compensation and Support Authority in collaboration with the Swedish Paediatric Society and the Uppsala University Children's Hospital. Lecturers from the UK and US participated: Dr Sabine Maguire and Dr Christopher Greeley [22].

The Swedish parliament was also targeted with information. In 2012, Dr Otterman, the leading promoter of the SBS/AHT theory in Sweden, served as a convener at a conference to present medically led child protection teams at a seminar jointly hosted with the Center Party in the parliament [7]. Dr Randell C. Alexander, a member and former chair of the section on Child Abuse of the American Academy of Pediatrics and the American Professional Society on the Abuse of Children, also participated in the seminar. In 2013, The Committee on Health and Welfare of the Swedish parliament held a hearing about the responsibility of healthcare in child protection. The participants included those already mentioned [7], as well as a representative of Save the Children and the President of the Ray E. Helfer Society, then a guest researcher at Uppsala University [23].

In 2014, Dr Christian, a member of the section Child Abuse and Neglect of the American Academy of Pediatrics, held a lecture entitled *The medical home for maltreated children in the US and child protection teams in hospital settings* at three Swedish university hospitals in Sweden [24]. Uppsala University–affiliated Dr Dubowitz, a professor of paediatrics in the US, member of the section Child Abuse and Neglect of the American Academy of Pediatrics, and President of the Ray E. Helfer Society, contributed to research on child protection and to foresee the leading role of Sweden in promoting child protection in Scandinavia and Europe [25].

In 2014, the governmental National Board of Health and Welfare issued guidelines entitled *Children being abused or at risk of being abused: Guidelines for healthcare and dental care for notification and liability*. The guidelines underlined health professionals' duty to report child physical abuse, with special attention paid to AHT (SDH, rib fractures, and classic metaphyseal lesions) [26]. Also in 2014, the *Swedish Medical Journal* published an overview on child abuse, evidence-based knowledge, and guidelines on how to detect child abuse. Abusive head trauma was specifically targeted by referring to US scholars and stating an incidence of 20–30 per 100,000 infants based on international literature [27].

23.2.3 The Period of Sustainability

In 2019, the Swedish Paediatric Society presented updated guidelines on investigation, action, and follow-up when child abuse is suspected, while SBS/AHT was not mentioned. Actions were recommended including skeletal x-ray, fundoscopy, and neuroimaging, without any interpretation on which radiological or ophthalmological findings would indicate abuse, making it mandatory to call social services and the police or block parents' access to electronic medical records [28]. The Swedish Society of Paediatric Radiology [29] and the

Swedish Society of Ophthalmology [30] also published guidelines on investigation of suspected abuse.

23.3 Shaken Baby Syndrome/Abusive Head Trauma and Out-of-Home Care

Swedish welfare law mandates all professionals report to social services any harmful domestic condition that may expose a child to risks. For child maltreatment welfare, interventions involve out-of-home care in foster families or residential care; such measures can be voluntary under the Social Services Act or compulsory under the Care of Young Persons (Special Provisions) Act. Decisions of voluntary measures are made by social services; decisions of compulsory measures can be appealed to family/administrative courts – the Administrative Courts, the Administrative Courts of Appeal, and the Supreme Administrative Court.

23.3.1 The Incidence of Out-of-Home Care

The overall incidence of any out-of-home care was 402 per 100,000 infants (n = 7,455) during the years 1997–2014 in Sweden, lower than rates reported from England, the US, or Manitoba (Canada): 696, 631, and 2,913, respectively [31]. Most out-of-home care is provided for social reasons and healthcare is not involved. Those coming from healthcare, having a medical diagnosis, are in a minority. In 1997–2014, the incidence of out-of-home care for infants having any findings of SDH, RH, rib fracture, or long bone fracture was 9.83 per 100,000 infants (n = 182). This incidence increased during this period. The mean age at entry into out-of-home care was 3.3 months; a majority were boys, had a twin, and/or were preterm-born or small-for-gestational age (SGA).

We have no systematic information on the number of cases of SBS/AHT processed in family/administrative courts. The National Association for Family Rights (RFFR)[1] , a non-governmental organisation (NGO) created by parents accused of SBS/AHT, supported six parents in family/administrative courts during 2014–21. In three cases, the children were returned to their families; in one of those cases, this required repeated decisions by the courts, as social services denied execution of court orders. In four cases, the matter never went to a family/administrative court and the children were returned to their parents following decisions from social services.

In 2018, the Swedish Supreme Administrative Court heard a case where a father was refused custody of his son because of suspected shaking [32]. The case never reached a criminal court because the police investigation was closed as no crime could be proven. The father regained custody by a decision of the Swedish Supreme Administrative Court. The court referred to the SBU's report that findings of the triad have limited scientific support [33]. The court stated,

> As regards suspicion of physical abuse of a child, when the assessment is based only on the existence of certain symptoms in the child, a prerequisite for mandatory intervention should be that there is clear scientific support for a causal connection between the medical findings and the presumed violence . . . If there is no clear scientific support for a causal connection, the absence of other possible explanations for the injuries cannot in itself be considered to make it likely that the injuries have been caused by violence.

1 www.rffr.se

23.4 Nationwide Annual Figures for Shaken Baby Syndrome/Abusive Head Trauma

In the US, the incidence of AHT, applying the International Classification of Diseases (ICD)-9 M, has been estimated to be 32 per 100,000 children and comparable figures have been reported from the UK. Shaken baby syndrome/abusive head trauma has no specific code in the ICD-10. In the Swedish National Patient Registry, SBS/AHT cases must instead be searched for among cases with ICD codes for abuse, maltreatment, battered-child syndrome or investigation for abuse (see also Chapter 16).

In 1987–2014, a total of 368 infants were diagnosed with maltreatment: 12.3 per 100,000 infants. Seven of the children diagnosed with abuse died – that is, 0.23 deaths per 100,000 infants, a case fatality rate of 1.9%. A 10-fold increase in diagnoses of infant abuse was observed from the start to the end of the period. The increase was slow, starting in 1996, and peaked in 2008–14. There was a doubling of the incidence of abuse diagnoses in 2008–14 compared with 1997–2007, from 12.0 to 26.5 per 100,000 infants. Of the 337 cases of infant abuse in 1997–2014, 137 (41%) had concomitant diagnoses of either SDH, skull fracture, cerebral contusion, traumatic brain injury, convulsions, RH, rib fracture, or long bone fracture. Subdural haematoma, rib fracture, RH, and skull fracture were the main drivers of the association with the probability for diagnosis of infant abuse in 1997–2014. During the peak period 2008–14, the incidence rates of maltreatment and SDH, RH, or rib fractures were 2.9, 2.3, and 2.5 per 100,000 infants, respectively [34].

The increasing incidence was geographically uneven. In Stockholm, cases of infant abuse began to rise steeply, eight-fold, concomitantly with the programme for 'mental vaccination' against shaking and the establishment of a child protection team at the Karolinska University Hospital in the early 2000s [34].

Fatal cases of AHT have been studied in a national study of *all* deceased infants 1994–2013 (n = 733) [35]. Of those, possible cases of AHT (n = 12) were scrutinised, with eight previously potentially diagnosed as AHT. Eight of them had perinatal vulnerabilities (preterm or twin). The incidence was found to be at least 10 times lower than in other Western countries [35].

A decline in the incidence of infant maltreatment diagnoses has occurred during the past years: 16% decline for infants born 2014 to 2019 and 25% for infants born 2017 to 2019 [36]. This can be interpreted as a burgeoning de-implementation process associated to the decision in Swedish Supreme Court (2014) [37] and the SBU report on traumatic shaking (2016) [33].

23.5 Prosecutions and Acquittals of Those Accused of Shaken Baby Syndrome/Abusive Head Trauma

According to the rule of law, the burden of proof for a criminal conviction is 'beyond reasonable doubt'. In 1992, the Swedish Supreme Court convicted a father of aggravated manslaughter because of traumatic shaking of his 5-week-old daughter resulting in SDH, RH, brain injury, and rib fractures. Another six parents were convicted of SBS in district courts or courts of appeal up to 2011 [38]. In convictions in SBS cases, expert opinions have had a high evidentiary value for the courts. In the aforementioned cases from 1992 to 2011, the courts based their convictions on medical conclusions that SBS/AHT had occurred [38].

For the period up to 2014, we have access to some information from the Pippigruppen and RFFR NGOs, created by parents accused of SBS/AHT (including classic metaphyseal lesions and fractures of ribs and long bones). During 2008–14, those NGOs provided support in 17 cases. Some of these 17 cases never went to criminal court because the police investigations were closed as no crime could be proved. In five cases, the father was convicted, one of whom was acquitted in the Court of Appeal. Two of the fathers petitioned the Supreme Court for new trials; in both instances, the cases were remanded to the respective Court of Appeal, which ultimately exonerated the fathers [39, 40]. In Sweden, the defence may bring medical experts to testify in court.

23.5.1 The Swedish Supreme Court Judgment of 2014

In 2014, the Swedish Supreme Court heard a case related to SBS/AHT. A father was convicted in the District Court and the Court of Appeal for shaking his twin-born son, who at 2 months of age developed convulsions and fell unconscious with findings of SDH/hygroma. The expert witnesses, both for the defendant and for the Legal Advisory Board of the National Board of Health and Welfare, questioned the scientific evidence for the SBS/AHT diagnosis, resulting in acquittal by the Supreme Court. The Supreme Court stated the following:

> For it to be considered beyond any reasonable doubt that the mere circumstance that certain physical injuries are at hand indicates that these injuries have been caused by someone in a certain criminal manner, the conclusion must be based on a scientific basis for which there is very strong evidence. At the same time, it must be more or less out of the question that there is any other conceivable explanation for the injuries. [37]

23.5.2 Changes in Case Law following the Supreme Court's Judgment

The judicial precedent by the Supreme Court in evaluating evidence of infant abuse was reflected in subsequent trials related to SBS/AHT. Systematic information is available only for the years 2014–18, retrieved from the Swedish Prosecutor's Office [41]. During the years up to 2018, 11 fathers accused of SBS/AHT (fractures included) were acquitted in District Courts or Courts of Appeal. In some of the acquittals, reference was made to the judgment of the Supreme Court and/or to the SBU report (see Chapter 10). One mother confessing to repeated impact head injury to her child was convicted in the Court of Appeal.

To conclude, Sweden has had a multi-sector child protection programme to prevent and detect child abuse executed by social service, healthcare organisations, and the judiciary for half a century. For two decades, Sweden has experienced the efficient implementation of SBS/AHT led by child protection teams at paediatric departments. Concomitantly, a steep increase in infant maltreatment diagnoses occurred, while during the past years a slow decline has been observed, possibly due to a decision of the Supreme Court and to the SBU report.

References

1. Sjölin S. [Social and legal actions, child abuse]. In [*Emergency pediatrics*]. 1st ed. S Sjölin, ed. Almqvist & Wiksell, 1976.
2. Ludvigsson J. [Social and legal actions, child abuse and sexual assault]. In [*Emergency pediatrics*] [Internet]. 4th ed. Almqvist & Wiksell, 1990.
3. Ludvigsson J, Sundelin C. [Social and legal actions, child abuse and sexual assault*]*. In *[Emergency pediatrics*]. 5th ed. A Larsson, ed. Liber, 1997.

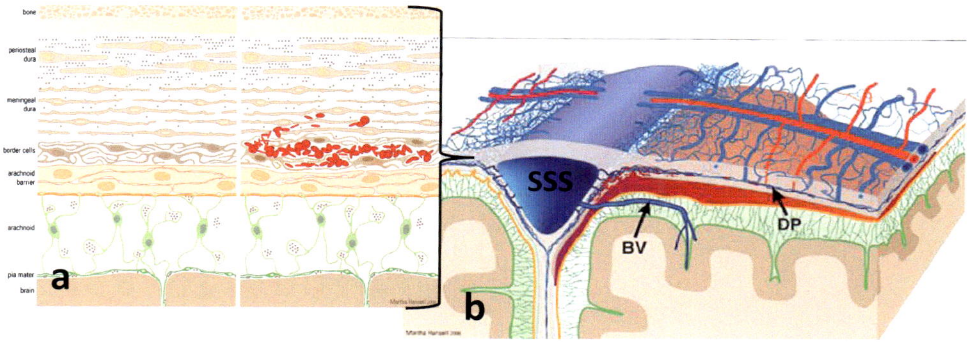

Figure 3.1 Diagrams of the meningeal membranes surrounding the brain and dural bleeding
a Diagram of detail of dural structure with blood in deep dural cell layers
b Anatomical diagram of the meninges and origin of subdural bleeding. A bridging vein (BV) drains blood from the brain, crossing the subarachnoid space and dura to enter the superior sagittal sinus (SSS). A thin film of blood leaking from the dural plexus (DP) between the dural leaflets spreads to split the dura from the arachnoid membrane. (Reproduced with kind permission [86])

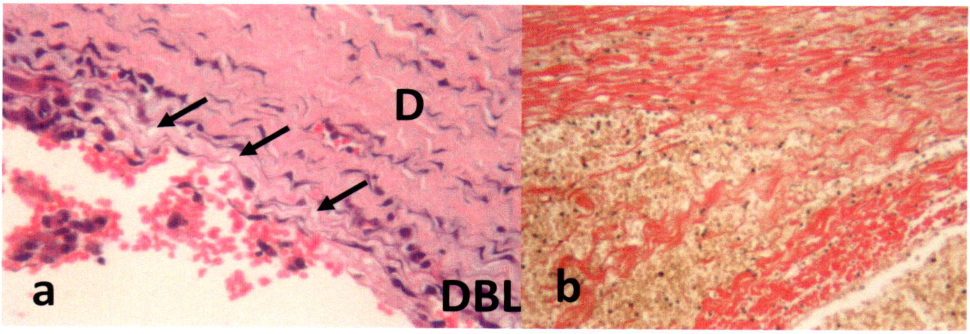

Figure 3.2 Microscopic images of infant dura
a Spinal dura (D). Note spaces between the loosely adherent cells of the deep dural border layer (DBL) (arrows). Red cells are seen between these dural cells and in the subdural compartment.
b Dura stained with Van Gieson stain; fibres of the dura are pink and red cells buff. Blood is extending between and spreading the fibres of the dura.

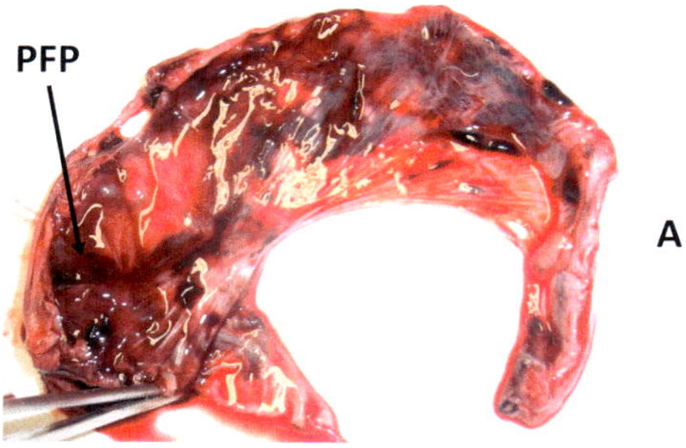

Figure 3.3 Falx at autopsy showing intense congestion. A = anterior. PFP = Posterior falcine plexus

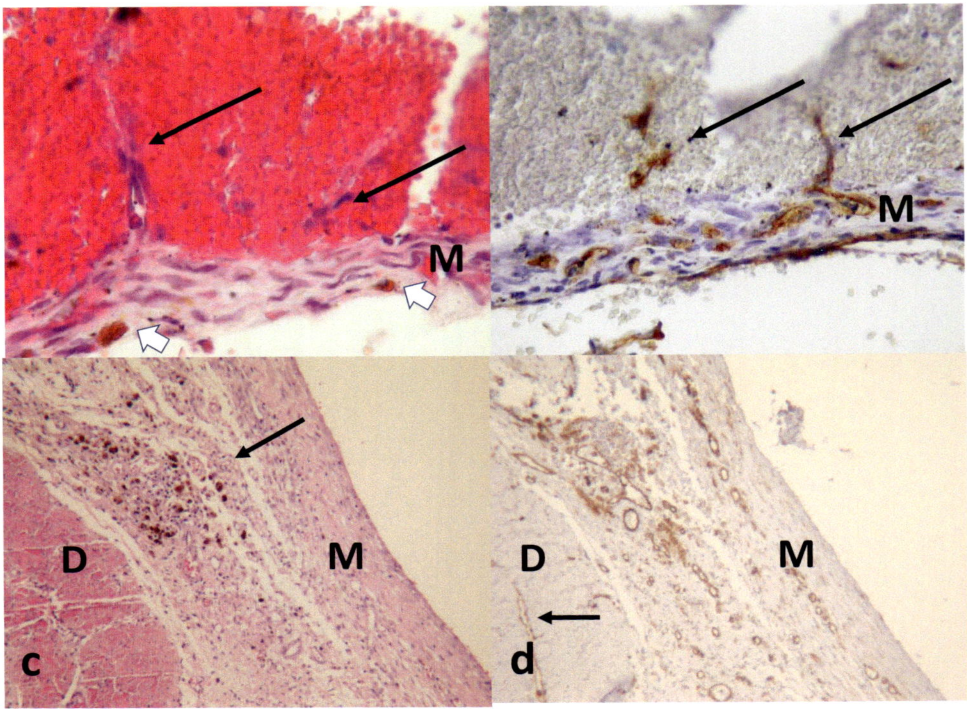

Figure 3.4 a A thin subdural membrane (M) about 6 cells deep and with a few macrophages containing brown haemosiderin (white open arrows). Blood vessels (black arrows) are growing into a mass of fresh blood above. H&E
b Same case, adjacent section stained with CD34, which stains blood vessels brown (a and b: Infant 3 months old, 3 days after trauma)
c Dura (D) bottom left with old, thick healing subdural membrane (M). The membrane is mainly fibrous but there is a patch of cells containing haemosiderin (brown) indicating more recent bleeding (arrow) H&E
d CD 31 stains blood vessels brown. Note the many rounded profiles of large, thin-walled blood vessels (sinusoids) in the membrane and the thin vascular plexus in the normal dura (black arrow) (c and d: Male 5 months)

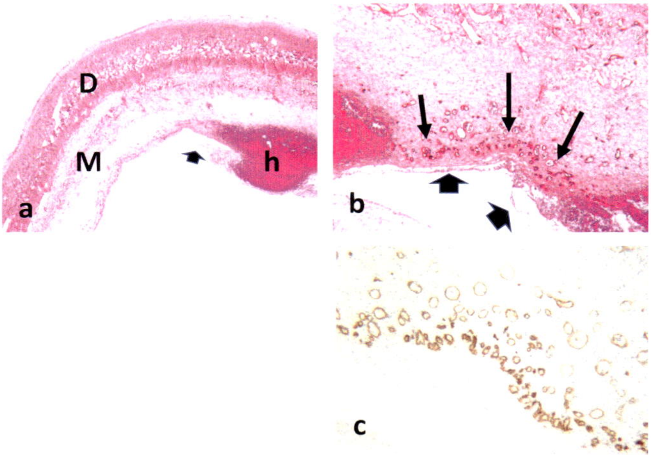

Figure 3.5 Female who had traumatic head injury at 3/12 and died in care at 7/12
a Section of dura (D) shows a thick chronic subdural membrane (M) which is pale pink and thicker than the dura itself, consistent with the 4 months since the original trauma. There is a small fresh haemorrhage (h) from the deep border of the membrane.
b Higher-power image of the edge of the membrane shows a thick layer of wide new blood vessels (arrows) which are the source of the bleeding. Fragments of deep dural border layer cells are seen adjacent to the blood clot (arrowheads).
c CD31 stain highlights the layer of new vessels close to the deep edge of the membrane. A is stained with H&E, b with H&E and CD31, c with CD31.

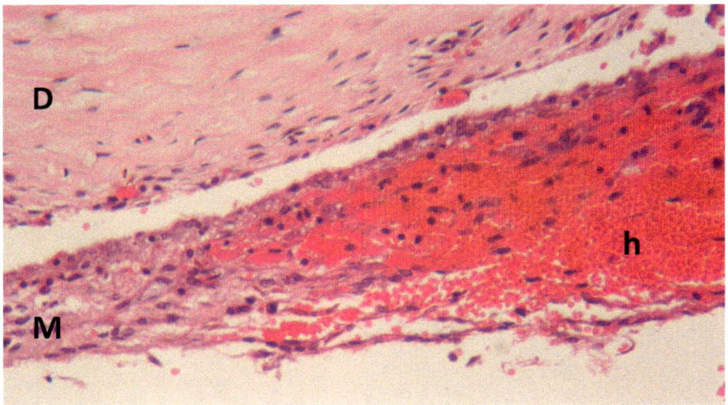

Figure 3.6 Subdural membrane (M) beneath the dura (D). The membrane has separated from the dura during tissue processing. The membrane is about 11 cells thick. There is a fresh haemorrhage (h) into the membrane.

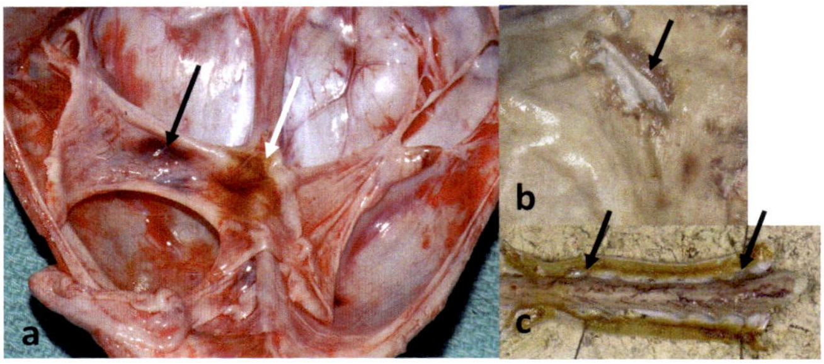

Figure 3.7 Old subdural haemorrhage
a Inner surface of the base of the skull at autopsy. The tentorium has fresh intradural bleeding (black arrow) and a patch of old, ochre-coloured subdural blood (white arrow).
b Fixed dura showing extensive pale brown subdural membrane which could easily be missed. There is a small tear (arrow) where the normal grey dura can be seen.
c Fixed infant spinal cord. The dura has been opened in the dorsal midline showing patchy yellow-brown discolouration at the thoracolumbar and sacral levels of the deep surface of the dorsal dura (arrows).

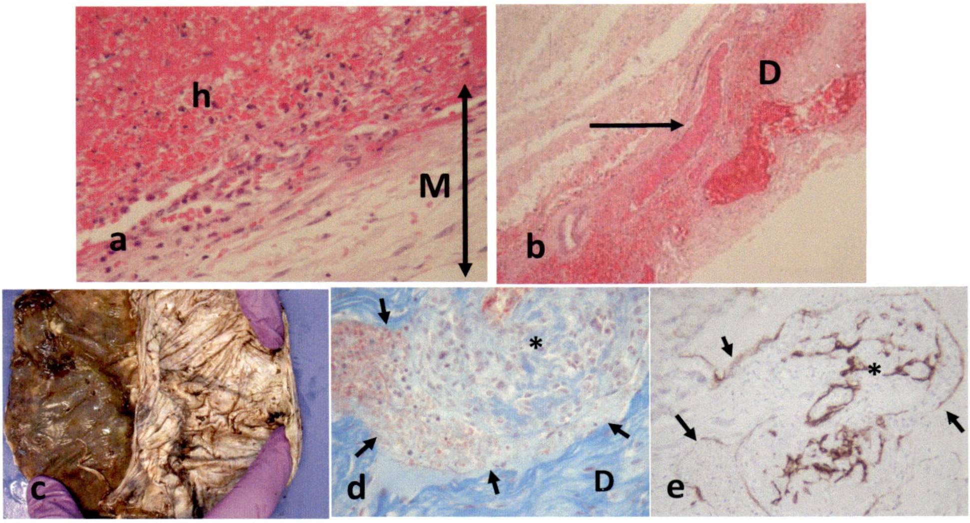

Figure 3.8 a and b: 2-month infant with venous thrombosis who collapsed 4 days following a fall and survived for 1 week
a Subdural membrane (M) and organising subdural haemorrhage (h)
b Thrombus within dural vessel (arrow). Note extensive fresh bright pink intradural bleeding. c, d, e Male 10 years with chronic subdural haemorrhage in association with arachnoid cyst
c Fixed dura with a fluid chronic subdural haemorrhage within a membrane on the left side
d Thrombosed vein within the dura (trichrome stain) D = dura. Small arrows indicate vessel wall. *= recanalising thrombus
e CD 34 stain delineates the blood vessel wall and new vessels in the recanalising thrombus

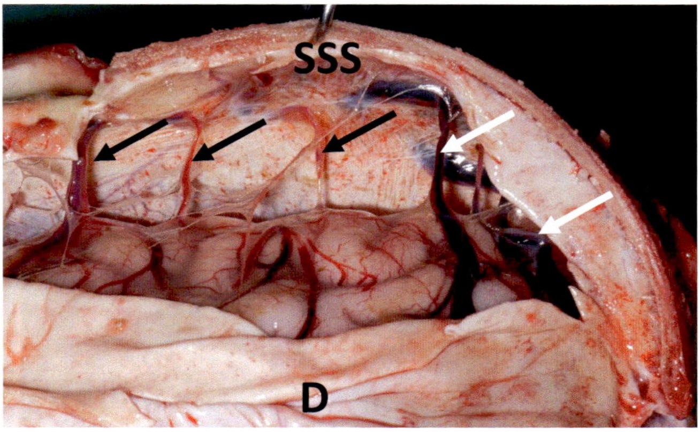

Figure 3.9 Bridging veins in infant with benign external hydrocephalus. The skull has been opened and the upper flap is lifted; the superior sagittal sinus is just below the bone (SSS). Below the dura has been folded back (D). Five bridging veins (arrows) pass from the brain surface, across a wide subarachnoid space to the SSS. The two white arrows indicate BV which are congested and possibly thrombosed. Note the acute angle as the BVs enter the SSS.

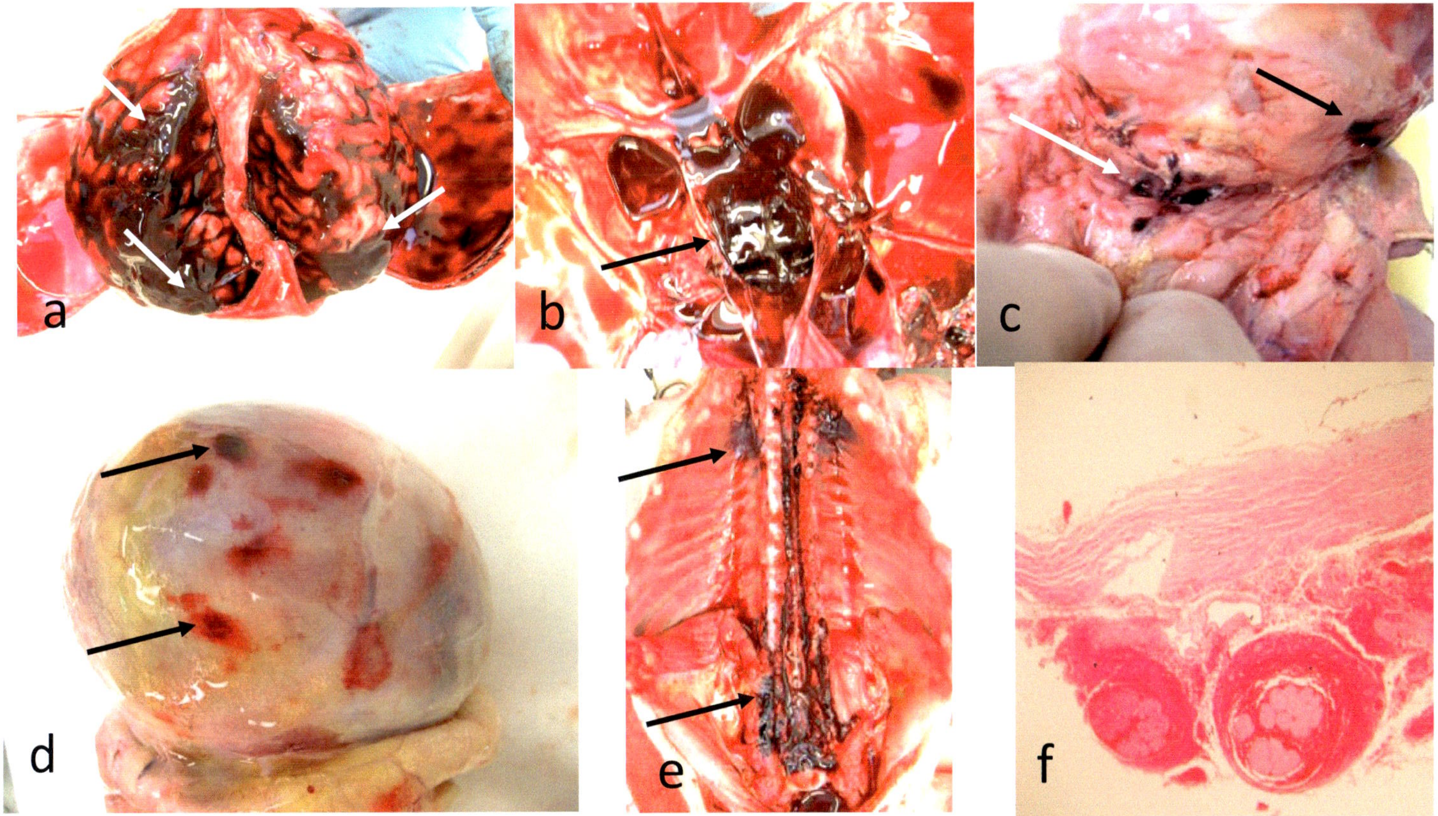

Figure 3.10 Newborn infant with displacement of the occipital bone and large cerebellar bleed following traumatic delivery
a Congested and dilated (varicose) surface and bridging veins (white arrows) over the cerebral hemispheres
b Blood clot (white arrow) occupying the posterior fossa
c The suboccipital sinus and internal vertebral venous plexus are dilated (white arrow). There is blood oozing from the right mastoid emissary vein (black arrow).
d Multiple subscalp blood patches over the vertex of the skull. Several are in sites of emissary veins (arrows).
e Extensive bleeding into nerve roots of cervical and sacral plexuses (arrows). There was no traumatic damage to adjacent soft tissues.
f Nerve roots are congested and haemorrhagic. There was no histological evidence of traumatic damage and no traumatic axonal injury.

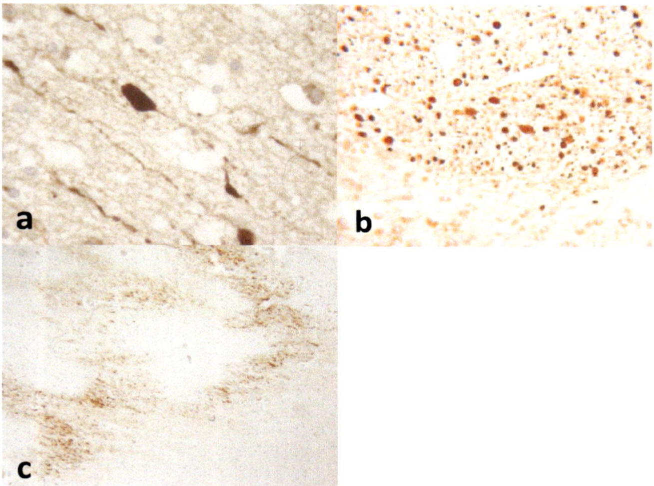

Figure 3.11 Axonal injury βAPP stain
a Single axonal swellings
b Traumatic axonal injury. A well-defined nerve fibre bundle contains many rounded, swollen axons. Note the lack of bleeding.
c Diffuse axonal injury. Irregular 'geographic' pattern of swollen axons

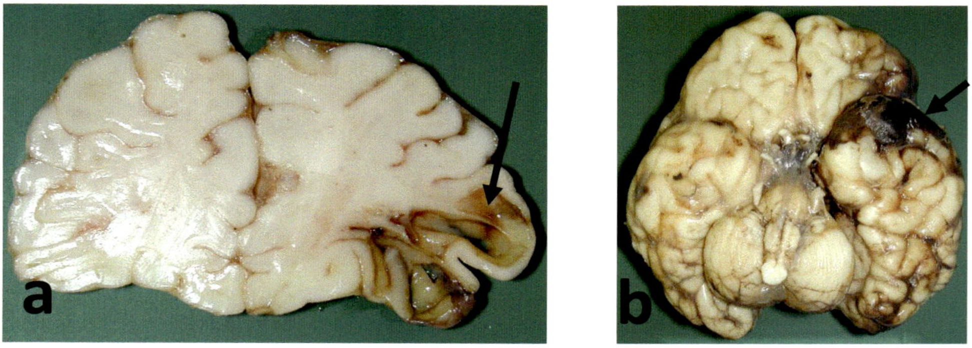

Figure 3.12 Infant brain: Subcortical cysts
a Coronal slice of fixed brain with smooth walled but blood-stained cyst (arrow) beneath an intact cortex
b Sub-pial bleed overlying the haemorrhagic cyst

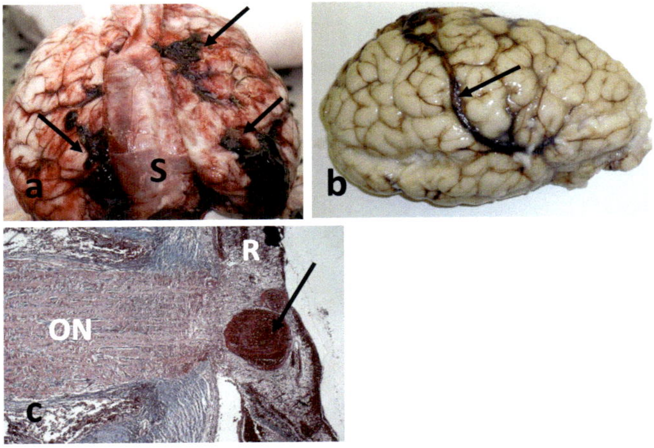

Figure 3.13 Cortical vein thrombosis in a 4-week-old baby who collapsed with seizures while in a public park
a Fresh brain with several congested, dilated, varicose veins (arrows). A midline strip of dura overlying the superior sagittal sinus (S) remains in situ
b The brain after fixation demonstrating a thrombosed superficial vein
c Central retinal vein showing a large thrombus at the optic nerve (ON) head (arrow). (R = retina)

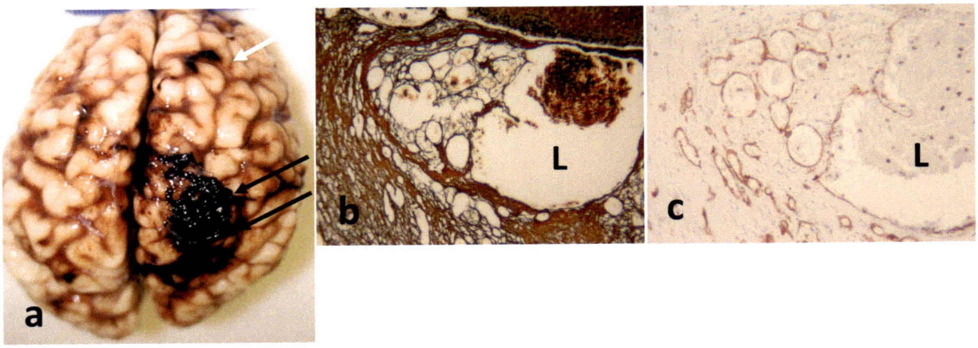

Figure 3.15 a Thrombosed surface veins. A single thrombosed vein (white arrow) and a mass of tortuous, congested, varicose veins (black arrows) are indicated.
b Thrombosed vein with organisation and recanalisation. The lumen of the vessel remains partly patent (L). The left half of the lumen is occupied by profiles of newly formed vessels which replace the original thrombus (reticulin stain).
c CD31 stains the walls of the new blood vessels brown.

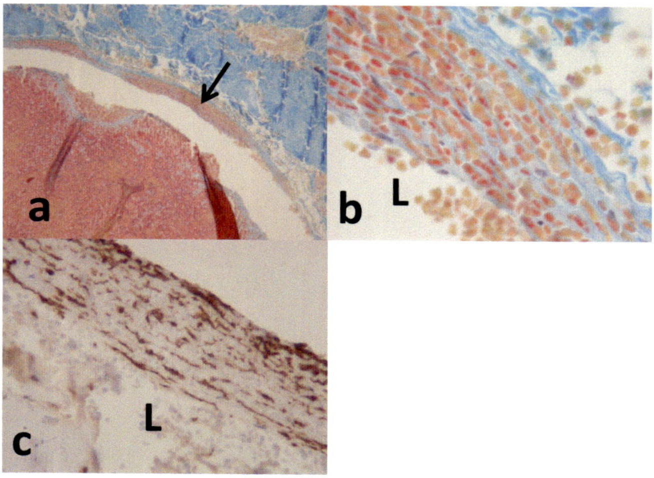

Figure 3.16 Cortical vein thrombosis – diapedesis
a Trichrome stain. Thrombus in a vein is stained pink. The clot has shrunk from the vein wall and cracked during tissue processing. The arrow indicates a point where red cells (buff colour) are passing between the cells of the vein wall (blue) to leak into the dura (intradural haemorrhage).
b Higher power shows the red cells (stained buff) between the cells of the vein wall (blue).
c Cells of the vein wall stained with smooth muscle actin (SMA) showing their separation by red cells (pale grey) lumen (L)

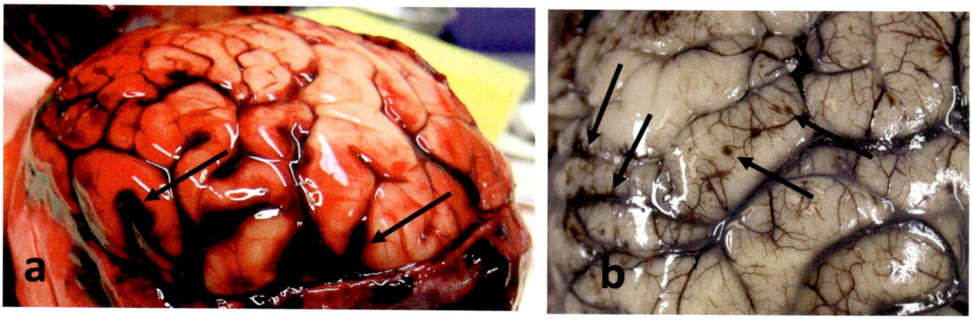

Figure 3.17 Cortical vein thrombosis – sub-pial bleeding
a Surface of fresh brain showing thin diffuse film of subarachnoid blood and well defined perivenous sub-pial blood
b Surface of fixed brain showing discrete rounded spots of sub-pial blood and localised perivenous blood (arrows)

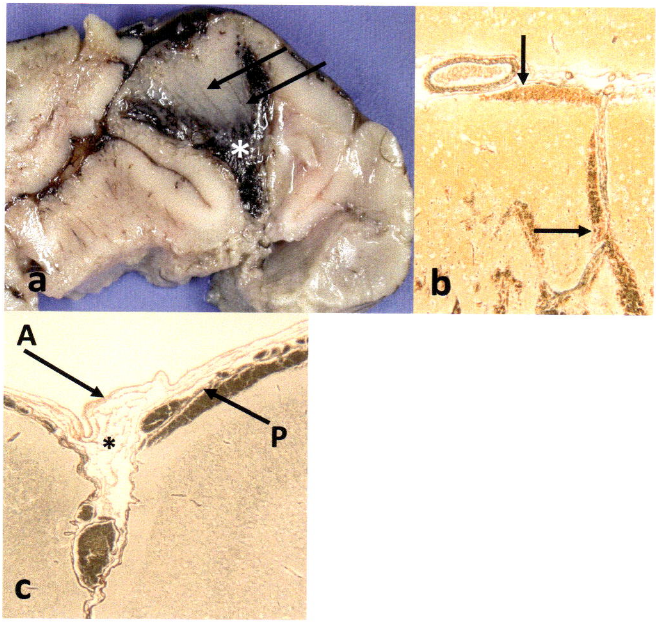

Figure 3.18 Cortical vein thrombosis – sub-pial bleeding
a Part of a slice of a fixed brain of a 3-month-old with venous thrombosis following a fall and skull fracture. There is a very thin surface sub-pial bleed. The cortex is mostly intact. Thin streaks representing veins (arrows) extend at right angles to the brain surface from a large subcortical haemorrhage (*).
b Brain surface showing blood around a vein in the subcortical white matter (arrows) tracking towards the surface. At the top a small collection of sub-pial blood (dark brown) lifts the fine pial membrane (arrow) (reticulin stain).
c Higher power of the sub-pial blood (dark brown). P = pia, A = arachnoid barrier membrane, * = subarachnoid space

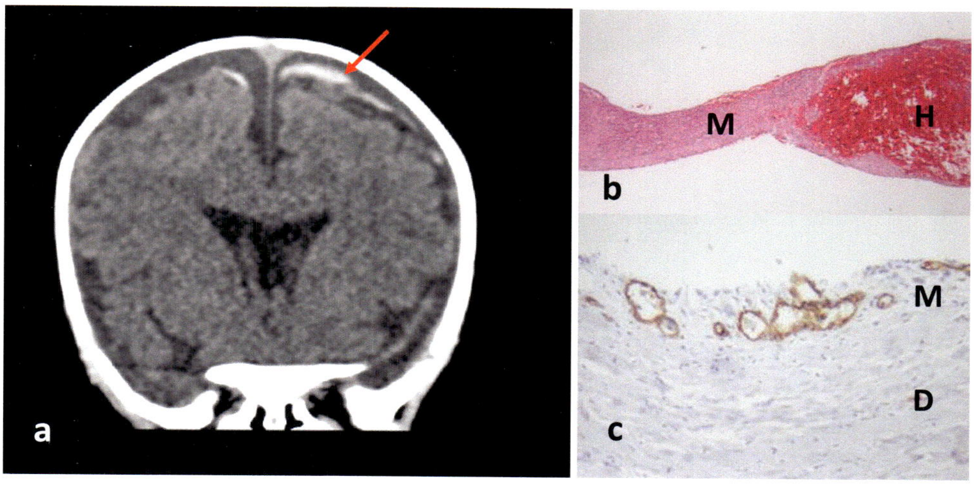

Figure 4.2 Bleeding from a subdural membrane
a CT scan showing bleeding from a neomembrane (red arrow) which was confirmed at pathology. The amount of haemorrhage is too small to have originated from bridging vein ruptures. Moreover, the blood is contained and not mixing with the surrounding fluid as would be expected if it represented free bleeding of a ruptured vessel into the subdural compartment.
b Haemorrhage (H, bright pink) from a thin subdural neomembrane (M, pale pink) which has separated from the dura during tissue processing
c An extensive thin membrane (M) adherent to the dura (D). CD 31 stain demonstrates multiple new blood vessels in the membrane as rounded brown profiles. a, b, and c are not the same case.

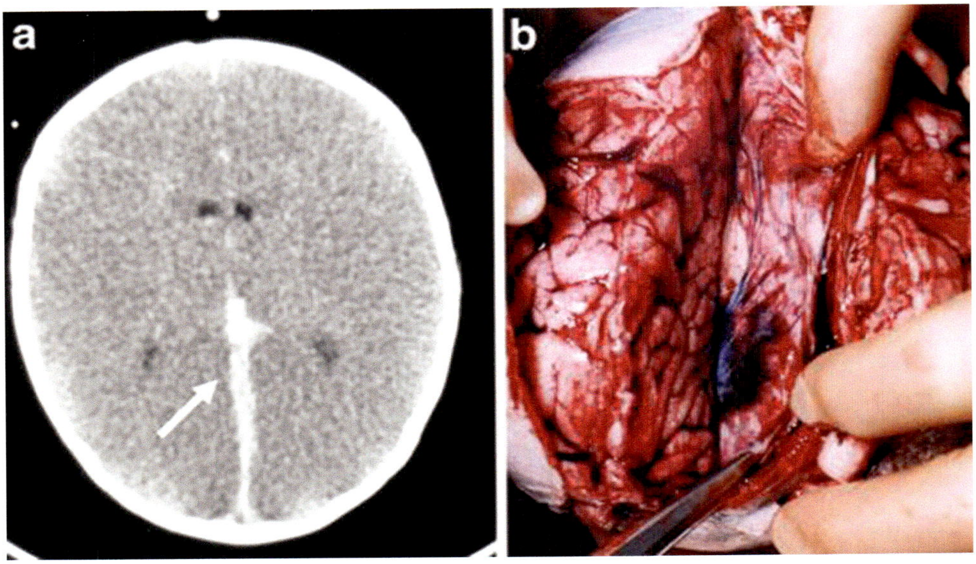

Figure 4.4 Infant 4 months. Sudden death, no trauma.
a CT scan showing thickened, dense falx (arrow) which was reported as SDH
b Autopsy showed the blood to be entirely intradural. There is no SDH (reproduced with permission from [34]).

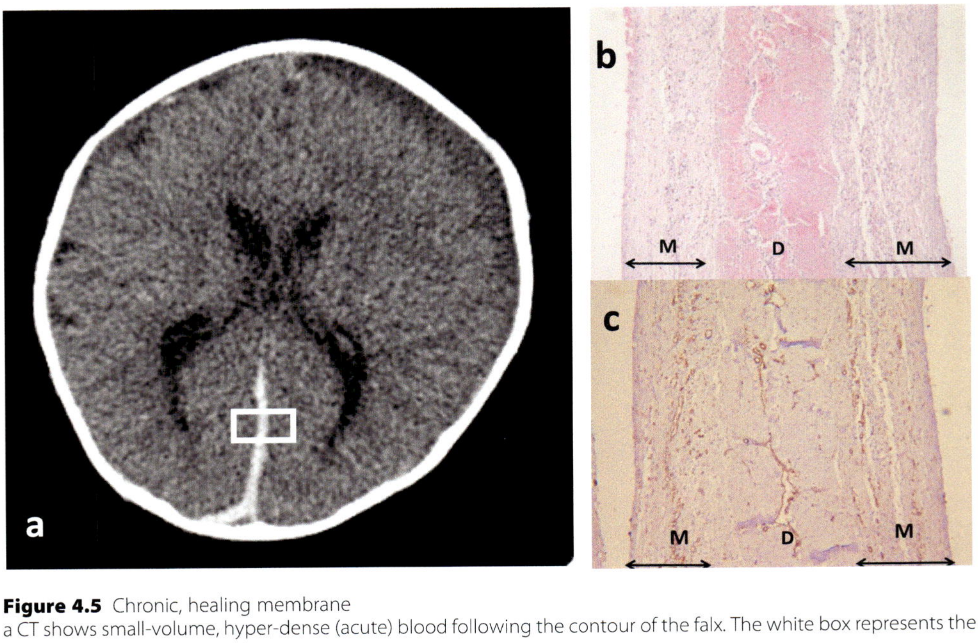

Figure 4.5 Chronic, healing membrane
a CT shows small-volume, hyper-dense (acute) blood following the contour of the falx. The white box represents the area shown in b and c.
b Same case. Sections from the falx showing subdural membrane (M) on each side of the dura (D), more than doubling its thickness (H&E). These could not be distinguished on the scan.
c CD31 stains the newly formed capillary blood vessels brown.

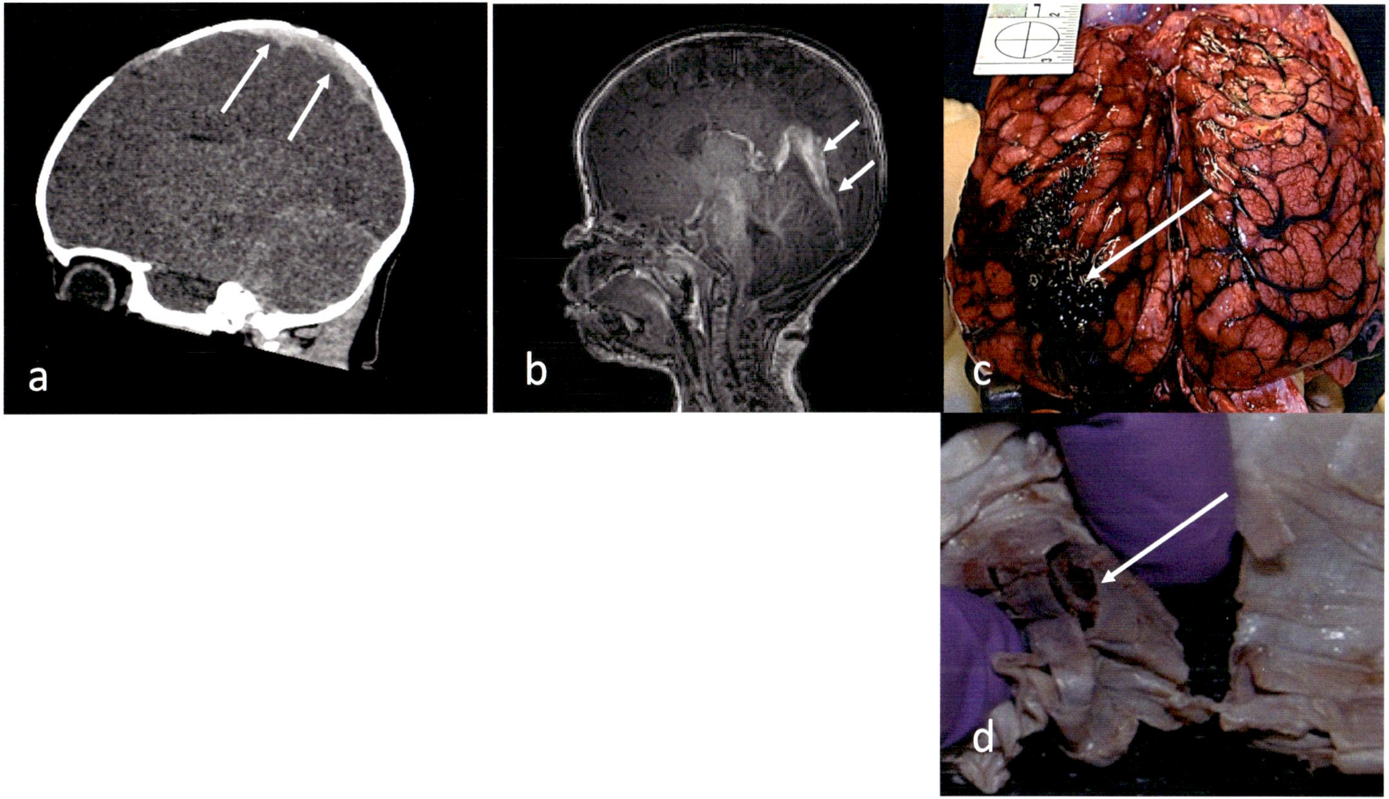

Figure 4.7 CVT in 3-month-old with several days of fever and progressive lethargy
a CT showed extra-axial parasagittal high density (arrows)
b T1-weighted MRI confirmed subacute thrombus ballooning the vein of Galen, straight sinus, and internal cerebral veins. The sagittal sinus also showed subacute thrombus, which was confirmed by pathology.
c Pathologic findings in another patient with confirmed sagittal sinus thrombosis. Dilated, tortuous, and clotted vessels on the surface of the brain were mistaken for SDH on initial CT exam.
d Fixed dura shows the solid clot (white arrow) in the superior sagittal sinus.

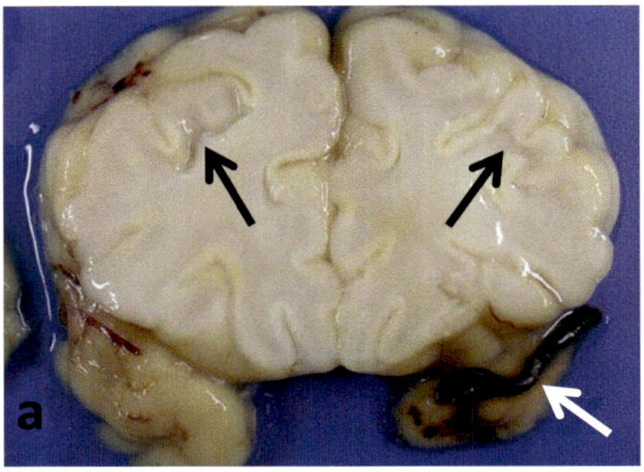

Figure 4.8 Coronal slice of fixed infant brain with thrombosed vein over the right temporal pole (white arrow). There is generalized brain swelling; the subcortical zone is oedematous. Clefts and cysts are developing in the immediate subcortical white matter (black arrows).

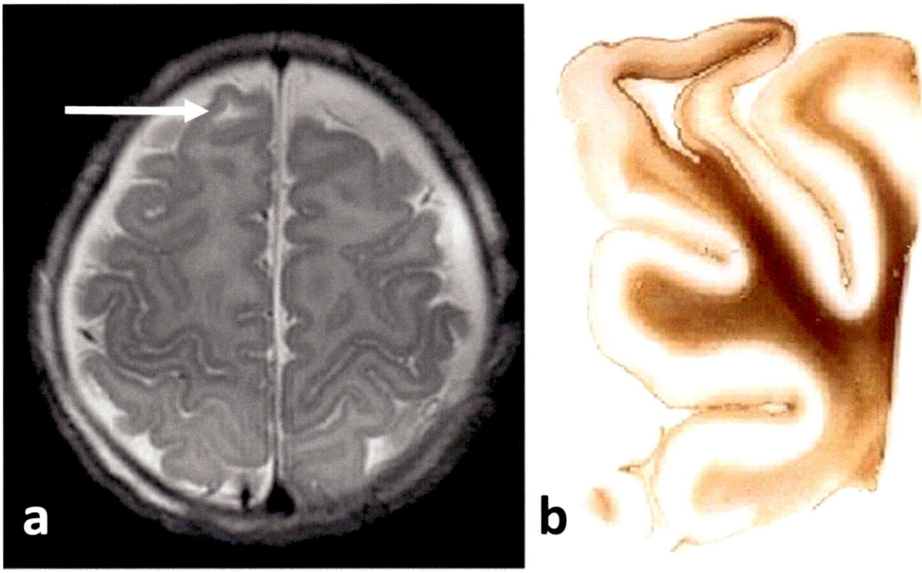

Figure 4.9 a MRI scan showing small cystic lesion beneath intact frontal cortex without evidence of associated swelling or haemorrhage
b Section of frontal lobe from a different case. A 3-month-old baby with bilateral parasagittal subcortical cysts. The section is stained for myelin proteolipid protein (PLP), which stains myelin brown. Note the thinning and aberrant myelination due to scarring of the overlying cortex, indicating the pathology is old.

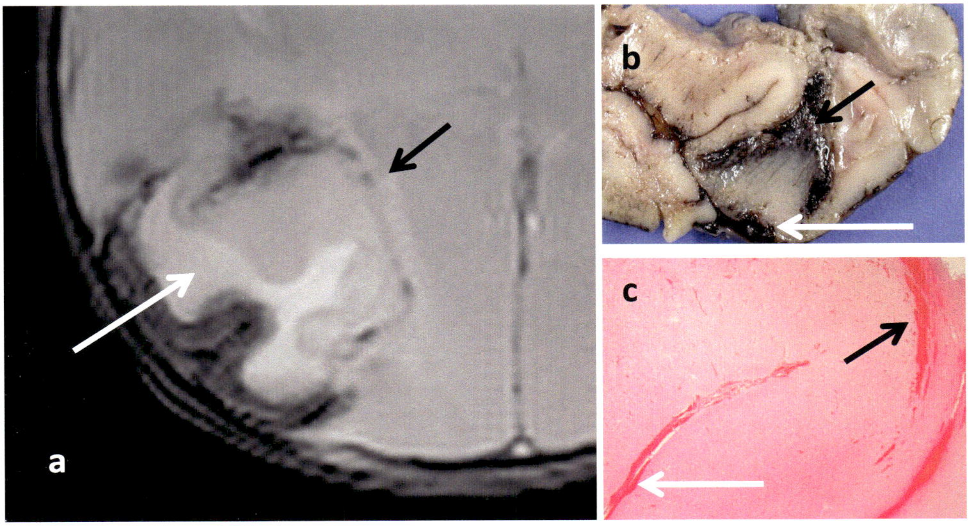

Figure 4.10 Sub-pial haemorrhage with associated subcortical haemorrhage
a MRI scan showing thick sub-pial bleed (white arrow) pushing the cortex away from the meninges. A hypo-dense linear bleed (black arrow) is seen beneath an apparently intact cortex.
b Fixed brain slice from baby with thrombosis of the sagittal sinus. Note thin sub-pial bleed (white arrow) and thick subcortical bleed (black arrow). The cortex is preserved.
c Section of brain from infant following a recent fall from a high bunk bed. There is a thin fresh sub-pial bleed (white arrow) and thin subcortical bleed (black arrow) following the deep cortical margin.

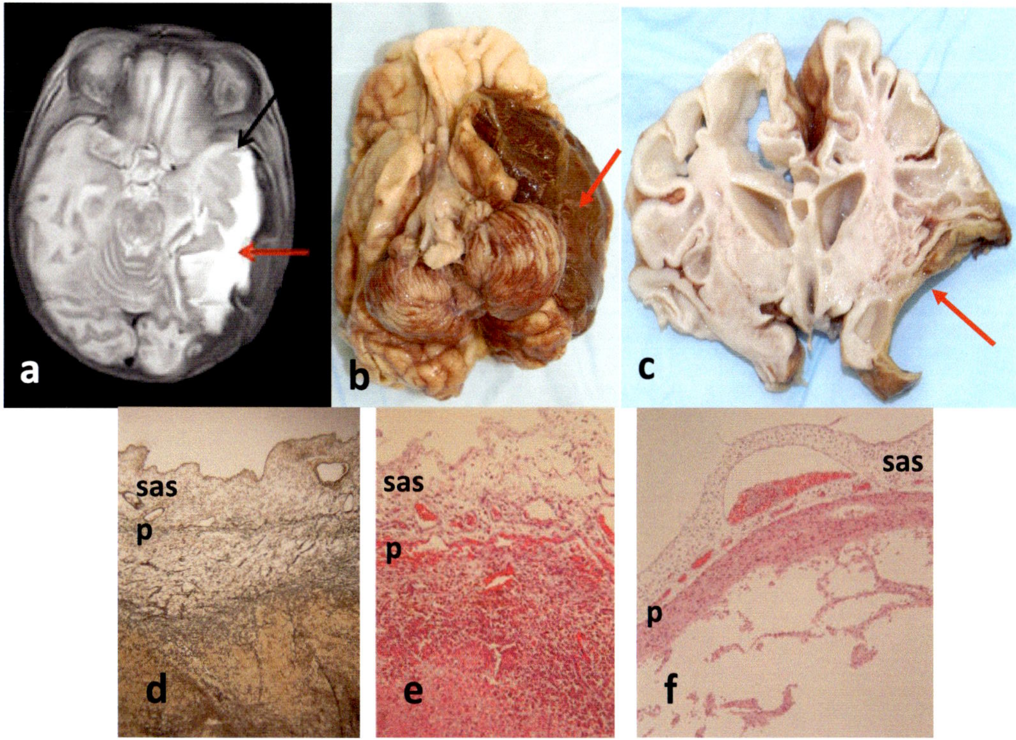

Figure 4.11 Temporal lobe CVT with sub-pial haemorrhage

a Admission brain scan showing right-sided sub-pial collection (red arrow). The cortex is relatively preserved and the right temporal lobe is pushed towards the midline by the extensive mass effect. Black arrow indicates tip of temporal lobe.

b Baby died three weeks after admission. The image shows the under surface of the fixed brain. The temporal lobe is shrunken and the gyri are not identifiable. The meninges are rust/red in colour due to old sub-pial bleeding.

c Coronal slice through fixed brain. The white matter shows established cerebral hypoxic-ischaemic injury (HII) and is reduced to a mass of clean-walled, non-haemorrhagic, predominantly subcortical cysts. The right temporal lobe has been compressed by sub-pial haemorrhage.

d Reticulin stain for collagen fibres showing the pia (p) and extensive destruction of the superficial cortex. The subarachnoid space is thickened and cellular.

e H&E stained section at higher power showing the pia and superficial cortex, which is necrotic and contains many cells staining brown due to their content of hemosiderin from old blood.

f Cortex distant from the sub-pial bleed showing deeper cortical destruction typical of HII. There was no sub-pial bleeding here and the pial surface is smooth and relatively preserved.

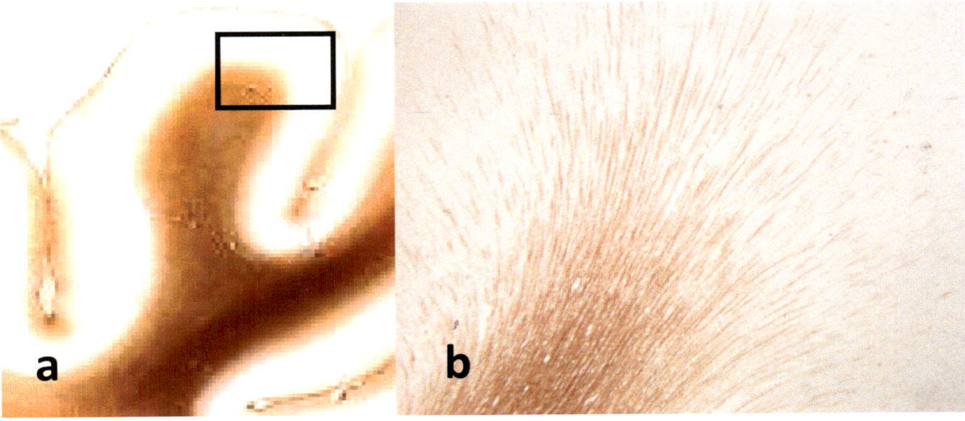

Figure 4.12 Junction of cortex and white matter. PLP myelin stain
a Low-power image showing dense myelinated fibres in the white matter contrasted with the cortex, which is almost devoid of myelin. The area in the box is represented in high power in b.
b Densely packed axons fan out from the white matter into the deep cortex, anchoring it firmly to the underlying white matter.

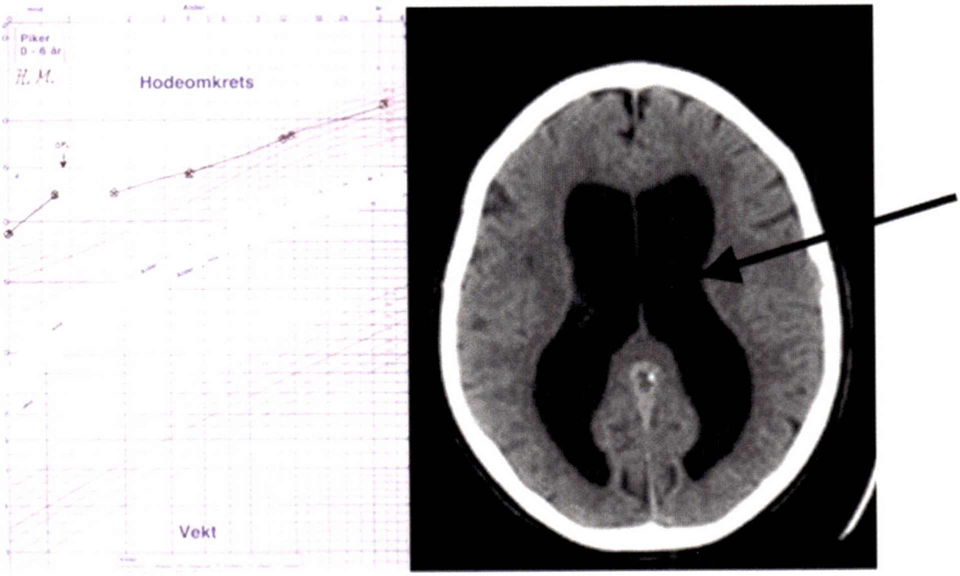

Figure 5.1 'Ordinary' hydrocephalus. Left: head circumference (HC) chart that shows an abnormally rapid (steep) growth. (Hodeomkrets (HC)) starting at birth, and a later normalisation after a neurosurgical procedure (OP = ventriculoperitoneal shunt) allowing permanent drainage of CSF to the abdomen. Right: CT image of a child with 'ordinary' hydrocephalus showing increased CSF (black) in the ventricles of the brain (black arrow). Normal amount of CSF outside the brain, unlike the image of external hydrocephalus (BEH/BESS) (see Figure 5.2)

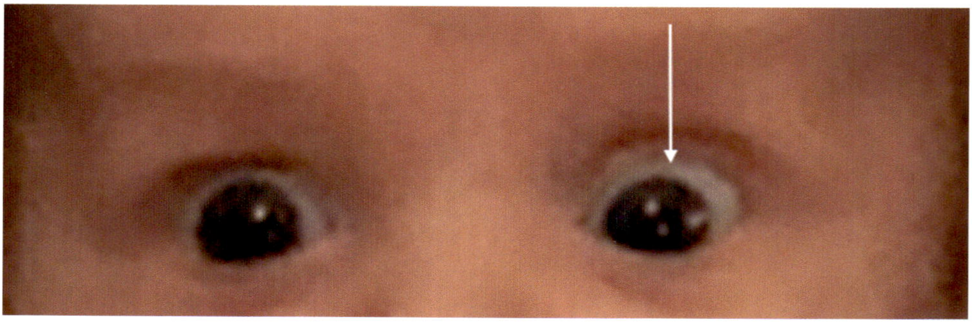

Figure 5.5 'Sunset gaze' resembles a setting sun and indicates increased intracranial pressure (ICP) in a 2-month-old infant. Note the typical rim of white sclera between the upper eyelid and the iris (arrow).

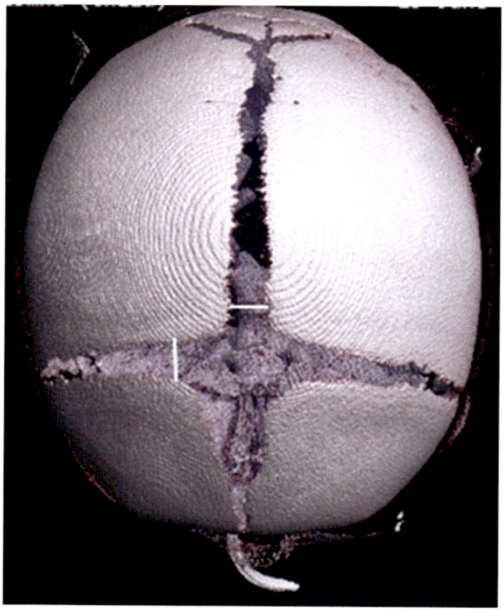

Figure 5.8 Reconstructed CT 3-D image showing suture diastasis (white lines) in infantile external hydrocephalus. Face at lower edge of image

4. Svedin G. [Neglect, abuse and sexual assault]. In [*Paediatric medicine*]. H Lagercrantz, ed. Studentlitteratur, 1999, pp. 180–96.
5. Hedbäck S. [Guideline on child abuse forces the doctor to act, interview*]. Swedish Medical Journal.* 2003;100(10):822–3.
6. Flodmark O, Hirsch G, Tingberg B et al. [*Regional guideline: Care programme on suspicion of physical abuse of infant and toddlers*]. Stockholm County Council and Karolinska Institute, 2008.
7. Otterman G. Curriculum vitae. https://bit.ly/3UsPMrF.
8. [Government proposition to the parliament: Improved protection to children in vulnerable situations etc.]. Government proposition to the parliament (2002).
9. Ludvigsson J, Stinzing G. [Children who are abused] In [*Emergency paediatrics*]. 6th ed. A Larsson, S Norgren, B Lindquist, eds. Liber, 2005.
10. Otterman G. *Course director: Graduate medical education course on child maltreatment (2006–2010)*. Ipuls AB, 2006.
11. Flodmark O. [*Physical abuse of small children, one often missed diagnosis: On the immediate care and the clinical result. National graduate medical education course on child maltreatment*]. Ipuls AB, 2006.
12. Flodmark O, Åström E, Blennow M et al. [Symposium about child abuse: The irresponsible expert testimony]. In *Neuroscience*. Karolinska Institute, 2007.
13. Tegern G, Tinghög P, Flodmark O. [*Prevention of shaken baby syndrome, report from an educational programme on 'mental vaccination'*]. Karolinska Institute and Linköping University, 2012.
14. Erlingson M, Tingberg B. [Risks of shaking infants]. In *1177 vårdguiden* [Internet]. Inera AB, 2013.
15. Janson S, Svensson B. [*Physical punishment and violation of children in Sweden: A national survey 2006–2007 & 2011*]. Allmanna Barnhuset and Karlstad University, 2007, 2011.
16. Jernbro C, Janson S. [*Physical punishment and violation of children in Sweden: A national survey 2016*]. Children's Welfare Foundation, 2017.
17. Tingberg B. Child abuse: Clinical investigation, management and nursing approach. PhD thesis. Karolinska Institute, 2010.
18. Tingberg B, Bredlov B, Ygge BM. Nurses' experience in clinical encounters with children experiencing abuse and their parents. *Journal of Clinical Nursing*. 2008;17(20):2718–24.
19. Tingberg B, Falk AC, Flodmark O, et al. Evaluation of documentation in potential abusive head injury of infants in a paediatric emergency department. *Acta Paediatrica*. 2009;98(5):777–81.
20. [Clinical management overview of child physical abuse] [Internet]. Internetmedicin.se. 2012. https://internetmedicin.se/page.aspx?id=3623.
21. Lucas S. [Signs that children are being abused]. In *The national handbook for child health services* [Internet]. Inera AB, 2013.
22. Otterman G, Maguire S, Greeley C, et al. [Physical abuse of the young child, medical and legal challenges: What does the science tell us?]. Swedish Crime Victims Compensation and Support Authority in collaboration with the Swedish Paediatric Society and Uppsala University Children's Hospital, 2013.
23. [Hearing: The responsibility of health care for child protection (Howard Dubowitz, Martin A. Finkel, Gabriel Otterman, et al.)]: Hearing before The Committee on Health and Welfare, Swedish Parliament (15 May 2013).
24. Christian CW. Curriculum vitae. https://bit.ly/3t1HE5E.
25. Lucas S. [*Application to invite Howard Dubowitz as guest researcher at Uppsala University*]. Uppsala University, 2013.
26. Danon A. [*Children being abused or at risk of being abused: Guidelines for health care and dental care for notification and liability*]. National Board of Health and Welfare, 2014.

27. Otterman G, Tindberg Y. [Injuries from violence in young children: Signs, management and diagnostics]. *Swedish Medical Journal.* 2014;111:CZYR.

28. Van Agthoven G. [*Medical routine, management of suspected infant abuse*]. Swedish Paediatric Society, 2019.

29. Wiksell Å, Caisander H. [*Guidelines for radiology during investigation of suspected child abuse*]. Swedish Society for Paediatric Radiology, 2018.

30. Hellgren K, Löfgren S, Lidén U, et al. [Retinal haemorrhage in violence to the head in young children: Proposal for clinical management support*]. Swedish Medical Journal.* 2019;117:19239.

31. Högberg U, Sennerstam R, Högberg G et al. Medical diagnoses among infants at entry in out-of-home care: A Swedish population-register study. *Health Science Report.* 2019;2(8):e133.

32. Swedish Supreme Administrative Court. Decision 991-7. 2018.

33. Swedish Agency for Health Technology Assessment and Assessment of Social Services (SBU). *Traumatic shaking. The role of the triad in medical investigations of suspected traumatic shaking: A systematic review.* Swedish Agency for Health Technology Assessment and Assessment of Social Services (SBU), 2016.

34. Högberg U, Lampa E, Högberg G et al. Infant abuse diagnosis associated with abuse head trauma criteria: Incidence increase due to overdiagnosis? *European Journal of Public Health.* 2018;28 (4):641–6.

35. Andersson J, Thiblin I. National study shows that abusive head trauma mortality in Sweden was at least 10 times lower than in other Western countries. *Acta Paediatrica.* 2018;107 (3):477–83.

36. Högberg U. Transfer of knowledge to diagnose infant abuse and its incidence: A time-series analysis from Sweden. *Implement Science.* 2022;17(1):15.

37. Swedish Supreme Court. Acquittal decision B 3438-12. 2014.

38. Arvidson V. [*Legal certainty around medical expert opinions in cases of child abuse*]. Stockholm University, 2015.

39. Swedish Supreme Court. Decision, Case No. Ö1860-12 (in Swedish). 2013.

40. Swedish Supreme Court. Decision, Case No. Ö2345-12 (in Swedish). 2013.

41. [Abusive head trauma and other aggravated assault against small children, legal PM]. RättsPM 2016:3, Utvecklingscentrum Göteborg, updated October 2018. Gothenburg, Prosecutor's Office, 2016 and 2018.

Chapter 24

Shaken Baby Syndrome/Abusive Head Trauma in Japan

Kana Sasakura

24.1 Introduction

This chapter describes the history of child abuse detection and prevention in Japan and how the fight against child abuse became a social agenda especially during the 2000s. The shaken baby syndrome/abusive head trauma (SBS/AHT) hypothesis became a commonly accepted notion during the same period and was used in criminal cases to prosecute the carers and in administrative cases to separate them from their children in order to 'protect' them.

However, as we shall see in this chapter, the SBS/AHT hypothesis has become a controversial topic of debate and a number of court decisions in criminal cases since 2018 have questioned the hypothesis or diagnoses based on it. This chapter will overview these developments and show the current status of debate around SBS/AHT in Japan with an emphasis on criminal cases.

24.2 Growing Interest in Child Abuse Detection and Prevention

The interest in child abuse detection and prevention is not a new phenomenon in Japan. The first effort to detect abuse and protect children from it was launched in the beginning of the twentieth century by Taneaki Hara, the head of Tokyo Rehabilitation Facility. He provided shelter to abused children. In 1922, Gunpei Yamamuro founded the Child Abuse Protection Division of the Salvation Army. When the Salvation Army heard reports of abuse, it investigated and protected the child. The project had to halt because of the Great Kanto Earthquake in 1923. The next year, the first child abuse prevention law was enacted. This legislation focused on preventing forced labour of children. Child abuse was linked with poverty, forced labour, and social defence in this period [1, 2].

The second wave of child abuse detection and prevention came in the 1970s, led by doctors influenced by Western research. Henry Kempe and his colleagues had already published their article 'The Battered Child Syndrome' [3]. The article quickly became influential among paediatricians, not only in the United States but also in other countries, including Japan (see Chapter 18). Paediatricians in Japan quickly introduced the syndrome and several medical articles focusing on child abuse were published in the 1970s, including some of the first case studies on child abuse [2].

These articles pointed out that Japanese paediatric studies were 'lagging behind' those of Western societies. They also indicated that, because there was a delay in introducing the notion of the battered child syndrome to Japan, the diagnosis of child abuse was inadequate, overlooking many cases of abuse. Doctors interested in child abuse in the 1970s either studied in the United States or were heavily influenced by English-language publications.

They 'discovered' child abuse in Japan, not through clinical practice, but by studying Western research. However, their discussions were confined to their small community during this period [1, 2].

During the 1990s, child abuse emerged as a social issue. Not only paediatricians but also scholars in psychiatry, nursing, social welfare, psychology, education, law, and so forth introduced the Western discussions on child abuse and its prevention. Japan ratified the Convention of the Rights of the Child in 1994 and the subject caught the attention of scholars as well as politicians, law enforcement, media, and the public.

In 1996, the Study Group for Prevention of Child Abuse and Neglect (later the Japanese Society for Prevention of Child Abuse and Neglect (JaSPCAN)) was founded. The group had strong ties with the International Society for the Prevention of Child Abuse & Neglect (ISPCAN), established by Kempe and others [1, 2, 4]. Moreover, the Act on the Prevention, etc. of Child Abuse came into effect in 2000. The Act made it obligatory for persons who had witnessed child abuse to alert a Child Consultation Centre (CCC) (or Child Guidance Centre [Jidou-Soudan-Jo]). In 2004, the obligation was expanded to cases of suspected child abuse.

It is also important to note that the first edition of the *Handbook for Responding to Child Abuse* [*Kodomo Gyakutai Taiou no Tebiki*], which focused on establishing guidelines for the assessment and prevention of child abuse, was published in 1999 by the Ministry of Health, Labour, and Welfare (MHLW). The *Handbook*'s latest version, revised in 2013, is still the most basic handbook on child abuse detection and prevention.

The most reliable data which indicate the extent of child abuse in Japan come from CCCs located nationwide. The CCCs serve as the primary agencies dealing with child abuse. Japan does not record statistics on the actual number of cases of child abuse but does document the number of consultation cases reported to CCCs. It was only from 1990 that the MHLW started keeping these numbers. In 1990, 1,010 cases were reported to CCCs, but the number grew dramatically to 2,722 cases in 1995, 17,724 cases in 2000, 34,472 cases in 2005, 56,384 cases in 2010, 103,286 cases in 2015, and 207,659 cases in 2021 [5]. It is important to note that these numbers do not indicate the number of *actual* cases of abuse. The most we can conclude from these numbers is that society's interest and responses towards child abuse has grown in the past 20 years [6]. It was during this period that SBS hypothesis was introduced to Japan. In 1991, when society's interest in child abuse was just emerging, Masahiro Ito introduced the notion to the Japanese medical community [7].

24.3 Nakamura Type I (Infantile Acute Subdural Haematoma)

Thirty years before the introduction of SBS in Japan, Norio Nakamura, a neurosurgeon at the University of Tokyo, co-authored an article describing special aspects of head injuries in infants and children [8]. The article studied six cases of acute and three cases of subacute subdural haematoma in the neurosurgical department of the University of Tokyo Hospital. Six patients out of nine were younger than 2 years of age.

Nakamura concluded that (1) the severity of trauma was moderate or slight; (2) impact was mainly to the occipital region of the head; (3) although the trauma was slight, in three cases, patients lost consciousness and deteriorated rapidly and two died from the injury; (4) retinal haemorrhage was found in six cases, thought to be associated with subdural haematoma; and (5) the prognosis of survivors was generally excellent. In eight of the nine cases, the injuries were minor to moderate, and they were all caused by accidents with minor force such as falls from beds or falling occiput-first to the floor. Nakamura called this acute subdural haematoma due to apparently minor trauma a 'grade I (mild) acute subdural hematoma', later called 'Nakamura type I' in the Japanese medical community [9, 10].

Characteristics of Nakamura type I are as follows: (1) 6–10-month-old infants; (2) mostly boys (80%); (3) minor head injury at home (falling backwards, short falls with occipital impacts onto a soft surface such as tatami mats); (4) the impact is mainly to the occipital region of the head; (5) initial symptoms are convulsion and minor disorder of consciousness; (6) retinal haemorrhage is present in many cases, mostly minor but sometimes serious; (7) no brain parenchymal injury; and (8) 90% have a good prognosis [11, 12].

Several studies followed the Nakamura article, all describing the same phenomenon (see Chapter 15).[1] In 1984, Aoki and Masuzawa introduced infantile acute subdural haematoma (IASDH) as the English name for Nakamura type I [14]. They defined IASDH as 'an acute subdural hematoma due to apparently minor head trauma without loss of consciousness that is not associated with cerebral contusion in infants' which 'differs in pathology from the acute subdural hematoma due to high-grade impact injury seen at all ages'.

They described 26 cases of IASDH, the average age of the patients being 8.1 months, with none having a significant medical history or being victims of child abuse before the trauma. The most common cause of trauma was a fall backwards while sitting or standing or hitting the head against a soft item such as a tatami mat (16 out of 26 patients). They concluded that 'this disorder has a good prognosis when appropriate therapy is given early; however, if it is overlooked or the hematoma is not removed, it may progress to chronic subdural hematoma or multicystic encephalopathy and such cases may be fatal', so physicians should 'bear in mind the age at which the disease frequently appears, the typical clinical course, and the consistent presence of retinal and preretinal hemorrhage'.

Aoki and Masuzawa's publication encountered harsh criticism from the American paediatric community. For example, Rekate wrote in a letter to the editor:

> [The Aoki and Masuzawa article] failed to recognize that most, if not all, of these babies suffered from the 'whiplash shake syndrome' and are victims of child abuse. While not totally pathognomonic of shaking, the constellation of SDH and retinal hemorrhage in the context of a historically trivial injury should be regarded as whiplash shake syndrome unless another etiology can be determined. When dealing with trauma in infants it is essential to maintain a degree of skepticism with regard to the trivial nature of the injury. It is inconceivable that bilateral SDHs with retinal hemorrhages could result from such minor head injuries. [15]

In response to these criticisms, Aoki and Masuzawa published another case series report in 1986 [16]. They pointed out the differences between the discussions in the United States and Japan regarding the constellation of retinal haemorrhages and subdural haematomas – in the United States, IASDH may be erroneously identified as child abuse.

Members of the Japanese paediatric community echoed Rekate's scepticism. They described Nakamura type I as an old theory which does not recognise the possibility of abuse and noted that a minor head trauma will not cause subdural haematoma or become severe. Although papers, mainly by neurosurgeons, continued to recognise the presence of

[1] According to Aoki, as of 2011, there were 14 papers describing more than 200 cases of IASDH in the Japanese literature. However, among the studies in the United States, only 2 papers on 41 cases written in English were cited [12]. In 2018, cases with similar findings were reported in the United States [13].

Nakamura type I [11, 12, 17–19], the mainstream academia came to rely on SBS/AHT hypothesis in the 2000s (see, e.g., [20–22]). As calls heightened for a 'child-first' model of abuse detection and prevention, Nakamura type I was superseded by SBS/AHT.

24.4 The Ministry of Health, Labour, and Welfare Handbook on Child Abuse

The *Handbook for Responding to Child Abuse* published by the MHLW, which provides the most basic guidelines for treatment of child abuse for CCCs and other specialised agencies, was revised in 2013 [23].[2] This latest edition states:

> The diagnosis of SBS is made based on three main features: (1) subdural haematoma or subarachnoid haemorrhage, (2) fundus haemorrhage and (3) parenchymal brain damage such as cerebral oedema. There may also be pressure marks on the body surface from shaking, minor trauma, rib and limb fractures . . . Except for diseases with a tendency to bleed, some metabolic diseases and obvious traffic accidents, subdural haemorrhage is rarely caused by a fall from less than 90 cm. Therefore, SBS should always be the first consideration when a subdural haematoma with an unknown cause is seen in infants and the primary explanation is a fall. Extensive, multilayered fundus haemorrhages are rare outside of SBS. If a tendency to bleed is ruled out, they provide the basis for a diagnosis of SBS.[3]

It obviously relies on the SBS/AHT hypothesis.

Similarly, a group of physicians who have strong ties with MHLW and led the dissemination of SBS/AHT hypothesis in the 2000s published a manual for medical practitioners in 2011.[4] The manual states that 'about 5% of subdural haematomas in infants are caused by unintentional accidents, such as falls or road traffic accidents, but the majority are caused by abuse, particularly violent shaking' and that 'if the triad is present and there is no evidence of a high fall from more than 3 meters, it is very likely to be an SBS even without a confession' [24].

As can be seen from these guidelines, the SBS/AHT hypothesis had already become a commonly accepted dogma and implemented in society. Prevention efforts also spread during this period. The MHLW launched a prevention programme in 2013 on its website named 'The Baby Does Not Stop Crying' (https://www.mhlw.go.jp/stf/houdou/0000030718.html). The video on the website was 'designed to help the viewers understand the characteristics of crying babies and what to do when they won't stop crying' and it specifically states that 'one shouldn't shake them too hard or cover their mouths to make them stop crying'. It emphasises the effect of violently shaking the baby to force the baby to stop crying, the mechanism of SBS (explained using computer graphics and dolls), and the 'effects of violent shaking on infants'.

---

2 The *Handbook* was first published in 1999 and was revised in 2000, 2004, 2007, 2008, and 2013.

3 The MHLW's website retains an older version of the *Handbook* which states that '95% of subdural haematomas in infants before they start walking are said to be abusive'. See www.mhlw.go.jp/bunya/kodomo/dv12/04.html.

4 The project 'Research on the role of medical institutions (prevention, medical assessment) in abuse response collaboration' was a sub-project of the main project, 'Research to ensure a system of medical treatment for children's mental health and to train professional personnel', which the MHLW funded from 2010 to 2012. The director of this research group was Makiko Okuyama, a psychiatrist at the National Centre for Child Health and Development. The co-authors of this manual were Fujiko Yamada and Fumitake Mizoguchi.

The *Maternal and Child Health Handbook* [*Boshi-Techou*], which is distributed by the local government when pregnancies are registered, also has a section on preventing SBS/AHT. It describes the mechanisms of SBS/AHT and how mothers should handle the crying baby [25].

> If you shake your baby violently, it can cause a concussion because the muscles in the baby's neck are undeveloped. This can cause serious brain injury or, in some cases, loss of life (i.e. shaken baby syndrome). Any parent will at some point become irritated because their baby will not stop crying, but never shake a baby. If you do happen to violently shake your baby, have the baby examined at a hospital or clinic right away and explain what happened.

These documents all suggest that the SBS/AHT hypothesis was implemented, promoted, and has become an accepted dogma in the paediatric community, but it has also become a part of the MHLW's policy.

24.5 Prosecution of and Challenges to Shaken Baby Syndrome/Abusive Head Trauma

The SBS/AHT hypothesis gained support in the 2000s. A number of SBS/AHT cases have been subject to criminal investigation and prosecution since around 2010. An increasing number of caregivers have been arrested, prosecuted, and convicted, mainly on the basis of medical opinion. The 'triad' of SBS was an essential part of the medical determination in these cases [26]. In fact, a prosecutor who has handled several SBS/AHT cases wrote in 2014 that, 'when diagnosing SBS, the triad of SBS (1) acute subdural haematoma, 2) cerebral oedema, and 3) retinal haemorrhage) should be confirmed by head CT and MRI' [27].

The 'victims' in SBS/AHT cases are typically children aged between 0 and 2 years, who are unable to give their own statements. Sudden deterioration of infants often occurs in a closed-door household with no security camera footage or third-party witnesses. Even if there were eyewitnesses, they are not seen as reliable since they are related to the accused. In SBS/AHT cases, there is no direct evidence to establish the circumstances of an infant's collapse. Medical findings are used to do so. Proving these circumstances involves going back to the injury (SDH, RH, parenchymal brain damage, etc.) and considering the mechanism and timing of the injury. However, results of the injury itself must be deduced from the CT/MRI images and/or symptoms, so the structure of the proof must be based on inference after inference.

In addition, in SBS/AHT cases, it is inferred from the medical findings that the injury was caused by an intentional act of assault. Moreover, the terms 'SBS' and 'AHT' themselves presuppose that the injury was the result of 'shaking' or 'abuse' and so were the result of an intentional act. Thus, in these cases, the proof is dependent upon medical evidence, namely opinions and testimonies of doctors.

Although there is no official statistic, there is a report that from 2000 to 2018, at least 151 carers had been considered for prosecution for SBS (assault, manslaughter, or attempted murder), with 72 convicted, 9 acquitted, and 31 not prosecuted. Prosecutions were especially numerous in the Osaka area (44 cases in Osaka, 9 in Tokyo, and 8 in Kanagawa) [28]. There have also been an unknown number of cases where the carers were not prosecuted but were separated from their children because of medical determination based on SBS/AHT hypothesis. According to a study commissioned by MHLW in 2020, in a survey sent to 220

CCCs throughout the country, 243 cases of suspected AHT were reported in 2019, of which children were temporarily taken into protective custody in 125 cases [29].

According to a recent study on the number of prosecuted SBS/AHT cases obtained through databases of court decisions, there were 64 cases in which the accused were prosecuted for causing death or injury to an infant by assault to the head. Of these, 13 resulted in acquittals and 51 in convictions [30]. The number of acquittals in SBS/AHT cases is quite high since usually more than 99.8% of criminal cases result in convictions [31].

The SBS/AHT acquittals can be divided into two groups: those in which a defendant was acquitted by denying a crime ever occurred (9 cases where medical determinations of SBS/AHT themselves were contested) and those in which a defendant was acquitted by denying he/she was the culprit (4 cases where medical determinations of SBS/AHT were not contested, but the perpetrator of the crime was contested). All but one of the cases in which the defendant was acquitted by denying that a crime ever occurred were decided after 2018.

One of the reasons behind the sudden increase in the number of acquittals after 2018 was that, in 2017, the SBS Review Project was launched by attorneys and scholars.[5] The project introduced the existing serious controversy around the SBS/AHT hypothesis around the world through its website, blog, and articles in professional magazines [32, 33].[6] The project also defended or helped to defend SBS/AHT cases. This led to a vigorous defence and eventually acquittals [34].[7] At the same time, there was a movement by neurosurgeons to raise awareness once again of Nakamura Type I acute subdural haemorrhage [11, 17].

---

[5] The co-directors are Masashi Akita (Osaka Bar Association) and Kana Sasakura (Konan University). The executive director is Hiroyuki Kawakami (Osaka Bar Association).

[6] The SBS Review Project has also hosted a number of symposia and other seminars. For the international symposia in 2018 and 2019, it invited several international speakers, including Waney Squier, Keith Findley, Kate Judson, and Anders Eriksson. See www.nichibenren.or.jp/library/pdf/activity/criminal/reforming/sbs_kiroku.pdf for a report of the 2019 events.

[7] The following is a list of nine acquitted cases in which the SBS Review Project was involved. All were handed down after 2018.

(1) Osaka District Court decision on 14 March 2018 (*Hanrei-Jihou* 2395 at 109). Upheld by Osaka High Court decision on 28 January 2020 (LEX/DB25564741). There was no proof of intentional assault and the defendant was acquitted. (2) Osaka District Court decision on 20 November 2018 (LEX/DB 255561710). Upheld by Osaka High Court decision on 13 March 2020 (LEX/DB 25570859). The district court found no proof of intentional assault but the appellate court upheld the acquittal by denying the defendant was not the culprit. (3) Osaka District Court decision on 11 January 2019 (LEX/DB25562102). Held that the cause may have been a sudden apnoea. (4) Osaka High Court decision on 25 October 2019 (*Hanrei-Jihou* 2476 at 110). A case in which the defendant was acquitted on the grounds that there was a possibility of venous sinus thrombosis. (5) Osaka High Court decision on 6 February 2020 (*Hanrei-Jihou* 2476 at 128, Finalized by the Supreme Court Decision on 30 June 2021 (LEX/DB 25506577)). The Osaka District Court decision on 13 March 2018 sentenced the defendant to 3 years imprisonment (5 years with probation). The High Court acquitted on the basis that a short fall, pre-existing medical condition, and choking due to aspiration of milk may have been involved. (6) Tokyo District Court Tachikawa Branch decision on 7 February 2020 (LEX/DB 25564820), acquitted and confirmed by Tokyo High Court decision on 28 May 2021(LEX/DB 25590699). A case in which the defendant was acquitted on the ground that there was a possibility of a sudden death. (7) Gifu District Court decision on 25 September 2020 (*Hanrei-Jihou* 2491 at 99). Nagoya High Court decision on 28 September 2021 (LEX/DB 25506578) affirmed. A case in which the defendant was acquitted on the ground that there was a possibility of a short fall. (8) Osaka District Court decision on 4 December 2020 (LEX/DB 25571223). The

24.6 Recent Court Decisions

This section will overview the recent successive acquittals in SBS/AHT cases (see [33] for a thorough discussion regarding this section and the following section). In some of these cases, the court decided that the cause of the child's injury or death was unknown and there was a reasonable doubt it was abuse. In others, the court pointed out that it was possible that the infant's injury could have come from other causes such as a fall from a low height, hypoxia due to venous sinus thrombosis, or aspiration. In these cases, it was also found that physicians who diagnosed SBS/AHT could not distinguish abuse and non-abuse cases.

For example, in the case of the Osaka High Court decision on 25 October 2019, a grandmother was accused of shaking her 2-month-old granddaughter to death [35–37]. The baby was found to have 'acute subdural haematoma, multiple subarachnoid haemorrhages, cerebral oedema secondary to diffuse brain injury and extensive multi-layered retinal haemorrhages in both eyes' – the typical 'triad' of SBS – and the defendant was prosecuted.

The Osaka District Court (decision on 2 October 2017) concluded that the prosecution's expert witnesses, Dr M (a paediatrician), and Dr K (a pathologist), were 'both doctors with extensive medical knowledge and experience', and that their testimonies were credible because they had analysed the relevant materials in the case and provided reasonable explanations based on their medical knowledge, and also because their statements were generally consistent with each other. The defendant was sentenced to 5 years and 6 months in prison with labour. However, on appeal, two neurosurgeons testifying for the defence pointed out that the baby's symptoms could have been caused by venous sinus thrombosis. The grandmother was acquitted on appeal.

The High Court ruled that the testimony of M,

> which goes so far as to say that it is common knowledge in diagnostic imaging that venous stasis and engorgement never appear white . . . is inconsistent with medical literature. It is questionable whether M has accurate professional knowledge of reading CT images and whether, in the context of this case, he can make an accurate differential diagnosis as to whether the white area is a bleeding such as subdural haematoma, or whether there are other possibilities . . . In light of the categorical nature of M's testimony, it is necessary to examine carefully whether he is taking his own views for granted and takes a one-sided view . . . M's testimony in court is not consistent with the original paper he relied on. It must be said that the paper on which M relied (which M himself translated) was quoted in bad faith. It is suspected that it was used to mean the exact opposite of the original paper.

We can see that the High Court criticised M's opinion, which was viewed as highly credible in the first instance and was used as the basis for the conviction. This suggests that the opinions of experts who cannot perform even a basic reading of CT and MRI images were relied upon in other cases and were used to convict in past cases. It is also clear from this case that the presence of the triad has led to convictions in the past. The fact that venous sinus thrombosis was overlooked in this case shows that differential diagnosis was not carried out properly and alternative causes of the triad were falsely ruled out.

Other recent acquittals have also addressed the problems inherent in the SBS/AHT hypothesis and cautioned the nature of fact-finding in this type of case. Firstly, the Osaka

---

defendant was acquitted on the ground that a pre-existing medical condition and minor bounce by bicycle ride may have played a role. (9) Niigata District Court decision on 9 May 2022.

High Court decision on 25 October 2019, commented on the danger of fact-finding based on the SBS hypothesis, stating that,

> in the present case, the existence of (1) subdural hematoma, which is usually caused by the rupture of bridging veins, cannot be confirmed, and (2) brain swelling and (3) fundus haemorrhage, even if the symptoms are recognised, could have developed by other causes ... This case shows the danger of fact-finding based on the SBS theory: if the SBS theory is simply applied, it may lead to a very mechanical and stereotypical finding of facts, and in conclusion, there is a risk of factual error.

The High Court also pointed out that the District Court

> adopted the so-called elimination method of identifying the culprit on the premise that B's [the baby's] symptoms were caused by external force [and not by a disease such as venous sinus thrombosis] ... It is true that such a method of fact-finding is generally employed in criminal trials. However, this case shows that there is an inherent risk of error. The elimination method is a method which, except under certain conditions, identifies the accused as the perpetrator even if there is no positive evidence or facts to show that he/she is. Thus, when facts, at a first glance, appear to have a sufficient objective ground, the accused will be found to be the perpetrator. Furthermore, especially in cases where the accused's culpability is the only issue ... the accused's rebuttal evidence will be rendered ineffective, and a finding of guilt will be inevitable without a proper hearing. This raises an extremely serious problem in the fact-finding process of criminal trials.

Secondly, in the Osaka High Court decision on 6 February 2020, the court cited the problem inherent in fact-finding of SBS cases [38].[8] It ruled that: (1) in this case where no craniotomy was performed, the existence of diffuse axonal injury and acute subdural hematoma had to be confirmed by inference from CT scans or symptoms; (2) shaking was then deduced from the presence of diffuse axonal injury and acute subdural hematoma; and (3) in conclusion, it was inferred that the defendant must have shaken the baby. The court pointed out that this structure of fact-finding was built upon inference after inference.

Recognising the danger of the structure of the SBS hypothesis, which consists of inferences, the court cautioned as follows: 'when a criminal case is prosecuted and a trial is held to determine the guilt or innocence of the accused, judges must keep in mind that the fact-finding is based on this misleading structure, and must pay particular attention to the circumstances that prevent inferences from being made, and carefully consider whether such circumstances can be excluded as unreasonable'.

The court further stated that, when the opinion of an expert is an important source of evidence in the process of inferring guilt, 'it is particularly necessary to examine carefully whether there is any doubt as to the opinion of the physician who denies the circumstances which prevent this inference of guilt, and even more so when there is an opinion of another physician who points out to the circumstance preventing the inference'. When examining the doctor's opinion, it is necessary to 'consider whether there are any logical inconsistencies or defects such as overlooking important objective data, or whether there is too much reliance on unreliable hearsay evidence in the absence of direct experience'.

8 A mother was accused of shaking her 1.5-months-old daughter to death. The baby had acute subdural haemorrhage and brain swelling. The High Court ruled that it was possible that the 2.5-year-old brother had dropped the baby from a low height combined with the baby having milk aspiration.

In this case, Dr M (the same expert witness for the previous case), who testified as a witness for the prosecution, misread CT images and relied on hearsay evidence (foreign literature) in his testimony. The court emphasised that 'the professional knowledge and expertise of a doctor often has a serious impact on the fact-finding in a criminal trial, and it is for this reason that we must return to the basics: requiring proof that leaves no reasonable doubt in the trial and judgment. A strict examination of the doctor's opinion is required'.

Thirdly, the Tokyo High Court decision on 28 May 2021 gave an important judgment on the 'comprehensive diagnoses' in an AHT case.[9] The District Court in this case found that each of the injuries (multiple acute subdural haematomas, injuries to the medulla oblongata and cervical vertebrae, cerebral oedema, multiple retinal haemorrhages, and multiple rib fractures) could have occurred from causes other than abuse and acquitted the defendant.

The prosecutors argued on appeal that the District Court was in error when it did not take into account the fact that these multiple injuries occurred at the same time. They argued:

> In paediatric medicine, when multiple injuries occur in infants, it is common understanding ... that a comprehensive diagnosis should be made on the assumption that they were triggered by a single cause ... It is medically unreasonable to assume that the three symptoms of (1) multiple subdural haematomas, (2) cerebral oedema and (3) fundus haemorrhage were caused by a combination of different causes. It is medically reasonable to conclude that the only reasonable explanation for these symptoms is abusive head trauma, namely shaking, and this is the consensus of the medical community supported by medical and other literature evidence.

The Tokyo High Court dismissed the prosecution's appeal, upholding the acquittal:

> In deciding the issues in this case, the District Court did not assume that each of the injuries in question occurred coincidentally on the same occasion or that they were caused by a single cause. This was legitimate. Even though a certain cause may produce a certain result, it does not follow that the cause and the result can be reversed, so far as the same result may be produced by other causes, and that the cause in question can be naturally inferred from the result. This structure remains basically the same in the case of three results from one cause. Even if it is possible to explain rationally the mechanism by which three symptoms result from shaking, unless the reasonable possibility that these symptoms can be produced by other causes can be excluded, the existence of the three symptoms does not mean that they can be traced back to a single cause, namely shaking. The prosecution's argument that it would be 'medically unreasonable' to assume that the aforementioned three symptoms happen to occur coincidentally obscures the aforementioned logical structure and overlooks the prosecutor's burden of proof regarding the fact that no other cause can reasonably be considered for the occurrence of these symptoms ... it is a leap of logic to assume the existence of an unproven injury in the process of retrospectively inferring a cause, and in this sense, it must be said that it is a view which cannot be adopted in this case.

The court sharply points out the problem of the conventional understanding of SBS/AHT, in which the diagnosis of SBS is made if certain symptoms are present, without a proper exclusion of other causes or differential diagnosis.

---

9 This was a case of a father whose 1-month-old daughter had bruising, acute subdural haemorrhage, brain swelling, multiple rib fractures, retinal haemorrhage, and injury to the medulla and cervical spinal cord. The court found that it was possible that the triad of symptoms came from cardiac arrest together with milk aspiration and the fractures could have come from resuscitation.

Lastly, the Nagoya High Court judgment on 28 September 2021 stated that

> It is the prosecutor who bears the burden of proof in a criminal trial. It is obvious that even if it is correct to say that 'a particular injury occurs if there is a shaking', we cannot conclude that 'there was shaking because the existence of a particular injury is there', unless there is a condition that 'a particular injury does not occur due to any other cause'.[10] Even if, as the prosecutor says, we should examine from the point of view that 'if the cause was not shaking, whether each injury which occurred coincidentally in the same period can be explained consistently and rationally', the prosecutor must prove a beyond reasonable doubt that 'each injury could not have occurred in the same period from any cause other than the shaking'. The prosecutor argues that the defence should argue and prove that each injury was caused by a specific cause which can be reasonably explained medically other than shaking. This argument is unacceptable.

Here again, as in the Tokyo High Court's decision, the burden of proof of the prosecutor is mentioned, showing the courts' awareness of the limitations of differential and exclusionary diagnosis in SBS/AHT cases.

24.7 Rebuttal to the Acquittals

The successive acquittals in SBS/AHT cases in Japan and other countries have been challenged nationally and internationally by those who have studied the issue of abuse. In 2018, proponents of the SBS/AHT hypothesis issued the 'Consensus Statement on Abusive Head Trauma in Infants and Young Children' [39]. The Consensus Statement was supported by a number of professional societies including the Society for Pediatric Radiology, European Society of Paediatric Radiology, and American Academy of Pediatrics. The Japanese Paediatric Society also joined.

The Consensus Statement criticises the 'denialism' of child abuse and addresses the 'misconceptions and misrepresentations about the diagnosis of abusive head trauma'. It also states that when AHT 'is diagnosed, it signifies that accidental and disease processes cannot plausibly explain the etiology of the infant/child's injuries'. The purpose of the Consensus Statement was to pressure the courts, media, and public and to delegitimise those who criticise or challenge the SBS/AHT hypothesis, denying there is any debate at all about its reliability [40].

In 2020, the Japanese Paediatric Society published an opinion on AHT [41]. The opinion was basically in line with the Consensus Statement. It stated: (1) AHT was established by medical evidence and its scientific validity has been agreed upon by many academic societies around the world. (2) Paediatricians and other healthcare providers who work with children make a careful differential diagnosis of AHT. (3) All healthcare professionals working with children need to act on behalf of children and uphold the principle of 'child first'.

In a recent article, a paediatrician who has appeared as a witness for the prosecution in several cases expressed his sense of crisis, saying that he had never heard of any other country where acquittals were handed down so numerously and consecutively as in Japan. He pointed out that, not only the police and prosecutors, but also CCCs were becoming ineffective in dealing with AHT cases and that there had been a series of cases where parents

---

10 A mother was accused of shaking her 3-month-old son. Acute subdural haemorrhage, brain swelling, and retinal haemorrhage were found. The mother argued that the baby had fallen from a sofa. The court agreed that this could have been possible.

who had confessed to abuse in clinical settings were not prosecuted because their attorneys had forced them to remain silent [42].

An ophthalmologist, who was also the prosecution's witness in several cases, said that, if there is no convincing evidence or symptoms of abuse, the case would not have been treated by doctors in the first place and that cases that go to trial are limited to those where there are sufficient grounds for abuse, implying that the acquittals were wrong. 'I am worried that we are being swamped by inaccurate defence arguments' [43]. Another paediatrician commented that 'the recent developments regarding the "false accusations" of AHT have been biased and have been exacerbated by some media reports' (quote by Dr Maibara in [44]).

Prosecutors and former prosecutors are also increasingly becoming concerned about these acquittals. They basically take the same position as these doctors. Kunihiko Sakai, a retired prosecutor who worked tirelessly on the issue of abuse during his tenure, has criticised the 'SBS denialists'. He points out that these attorneys subject prosecution witnesses to cross-examination in which they 'ask questions to surprise witnesses' in an attempt to create 'a reasonable doubt' and 'confuse' the judges and juries in order to acquit the case [45].

Kazuko Tanaka, a prosecutor and author of a book on sex crimes and abuse, has handled the trial of several SBS/AHT cases in the past. She says that the acquittals were due to the fact that:

> [I]n a jury trial, important objective evidence such as medical records of the victim child, autopsy records, and photographs of bruises were not permitted as evidence because they were too difficult or provocative for the lay judges. In addition, various indirect facts, which in Europe and the United States are considered to be important prosecution evidence for proving AHT, are uniformly excluded by the courts as being 'irrelevant' [44].

These publications point out that the reasons for these successive acquittals were defence litigation tactics which proved effective and because courts did not allow prosecution evidence. They do not mention the fact that these decisions pointed out basic problems such as misinterpreting CT/MRI images and inaccurate medical determinations by witnesses for the prosecution.

Another publication by a prosecutor points out that the 'common denominator' of these acquittals was that 'the main issues in these cases were the appropriateness of medical diagnoses, whether or not it was possible to infer deliberate external force from these diagnoses, and whether or not the other causes could be ruled out'. Also, 'when there is a disagreement among experts, the courts heavily weigh the expertise of the neurosurgeons, and recognize the high credibility of their opinion. Also, on the grounds that medical proof inevitably involves a multi-step process of inference, courts carefully consider whether or not alternative causes can be ruled out' [46].

This shows the recent attitude of the public prosecutor's office towards SBS/AHT. The prosecution, who, in the past, has sought expert opinions from paediatricians and other medical experts specialising in abuse, has shifted their focus to neurosurgeons. However, the question is not whether to have a paediatrician or a neurosurgeon as a witness. These acquittals emphasised whether there was evidence for each doctor's opinion and whether it was accurate and scientific.

However, there has not yet been any move by physicians or prosecutors who have traditionally promoted the SBS/AHT hypothesis to take these acquittals seriously and conduct a full review of the way in which SBS/AHT cases have been investigated and prosecuted. In February 2021, the Supreme Public Prosecutor's Office and eight high public prosecutors' offices, in response to these acquittals, established a system in which each office appoints one prosecutor in charge of child abuse cases, with the aim of consolidating investigations in their cases and sharing their expertise with district public prosecutors' offices across the country. However, since prosecutors' offices have not officially reviewed the causes of wrongful prosecutions in these recently acquitted cases and made fundamental reforms in the way they investigate and prosecute, this system, even if implemented, will not prevent further wrongful accusations.

24.8 Conclusion

It is often said that the Japanese criminal justice system is infected with a 'culture of denial'. A prominent scholar of Japanese law, David T. Johnson, once wrote: 'Japan continues to have problems with wrongful conviction, and the most serious problem involves a culture of denial that makes it difficult for police, prosecutors, and judges to acknowledge their own mistakes and for the media and other external agents of accountability to conduct rigorous investigations' [47]. The exact same can be said for SBS/AHT cases.

An official and scientific review of recent SBS/AHT acquittals is vital. For 'comprehensive diagnoses', the cooperation of experts in the many specialties involved in SBS/AHT cases (neurology, forensic medicine, radiology, ophthalmology, perinatology, haematology, pathology, cardiology, infectious and respiratory diseases, epidemiology, physics, bioengineering, etc.) is needed [48]. Research on SBS/AHT in Japan to date was led by paediatricians and other physicians specialised in abuse. A review by independent experts who are not involved in the controversy is crucial [49]. Without a serious objective review of these acquittals and the problems of the SBS/AHT hypothesis, it is impossible to learn from our mistakes and prevent further wrongful convictions. Also, in light of these recent acquittals, a full review of cases that were convicted in the past is essential.

The successive acquittals in criminal cases in Japan suggest fundamental problems with medical determination of SBS/AHT. This raises concerns not only in criminal cases, but also in administrative/family court cases where children are separated from their carers by CCCs. The MHLW should also conduct a comprehensive review on this matter. So far, the MHLW has made no move to review its current guidelines on abuse diagnosis. The *Handbook* should also be revised based on the most current scientific knowledge.

References

1. Ueno K. *Gyakutai risuku: Kouchiku sareru kosodate hyojun kazoku [Child abuse risk: Constructing a 'normal' childrearing family]*. Seikatsu-Shoin, 2022.
2. Ueno K. Jido-gyakutai no hakken houhou no henka [The change in ways to detect child abuse]. In *Jido-gyakutaino politikkusu [The politics of child abuse]*. K Ueno, ed. Akashi-Shoten, 2006.
3. Kempe H, Silverman F, Steele B, Droegemueller W, Silver H. The battered child syndrome. *JAMA*. 1962;181(1):17–24.
4. Ueno K. *Jido-gyakutai no shakai-gaku [The sociology of child abuse]*. 1996. Sekai-Shiso-Sha, 1996.
5. Ministry of Health, Labour and Welfare. Reiwa 3 nendo jidou-soudan-jo deno jidou-gyakutai-taiou-kensuu [Number of child abuse consultation cases to CCCs in fiscal year 2021]. www.mhlw.go.jp/content/000863297.pdf.
6. Uchida R. *'Jidou-gyakutai' he no manazashi: Shakai genshou ha dou katarareru-noka [Looking at 'child abuse': How social*

phenomena are described]. Sekai-Shisou-Sha, 2009.

7. Ito M. *Yusaburarekko shoukougun to kodomo no jiko [Shaken baby syndrome and children's accidents*]. Ootsuki Shoten, 2003.
8. Nakamura N, Kobayashi S, Hirakawa K, Yamada H, Jinbo M. Shouni no toubugaishou to zugainai kesshu no tokucho [Special aspects of head injuries in infants and children]. *No to Shinkei*. 1965;17(8):785–94.
9. Nakamura N. *Toubu gaishou: Kyuuseiki no mekanizumu [Head injuries: Mechanisms in the acute stages]*. Kobun-Do, 1986.
10. Aoki N, Masuzawa H. Nyuuyouji mansei koumakuka kesshu: Nyuuyouji kyuusei koumakuka kesshu (nakamura I gata) no yakuwari [Infantile chronic subdural hematoma: Etiologic significance of infantile acute subdural hematoma]. *Neurologia medico-Chirurgica (Tokyo)*. 1981;21:595–9.
11. Fujiwara K, Nishimoto H, Sakurai K, Kiyosawa M. *Akachan wo korobasenaide: Nakamura I gata wo shiru [Do not let the baby fall: Knowing about Nakamura Type I]*. Sanseido Shoten, 2021.
12. Aoki N. Nyuuyouji kyuusei koumakuka kesshu ha gyakutai ni yorunoka keibina toubugaishou ni yorunoka? [Infantile acute subdural hematoma: Caused by abuse or minor head trauma?] *Nervous System in Children*. 2011;36(3):326–30.
13. Atkinson N et al. Childhood falls with occipital impacts. *Pediatric Emergency Care*. 2018;34(12):837–41.
14. Aoki N, Masuzawa H. Infantile acute subdural hematoma: Clinical analysis of 26 cases. *Journal of Neurosurgery*. 1984;61:273–80.
15. Rekate HL. Subdural hematomas in infants. *Journal of Neurosurgery*. 1984;61:316–17.
16. Aoki N, Masuzawa H. Subdural hematomas in abused children: Report of six cases from Japan. *Neurosurgery*. 1986;18 (4):475–7.
17. Nishimoto H, Fujiwara K. *Akachan ga atamawo utta, doushiyou? [The baby bumped their head. What can we do?]*. Iwasaki Shoten, 2018.
18. Nishimoto H, Kurihara J. Kateinai no keibi na gaishou ni yoru nyuuyouji kyuusei koumakuka kesshu no saihyouka [Re-estimation of acute subdural hematoma in children caused by trivial household head trauma]. *Shouni no Noushinkei*. 2006;31(3):215–23.
19. Shimoji K, Suehiro E. Matsuno A, Araki T. Abusive head trauma in Japan. *Child's Nervous System*. 2022; DOI: 10.1007/s00381-022-05692-4.
20. Konuma T. Gyakutai ni yoru toubu gaishou [Abusive head trauma]. In *Kodomo gyakutai no rinshou [Clinical practice of child abuse]*. S Sakai, Okuyama M, Inoue N, eds. Nanzan-Dou, 2005.
21. Okuyama M. Shaken baby syndrome [in Japanese]. In *Kodomo gyakutai no rinshou [Clinical practice of child abuse]*. S Sakai, M Okuyama, N Inoue, eds. Nanzan-Dou, 2005.
22. Fujiwara T, Okuyama M, Matsumoto T. Nisai miman ji no gyakutai ni yoru toubu gaishou no shindan kijun no teian [Proposed diagnosis criteria for inflicted head injury of children younger than two years of age]. *Journal of the Japan Paediatric Society*. 2008;112(4):704–12.
23. Ministry of Health, Labour and Welfare (MHLW). *Kodomo gyakutai taiou no tebiki [Handbook for responding to child abuse*]. Ministry of Health, Labour and Welfare, 2013. www.mhlw.go.jp/seisakunitsuite/bunya/kodomo/kodomo_kosodate/dv/dl/120502_11.pdf.
24. Okuyama M, Yamada F, Mizoguchi F. *Kodomo gyakutai taiou ishi no tameno kodomo gyakutai taiou/igaku shindan gaido [Pocket manual for responding to child abuse: Child abuse handling and medical diagnostic guide for doctors]*. 2011.
25. Centre for Maternal and Child Health Promotion. Maternal and child health handbook, English version, obtainable at http://bosui.or.jp/.
26. Sasakura K. Nyuuyouji yusaburare shoukougun (SBS) wo meguru giron no genzaichi [The present discussions on

shaken baby syndrome]. *Kikan Keiji Bengo.* 2020;103:53–9.

27. Tanaka K. *Sei hanzai jidou gyakutai sousa hando bukku [Handbook on sex crimes and child abuse]*. Tachibana-Shobou, 2014.
28. Kyodo News Service. 'Nyuuyouji yusaburi': Gyakutai ka enzai ka ['Shaken baby': Abuse or wrongful accusation]. 10 September 2019. www.47news.jp/3981900.html.
29. PwC Consulting Group. Jidou soudan jo niokeru gyakutai ni yoru nyuuyouji toubu gaishou jian heno taiou ni kansuru chousa kenkyuu jigyou houkoku-sho [Research and study on the response to cases of abusive head trauma in children's consultation centres: Project report]. www.pwc.com/jp/ja/knowledge/track-record/assets/pdf/r2cc-report-32aht.pdf.
30. Nakatani Y. Gyakutai ni yoru nyuuyouji toubu gaishou (AHT) wo meguru saibanrei no bunseki [Analysis on court decisions concerning abusive head trauma]. *Keijihou Journal.* 2021;70:33–61.
31. Murai T, Muraoka, K. (interview). Order in the court: Explaining Japan's 99.9% conviction rate. www.nippon.com/en/japan-topics/c05401/order-in-the-court-explaining-japan%E2%80%99s-99-9-conviction-rate.html.
32. SBS Review Project. https://shakenbaby-review.com/index_e.html.
33. Sasakura K. SBS/AHT to enzai [SBS/AHT and wrongful accusations and convictions]. *Hanzai to Keibatsu.* 2022;31:57–82.
34. Naruse G. Gyakutai ni yoru toubu gaishou (AHT) jiken no genjou to kadai [Present status and problems of abusive head trauma (AHT) cases]. *Kenshu.* 2021;876:7–14.
35. Sasakura K. Nyuuyouji yusaburare shoukougun (SBS) jiken to enzai [Shaken baby syndrome (SBS) cases and wrongful convictions]. *Konan Hougaku.* 2020;60(1–4):217.
36. Akita M. Nyuuyouji yusabrare shoukougun (SBS) kasetsu to enzaijiken: 2 tsu no gyakuten muzai hanketsu kara manabubeki koto [Shaken baby syndrome (SBS) hypothesis and wrongfully convicted cases: What we should learn from two overturned convictions]. *Enzai Hakusho.* 2020;2.
37. Kawakami H. Naze genshin ha ayamatte yuuzaihanketsu wo kudashi, kousoshin ha gyakuten muzai to shita noka [Why was the first instance convicted and the second instance acquitted?] *Iryou Hanrei Kaisetsu.* 2020;86:70.
38. Akita M. Teiirakka niyoru kanousei wo mitomete gyakuten muzai toshita jirei [The case where the possibility of short falls was recognized and the conviction was overturned]. *Kikan Keiji Bengo.* 2020;103:47.
39. Choudhary K, Servaes S, Slovis TL et al. Consensus statement on abusive head trauma in infants and young children. *Pediatric Radiology.* 2018;48:1048–65.
40. Findley KA, Risinger M, Barnes P et al. Feigned consensus: Usurping the law in shaken baby syndrome/abusive head trauma prosecutions. *Wisconsin Law Review.* 2019;4:1211–68.
41. Japanese Paediatric Society. Gyakutai ni yoru nyuuyouji toubu gaishou (Abusive head trauma in infants and children) ni taisuru Nihon Shounika Gakkai no kenkai [Opinion of the Japanese Paediatric Society on abusive head trauma in infants and children]. 2020. www.jpeds.or.jp/uploads/files/AHT_kenkai.pdf.
42. Mizoguchi F. AHT kyousoukyoku [AHT rhapsody]. *Child Abuse and Neglect.* 2020;22(3):351–6.
43. Nakayama Y, Sakai K. Jidou gyakutai ni tsuite (shouni ganka) [On child abuse (paediatric ophthalmology)] *Keisatsugaku Ronshu.* 2021;74(2):68–75.
44. Tanaka K. Gyakutai ni yoru toubu gaishou (AHT) jiken no kisochishiki [Basic knowledge on abusive head trauma cases]. *Keisatsugaku Ronshu.* 2020;73(9):142.
45. Sakai K. Kodomo gyakutai boushi wo meguru shihou no shiren to chousen [Tests and challenges of the judiciary on child abuse prevention]. *Kenshu.* 2020;860:22–8.

46. Shirai M. AHT jian ni okeru tekisetsu na rissho wo kakuho surutame no housakutou: kensatsu no tachiba kara [Ways to ensure appropriate presentation of evidence in AHT cases: from a prosecutor's perspective. Keijihou Journal.2021; 70:62-69.

47. Johnson DT. *The culture of capital punishment in Japan.* Palgrave, 2020. https://link.springer.com/content/pdf/10.1007%2F978-3-030-32086-7.pdf.

48. Akita M. Aitsugu SBS muzai hanketsu ga toumono [What successive SBS acquittals tell us]. *Keijihou Journal.* 2021;70 70–78.

49. Guthkelch N. Problems of infant retino-dural hemorrhage with minimal external injury. *Houston Journal of Health Law and Policy*. 2012;12:201–8.

Chapter 25

Shaken Baby Syndrome in Australia

Chris Brook and Michael Nott

25.1 Australia: Decades of Orthodoxy

In 1995, an infant was admitted to an Australian hospital with cerebral oedema and hypoxic brain damage, subdural haemorrhages, and bilateral retinal haemorrhages. The pathologist in this case reported a lack of external signs of injury. It was asserted that the trauma to the head causing the types of intracranial and ocular damage seen in this baby was a shaking injury. Elucidating further, it was argued that the mechanism of traumatic damage was associated with changes in the rate of velocity of the head by acceleration and deceleration forces, which resulted in shearing forces applied to the bridging veins around the brain and its surrounding membranes. It was asserted that these forces tore or ruptured blood vessels, leading to subdural haemorrhages.

The pathologist further reported that the post-mortem examination showed no evidence of a significant natural disease that would have contributed either directly or indirectly to cause the child's death. The reasoning and conclusions in this case were strikingly similar to cases prosecuted today in Australia under the 'diagnostic' label of 'shaken baby syndrome' (SBS) and/or 'abusive head trauma' (AHT) in both criminal and child protection courts.

The number of accusations in Australia that have led to convictions and/or child removal is difficult to calculate precisely, particularly because child protection courts do not publish relevant details. However, there are almost certainly scores of cases over the past three decades, likely hundreds.

In the criminal context, two levels of charges are available if an infant has died: child homicide/manslaughter and murder. Conviction for child homicide or manslaughter generally results in a sentence of 7 to 10 years or more,[1] while conviction for murder could result in 20 to 30+ years.[2] For this reason, defendants often take a plea deal on a child homicide or manslaughter charge rather than risk a murder conviction.[3] In cases where the child does not die, a parent may be charged with assault or grievous bodily harm. In the child protection context, prospects of successfully fighting the removal of children from their parents are low, rules of evidence generally do not apply, there is a lower burden of proof (on balance of probabilities), and there is less visibility and

1 For example, *R v Rowe* [2018] VSC 490 (31 August 2018), *R v Harvey* [2018], The *Queen v Vinaccia* [2019] VSC 683 (14 October 2019).

2 In the case of *R v Nicholas Baxter* in 2017 when Baxter, at the first trial, was found not guilty of murder by a jury but guilty of manslaughter, he was sentenced to 9 years in jail. Baxter was successful in appealing the manslaughter conviction and in retrial found not guilty by judge alone on 6 April 2021; as an example, Duane Lindsey received a 34-year sentence.

3 For example, Cameron Staples, who maintains his innocence after pleading guilty to child homicide and receiving a 9-year sentence.

scrutiny due to strict privacy rules surrounding the child protection courts (unless there is an appeal to higher courts).[4] In both criminal and child protection cases, the resource mismatch between the state and the accused is immense. Often parents who wish to defend a shaken baby allegation do not have the financial resources to do so.

A significant issue has been the currency of the shaken baby hypothesis in Australia, based on the SBS 'triad' as definitive of child abuse. It has gained almost blanket acceptance, without critique, within multiple institutions such as official investigative bodies, child protection units in hospitals, forensic medical institutions, and the judiciary. However, as outlined further in this chapter, when we consider a number of recent judicial decisions, institutionalised acceptance of the theory has recently shown signs of a shift. Nevertheless, despite recent cases questioning the diagnosis in Australian courts, there is evidence that the shaken baby hypothesis still carries significant weight in Australian institutions.

In Victoria, senior members of the top forensic medicine institute have provided opinions of shaking following orthodox diagnostic methods, similar to the example just provided. In the State of Queensland, the state's official corruption body, the Crime and Misconduct Commission (CMC), can investigate cases of suspected homicide, grievous bodily harm, and torture where the victim is under 16 years of age. The CMC can investigate cases where conventional practices have not proven effective, having the power to conduct hearings that require witnesses to attend and give evidence.[5] Witnesses in these hearings have no right to silence and cannot claim privilege against self-incrimination.[6] Evidence from these hearings can be utilised in later criminal trials. The CMC appears to consider the shaken baby hypothesis a valid medical diagnosis, stating that 'the most common cause of death resulting from child abuse is shaken baby syndrome'.[7] However, the CMC also acknowledges some of the challenges to SBS and the recent studies which have cast doubt on the SBS triad as definitive of child abuse.[8]

Likewise, the diagnosis, based on the triad, carries weight in the children's courts. For example, the former head of the Children's Court in New South Wales discussed at a 2012 seminar an appeal to a case of alleged non-accidental abusive head injury causing severe brain damage.[9] The parents contended that the medical conclusion of a 'shaken baby' was based on unsafe foundations and submitted that the existence of alternative hypotheses, together with the 'circular reasoning' of the 'science', meant that the Court could not comfortably be satisfied of the case against the parents.

Two doctors from the United States advanced alternative hypotheses as to the cause of the baby's brain damage, including meningitis or a congenital condition. The judge described them as professional expert witnesses who were nothing more than 'hired guns'

4 For example, the head judge of the NSW child protection court told an NSW Upper House parliamentary inquiry in 2017 that 99% of all cases (including shaken baby matters) are resolved in favour of the child protection agency on the first mention, which means that the child is removed from their parents.

5 See Crime and Misconduct Commission Research and Issues paper number 10, June 2013. This paper has not been updated since 2013.

6 See www.ccc.qld.gov.au/about-us/our-powers.

7 See Crime and Misconduct Commission Research and Issues paper number 10 June 2013, page 7, referencing Blumenthal 2002.

8 See Crime and Misconduct Commission Research and Issues paper number 10 June 2013, page 7.

9 *SS v Department of Human Services* [2010] NSWDC 279.

whose evidence was not directed at discovering the true cause but instead designed to create doubt as to the child protection agency's hypothesis of SBS. The judge said this doubt may be appropriate for a criminal standard of beyond reasonable doubt, but not a child protection standard of balance of probabilities. The judge further stated that cases involving suspected non-accidental head injury often rest entirely upon forensic evidence.[10] In other words, there are often no witnesses or other evidence to substantiate abuse. The New South Wales (NSW) Judicial Commission's *Children's Court of NSW Resources Handbook* restates this judge's comments.[11]

The currency of the hypothesis is further demonstrated by the Sydney's Children's Hospitals Network which states that AHT is a form of non-accidental brain injury and that SBS is a type of AHT.[12] This position was further consolidated with the Sydney Children's Hospital network supporting the international National Centre for Shaken Baby Syndrome Conference in 2019. Significant numbers of Australian participants attended from healthcare, child protection, law enforcement, and prosecution to learn what could be called the orthodox approach. In one instance, participants were advised that attacks on the SBS/AHT theory were 'largely not driven by science'.[13] The event was financially supported by the state of NSW's premier children's hospital network board and a unit of a department of the NSW Ministry of Health.[14]

25.2 Disruptions to the Orthodoxy

It has not, however, always been business as usual for the shaken baby orthodoxy in Australia. Indeed, there have been some remarkable disruptions in this 'same as it ever was' story. In 2001, Stuart Lee appealed to the Supreme Court of the Australian Capital Territory against his conviction for having shaken his 3-week-old daughter.[15] The appeal was heard by Justice Crispin, who overturned the conviction. The arguments addressed by Crispin J two decades ago are similar to the arguments put forward by shaken baby proponents today. Crispin J engages these arguments in detail, having determined that

> issues were raised as to whether certain witnesses were expert in the resolution of issues as to whether or not injuries had been caused to babies and/or young children by shaking. Such claims of expertise seem to have assumed some credibility within the medical profession, and at least one witness said that he would defer to baby shaking experts on some matters. However, that does not absolve the Court of the need to critically examine the relevant issues.

Crispin J found that '[t]he evidence revealed a paucity of empirical research on potentially critical issues':

> I accept that the medical witnesses have generally expressed scepticism about the possibility of the constellation of injuries occurring without a blow to the head or an episode of

[10] NSW Judicial Commission's *Children's Court of NSW Resources Handbook*, pages 408–20.

[11] NSW Judicial Commission's *Children's Court of NSW Resources Handbook*. See www.judcom.nsw.gov.au/publications/benchbks/children/CM_Forensic_evidence.html.

[12] See www.schn.health.nsw.gov.au/fact-sheets/abusive-head-trauma-aht.

[13] See Brian Holmgren [retired prosecutor], paper to the 2019 SBS international conference 'Legal and Medical Controversies surrounding SBS/AHT', September 2019.

[14] See https://dontshake.org/past/item/415-2019-sydney.

[15] *R v Lee* [2001] ACTSC 133 (21 December 2001).

shaking. However, I am not satisfied that such scepticism is warranted. The mere fact that a number of people, even a number of experts, believe something, does not warrant the conclusion that it must be true. The need for great force has not been demonstrated by empirical research, and for the reasons already given, I am not satisfied that it has been otherwise established.

Regarding the medical experts' reliance on a 'constellation' of findings, Crispin J remarked that

[t]he proposition that there is only one explanation for a constellation of injuries is obviously significant only if all of the injuries were caused in the same manner or, to put it another way, that all of the stars belong in that constellation. Yet many, if not all, of the medical opinions relied upon to exclude competing hypotheses seemed to betray an assumption that the injuries which [the child] had suffered must have been caused by shaking unless there was some other single cause capable of accounting for the whole constellation. Such an approach could obviously be justified only if the injuries had all been inflicted at the same time, or at least as a consequence of the one mechanism. However, that assumption is not necessarily, or in my opinion even probably, valid.

During the trial, as reported in the *Lee* appeal,

[s]everal of the medical experts referred to a paper apparently written in 1990, based upon interviews with people who had admittedly shaken babies. It was suggested that this study provided a basis by which the type of injuries caused by such actions could be determined. Some witnesses referred to the 'classic' pattern of injuries sustained in that manner and sought to draw, or at least support, conclusions as to the degree of force required to cause them, from the descriptions given by the admitted perpetrators.

Expert witness for the Crown Dr Packer referred to these confession-based studies as 'the best range of indicators we can get'. In regards to such confession evidence, Crispin J remarked that

[i]t would plainly be possible for a medical practitioner to read an account of injuries caused by people who admitted shaking their babies and to assume that any subsequent cases of similar injuries which he or she encountered during the course of his or her medical career had been similarly caused. In such circumstances a medical practitioner might later be able to assert that he or she had never seen a case in which injuries of that nature had been caused in any other manner. However, the conclusion would have been based upon circulatory reasoning and the accretion of experience would not have lent validity to it.

Regarding the difficulty of undertaking studies in this area, Crispin J states that '[t]he fact that it may be difficult to ascertain the truth does not relieve the Crown of the need to prove the defendant's guilt beyond reasonable doubt, nor does it permit the Court to act upon some lesser standard determined by reference to the quality of evidence available'.

On the difference between the evidence base for the assertion that shaking can cause these injuries and the evidence base that shaking can be diagnosed by reference to these injuries, Crispin J

was satisfied that evidence was admissible as to the opinions of each of the relevant experts that the injuries *could have been* caused by either a blow or by the baby being vigorously shaken. On the other hand, I find that the evidence was not admissible to the effect

> that the injuries were caused in that manner, whether by the accused or otherwise, or that they *could only have been* caused in that manner. The evidence suggests that such opinions would not be based wholly or even substantially on the expert's specialised body of knowledge as a paediatrician but, as in *HG v R*, on a combination of speculation, inference, and a process of reasoning beyond the relevant field of expertise.

Crispin J further stated that he did '*not accept that there is any adequate body of expertise extending to the degree of force required to cause particular injury or injuries beyond that basic proposition*', suggesting that he would have disallowed the evidence concerning force as it was '*unfairly prejudicial to the accused, misleading or confusing, or caused or resulted in an undue waste of time*' (emphasis added).

Further disruption occurred to the shaken baby orthodoxy in 2003, when Australian general practitioner Dr Mark Donohoe published an *Evidence Based Medicine* review of the SBS literature [1]. Donohoe described the vast majority of SBS literature as 'poor-quality original research, retrospective in nature, and without appropriate control groups', remarking that 'repeated opinions based on poor-quality data cannot improve the quality of evidence'. Donohoe concluded that 'the commonly held opinion that the finding of SDH [subdural haemorrhage] and RH [retinal haemorrhage] in an infant was strong evidence of SBS was unsustainable, at least from the medical literature'.

The shaken baby community dismissed Donohoe's findings, claiming they were 'poor scholarship' that 'failed to capture the breadth of SBS/AHT medical research' [2]. Yet they did not point to any studies he had missed that would provide the evidence Donohoe found lacking. Nor did they address the substantive issues of poor research methods Donohoe identified. Articles continue to be published without relevant control groups. The conclusions of Donohoe closely mirror those of the later Swedish SBU report (see Chapter 10). Likewise, the reaction of the SBS community to Donohoe's conclusions closely mirrors their reaction to the SBU report.

In 2008, Tomas Klamo was charged and convicted of manslaughter by an unlawful and dangerous act after the death of his 4-week-old son.[16] The cause of death had been reported from autopsy as subdural haemorrhage, which had two components – recent and old. The main part of the haemorrhage occurred within 24 hours before the death and underlying this was a small, older haemorrhage which occurred between 3 days to some weeks prior.

The Crown claimed that Klamo had shaken his 4-week-old son 2 weeks prior to his collapse and death and had further shaken the child hours before death. Klamo admitted to 'shaking' the baby in the first instance but claimed this had not been violent. Klamo won his appeal with Justice Maxwell, President of the Court of Appeal, finding that the medical evidence had left open possibilities of shaking or other trauma causing the older and recent haemorrhages, but also that there was no medical evidence positively indicating that either of these events had actually occurred. In other words, other possible causes had not been ruled out. Maxwell concluded that 'I am not persuaded that there was any other evidence which could have justified the jury in reaching an affirmative conclusion, beyond reasonable doubt, that the cause of the death was either a re-bleed or a fresh shaking.'

What was remarkable about the *Klamo* case were the efforts of the pathologist, Prof. Steven Cordner, to inform the Court of Appeal about his concern with the guilty verdict and the manner in which his evidence had been misunderstood at the trial [3]. According to

---

16 *R v Klamo* [2008] VSCA 75 (9 May 2008).

Cordner, he 'was never asked, and did not explicitly say, that the subdural haemorrhage (whether the older one or the more recent one) *must* have been the result of inflicted trauma' and he had left 'open the possibility it was related to birth trauma' [3]. Cordner and Justice Maxwell jointly used the failings of the trial as a launching pad for improving the way in which forensic evidence is presented in Victorian courts, leading to the creation and the establishment of a Practice Note entitled 'Expert Evidence in Criminal Trials', which came into force in 2014, providing a set of guidelines for the manner in which forensic evidence should be admitted in court [4]. Cordner warned that 'a category we have to be careful of is the diagnosis – or coming to conclusions of any sort – by exclusion' [3].

25.3 Admissibility of Expert Evidence in Australia: 'Specialised Knowledge' and Circumstantial Evidence

Despite these disruptions, shaken baby orthodoxy in Australia continues to be widely accepted and invoked, with its admissibility in criminal and children's courts routinely unchallenged. In Australia, expert opinion in the criminal jurisdiction is governed by the rules of evidence of each particular state (see also Chapter 19). Adherence to the rules of evidence can be highly variable and are often interpreted liberally by the courts and lawyers. Most states admit evidence under a uniform Evidence Act, although some states continue to use the common law rules, drawing from English jurisprudence.

The key factor is that an expert's opinion must be wholly or substantially based upon the expert's 'specialised knowledge' [s 79 (1) Evidence Act 1995 NSW]. An essential precondition of this specialised knowledge is that it is the product of 'study, training or experience'. If the expert has undertaken some study or training in relation to that particular issue, then other conditions come into play. One of these other conditions is that the expert's opinion has to be derived from facts which have been or will be proven in evidence.

The expert opinion evidence rules were focused in the decision of (then) Heydon JA in *Makita (Australia) Pty Ltd v Sprowles* [2001] NSWCA 305b. In short, this decision noted that, if evidence tendered as expert opinion evidence is to be admissible, it must be agreed or demonstrated that there is a field of 'specialised knowledge'; there must be an identified aspect of that field in which the witness demonstrates that, by reason of specified training, study, or experience, the witness has become an expert; the opinion proffered must be 'wholly or substantially based on the witness's expert knowledge'; so far as the opinion is based on facts 'observed' by the expert, they must be identified and admissibly proved by the expert and so far as the opinion is based on 'assumed' or 'accepted' facts, they must be identified and proved in some other way; it must be established that the facts on which the opinion is based form a proper foundation for it; and the opinion of an expert requires demonstration or examination of the scientific or other intellectual basis of the conclusions reached. That is, the expert's evidence must explain how the field of 'specialised knowledge' in which the witness is expert by reason of 'training, study or experience' and on which the opinion is 'wholly or substantially based' applies to the facts assumed or observed so as to produce the opinion propounded.

Later in the High Court Heydon J in *Dasreef Pty Ltd v Hawchar* [2011] at [91], further addressed this final point concerning the statement of reasoning rule, affirming that '[a]t common law there is no doubt that an expert opinion is inadmissible unless the expert states in chief the reasoning by which the expert conclusion arrived at'. The 'reasoning must be stated', Hayden J noted, and '[t]he opposing party is not to be left to find out about the expert's thinking for the first time in cross-examination'.

Justice Heydon in *Dasreef* noted that Sir Owen Dixon, speaking extrajudicially, said: 'courts cannot be expected to act upon opinions the basis of which is unexplained'. Further, in *R v Jenkins; Ex parte Morrison*, Fullagar J quoted that specific statement with approval and added that expert scientific witnesses should be asked to 'explain the basis of theory or experience' on which their conclusions rest. He also articulated that, on appeal, Rich and Dixon JJ approved what Fullagar J had said and stated that the witness must explain the basis of theory or experience because the court is not limited to examining the conclusion or the expertise of the expert witness. It must look to the 'substance of the opinion expressed'. They said, since choosing between conflicting experts depends in part on 'impressiveness and cogency of reasoning', their 'processes of reasoning' must be identified. Additionally, he referred to the Victorian Court of Appeal (Winneke P, Charles and Chernov JJA), which stated in *R v Juric* [2002] VSCA 77 (29 May 2002): '[t] he jury must be able to evaluate the strength of [expert opinion] evidence by reference to its factual or scientific basis'.

The link between facts and the opinion should be in accordance with established scientific principles. The existence of established scientific principles should be supported by references in the scientific literature, which will refer to the studies which have established those principles. It is also a requirement in mandatory codes of conduct for expert witnesses to provide any literature or other materials utilised in support of any opinions. Without those facts and scientific principles being in play, the apparent inference or opinion is no more than 'speculation', which cases such as *Straker* and *Wood* have shown to be inadmissible.[17]

Unlike other countries, a 'reliability' test is not imposed or required in Australia. Indeed, a requirement of scientific reliability has been expressly rejected by the High Court in *Honeysett* [2014]. Attempts to legislate to include a reliability standard have not occurred. At least theoretically, this leaves experts more room to provide unsubstantiated opinions than in the United States, where *Daubert* or *Frye* standards apply. However, a study comparing the admission of forensic evidence in the United States, the United Kingdom, Canada, and Australia, found that, once an expert demonstrates their training, studies, and/or experience, then 'there is almost no expert testimony so threadbare that it will not be admitted if it comes to a criminal proceeding under the banner of forensic science' [5]. A leading expert on admissibility rules for forensic science in Australia, Prof. Gary Edmond, writes that 'in *Dasreef* v *Hawchar* the High Court indicated that "in many, perhaps most, cases" the requirements of s 79(1) of the Evidence Act can be satisfied "very quickly and easily . . . once the witness has described his or her qualifications and experience, and has identified the subject matter about which the opinion is proffered. This approach – really a "short cut" – has been applied to many types of forensic science and medicine evidence'. However, Edmond advised where reliability is a serious issue some courts use it implicitly in their application of s 79(1) or s 137 of the Evidence Act 1995 NSW.[18]

Therefore, despite the rules of evidence, courts in Australia are very liberal in allowing opinions to be expressed by an expert. It is left to the opposing legal teams to challenge the

[17] Straker v Queen (19770 51 ALJR 690, Wood v R [2012] NSWCA 21[see also: *Dasreef Pty Ltd v Hawchar* [2011] HCA21at 91]).

[18] Personal communication with Michael Nott, Monday, 27 April 2020.

opinions. If the opinion is not challenged, it remains in evidence. Experts who are well credentialed, such as medical doctors, are generally very free to express opinions without having to show that they are based on reliable science. Professor Edmond notes that it is increasingly obvious over the past decade that the manner in which Australian courts admit, present, and evaluate scientific, technical, and medical evidence, is in many ways inconsistent with the recommendations and advice of peak scientific and technical organisations [6].

The steps outlined in the uniform Evidence Act are no more than a simple checklist, but as noted, are often ignored by experts and the prosecution in shaking baby cases. Experts have provided orthodox shaken baby testimony for decades in Australia. More often than not, the testimony stands without being challenged and without experts being called by the defence, who most often concede that abuse occurred and base their defence on identity (e.g., *R. v Harvey* 2018) or uncertainty surrounding degree of force (e.g., *R v Vinaccia* 2019).

The assumed or the primary facts used by an expert when they form their opinion must be proven – in other words, the expert opinion must be supported by the primary evidence.[19] This aspect of admissibility was used successfully by the defence in the 2021 Townsville shaking baby case of *Baxter*, who had been charged with manslaughter of his 6-week-old son, allegedly by shaking. The prosecution experts were found by North J to have made 'falsified assumptions' that were 'fatal' to the prosecution (*R v Baxter* [2021] QSC 70 at 254, 256).

The prosecution had relied upon a series of links in a circumstantial case, each link necessary to establish the case. In a circumstantial case, the prosecution must prove every link in the chain of evidence beyond reasonable doubt (see *R v Baxter* [2021] QSC 70 at 255). The key issue in Baxter was the matter of rupture or tearing of the bridging veins. The prosecution alleged that the rupture or tearing of the bridging veins was caused by the child being subject to acceleration/deceleration and/or circular rotational forces and that this process precipitated the medical findings in the deceased child. However, there was no provable evidence that the bridging veins were ruptured or torn, as asserted by the prosecution's expert radiologist and paediatrician. Justice North reverted to the opinion of the prosecution neuropathologist, who examined the child's brain and noted 'there was no evidence of any torn bridging vein or venous source either on the surface or localised subarachnoid haemorrhage'. This evidence contradicted the radiologist's hypothesis of torn bridging veins, which was an essential inference to his hypothesis. Justice North stated, '[m] y finding that there were no torn bridging veins within [the child's] brain is contrary to one of the essential links in the circumstantial case propounded by the Crown. It is trite law that each link in such a circumstantial case must be proven beyond reasonable doubt' (see *R v Baxter* [2021] QSC 70 at 255). Justice North entered a verdict of not guilty.

In addition to the fact that the tearing of bridging veins is assumed, rather than proven, it also needs to be remembered that the hypothesis that the tearing of bridging veins is the mechanism underpinning SBS has not been validated scientifically and has no measure of reliability. Additionally, assertions by prosecution experts regarding degree of force, which were rejected in 2001 by Justice Crispin in *Lee* as lacking an evidence base, are still made today and accepted by the courts. In the evidence of the expert witness for the prosecution in the Victorian Supreme Court of Appeal in November 2021, it was stated: 'We just simply don't know the force required' (*Vinaccia v R*, S EAPCR 2020 0184 25 November 2021).

---

19 *Dasreef Pty Limited v Hawchar* [2011] HCA 21 per Hayden J at 90.

Thus a question arises: if it is not known what level of force is required, then there is no scientific foundation or 'any adequate body of expertise' surrounding a fundamental issue required for the prosecution to proceed in an allegation of SBS. As Professor Cordner suggested to the court in the 2008 *Klamo* case, there is no evidence base that allows an answer to the question 'Is it always the case that the shaking has to be so severe that the person doing it would have some understanding that some harm might result?' Thus expert opinion concerning acceleration/deceleration and/or circular rotational forces is not a proper matter for expert opinion (see *Makita*, *Dasreef*, and *Sanrus* and opinion evidence asserting acceleration/deceleration forces causing injuries *should be* inadmissible).[20] However, most often, such opinions are not ruled inadmissible and the consequence is that many defendants in Australian criminal cases are found guilty of shaking the infant. Similar assertions are also still being provided to the child protection courts, without the scientific line of reasoning as required by evidence law.

References

1. Donohoe M. Evidence-based medicine and shaken baby syndrome part I: Literature review, 1966–1998. *American Journal of Forensic and Medical Pathology*. 2003;24:239–41.
2. Narang S. A Daubert analysis of abusive head trauma/shaken baby syndrome. 11 *Houston Journal of Health Law and Policy*. 2011;11:505–7, 539–60.
3. Cordner S. *R v Klamo*: An example of miscommunication and misunderstanding of expert evidence where the conviction was overturned. *Australian Journal of Forensic Sciences*. 2012;44(4):323–31.
4. Maxwell C. *R v Klamo*: An example of miscommunication and misunderstanding of expert evidence where the conviction was later overturned. *Australian Journal of Forensic Sciences*. 2014;46(1):4–7. https://doi.org/10.1080/00450618.2013.784359.
5. Edmond G, Cole S, Cunliffe E, Roberts A. Admissibility compared: The reception of incriminating expert evidence (i.e. forensic science) in four adversarial jurisdictions. *University of Denver Criminal Law Review*. 2013;3(1):31–109.
6. Edmond G. Regulating forensic science and medicine evidence at trial: It's time for a wall, a gate and some gatekeeping. *Australian Law Journal*. 2020;94:427–43.

[20] *Makita (Australia) Pty Ltd v Sprowles* (2001) NSWLR *705* at [85]; *Dasreef Pty Ltd v Hawchar* (2011) 243 CLR 588 [69]; and [91]–[94]; Sanrus *Pty Ltd & Ors v Monto Coal 2 Pty Ltd & Ors* (No 5) [2019] QSC 210 at [45]–[52]; see also *R v Ping* [2005] QCA 472 at [43]–[46].

Chapter 26

Shaken Baby Syndrome around the World

Multiple Authors

This chapter describes how countries around the world are addressing alleged child abuse and/or shaken baby syndrome/abusive head trauma (SBS/AHT). It includes contributions from the following countries: China, India, Israel, Luxembourg, Norway, New Zealand, South Korea, Spain, Taiwan, Ecuador, Peru, Argentina and Costa Rica, with the last four countries responding via a collective interview conducted with a group of medical examiners and a neurosurgeon from those countries. Separate chapters in the law and international sections of this book cover the United States (Chapters 18–20), Great Britain (Chapter 21), France (Chapter 22), Sweden (Chapter 23), Japan (Chapter 24), and Australia (Chapter 25).

The same set of questions were asked to each contributor in order to compare the answers. The answers were then edited and combined to form this chapter. The questions asked were the following:

1. How prevalent is child abuse in your country? Please briefly describe the history/development of child protection guidelines in your country. Most importantly, do you have mandatory reporting of suspected abuse to authorities?
2. Please briefly describe the history/development of SBS/AHT hypothesis and medical determinations in your country, if any. Can you provide an approximate timeline regarding when SBS/AHT medical determinations started to be made in your country? Is the sole presence of components of the triad (subdural haemorrhage (SDH) and retinal haemorrhage (RH), brain swelling) sufficient to make a medical determination of SBS/AHT?
3. How has case law and legislation (if any) concerning SBS/AHT cases developed? What are the legal standards for scientific evidence in criminal cases? Are you aware of any important court decisions in your country in these cases?
4. Have there been any government-sponsored reviews of the science underlying SBS/AHT? (e.g., the systematic Swedish review of SBS/AHT published in 2016 by the Swedish Agency for Health Technology (SBU)).
5. Is the defence allowed to bring its own medical experts? If so, have there been any difficulties in getting these experts to testify in court? Are these defence experts from your country or from abroad?
6. Is SBS/AHT used as a basis to remove babies from their families in family/administrative courts in your country? If so, by which process?
7. Do you have any idea of the approximate nationwide annual number of:
   (a) medical determinations of SBS/AHT,
   (b) prosecution of SBS/AHT cases,
   (c) acquittals/exonerations of defendants in SBS/AHT cases?

As the readers go through this chapter, they will see how different countries have employed diverse strategies to fight child abuse and SBS/AHT. The prevalence of SBS/AHT hypothesis also appears to differ from country to country: indeed, in some countries the SBS/AHT hypothesis has not been implemented at all, while in others it has already gained the full attention of the medical community as well as academia, not to mention public agencies and law enforcement, sometimes as early as the 1990s. Several countries report criminal/ family (or administrative) court cases of SBS/AHT, while others report none at all. Then, some countries have seen several exonerations in criminal cases in which the defendants have vigorously challenged the SBS hypothesis, whereas in others the accusation virtually always leads to conviction. The information collected in this chapter and in the other chapters in Section 5 of this book (Chapters 21–25) reveal some of the possible causes behind these major differences and raise many interesting questions.

This chapter would not have been written had it not been for the contributions of dedicated authors from each country. We truly thank the contributors: Amy Gao (China), Aiyar Suranya (India), Irit Shlesinger-Zribi (Israel), Michael Mittelbronn (Luxembourg), Knut Wester (Norway), Felicity Goodyear-Smith (New Zealand), Guadalupe Blanco Velasco and Maria Cabezas Garcia (Spain), the Innocence Project Taiwan (Taiwan), and Myeonki Kim (South Korea). We would also like to thank the five medical examiners from Argentina, Ecuador, and Costa Rica, as well as Maria José Hidalgo and Lisset Hechavarria Andrial (Ecuador), Hugo Llerena Miranda (Peru), Jorge Perez (Costa Rica) and Juan Carlos Toulouse, Inés Aparici, Jorge Pereyra, and Maria Beatriz Vazquez (Argentina), all of whom provided answers to an interview conducted by Dr Marta Cohen.

26.1 Prevalence of Abuse by Country

While no country disputes the existence of child abuse, its definition – in particular the sometimes fine line that separates discipline or simply traditional behaviour from abuse – differs widely from country to country. **India**, which established a basic charter on child welfare as early as the 1950s, has no statistics on child abuse, and a United Nations International Children's Emergency Fund (UNICEF) report estimating that one in five children experience abuse is considered exaggerated and misleading by some. In particular, the UNICEF report may interpret as abuse practices that are viewed as legitimate and positive in Indian society, concerning, for example, filial obedience and duty, while the increasingly frequent practice of protecting children from physical punishment may be perceived in India as an attack on the family unit.

The Ministry for Women and Children was created in 2006, but some of its activities (such as rounding up street children in Delhi and placing them in state care) came to be understood as cruel and the Ministry was abandoned. Recent initiatives in India have made reporting mandatory in cases of sexual abuse and have instituted hotlines that children themselves may call in case of abuse. However, no form of mandatory reporting exists for general child abuse and indeed family doctors tend to prefer to help the family. One notable particularity of Indian society is that extended families live together and mothers are rarely alone with their children, leading to a higher level of help for exasperated parents and a higher level of surveillance for mobile babies, and significantly diminishing opportunities for unwitnessed child abuse.

In **China** also, a long tradition of respect for discipline and the family unit has slowed the development of child protection laws. No national statistics are available on the incidence of child abuse, although small-scale studies have shown it to be extremely prevalent, but, then again, the prevalence depends strongly on the definition; in one study, as many as 62% of children aged 9–12 were victims of some form of physical abuse. Sexual abuse and trafficking are the forms of abuse most frequently addressed in Chinese law, with tens of thousands of cases prosecuted each year.

Although a law prohibiting abuse of minors has existed since 1991 and has been revised and updated several times, and a new law against abuse of individuals in care was passed in 2015, China has no explicit law against child abuse. However, a law has been proposed that would explicitly criminalise child abuse and implement a mandatory reporting system. This law would expose to sanctions anyone who would fail to report any suspicion of child abuse.

The notion of mandatory reporting does exist in China, and reporting is encouraged although it is not yet legally mandatory. Such reporting is considered to have brought a large number of cases to light.

Persons hired to work with children in China must undergo a mandatory background check and a database of offenders is available for consultation by employers. However, concerning parents and guardians, it is notable that reporting does not lead to immediate removal of the child. Rather, the accused guardians' failure, whether it consists in insufficiently supervising or actually victimising the child, leads to a custody supervision of the guardians that is intended to motivate them and give them a chance to improve their behaviour before losing custody.

Twenty years ago, child abuse was considered in **South Korea** as a purely domestic affair concerning parents' choice of discipline. This situation has changed considerably since then, partly due to an explosion in cases reaching hospitals; the large majority of cases are due to parental abuse (82%), with a minority due to abuse by other caretakers. The duty to report was legally established in 2000 along with the creation of 17 centres for child protection, a number that has since quadrupled.

The rate of reported child abuse in 2020 in South Korea was about 373 cases per 100,000 children, leading to child abuse being deemed a major problem today. Mandatory reporting has been instituted for all medical personnel, teachers, public officials, and persons involved in child protection. Mandatory reporting is considered to be responsible for identifying about 28% of known cases.

Taiwan also has a high rate of reported child abuse cases – nearly 400 out of 100,000 children on yearly average since 2012. Mandatory reporting was initiated quite early in Taiwan, with a 1993 law requiring reporting of all suspected cases by medical personnel, social workers, educators and day care staff, police, and any other individual dealing professionally with children. The law was updated in 2003 to specify new methods of reporting. In 2011, reporting was made mandatory for officials at the village level, and, in 2015, it was extended to preschool educators and immigration personnel. All mandatory reporting must take place within 24 hours. The yearly data show relatively stable numbers since 2015.

Spain has a somewhat lower official prevalence of child abuse with 235 confirmed cases per 100,000 in 2019, although, depending on the definition, some studies show that up to 25% of children suffer some form of maltreatment. The first law on protection of children in Spain appeared in 1904 and concerned the welfare of abandoned children. This attitude of concentrating protection on abandoned children continued through the Spanish Civil War.

Following the war, a social aid organisation was created to help children whose lives had been devastated by the war; unfortunately, the organisation was suspected of removing children from their homes to have them adopted by families in line with the political dictatorship. Only after the dictatorship came to an end in 1978 did the new Spanish constitution refer explicitly to the need to protect all minors. In 1981, the Civil Code was modified to confer full individual rights on minors and, in 1987, a law was passed giving parents/guardians and the state joint responsibility for protecting children. A new law in 1996 stressed the paramount interest of the child and, in 2000, laws appeared regulating the protocol in case of offences against minors. The latest reforms, in 2021, address child sexual abuse and pornography and institute mandatory reporting of any crime against children.

In **Israel**, child abuse is treated with severity and is subject to harsher punishments than abuse of non-minors; sanctions are particularly severe in the case of abuse by anyone who has legal responsibility for the child (parents, teachers, carers, social workers, etc.). Reporting of suspicion has been mandatory for a specific set of professionals (doctors, teachers, social workers, psychologists, etc.) since 1989 and failure to report is a criminal offence.

Israel prefers to place children removed from the home in residential centres or boarding schools rather than foster care, which is considered a risk to the family unit, whereas a child at boarding school is protected but still belongs to his or her own family. When the choice is made to place a child at a centre, social workers' main concern is to re-establish family relations.

Because of the kibbutz-like nature of residential care, it was viewed quite positively in the past, but is less so now. From a placement rate of about 380 children in 100,000 in 2000, today that number has diminished to 340. There are many less absolute alternatives to placement for at-risk children, such as sending them to after-school day care centres; however, removing fewer children from the home does increase the number of at-risk children.

In **Luxembourg**, all professionals are required to report any suspicion of a crime and will suffer no consequences for unjustified reporting. Non-assistance to a person in danger is also criminal, so ordinary citizens themselves are also required to report if they have knowledge of a situation of danger for a child.

In **Norway**, the prevalence of child abuse and child protection cases is unknown as there is no national registry. In the period 2004–15, there were 17 criminal cases in the court registry (in a population of about 5 million and 55,000 live births each year), which amounts to one new case every year. Both lay and professional persons may report suspected child abuse. For professional persons, mainly in healthcare, this is mandatory according to the child protection law.

In **New Zealand**, no prevalence data are available due to the impossibility of finding an adequate definition of child abuse. The mortality rates are known; there were on average 1.2 deaths due to child abuse per 100,000 children during the 5-year period 1990–95. This situation has improved slightly, with an average of 1.01 per 100,000 in the 5-year period 2015–19 (11 deaths under 1 year, 19 deaths 1–4 years, 6 from 5–15). The director of a major child protection centre has called since the 1990s for mandatory reporting by generalists and other health professionals; however, it does not exist at present as there is a countermovement indicating the arbitrary nature of the decision and the risk of harm to innocent families. There is a form of mandatory reporting in hospitals; however, it leads to a concerted investigation plan, not to immediate removal.

Between 1950 and 1992, the Oranga Tamariki (Ministry for Children) of **New Zealand** removed more than 100,000 children from their homes and placed them in state care, where many assert that they were abused. While the number of removals has diminished since then, the Maori population is still targeted, which has led to political movements and demonstrations. In 2021, New Zealand announced that it will virtually halt removals of at-risk children.

Some South American countries declare a high prevalence of child abuse. **Ecuador** has regulations aiming at the protection of children, but the institutions do not adequately guarantee their application. There are unfortunate cases of neglect or re-victimisation due to lack of attention from the authorities. **Peru** also has a high level of violence towards children. There is a telephone hotline and media attention is given to the issue, as well as a system of mandatory reporting, but it continues. **Argentina** also has a high prevalence, although the country adheres to UNICEF good practice guidelines and to the Convention on the Rights of the Child as the constitutional basis for laws protecting children. Argentina also has a system of mandatory reporting, a hotline to denounce child abuse that was created in 2009, and a government bureau specifically dealing with public policies on childhood and adolescence, the Secretaría Nacional de Niñez, Adolescencia y Familia (SENAF). In **Costa Rica**, 1 out of 5 deaths of children was attributed to violence in 2019 and the number was revised upwards to 1 in 3 in 2020.

26.2 The History and Development of the Shaken Baby Syndrome/Abusive Head Trauma Hypothesis and Medical Determinations of Abuse

While a retrospective study covering the period 2013–21 revealed 48 cases of possible AHT from a review of medical files, the diagnosis is not officially used at present in **India**. One of the reasons for this is cultural, as babies are raised by extended families, and in rural areas and slums life takes place largely outdoors. Furthermore, the poor tend to spend time on the floor as opposed to furniture while the middle class and the wealthy almost always have maids to help with housework and childcare. Thus, in the Indian lifestyle, mothers are rarely alone with their babies, which diminishes the stress and exasperation in moments of inconsolable crying and also provides witnesses to health events. Fathers generally participate little in childrearing, all of which reduces many typical opportunities for abuse.

Similarly, although pathologists in **China** perform complete autopsies in all cases of death due to suspected child abuse, SBS/AHT is not well known and the diagnosis is never made. The media is just beginning to make the public aware of the dangers of shaking and tossing babies, using information provided by hospitals, but the purpose of these reports is preventive, to warn parents of the danger. Preventive education of new mothers is increasing, although only 5% of new mothers have heard about the danger of shaking at present.

In **South Korea**, SBS has been the object of a few medical publications since 2003 which examine a handful of cases. Following the European examples, these articles conclude that the triad indicates violent shaking. However, the diagnosis remains purely scientific and has not been established as a criminal act of child abuse.

In **Taiwan**, diagnoses of SBS or non-accidental trauma from SDH, RH, and so forth have been made since 2002, although the number of cases remains very small. Instead of the brain swelling usually associated with the triad, Taiwan identifies delirium as the third symptom of SBS. A 2020 paper published by a medical examiner asserts that the isolated symptoms are not sufficient to conclude that shaking has taken place and that accidental trauma can also be a cause.

Spain has used the term 'SBS' in court in 58 trials since 1997. However, the definition varies and there is a lot of disagreement, especially as to whether the isolated triad suffices to conclude that shaking has taken place; generally, further signs are sought and there is an extended search for differential diagnoses.

The situation in **Israel** corresponds closely to that in the United States and Western Europe, in that Israeli common law has recognised SBS/AHT since the early 2000s, in part according to medical protocols applied in hospitals which sees signs of the triad as grounds for suspecting abuse. Doctors in Israel are ordered to report to the police or social services cases in which there are no other explanations (such as traffic accidents) for observed triad signs. Most medical experts in Israel agree that the presence of the triad is sufficient for a medical diagnosis of SBS/AHT.

The situation in **Luxembourg** is not as rigid; one doctor reports: 'for me, the triad (SDH, RH, and brain swelling) is definitely not enough to diagnose SBS/AHT'. In order to justify the diagnosis of SBS/AHT, he further considers intracerebral haemorrhages (localisation, potential temporal course), diffuse axonal injury (with a special focus on APP) and the morphology (axon positivity, axonal swelling, axonal constriction, axonal bulb/spheroid formation, and orientation in 3D), and often associates the result with a focal trauma (external injury and internal coup/contrecoup), in contradiction with many doctors in Western Europe who consider multifocal SDH an automatic indicator of shaking. Shaken baby syndrome as a diagnosis exists, but it is not automatic, and therefore the triad does not lead to automatic mandatory reporting since it can be found by doctors without suspicion of child abuse.

In **Norway**, the term 'shaken baby syndrome' has probably been in use since 2001–03, when it was imported from Sweden shortly after it was introduced there from the United States. The 'diagnosis' is made on the basis of components of the triad.

Shaken baby syndrome has been a recognised diagnosis in **New Zealand** from the 1990s. A public website warns parents about the dangers of shaking, describing the possible effects as seizures, drowsiness/lethargy, inability to feed, and so forth, as well as serious complications such as paralysis, blindness, developmental delays, and broken ribs. An article appeared in 2020 specifically advising ophthalmologists who find RH in babies to diagnose shaking, stating that 'RHs are exceedingly rare in accidental head trauma'. In the same article, ophthalmologists are warned that saying their observations are 'consistent with non-accidental head trauma' is insufficient; they need to go further and explain exactly why their findings are not consistent with accidental trauma or any other explanation, a piece of advice which might seem to encourage the search for differential diagnoses, except that most of these are ruled out in the same paper as possible causes for RH. A 10-year review of 519 children with structural head injury noted a large number of infants < 6 months with SDH and no atraumatic explanation (i.e., disease), and concluded that 'it must be seriously considered that the history is false'.

In **Ecuador**, the elements of the triad may be considered sufficient to make a medical determination of SBS/AHT, but not necessarily; there is no obligation and no action that must be taken. The prevailing information is drawn from international scientific articles. There have been no Ecuadorian studies on the subject apart from bibliographical reviews of the literature. In Peru, the presence of the triad is sufficient to make a medical determination of SBS/AHT, and such determinations have been made since the 1990s and increasingly since 2010 with media support. Children with suspected AHT are given prompt and full support.

The case of **Argentina** is interesting, as it was held in the past that the triad was sufficient to diagnose SBS/AHT, but today it must be part of a set of findings in a criminal context. While SBS garnered a lot of attention especially between 2000 and 2010, leaving a strong imprint on the courts, the idea has now spread that the sole presence of components of the triad is not necessarily indicative of shaking. In particular, RH, previously considered pathognomonic for abuse, is no longer thus considered and other causes are recognised as possible; there are some Argentinian publications on this topic. In **Costa Rica**, while the presence of the triad commonly raises suspicion of abuse, most forensic pathologists do not consider it pathognomonic for shaking.

26.3 Case Law and Legislation on Shaken Baby Syndrome/Abusive Head Trauma

There are no cases of SBS in **India**. In **China**, while there is no specific SBS/AHT case law, there are some criminal cases in which shaking contributed to a child's death in conjunction with other acts of violence. It seems there have been no cases based on elements of the triad alone with no external injuries. Nanny cams (cameras monitoring nanny behaviour) have been responsible for uncovering numerous cases of nannies shaking and otherwise abusing children, which are reported in the media; however, none of these cases have led to serious injury or SBS. These cases are prosecuted and frequently encounter a defence of the type 'This is the common way to care for babies where I come from', and 'lightly shaking or tossing babies is a good way to put them to sleep or stop them crying'. Expert witnesses are allowed in Chinese courts and the value of their evidence is judged by the court according to criteria such as the expert's credentials, the chain of custody of the evidence, and conflict with the opinions of other experts.

In **South Korea**, while SBS has been mentioned in court cases since 2010, there seem to be no cases founded on SBS or on the triad alone; virtually all cases, at least those that are made public, show obvious external trauma (such as when a child falls after being tossed). The standard for expert evidence in South Korea is quite similar to the American *Daubert* standard (the scientific evidence is probative when 'an expert with sufficient ability draws a conclusion by using standard techniques and all premises are true and the method of inference is scientifically justified'). However, the Korean Supreme Court did not clearly state whether these factors were the standard for the admissibility issue or probative value issue. This is because most criminal trials in South Korea are bench trials, so the admissibility of evidence is not as strict.

There have been only 12 cases in **Taiwan** since 2001 explicitly mentioning SBS, but it is doubtful whether any of them were based on the triad symptoms alone. Presiding judges may select expert witnesses among individuals possessing the requisite expert knowledge.

There appear to be no specific laws or important court decisions in **Spain** directly addressing SBS. Expert reports and forensic evidence are not binding for the judge or the court. Based on Spanish legislation, the judge assesses everything based on their 'sana crítica' (sound judicial discretion). This concept is not regulated, but the Supreme Court judgments state that it is an 'integrated system under logic, scientific, and experience rules', paying attention to elements such as the sturdiness of conclusions, details, and accuracy of arguments, operations, and means used to support conclusions or experts' competency.

Similarly, there are no laws in **Israel** pertaining specifically to SBS/AHT. Legal development on the issue has occurred mainly through court rulings on SBS cases; however, there have been few of these and, in all of them, infants were observed to have suffered from additional injuries besides brain damage, which strengthened the suspicion that violence was used. It seems there have been no cases based on elements of the triad alone and the validity of the triad to diagnose shaking has not arisen in court.

The most substantial case in Israel concerned a father convicted of shaking his two children, leading to the death of one. As part of his appeal, the court did discuss the defence claim that there are other explanations for the observed triad components and produced various experts who challenged the triad's exclusivity. The Supreme Court stated that there is scientific debate regarding SBS/AHT but that this debate was not relevant in the specific case since there was other external evidence beyond the triad on which to base the father's conviction. Israeli law has yet to rule on the scientific disagreements surrounding the triad.

In **Luxembourg**, the issue appears not to have come yet before the courts, but in **Germany**, there have been several cases including at least one very high-profile case (Baby Nils). Decisions in Germany are mainly based on expert opinion; there are no national guidelines and therefore experts are all reading the primary sources. In **New Zealand**, there have been several high-profile cases. In one particular case from 2006, extremely premature 2-month-old twins became unresponsive while in the care of their 21-year-old father; they were brought to the hospital where they both died. The medical examination concluded that they had all the classic signs of SBS but further signs of direct blows or impacts with a hard surface. Although the coroner concluded that the injuries were inflicted on the twins at home during a certain time period when they were alone with their father, he was nevertheless acquitted. This case led to strong recommendations for new legislation aimed at identifying and protecting at-risk children and instituting mandatory reporting for health professionals.

In **Norway**, there appear to be no standards for scientific evidence in criminal cases. The term 'SBS' was incorporated into the existing child protection law on physical child abuse. Out of 17 cases between 2004 and 2015, research has suggested that the *intracranial* findings are compatible with a non-traumatic aetiology in 16.

In **Ecuador**, there is no legal standard for scientific evidence in SBS cases, whereas, in **Peru**, there is jurisprudence and specific legislation. In **Argentina**, although there is no specific legislation for SBS cases, specialists are called into court as expert witnesses. The standards are based on scientific papers, personal experience, and validated study methodology. Court verdicts are rarely shared with the experts. In two cases in Tierra del Fuego, a family member was imprisoned although rickets is endemic in that region and could have been a differential diagnosis. On the other hand, short falls were accepted as differential diagnoses for SBS-like symptoms in two other cases.

26.4 Government-Sponsored Reviews of the Science Underlying Shaken Baby Syndrome/Abusive Head Trauma

India and **China** have no government-sponsored reviews. Shaken baby syndrome/abusive head trauma is not a recognised scientific discipline and there is no community of 'experts'.

Since SBS/AHT is not a very serious social problem in **South Korea**, there has not been any government-funded research focusing solely on SBS/AHT. However, as interest in child abuse in general grew, the South Korean National Forensic Research Institute was awarded a government grant to study all child abuse death cases that were autopsied. There exists also a single medical report in Taiwan which devotes three pages to SBS, written after the author, the chief medical examiner of the Institute of Forensic Medicine of the Ministry of Justice, had completed training in the United States.

To date, **Spain**, **Israel**, **Luxembourg**, **Norway**, and **New Zealand** have produced no government report dealing with SBS/AHT. However, a literature review of publications discussing AHT was published in New Zealand, albeit in a non-systematic manner with no explicit method for locating and assessing the literature. This review, covering the diagnosis in the United States as well as international epidemiological studies, legal processes, and outcomes in selected countries, was published in New Zealand, which explicitly includes shaking alone as one possible mechanism of injury. The report concludes quite strongly in favour of the SBS diagnosis.

> Diagnosis, legal interventions and outcomes and ultimately prevention depend upon the medical resources and training of medical professionals in that country, and level of recognition of the problem. Many Western countries are faced with challenges to the diagnosis in the legal system that have not served the interests of abused children. Such challenges have only increased the adversarial nature of proceedings. Highly paid defence experts, mostly from the US and the UK, travel internationally to refute and challenge a diagnosis that has a strong history and evolution of research to support its basis.

South American countries document no government report on SBS/AHT at all.

26.5 Defence Experts

In principle, defence witnesses may be brought in **India**, although the situation has not yet occurred in the context of SBS/AHT. In **South Korea**, it is normal for the accused to present a medical professional as an expert witness; however, the testimony of such a witness is not evaluated as rigorously as the evidence of the prosecution. Also, it is sometimes difficult to find an expert in the specific field and the expert's fee is in many cases excessive for defendants without means. In major criminal cases, where defendants are wealthy, foreign experts are sometimes introduced as expert witnesses for the defence.

Similarly, in Israeli law, the defence is allowed to bring in an expert of their own to testify; in the SBS cases which have occurred in **Israel**, the defence brought in both local and foreign professionals to testify on multiple occasions. However, again, finding local experts is difficult due to most medical professionals being in support of the triad approach. Even if some medical professionals do criticise the triad, they are generally perceived as unprofessional or even strange by their colleagues, so they may hesitate to testify and, if they do, their testimony has less weight.

In **Spain** also, defence lawyers are allowed to bring their own medical experts, although they sometimes must rely on the text of the official and public report in order to avoid 'secondary victimisation', which limits the evaluation. According to Spanish civil procedural law, any expert with an official title or expertise in the topic can testify. They are mostly from Spain, although the law does allow for experts from abroad.

In **Germany**, the defence may bring its own defence medical experts, but sometimes this leads to an endless pro and contra 'army' of experts. Often defence experts face a hostile atmosphere. Furthermore, the judge has the authority to reject any expert that he does not wish to hear for whatever reason (e.g., 'not suitable'). Foreign experts rarely or never testify in Germany, probably mainly due to language. In **Norway**, the defence may also bring its own defence medical experts. They are generally Norwegian, although foreign experts have started to come in recent years.

In **New Zealand**, the Crown calls expert witnesses, but medical experts are also allowed for the defence. Again, the pool is small; there are few or none from New Zealand with the expertise and inclination to take on this work. There is a single recognised SBS expert in New Zealand (the author of the aforementioned report), who is nearly always called as the expert witness for the Crown. Extended 'voir dire' challenges to a witness's credibility and long aggressive cross-examination by Crown lawyers make appearing for the defence unattractive to many professionals. The defence may engage an expert from overseas. Defence counsel is entitled to funding for expert witnesses under legal aid, but this is limited. The Crown's chief SBS witness and his colleagues are scathing of 'highly paid' overseas defence experts who 'refute and challenge a diagnosis [SBS] that has a strong history and evolution of research to support its basis'.

In **China**, the defence may not bring an expert of its own; however, criminal procedure law does allow the defence to request a new witness to be called to the court, new physical evidence submitted, or a new forensic evaluation conducted. Both the prosecution and the defence may also request the court call a 'person with specialised knowledge', usually from China, to appear before the court to offer an opinion on the expert opinion of the forensic expert. However, the court can make the final decision whether to grant these requests. When the expert evaluation is in dispute, the forensic examiner may be notified to testify in court. It is always up to the court to decide whether an expert or person with specialised knowledge needs to testify. There are cases where experts or persons with specialised knowledge retained by the defence provide written or in-court testimonies in support of the defence's case. There have been cases (not SBS) where the contradictions between the forensic report and the testimonies of persons with specialised knowledge ultimately led to the exoneration of the defendant.

Defendants in **Taiwan** are not allowed to bring their own medical experts. They must ask for the permission of the courts and the prosecution; then those experts are summoned by the courts, not by the defence. Hence, a defendant in an SBS case needs to obtain the court's permission to bring in any defence medical experts.

In **Ecuador**, **Peru**, **Argentina**, and **Costa Rica**, the defence may bring its own expert witnesses and there has been no difficulty in doing so; in particular there are doctors in each country willing to testify for the defence, so there is no need to bring in international defence witnesses.

26.6 Removal of Babies from Their Families in Family or Administrative Courts Based on Shaken Baby Syndrome/Abusive Head Trauma

Removal of babies does not occur in **India**. There have been no specific SBS cases in **China**, but, in general, when parents are accused of maltreatment, their custody of their child is not necessarily revoked (although this may happen in serious cases). Rather, the government will attempt to find a family member to take in the child or, failing that, a government-organised neighbourhood committee or a child welfare centre, but this is temporary while the parents undergo supervision and training while having the right to supervised visits with their child.

In **South Korea**, public officials and investigative agencies dispatched to the scene may take emergency measures if child abuse is confirmed, including isolating child abusers from victimised children and taking victimised children to child abuse-related protection facilities or medical institutions. Such emergency measures may not exceed 72 hours and require the permission of a judge. Shaken baby syndrome/abusive head trauma is not explicitly mentioned in the statute, and it is up to public officials whether to enforce these measures.

In **Taiwan**, municipal or county competent authorities are required by law to provide children and youth with protection, placement, dispensation, or emergency placement as needed. If there is suspected physical or mental abuse of a child or youth, the authorities consider the best interests of children and youth and reinforce necessary protection, placement, emergency placement, or necessary dispensation after multiple assessments. The authorities may place children and youth in foster families or turn them over to suitable relatives, third parties, children and youth welfare institutes, or other placement institutions. Therefore, if any child shows symptoms of SBS suspected of being caused by abuse, the authorities and prosecutors apply dispensation for the child; however, since decisions concerning children are not made public, it is impossible to know whether SBS has actually ever been invoked to remove a baby from its family.

In **Spain**, if there is a suspicion of child abuse and the child is considered at risk, authorities can initiate a process regardless of the hypothetical intention of the harm. There are slight differences between autonomous communities, but they need to report to social services at their hospital if the danger is less than moderate. When a physician suspects grave danger to a child, he or she must write a report together with a social worker and notify the Service for the Protection of Minors and the judge on duty, explaining the child's injuries. In the absence of another family member who can take in the child, the Service will assess possible consequences for the child and focus on making the best possible decision for him or her. Shaken baby syndrome has not yet been invoked in Spain in this context.

Similarly, in **Israel**, child abuse may result in taking children away from their parents' care. In extreme cases, where there might be immediate danger to a minor's life, social services may issue an executive order to temporarily remove the minor from the home without prior notice until the appropriate legal proceeding can take place. However, these executive actions and resulting legal proceedings are subject to appeal.

In **Norway**, children may be removed from the home by a decision from the local child protection authority, with a possibility to appeal the decision to a higher child protection authority. Only thereafter will it be possible to take the case to court at two levels.

In **New Zealand**, as soon as abuse is suspected after assessment of a child at a public hospital, the clinical team, Oranga Tamariki social workers, and the police will meet within 24 hours. At this meeting, a detailed multi-agency management plan is developed to address safety, support needs, whether a watch is required, named person access, and any other necessary matters. The meeting also considers the risk to siblings and other children living in the home and develops an agreed plan of management and investigation for the child in hospital and for any other children at risk. This plan is incorporated into the clinical file. There may be additional measures such as a place of safety warrant or a declaration that the child is in need of care and protection. The child and/or siblings may be removed from the family under the Children, Young Persons, and Their Families (Oranga Tamariki) Legislation Act 2017 and placed into care.

In **Ecuador**, children have not been removed from their parents due to accusations of SBS, but, in **Peru**, civil courts have removed children from families. Family courts can also make this decision in **Argentina** and **Costa Rica**, depending on forensic opinion.

26.7 Shaken Baby Syndrome/Abusive Head Trauma: the Numbers

India and **China** seem to have reported no SBS cases, and no information on these numbers is available in **South Korea** or **Israel**. No general statistics on SBS prevalence are available in **Taiwan**, but a single case of SBS was prosecuted in 2020, ending in acquittal.

In **Germany**, there are 100–200 cases each year. In **Norway**, there is approximately one criminal case per year, with an acquittal in 10–15% of the cases. In **Spain**, although official numbers are not published, records of 57 cases of SBS accusation were found, all ending in conviction. One of these was subsequently reversed after the expert who had testified retracted his testimony after having studied recent literature.

New Zealand, having a Crown expert specialist in SBS, does have some published reports: from 1988 to 1998, there were 64 cases of children with SDH at the main children's hospital, of which 39 were assessed as cases of non-accidental head injury (by criteria that are unclear). Of these, 6 died and 9 were removed permanently from their homes; 18 cases led to charges, 15 of which came to trial (the others did not because the accused fled the country), ending in 14 convictions and 1 acquittal.

No statistics seem to be available in **Ecuador**, **Peru**, **Argentina**, or **Costa Rica**. The general opinion is that the number is quite high. During the week this interview took place, there were two ongoing cases in Costa Rica.

26.8 Other Countries

To conclude, we provide a few observations about other countries. In **Canada**, the attorney general of Ontario assembled in 2008 a committee of experts to review criminal convictions based on medical determinations of SBS/AHT.[1] The Committee recognised, as did the Royal College of Pathologists in the United Kingdom [1], an evolution in the science of SBS/AHT. While maintaining that the triad continued to be a 'strong pointer to abuse', it also declared that 'many professionals do not accept the triad as a definitive diagnosis of abuse' while 'some experts [believe] that retinal hemorrhages are not necessarily diagnostic of abuse'. The Committee also acknowledged the existence of a lucid interval between head trauma and loss of consciousness in some cases. A non-systematic literature search showed that triad-based medical determinations of SBS/AHT appear to exist in **Mexico** [2, 3], **Brazil** [4], **Chile** [5, 6], **Colombia** [5], **Switzerland** [7], **Turkey** [8], **Saudi Arabia** [9], and **Estonia** [10].

In contrast, this diagnosis does not yet seem to be widely implemented in **Portugal** [11] or **South Africa** [12]. A review published by authors from **Romania** cautioned against systematic 'diagnoses' of abuse based on an isolated triad [13]. A study from **Denmark** identifying cases of fatal inflicted head injury in infancy did not rely solely on the triad to

1 https://wayback.archive-it.org/16312/20210403180210/https://www.attorneygeneral.jus.gov.on.ca/english/about/pubs/sbdrt/sbdrt.html.

make determinations of abuse [14]. A study from **Vietnam** found that most healthcare professionals participating in a training programme had never heard of SBS [15].

References

1. The Royal College of Pathologists. Report of a meeting on the pathology of traumatic head injury in children. 10 December 2009. www.rcpath.org/Resources/RCPath/Migrated%20Resources/Documents/S/sbs_meeting_report_final.pdf.
2. Díaz-Olavarrieta C, García-Piña CA, Loredo-Abdala A et al. Abusive head trauma at a tertiary care children's hospital in Mexico City: A preliminary study. *Child Abuse and Neglect*. 2011;35(11):915–23.
3. Loredo-Abdalá A, Casas-Muñoz A, Villanueva-Clift HJ et al. Pediatric abusive head trauma: Multicentric experience in Mexico. *Journal of Interpersonal Violence*. 2020;0886260520916283.
4. Paiva WS, Soares MS, Amorim RLO et al. Traumatic brain injury and shaken baby syndrome. *Acta Medica Portuguesa*. 2011;24(5):805–8.
5. Cooper M, Townsend ES, Darden PM. Abusive head trauma in Spanish language medical literature. *Child Abuse and Neglect*. 2016;58:173–9.
6. López F, Parra P, Troncoso M et al. Síndrome del niño sacudido en Chile: Una forma más de maltrato infantil. *Revista chilena de neuro-psiquiatría*. 2009;47(4):279–85.
7. Fanconi M, Lips U. Shaken baby syndrome in Switzerland: Results of a prospective follow-up study, 2002–2007. *European Journal of Pediatrics*. 2011;169(8):1023–8.
8. Oruç M, Dündar AS, Okumuş H et al. Shaken baby syndrome resulting in death: A case series. *Turkish Journal of Pediatrics*. 2021;63(1):31–6.
9. Alanazi FS, Saleheen H, Al-Eissa M et al. Epidemiology of abusive head trauma among children in Saudi Arabia. *Cureus*. 2021;13(10):e19014.
10. Talvik I, Metsvaht T, Leito K et al. Inflicted traumatic brain injury (ITBI) or shaken baby syndrome (SBS) in Estonia. *Acta Paediatrica*. 2006;95(7):799–804.
11. Pereira S, Magalhães T. Shaken baby syndrome: Fact or fiction in Portugal? *Acta Medica Portuguesa*. 2011;24:369–78.
12. Mattes FMG, Chibamboa VS, Nefdt KC, Van As AB, Ward CL. Does 'shaken baby syndrome' occur in South Africa? A review of emergency room and inquest records in Cape Town. *Vulnerable Children and Youth Studies*. 2021:1–10.
13. Duncea RM, Apostol I, Calota RG, Belis V. Forensic and clinical diagnosis in 'shaken baby syndrome': Between child abuse and iatrogenic abuse. *Journal of Mind and Medical Sciences*. 2017;4(1):13–18.
14. Flugt A, Frost L, Søndergaard C, Milidou I. Lethal abusive head trauma in infancy in Denmark from 2000 to 2011. *Danish Medical Journal*. 2021;68(4): A08200604.
15. Fraser JA, Flemington T, Doan TND et al. Prevention and recognition of abusive head trauma: Training for healthcare professionals in Vietnam. Acta paediatrica. 2017;106(10):1608–16.

Chapter 27 Conclusion

In 1971 Dr Norman Guthkelch hypothesised a causal link between shaking infants, a relatively common practice in the UK at the time, and findings of retinal and subdural haemorrhage with no or minimal evidence of trauma (see Chapter 2). The link between shaking and a 'triad' of retino-dural haemorrhage and encephalopathy would come to be known as shaken baby syndrome (SBS). This book has taken a broad overview and analysis of the state of SBS, addressing global medical, scientific, social, and legal aspects of the determination.

Perhaps the most significant observation of this book is that, some 50 years after Guthkelch suggested shaking as a cause for these findings, this hypothesis still lacks a scientific evidence base.

Decades of experimental and observational research, most notably in neuropathology (Chapters 3 and 4), have failed to verify the hypothesis. The triad has never been fully reproduced in animal, biomechanical (Chapter 14), or computer-based models. To date virtually no truly independent observations of shaking without impact have been reported to result in the triad (Chapter 3). Meanwhile the clinical literature continues to be plagued by methodological flaws (Chapter 10). Population studies supposedly comprising 'shaken babies' lack a suitable control sample: many cases classified as having been shaken may not have been, as such classifications have relied upon the very assumptions the research is attempting to verify. It has been shown that some population studies contain many false positives – children labelled with SBS but who have medical conditions responsible for the triad and for whom the justice system has ruled out abuse (see Chapter 22). Algorithms and artificial intelligence methods based on flawed data are inherently unreliable and relying on them for 'diagnosing' abuse is not appropriate.

Videotaped, or independently witnessed cases, which would provide a reliable control sample, are conspicuously lacking. When they do exist, the triad is typically not observed (see Chapters 3 and 5). The use of confessed cases as a control sample has been shown by extensive scientific literature to be unreliable (see Chapters 11 and 12). In particular, confessions are gained *after* shaking has been assumed and asserted by authority figures – either police or doctors – leading to the real risk that the interrogations are suggestive and coercive. When confessions are spontaneous and gained *before* diagnosis, the triad is virtually never observed (see Chapters 5 and 12). The extent of injuries caused by shaking remains unknown and probably depends on many risk factors, including pre-existing medical conditions that could lead some children to be more vulnerable than others. Of course, violent shaking is never acceptable. Perpetrators of child abuse should always be held accountable, no effort at education should be spared, and appropriate measures must be taken to ensure that children are protected.

Meanwhile, research has found dozens of medical (Chapters 3–9) and accidental (Chapters 14 and 15) causes for the components of the triad and all other findings sometimes relied upon to 'diagnose' abuse. Neuropathological studies have shown that trauma is not their only cause (Chapter 3). Radiological imaging allows us to observe the intracranial changes but their accurate interpretation depends on pathological correlation (Chapter 4).

While an inability to conduct case control studies and the inability of infants to provide information make research in this area challenging, this does not justify a failure to apply the highest standards of modern science to the analysis and investigation of infant head injury. Attempts by clinicians to circumvent these challenges have too often employed methods from outside their field of expertise and done so without partnering with experts from other disciplines who could provide invaluable input. For example, confession-based studies, widely quoted as proving an evidence base for the shaken baby hypothesis (see Chapter 12), have been made without regard to, and ultimately in direct conflict with, well-established literature regarding the psychology of interrogations and confessions (see Chapter 11). Lack of awareness of their own cognitive biases make some medical experts prone to systematic errors (Chapter 13). Similarly, using defective, poorly collected data, or applying erroneous analysis even to perfectly good data, will yield no results of value; doctors would be well-advised to consult with professional statisticians in publishing epidemiological studies (Chapter 17).

Despite the enduring lack of a reliable scientific evidence base, widespread belief in an unsubstantiated causal link between shaking and the triad is used more than ever to convict carers for crimes of abuse against infants, which carry long prison sentences and are considered some of the worst crimes in our society (see Chapter 20). The associated wrongful removal of babies from families has emotional and social consequences which are potentially far greater and almost invariably ignored (see Chapters 16 and 22).

Proponents refute the idea that the triad is ever used as a marker for shaking, contradicting decades of publications, courtroom testimony, and case law (Chapter 10). They assert that they first exclude other known causes. Yet such a 'diagnosis by exclusion' is circular, often involving a multidisciplinary team who ultimately rely on the triad of injury to infer that shaking or abuse has occurred. It is a vain hope that all potential causes of the triad can be excluded. On a clinical level this is not only precluded by resources and time but takes no account of the 'known unknowns'. For these reasons a list of causes of the triad is not found in this book. The legal difficulties with 'differential diagnosis' are discussed in Chapter 19. Without an independent measure of accuracy, there is no way of knowing the reliability of the 'diagnoses' of shaking or abuse.

Proponents also point to details of the triad, such as particular patterns of retinal haemorrhages, to claim that general reference to the triad is misleading and that their approach is more complex and sophisticated than critics proclaim. However, problems with research methods apply to all manifestations of the triad. For example, the purported causal link between shaking and extensive, 'too numerous to count' retinal haemorrhages, or other retinal findings such as retinoschisis and retinal folds, suffers from the same methodological flaws, including a lack of an independent control group.

Although shaking, or the application of acceleration/deceleration forces, is routinely invoked as an explanation for the triad (or particular manifestations thereof) the use of the term 'shaken baby syndrome' has also been largely disavowed, replaced by the more general 'abusive head trauma' (AHT). This umbrella term encompasses traumatic injuries inflicted to the head, including cases with impact where no shaking is being asserted. There is no controversy about the nature of injuries following *impact*: the controversy is specifically about *shaking* and about whether any constellation of non-specific findings like the triad can be used reliably to distinguish between natural or accidental aetiologies and deliberate shaking or shaking with impact. Using an umbrella term for a specific condition makes debate difficult, adding an unnecessary level of obfuscation and confusion.

This book has emphasised that the triad is better referred to as retino-dural haemorrhage of infancy (RDHI), as suggested by Dr Norman Guthkelch, attaching no presumptions regarding the aetiology of findings widely accepted to have a range of causes. This book has further demonstrated that significant gaps remain in our knowledge of these causes and further research is required. By adopting the neutral term RDHI, medical conditions that cause one or more elements of the triad are not considered to be 'mimics' of child abuse; they are considered causes of the triad. The cause in each particular case can then be explored without the prejudice of defaulting to an assumption of abuse.

Beyond the growing number of acquittals and exonerations in the past 20 years (Chapter 20), how many more of the thousands of diagnoses of shaking or abuse that have been made worldwide (Chapters 21–26) using flawed methods are incorrect? A definitive answer is impossible, but several observations may indicate a large number. The predominance of male children in SBS/AHT has never been explained but is also found in non-traumatic medical conditions known to cause the triad (Chapters 5–8). Spontaneous confessions of shaking are extremely rare and a proportion of false confessions is expected (Chapters 11 and 12), in contrast to the frequently given histories which are stereotypical of a medical cause. Finally, the failure of large-scale prevention campaigns in reducing the incidence of SBS/AHT may be explained by the lack of a robust causal link between shaking and RDHI (Chapter 10).

While this book challenges the SBS hypothesis and invites the medical community to improve its research and investigation standards, it does not deny the existence of abuse itself. Nor does it in any way obviate the need for child protection. The assertion that those who apply the principles of science to study RDHI are denying the existence of child abuse is a straw man argument that hampers rational discourse. Prevention of child abuse is a noble and necessary endeavour. However, we argue strenuously that there is no justification for the removal of children and for criminal convictions on the basis of unsound science propped up by poor methodology.

We hope this book will give lawyers, judges, doctors, social workers, and other health care professionals, as well as families, better insight into the unsupported foundations of SBS. We hope it will lead to more accurate medical diagnoses and that medical professionals will engage objectively in evidence-based scientific inquiry to better understand the pathophysiology of infant intracranial injury and associated findings. Such an objective approach will allow us to know and respect the limits of our medical and scientific knowledge. We hope the information in this book will lead to more scientifically-supported judicial decisions and to policy makers prioritising urgently needed reforms. Finally, we hope to see an end to attempts to villainise and silence critics.

Appendix: Frequently Repeated Claims concerning Shaken Baby Syndrome

In this appendix we review widely repeated but controversial – or disproven – claims concerning shaken baby syndrome (SBS)/abusive head trauma (AHT) and we refer to the relevant parts of this book where these statements are challenged.

A.1 The Shaken Baby Syndrome/Abusive Head Trauma Controversy

'SBS/AHT diagnoses never rely exclusively on the triad.'

'*Efforts to create doubt about AHT include the deliberate mischaracterization and replacement of the complex and multifaceted diagnostic process by a near-mechanical determination based on the 'triad' – the findings of subdural hemorrhage, retinal hemorrhage and encephalopathy*' [1].

'*AHT is not a diagnosis that is made, or excluded, based only on the presence of the three 'triad' factors, namely retinal haemorrhage, subdural haematoma and encephalopathy. Although these findings are commonly seen in AHT cases, to suggest that diagnostic processes simply rest on the presence or absence of the 'triad', without regard to the specific features and clinical circumstances of the findings, is, at best, misleading*' [2].

'*The diagnosis of abusive head trauma in children is not solely based on the findings of subdural hematoma, hypoxic–ischemic encephalopathy and retinal hemorrhage – it never has been*' [3].

The fact that the 'triad', or isolated SDH/RH, has long been used to 'diagnose' SBS/AHT, is well-documented in the clinical and legal literature [4, 5]:

'*Notwithstanding the protest in the Consensus Statement, it is a matter of easily confirmed historic fact that, for at least three decades, the triad findings served as the primary diagnostic criteria for SBS/AHT . . . SBS proponents argued and testified that the notion that almost anything else could explain the triad findings in a young child was 'foolish''* [5].

The literature predating the 2000s is replete with citations proving extensive reliance on the triad or some of its components for medical determinations of SBS/AHT:

'*SBS usually produces a diagnostic triad of injuries that includes diffuse brain swelling, subdural hemorrhage, and retinal hemorrhages. This triad must be considered virtually pathognomonic of SBS in the absence of documented extraordinary blunt force such as an automobile accident*' [6].

'*The shaken baby syndrome (with or without evidence of impact) is now a well-characterized clinical and pathological entity with diagnostic features in severe cases virtually unique to this type of injury –*[1] *swelling of the brain (cerebral edema) secondary to severe brain injury,* [2] *bleeding within the head (subdural hemorrhage), and* [3] *bleeding in the interior linings of the eyes (retinal hemorrhages). Let those who would challenge these diagnostic features first do so in the peer-reviewed literature, before speculating on other causes in court*' [7].

'The expert who acknowledges the classic findings of SBS include subdural hematoma, retinal hemorrhage and edema, but chooses to ignore this constellation in favor of an alternative hypothesis will appear foolish' [8].

'According to all credible studies in the past several years, retinal hemorrhage in infants is, for all practical purposes, conclusive evidence of shaken baby syndrome in the absence of a good explanation' [9].

In France, for example, national guidelines to healthcare professionals published in 2017 state that SBS is 'certain' when a child has unexplained bilateral subdural haemorrhage (SDH) and RH, two of the three components of the triad (see Chapter 22). See also Chapters 2, 10.4.1.1, and 23.4.

'There is no legitimate controversy on SBS/AHT.'

'AHT is a scientifically non-controversial medical diagnosis broadly recognized and managed throughout the world' [1].

'The denialists have tried to create a medical controversy where there is none' [1].

The tenets of SBS/AHT have been challenged by doctors, scientists, and scholars from all relevant disciplines [4]. This is shown in all chapters throughout this book.

'SBS/AHT reliability is supported by an extensive clinical literature.'

'Currently, the medical literature and overwhelming clinical experience and judgment demonstrate that AHT can be caused by shaking alone, shaking with impact, or blunt impact alone' [1].

'The diagnosis of AHT is supported by at least 700 peer-reviewed, clinical medical articles comprising thousands of pages of medical literature . . . [S]uch literature [is] scientifically valid, and consequently [provides] the clinician with sound scientific basis for arriving at diagnosis of AHT' [10].

A large-scale systematic review of the clinical literature on SBS/AHT by an independent Swedish governmental panel, examining more than 3,000 articles, has found that there was 'insufficient scientific evidence on which to assess the diagnostic accuracy of the triad in identifying traumatic shaking' [11]. Although criticised by SBS/AHT proponents, this review has shown deep and pervasive methodological flaws across the literature. A similar literature review from 2003 came to similar conclusions. See Chapters 2, 10, and 19 [12].

'SBS/AHT challengers deny the existence of child abuse and claim shaking is safe in infants.'

'Denialism of child abuse is a huge problem that threatens the responsible care of children and families, and it is getting worse . . . Child abuse denialism has as its base a very small number of physicians who perpetuate false science while ignoring the bulk of the scientific literature and the experience of the overwhelming majority' [13].

'Defense attorneys and few medical witnesses who promulgate scientifically unsubstantiated theories about abuse 'mimics' in an effort to manufacture a scientific-sounding controversy run afoul of professional norms and standards, can distort the view of the relevant medical community, and create a grave public health risk by promulgating dangerous misinformation regarding safe infant and child care (i.e. infant shaking is safe)' [1].

The existence and danger of child abuse is not in question: child abuse exists and must be fought. Intentional head injury can harm and kill infants and perpetrators must be prosecuted. The claim that 'infant shaking is safe' is a straw man argument that, to the best of our knowledge, has never been made by those who challenge medical determinations of SBS [14, 5]. As shown across the entire book, the central controversy is whether the presence of RDHI alone suffices to make a reliable determination of abusive shaking (or shaking with impact). Promoting this unsupported theory in court leads to wrongful convictions and unjustified removal of children from their families.

'SBS/AHT is a preventable condition.'

'We still believe that AHT is, at least to some extent, a preventable condition, for which research on prevention strategies should be strongly supported' [15].

Although preventing child abuse is a noble and necessary endeavour, there is to date no robust evidence that large-scale prevention campaigns against shaking are successful in reducing the incidence of SBS/AHT [15, 16]. On the contrary, research collectively shows that 'do not shake' educational programmes for parents have an overall tendency of no effect, while preventive programmes addressing other aetiologies (e.g., position of infants in car seats, positioning infants on their backs while lying down, or verifying correct bath water temperatures) resulted in a significant decrease in the 'diagnosis' of AHT. This research suggests shaking may not be the true preventable cause in many of these cases. See Chapter 10.

'Wrongful determinations of SBS/AHT are an extreme rarity.'

'Responsible and reputable medical professionals are extremely careful in making the diagnosis of abusive head trauma and not misdiagnosing another condition as abusive head trauma. Appropriate differential diagnoses are always considered. Not infrequently, and probably more often than not, a diagnosis of abusive head trauma is excluded or remains uncertain due to lack of corroborative findings. Valid cases of misdiagnosis of abusive head trauma with reputable proof of another diagnosis are extremely rare' [3].

The high number of triad-based determinations, the rarity of confessions, and the failure of large-scale prevention campaigns to reduce the incidence of SBS/AHT suggest wrongful medical determinations of abuse are anything but rare. The overrepresentation of male children and perinatal complications in SBS/AHT suggests alternative medical causes and that appropriate differential diagnoses are not always considered in a meaningful way. The relatively small number of exonerations does not prove the rarity of wrongful convictions, but it does prove the extreme difficulty in getting them reviewed by the criminal justice system. See Chapters 5–7, 12, 16, and 20.

A.2 Mechanisms and Neuropathology

'Abusive shaking causes rupture of bridging veins and traumatic SDH.'

'*Subdural bleeding is a marker for a traumatic mechanism (i.e., acceleration/deceleration, rotational and shearing forces due to violent shaking) causing rupture of the bridging veins . . . Bilateral bridging vein rupture confirms violent shaking. Unilateral bridging vein rupture is suggestive of unilateral trauma*' [17].

'*Violent shaking of the infant can result in bridging vein rupture, either in the subarachnoid or subdural segment*' [20].

'*The inflicted injury (acceleration/deceleration +/− impact) can lead to tearing of convexity bridging veins at the junction of the bridging vein and superior sagittal sinus. Additionally, rupture of the arachnoid membrane allows cerebrospinal fluid to enter the subdural space, mixing with subdural blood (hematohygroma)*' [1].

The hypothesis initially proposed by Norman Guthkelch and John Caffey – that abusive shaking without impact can rupture bridging veins – has so far received no support from neuropathological, animal, biomechanical or modelling studies. There are virtually no independently witnessed or videotaped cases of abusive shaking without impact causing isolated RDHI. See Chapters 3.2, 4, 5.6, 9, 14, and 19.5.

'Radiological or pathological description of bridging vein thrombosis proves shaking.'

'*The existence of ruptured bridging veins confirms the traumatic nature of the subdural haematoma*' [18].

'*Demonstration of bridging vein rupture allows the unequivocal diagnosis of a traumatic mechanism*' [17].

'*The diagnosis of non-accidental head injury caused by shaking is certain in case of: multifocal SDH with blood clots at the convexity (vertex) evidencing ruptures of the bridging veins*' [19].

The evidence base for this hypothesis is weak [21]. Radiological signs of bridging vein thrombosis reflect blood clot within the vessel, not traumatic vessel rupture. Rupture of bridging veins cannot be demonstrated by imaging and can only be inferred from associated massive haemorrhage. It is virtually impossible to confirm ante-mortem rupture of bridging veins at autopsy without extremely careful techniques due to the artefact associated with autopsy procedure. See Chapters 3.6, 4.4.

'Most SDH in infants is caused by trauma.'

'*All cases of infantile subdural haematoma are best assumed to be traumatic unless proved otherwise*' [22].

'*(D)ata regarding the nature and frequency of head trauma consistently support the need for a presumption of child abuse when a child younger than [one] year of age has intracranial injury*' [23].

'Most (subdural bleeding) in infants is attributable to trauma' [24].

'Trauma is the most common cause of SDHs – based upon epidemiologic studies in young children, both prospective and retrospective, from multiple countries' [10].

Birth is the most common cause of SDH in the first months of life as almost half of newborns have SDH. There are many natural causes beyond trauma. See Chapter 3.2.

'SDH in birth trauma and SBS show distinct patterns.'

'Birth mechanical trauma is often associated with extensive lesions of the soft tissue and skull, and subdural bleeding typically located in the vicinity of the tentorium. Lesions in birth trauma and SBS thus show distinct patterns' [25].

Almost half of healthy asymptomatic newborn infants have subdural bleeding. Both accidental and birth-related SDH may be multi-compartmental and most common in the posterior inter-hemispheric fissure. See Chapter 3.

'Accidental and abusive SDH show distinct patterns.'

'The pattern of intracranial bleeding in SBS is clearly different from accidental trauma' [25].

'The findings in SBS are stereotyped, with a very specific constellation of lesions, not found in accidental trauma. These lesions are by themselves evidence of the trauma' [25].

These statements are undermined by their author and others:

'The pattern of bleeding in traumatic cases appears similar in inflicted head injury and accidental trauma' [26].

'Our study (comparing SDH from traffic accidents (TA) with non-accidental SDH) shows that supposedly suspect features (for non-accidental injury) are common after TA in infants, and are specific to the patient's age rather than the cause of trauma. Only RH is clearly more evocative of SBS than of accidental injury' [27].

'The mechanisms and resultant injuries of accidental and abusive head injury overlap' [28].

See Chapter 3.

'Abusive shaking causes RH.'

'The powerful association of severe hemorrhagic retinopathy with the unique repetitive acceleration-deceleration forces of SBS, as opposed to single-impact events, together with the findings of RH in areas of maximal vitreoretinal traction, strongly support causation by vitreoretinal traction' [29].

'This research, along with clinical experience, support the role of vitreoretinal traction sustained during the repetitive acceleration or deceleration mechanism that characterizes shaking as an important contributory factor in causing RH and macular retinoschisis' [30].

The 'vitreoretinal traction' hypothesis has a weak evidence base and has to date not been reproduced in animal or biomechanical models. See Chapters 2, 3.3, 9.2.3, 10.4.1, and 19.5.4.

'RH (or a particular pattern of RH) is almost diagnostic of abuse.'

'*Retinal hemorrhage in children under 3 with or without other evidence of injury is pathognomonic of the battered child syndrome*' [31].

'*The presence of retinal hemorrhages in the absence of a history of severe trauma is diagnostic of some type of shaken impact injury*' [32].

'*It must be embedded in the minds of the pediatric emergency room residents that retinal hemorrhage is associated with child abuse until proven otherwise*' [33].

'*Retinal hemorrhages in an infant without a history of severe accidental trauma constitute child abuse until proven otherwise*' [34].

'*Retinal hemorrhages in young children have almost become diagnostic of child abuse*' [35].

'*The presence of retinal hemorrhages is virtually diagnostic of the violently shaken infant in the absence of severe accidental trauma*' [36].

'*The specific pattern and extent of RH help to delineate the cause of the eye findings*' [37].

'*Multiple (too numerous to count), bilateral, and multilayered hemorrhages that extend to the periphery of the retina are highly specific for AHT*' [30].

'*RH are rarely found in accidental trauma, generally of high velocity; moreover, accidental RH are never as severe as in SBS*' [25].

The mainstream view according to which RH were nearly diagnostic of abuse changed around 2001: it is now claimed that only particular patterns of severe RH are virtually pathognomonic of abuse.

More recently the view softened further when Binenbaum effectively refuted previous claims for the specificity of RH for shaking, acknowledging that '*there is generally more overlap than appreciated between abusive and accidental retinal hemorrhages*' [38].

Some authors have recognised that circular reasoning undermines the correlation between RH and abuse. '*The importance of an RH for the diagnosis of child abuse is well established; however, the evaluation of its incidence in child abuse is almost impossible because the diagnosis of child abuse is in great part based on the presence of an RH, providing a circularity bias. In addition, RHs have been reported after indisputable accidental trauma such as traffic or household accidents, especially after a fall down a staircase*' [39]. See Chapters 2.2.1, 3.3, 9.2.3, 10.4.1, and 19.5.4.

'Spinal findings are common in SBS/AHT.'

'*(O)n MRI 78% of these infants (victims of AHT) have spinal findings, mostly ligamentous, and up to 75% have spinal subdural hematoma that tracks from the posterior fossa*' [1].

'*There is a high incidence of previously unsuspected spinal SDHs associated with intracranial collections in children with NAI*' [40].

'*Non-bony spinal abnormalities have, however, been identified in up to 2/3 of victims of AHT*' [41].

Spinal ligamentous findings have not been verified as traumatic by pathology and may be explained by non-specific soft tissue oedema. Spinal subdural bleeding is not evidence of independent trauma but is secondary to intracranial subdural bleeding of any cause. See Chapter 3.4.

'Brain lesions associated with SBS/AHT are traumatic.'

'Extensive clinical and experimental data have demonstrated that such rotational movements of the brain result in a type of injury referred to as shearing injury or diffuse axonal injury' [42].

Brain lesions in SBS are most commonly caused by an insufficient oxygen or blood supply, not by mechanical tearing of nerve fibres. This was demonstrated by Geddes in 2001 and has subsequently been accepted by SBS/AHT proponents. A major textbook on child abuse claimed that *'[i]t is becoming increasingly clear from both neuroimaging and post-mortem analyses of fatal cases that the widespread cerebral and axonal damage in cases of AHT are, in fact, ischemic rather than directly traumatic in nature'* [43]. See Chapter 3.5.

'There is no lucid interval between abusive shaking and the onset of symptoms.'

'There is no 'lucid' or asymptomatic period in infants following serious or lethal head injury' [6].

'If a history purports a lucid interval in a fatal head injury case that does not involve an epidural hematoma, that history is likely false and the injury is likely inflicted. The time of most fatal head injury events can be restricted to the time period after the last confirmed period of wellness for the child' [44].

'There is no evidence of a prolonged interval of lucidity between the injury and the onset of symptoms in children with acute subdural hematoma and brain swelling' [45].

'In all cases, symptoms occur immediately after shaking' [19].

The basis for the belief that shaking causes traumatic rupture of the nerve fibres of the brain which would lead to immediate loss of function has been shown by neuropathology to be incorrect.

'Recent evidence also shows that victims often suffer repeated shaking before being diagnosed, attesting that, in many instances of shaking, the child remains asymptomatic or paucisymptomatic' [25].

'The potential exists therefore, for hours or potentially days to pass between the injury event and loss of consciousness/collapse. This interval, during which the baby appears 'lucid' (appears to be functioning on some level), reduces the ability to pinpoint the timing of the injury and contradicts the belief that a baby will become unconscious immediately after having been shaken vigorously, a belief relied on previously to identify the perpetrator as the person with the baby at the time of collapse' [46].

'[I]n more than 1/4 of the cases, the interval from injury to the onset of severe symptoms is longer. In all cases in which the children were seen by an independent observer after injury, they were described as not normal' [47].

See Chapter 3.5.

A.3 Denial of Alternative Causes of Retino-dural Haemorrhage of Infancy

'Rare differential diagnoses are properly excluded before concluding abuse.'

'The HAS-SOFMER guidelines have defined the diagnostic methodology to be followed by a multidisciplinary team including a paediatric radiologist to eliminate all possible differential diagnoses and make the diagnosis of AHT through shaking, with or without impact' [48].

'When a conclusion is reached by the multidisciplinary team that an infant's injuries were likely to have been inflicted, it is a result that has carefully considered all the reasonable explanations and excluded conditions, such as leukaemia, bleeding diathesis or metabolic disease, that in rare cases may mimic some features associated with AHT' [2].

Many SBS/AHT cases, including acquittals or exoneration cases, have been described where alternative causes were not sought or undisclosed. The claim that all differential diagnoses can be excluded is within the realm of fantasy; the list of potential alternative differential diagnoses is endless and constantly growing. There are diagnoses that can only be determined after death, and others that can only be determined during life. There are also entire categories of medical conditions (more than 100 disorders of bleeding, for example) that could potentially lead to SDH. In neither situation can time and resources allow for all differential diagnoses to be tested for and excluded in each case. See Chapter 22.

'Cerebral venous sinus thrombosis does not cause SDH and RH.'

'There is no reliable medical evidence that the following processes cause the constellation of injuries associated with AHT: cerebral sinovenous thrombosis' [1].

'In concordance with the literature, our study also does not support the correlation of Intracranial Venous Thrombosis (IVT) with SDH. It remains an untenable position that, in a child who presents with a traumatic SDH and then subsequently develops IVT, IVT is the cause and not the result of the injury' [49].

'This study did not find evidence to support the claim that CSVT causes SDH' [50].

In general, it is difficult to establish causation between two conditions in medicine as there are always intermediary and predisposing factors to consider. Still, there are many descriptions of SDH *in association* with venous thrombosis. Multi-centre epidemiological studies of paediatric cerebral venous sinus thrombosis (CVST) have reported 10–20% of SDH among these children. Even if Anderst et al. do not recognise any causal link between CVST and SDH, their own data show abuse was not suspected in 18 of their 20 cases with CVST and SDH (among 216 children with CVST) [50].

'The causal link between CVT in sinuses or cortical/medullar veins and infantile SDH is now well recognized and documented in medical textbooks and recent diagnosis recommendations of the main research groups on infant stroke, and formally validated by reference medical societies such as the American Heart Association' [51].

See also Chapters 3.6, 4.4.2, and 8.9.

'Benign external hydrocephalus rarely causes SDH.'

'*Our numerical simulations suggest that the benign enlargement of the subarachnoid space may not be considered as a risk factor for subdural bleeding*' [52].

'*Only a small minority of the patients with enlargement of the subarachnoid spaces had SDH . . . In the absence of additional injuries, however, the presence of an unexplained SDH in the setting of enlargement of the subarachnoid spaces may be insufficient to support a diagnosis of nonaccidental trauma*' [53].

'*Subdural hematoma is uncommon in the setting of benign enlargement of the subarachnoid space, and when present, AHT should be considered in the differential diagnosis*' [1].

Benign external hydrocephalus (BEH) is a common cause of SDH in infants, and many SBS/AHT cases may have been misdiagnosed BEH cases. See Chapters 5, 6, and 8.6.

'Short falls almost never cause RDHI or death in infants.'

'*Short falls do not cause life-threatening serious injuries of the kind seen in SBS/SIS [shaken impact syndrome]*' [54].

'*[T]here are no literature cases of children under the age of one presenting both SDH and RH after a fall from a low height*' [55].

'*Review of the extensive literature informs us that mortality from short falls is extremely rare, and the majority of these are benign occurrences with no significant neurologic dysfunction*' [1].

Short falls can cause death or RDHI. Although rare, wrongful determinations of SBS/AHT have been made in babies who have suffered short falls. Multiple short-fall deaths presenting with the triad have now been reported in the medical literature, and even captured on video. The AAP has now dropped its previous assertion in official policy statements that had claimed that short falls do not cause this constellation of findings [56]. Moreover, the literature establishing the asserted rarity of short-fall deaths is marred by serious statistical and data-collection errors [57]. The argument that short falls can be disregarded as a cause of RDHI or death because they are rare erroneously applies statistical averages to individual case determinations. See Chapters 14 and 15.

A.4 Confessed or Witnessed Shaking

'Shaking is almost never filmed or independently witnessed.'

'*Accurate classification of trauma as being from abuse remains difficult, because the trauma is generally unwitnessed and denied by perpetrators*' [58].

'*To be selected, the actions that led to AHT had to be filmed or committed in front of a neutral witness and the chance of this happening is very rare*' [59].

'*The gold standard for certainty of abuse would be a video recording or the testimony of independent witnesses, which are almost always lacking*' [65].

Dozens of cases of witnessed or videotaped abusive shaking have been reported, but RDHI, the triad, and other findings considered specific for abuse are found extremely rarely [60]. Thiblin et al. described 2 out of 36 witnessed or filmed cases. Feldman et al. described 1 case of symptoms in a series of 19 witnessed shakings, and 5 cases from a different US series covering a period of 13 years [61]. The evidence appears to indicate that shaking is particularly dangerous when the child suffers from some predisposing factors. It is worth noting that nearly all the witnesses in these cases are family members, so they do not fulfil the conditions of 'independent witnessing' defined by Keenan [62] or Williams [63]. See Chapters 3.2 and 16.

'Innocent parents or caregivers have no reason to falsely confess to shaking.'

'*[T]he presumption that confession evidence consistent with infant injuries was coerced (in the two papers on confessions from France, in fact, the perpetrators were offered no reason to confess because leniency cannot be offered via French law). These arguments are repeatedly raised in court despite the fact that they have never been empirically substantiated or are patently false*' [1].

'*Our opinion is that the perpetrator confesses with the sole purpose of relieving his conscience. On the opposite, denial can become entrenched, especially if reinforced by lawyers or associations of 'victims of miscarriage of justice', to the point that it becomes sincere*' [65].

There are many reasons why innocent parents or caregivers may give false confessions, as reviewed in detail in Chapters 11 and 12. See also Chapter 22.5.

'The existence of confessions of shaking prove the validity of SBS/AHT determinations.'

'*Although admittedly imperfect from a purely scientific standpoint, the confessions of many perpetrators to having shaken an infant without an impact mechanism suggest that shaking alone can indeed cause some or even all of the components of shaken baby syndrome*' [64].

'*[C]onfessed shaking . . . **is** the evidentiary basis for shaking*' [43].

'*Confessional evidence is quite striking that shaking alone can cause AHT*' [1].

'*Generally, the diagnosis receives confirmation when the perpetrator confesses his actions*' [65].

'*The description of the true mechanism of abusive shaking comes from the perpetrators' confessions*' [65].

Extensive literature has shown that confessions obtained during the judicial process are highly unreliable, especially in situations where investigators are prone to exert various types of pressure. See Chapters 11, 12, and 22.

References

1. Choudhary AK, Servaes S, Slovis TL et al. Consensus statement on abusive head trauma in infants and young children. *Pediatric Radiology*. 2018;48.8:1048–65.
2. Lucas S, Bärtås A, Bonamy AE et al. The way forward in addressing abusive head trauma in infants: Current perspectives from Sweden. *Acta Paediatricia*. 2017;106(7):1033–5. https// :doi.org/10.1111/apa.13840.

3. Strouse PJ. Shaken baby syndrome is real. *Pediatric Radiology*. 2018;48(8):1043–7.

4. Findley KA, Risinger DM, Barnes PD et al. Feigned consensus: Usurping the law in shaken baby syndrome/abusive head trauma prosecutions. *Wisconsin Law Review*. 2019;1211–67.

5. Papetti R, Kaneb P, Herf L. Outside the echo chamber: A response to the consensus statement on abusive head trauma in infants and young children. *Santa Clara Law Review*. 2019;59:299–366.

6. Kirschner RH. The pathology of child abuse. In *The battered child*. 5th ed. ME Helfer, RS Kempe, RD Krugman, eds. University of Chicago Press, 1997, pp. 248–95.

7. Chadwick DL, Kirschner RH, Reece RM et al. Shaken baby syndrome: A forensic pediatric response. *Pediatrics*. 1998;101 (2):321–3. https//:doi.org/10.1542/peds.101.2.321.

8. Holmgren BK. Prosecuting the shaken infant case. In *The shaken baby syndrome: A multidisciplinary approach*. S Lazoritz, VJ Palusci, eds. Routledge, 2001.

9. Parrish R. *Battered child syndrome: Investigating physical abuse and homicide*. 4th ed. US Department of Justice, 2002.

10. Narang SK, Melville J, Greeley C et al. A Daubert analysis of abusive head trauma/shaken baby syndrome. Part II: An examination of the differential diagnosis. *Houston Journal of Health Law and Policy*. 2012;13:203–327.

11. Lynøe N, Elinder G, Hallberg B. Insufficient evidence for 'shaken baby syndrome': A systematic review. *Acta Paediatrica*. 2017;106(7):1021–7.

12. Donohoe, M. Evidence-based medicine and shaken baby syndrome. Part I: literature review, 1966–1998. *American Journal of Forensic Medicine and Pathology*. 2003;24(3):239–42.

13. Strouse PJ. Child abuse: We have problems. *Pediatric Radiology*. 2016;46(5):587–90.

14. Lynøe N, Eriksson A. Denialism preserves scientific controversies: A case study of abusive head trauma research. *Journal of Controversies in Biomedical Research*. 2020;6(1):1–6.

15. Dias MS, Cappos KM, Rottmund CM et al. Preventing abusive head trauma: Can educating parents reduce the incidence? *Pediatric Radiology*. 2021;51(6):1093–6.

16. Scott LJ, Wilson R, Davies P et al. Educational interventions to prevent paediatric abusive head trauma in babies younger than one year old: A systematic review and meta-analyses. *Child Abuse and Neglect*. 2022;134:105935.

17. Rambaud C. Bridging veins and autopsy findings in abusive head trauma. *Pediatric Radiology*. 2015;45(8):1126–31.

18. Adamsbaum C, Rambaud C. Abusive head trauma: Don't overlook bridging vein thrombosis. *Pediatric Radiology*. 2012;42 (11):1298–1300.

19. Adamsbaum C, Laurent-Vannier A. Shaken baby syndrome or non-accidental head injury caused by shaking. Update of the guidelines issued by the 2011 hearing commission. Haute Autorité de santé (HAS) and Société française de médecine physique et de réadaptation (SOFMER); 2017. https://bit.ly/3WK3zvJ.

20. Choudhary AK, Bradford R, Dias MS, Thamburaj K, Boal DKB. Venous injury in abusive head trauma. *Pediatric Radiology*. 2015;45(12):1803–13.

21. Zahl SM, Mack JA, Rossant C, Squier W, Wester K. Thrombosis is not a marker of bridging vein rupture in infants with alleged abusive head trauma. *Acta Paediatrica*. 2021;110 (10):2686–94.

22. Guthkelch AN. Infantile subdural haematoma and its relationship to whiplash injuries. *British Medical Journal*. 1971;2(5759):430–1.

23. Committee on Child Abuse and Neglect. Shaken baby syndrome: Inflicted cerebral trauma. *Pediatrics*. 1993;92 (6):872–5.

24. Matschke J, Voss J, Obi N et al. Nonaccidental head injury is the most common cause of subdural bleeding in infants < 1 year of age. *Pediatrics*. 2009;124(6):1587–94.

25. Vinchon M, Noulé N, Karnoub MA. The legal challenges to the diagnosis of shaken baby syndrome or how to counter 12 common fake news. *Child's Nervous System*. 2022;38(1):133–45.

26. Vinchon M, Defoort-Dhellemmes S, Desurmont M, Delestret I. Confessed abuse versus witnessed accidents in infants: Comparison of clinical, radiological, and ophthalmological data in corroborated cases. *Child's Nervous System*. 2010;26(5):637–45.

27. Vinchon M, Noizet O, Defoort-Dhellemmes S, Soto-Ares G, Dhellemmes P. Infantile subdural hematomas due to traffic accidents. *Pediatric Neurosurgery*. 2002;37.5:245–53.

28. Christian CW, Block R, Committee on Child Abuse and Neglect. Abusive head trauma in infants and children. *Pediatrics*. 2009;123(5):1409–11.

29. Levin AV. Retinal hemorrhage in abusive head trauma. *Pediatrics*. 2010;126:961–70.

30. Christian CW, Levin AV, Council on Child Abuse and Neglect et al. The eye examination in the evaluation of child abuse. *Pediatrics*. 2018;142(2): e20181411. https://doi.org/10.1542/peds.2018-1411.

31. Eisenbrey AB. Retinal hemorrhage in the battered child. *Child's Brain*. 1979;5(1):40–4. https//:doi.org/10.1159/000119800.

32. Bruce DA, Zimmerman RA. Shaken impact syndrome. *Pediatric Annals*. 1989;18(8):482–94.

33. Rosenberg NM, Singer J, Bolte R, Christian C, Selbst SM. Retinal hemorrhage. *Pediatric Emergency Care*. 1994;10(5):303–5. https//:doi.org/10.1097/00006565-199410000-00017.

34. Monteleone JA, Giardino AP, Brodeur AE. Identifying, interpreting, and reporting. In *Child maltreatment: A clinical guide and reference*. 2nd ed. JA Monteleone, AE Brodeur, eds. GW Medical, 1998, pp. 15–41.

35. Christian CW, Taylor AA, Hertle RW, Duhaime A-C. Retinal hemorrhages caused by accidental household trauma. *Journal of Pediatrics*. 1999;135(1):125–7.

36. Reichert KW, Schmidt M. Chapter six: Neurologic sequelae of shaken baby syndrome. *Journal of Aggression, Maltreatment and Trauma*. 2001;5(1):79–99.

37. Binenbaum G, Reid JE, Rogers DL et al. Patterns of retinal hemorrhage associated with pediatric cerebral sinovenous thrombosis. *Journal of the American Association for Pediatric Ophthalmology and Strabismus*. 2017;21(1):23–7.

38. Binenbaum G. 2021. https://bit.ly/3UutsOC.

39. Vinchon M, Defoort-Dhellemmes S, Desurmont M, Dhellemmes P. Accidental and nonaccidental head injuries in infants: A prospective study. *Journal of Neurosurgery: Pediatrics*. 2005;102(4):380–4.

40. Koumellis P, McConachie NS, Jaspan T. Spinal subdural haematomas in children with non-accidental head injury. *Archives of Disease in Childhood*. 2009;94(3):216–19.

41. Choudhary AK, Ishak R, Zacharia TT, Dias MS. Imaging of spinal injury in abusive head trauma: A retrospective study. *Pediatric Radiology*. 2014;44(9):1130–40.

42. Case ME Graham MA, Handy TC et al. Position paper on fatal abusive head injuries in infants and young children. *American Journal of Forensic Medicine and Pathology*. 2001;22(2):112–22.

43. Dias MS. The case for shaking. In *Child abuse and neglect*. Elsevier, 2011, pp. 364–72.

44. Willman KY, Bank DE, Senac M, Chadwick DL. Restricting the time of injury in fatal inflicted head injuries. *Child Abuse and Neglect*. 1997;21(10):929–40.

45. Duhaime A-C, Christian CW, Rorke LB, Zimmerman RA. Nonaccidental head injury in infants: The 'shaken-baby syndrome'. *New England Journal of Medicine*. 1998;338(25):1822–9.

46. https://bit.ly/3trhJVr.

47. Gilliland MGF. Interval duration between injury and severe symptoms in nonaccidental head trauma in infants and young children. *Journal of Forensic Science*. 1998;43(3):723–5.

48. Laurent-Vannier A, Bernard JY, Chevignard M. Abusive head trauma through shaking: Examination of the perpetrators according to dating of the traumatic event. *Child Abuse Review*. 2021;30(4):283–99.

49. McLean LA, Frasier LD, Hedlund GL. Does intracranial venous thrombosis cause subdural hemorrhage in the pediatric population? *American Journal of Neuroradiology*. 2012;33(7):1281–4.

50. Anderst J, Carpenter S, Frazier T et al. Subdural hemorrhage in a cohort with cerebral sinovenous thrombosis: Application to abusive head trauma. *Child Abuse and Neglect*. 2021;117:105119.

51. Sébire G. Subdural hematoma following cerebral veinous thrombosis in infants. In *Le syndrome du bébé secoué*. B Echenne, A Couture, G Sébire, eds. Sauramps, 2020, pp. 359–86.

52. Raul JS, Roth S, Ludes B, Willinger R. Influence of the benign enlargement of the subarachnoid space on the bridging veins strain during a shaking event: A finite element study. *International Journal of Legal Medicine*. 2008;122 (4):337–40.

53. McKeag H, Christian CW, Rubin D et al. Subdural hemorrhage in pediatric patients with enlargement of the subarachnoid spaces. *Journal of Neurosurgery: Pediatrics*. 2013;11(4):438–44.

54. Reece RM. Chapter eighteen: Controversies in shaken baby/shaken impact syndrome. *Journal of Aggression, Maltreatment and Trauma*. 2001;5 (1):367–88.

55. Laurent-Vannier A, Nathanson M, Quiriau F et al. A public hearing. Shaken baby syndrome: Guidelines on establishing a robust diagnosis and the procedures to be adopted by healthcare and social services staff. Scoping report. *Annals of Physical and Rehabilitation Medicine*. 2011;54(9–10):533–99.

56. Atkinson N, Van Rijn RR, Starling SP. Childhood falls with occipital impacts. *Pediatric Emergency Care*. 2018;34 (12):837–41.

57. Findley KA. The absence or misuse of statistics in forensic science as a contributor to wrongful convictions: From pattern matching to medical opinions about child abuse. *Dickinson Law Review*. 2021;125:615–52.

58. Bhardwaj G, Chowdhury V, Jacobs MB et al. A systematic review of the diagnostic accuracy of ocular signs in pediatric abusive head trauma. *Ophthalmology*. 2010;117(5):983–92.

59. Laurent-Vannier A, Adamsbaum C, Raul JS, Rey-Salmon C, Rambaud C. Flawed Swedish study on traumatic shaking is already being used by defence lawyers and its findings must be ignored. *Acta Paediatrica*. 2018;107 (12):2048–50.

60. Thiblin I, Andersson J, Wester K et al. Medical findings and symptoms in infants exposed to witnessed or admitted abusive shaking: A nationwide registry study. *PLoS One*. 2020;15(1):e0240182.

61. Feldman KW, Melville JD, Johnson KL et al. Abusive head trauma follows witnessed infant shaking. *Child Abuse Review*. 2022:e2739.

62. Keenan HT, Runyan DK, Marshall SW, Nocera MA, Merten DF. A population-based comparison of clinical and outcome characteristics of young children with serious inflicted and noninflicted traumatic brain injury. *Pediatrics*. 2004;114(3):633–9.

63. Williams RA. Injuries in infants and small children resulting from witnessed and corroborated free falls. *Journal of Trauma*. 1991;31(10):1350–2.

64. Dias MS. Inflicted head injury: Future directions and prevention. *Neurosurgery Clinics*. 2002;13(2):247–57.

65. Vinchon M, Karnoub M-A, Noulé N, Lampin ME. Confessed versus denied inflicted head injuries in infants: Similarities and differences. *Child's Nervous System*. 2022;38(1):147–52.

Index

Please note: page numbers in bold type indicate figures or tables.